Understanding Nursing Care

£16.95

Understanding Nursing Care

Understanding Nursing Care

EDITED BY

Anne M. Chilman

Director of Nurse Education,
North Lothian College of Nursing and Midwifery,
Edinburgh

Margaret Thomas

Former Principal Officer,
Committee for Clinical Nursing Studies,
Edinburgh

THIRD EDITION

EDINBURGH LONDON MELBOURNE AND NEW YORK 1987

CHURCHILL LIVINGSTONE
Medical Division of Longman Group UK Limited

Distributed in the United States of America by
Churchill Livingstone Inc., 1560 Broadway, New
York, N.Y. 10036, and by associated companies,
branches and representatives throughout the
world.

First edition 1978
Second edition 1981
Third edition 1987

ISBN 0-443-03040-5

British Library Cataloguing in Publication Data
Understanding nursing care. — 3rd ed.
  1. Pathology   2. Nursing
  I. Chilman, Anne M.   II. Thomas, Margaret
  616'.0024613   RT65

Library of Congress Cataloging in Publication Data
Understanding nursing care.
  Includes bibliographies and index.
  1. Nursing.   I. Chilman, Anne M.   II. Thomas,
Margaret. [DNLM: 1. Nursing Care. WY 100 U55]
RT41.U65   1986   610.73   85–24653

Produced by Longman Group (FE) Ltd
Printed in Hong Kong

Preface to the Third Edition

During the 10 years which have passed since the first edition of *Understanding Nursing Care* was prepared many changes have taken place in nursing practice. Alterations were made to the second edition but continuing developments point to the need for further amendments and amplifications. Sometimes only a slight change has been made in the text but the parallel changes in nursing care may be profoundly important. In some areas it has been thought necessary to revise whole sections or even a chapter, and new illustrations have been included where they were thought to be more helpful. Terms printed in *italics* within the text are included in the Glossary at the end of the book.

The purpose of the book remains unchanged: that is to help nurses to understand why certain treatments and nursing care are required and to foster a perceptive, sympathetic and empathetic approach to each patient and his relatives. Medical specialties proliferate and consequently nurses are required to learn and have the opportunities to acquire skills relevant to each specialty. Regardless of the technique required it should be remembered that they are used for, or on behalf of, an individual and adaptation of these skills to meet the special needs of an individual patient is a nurse's responsibility.

Once again we are grateful to several medical practitioners who have given willingly of their time and expert knowledge in revising some chapters. In particular we wish to thank Dr J.D. Mitchell, Senior Registrar, for his contribution to Chapter 3 and Dr N.C. Allan, Consultant Haematologist for his help in revising Chapter 8.

1987

Anne M. Chilman
Margaret Thomas

Preface to the First Edition

The contributors to *Understanding Nursing Care* believe that the panoramic view of nursing which a broadly based primary programme encourages should be supplemented by a guide with a similar breadth of view. The purpose of the book is to help nurses to understand more fully why certain treatments and nursing care are required and to foster a perceptive, sympathetic and empathetic approach to the patient and his relatives. No attempt has been made to replace specialized texts; they will still be necessary for those needing detailed knowledge of particular subjects.

It has been assumed that the reader has some knowledge of biological sciences, and Section A explains the relationship of common disorders of biological systems to nursing care. Section B contains descriptions of needs and resources that are of particular relevance to different age groups. Some titles for further reading appear at the end of each chapter, and suggestions for either written assignments or topics for discussion have been made for chapters in Section A.

Two words — 'patient' and 'reassurance' — appear repeatedly in any nursing textbook, and this is no exception. 'Patient' is a word which nurses and doctors find convenient to use, as a kind of shorthand, for an individual who is deemed to need their help. But each patient is essentially a person with experiences and needs that distinguish him from all other members of the human race. We have tried to emphasize throughout the book the nurse's responsibility to respect her 'patient's' individuality, even when performing the most routine of hospital procedures.

The second word, 'reassurance', is used here to mean restoration of courage or confidence. Possible approaches have been indicated in some chapters, but there are no words which are appropriate for all people and from all nurses, and words alone may not convey the right message. This important professional responsibility demands skills which come more easily to some nurses than others. Observation of experienced staff — from many disciplines — and perception of the various strategies used should enable the student to add to her own repertoire of supporting and encouraging tactics.

Patients are not the only people who have needs a nurse should meet and expectations she should learn to fulfil. Nursing and other health staff colleagues, relatives and friends of patients and men and women engaged in official and voluntary services all deserve willing help and a friendly response.

We have had much help and encouragement in preparing this book and are grateful to many medical practitioners and other experts who have given generously of their time and advice. Our thanks are due, too, to Miss Moira Alexander, Mrs Anne Davies, Miss M. Rea Johnston and Miss Kathleen Wright for their contributions.

There would, however, have been no book without the great assistance we received from the publishers, and we wish, in particular, to thank Miss Mary Emmerson and Mrs Ellen Green for their invariable support, professional advice and, most of all, for their patience with us. We thank them, too, for recruiting Mr Douglas Kirk to illustrate the book; his work has given us great pleasure and we are confident that his unique contribution will add to its usefulness. Finally, we wish to acknowledge the help of the staff of the Medical Photography Department of the Western General Hospital, Edinburgh.

1977   Anne M. Chilman
                                                                       Margaret Thomas

Contributors

Noelle I. Cairns RFN RGN SCM RCT RNT
Tutor, North Lothian College of Nursing and Midwifery

Anne M. Chilman RGN SCM RNT
Director of Nurse Education, North Lothian College of Nursing and Midwifery

Mary Clements RGN RSCN SCM
Former Clinical Teacher, North Lothian College of Nursing and Midwifery

Philip Darbyshire RSCN RNMH RNT DN (London)
Nurse Tutor, South Lothian College of Nursing and Midwifery

Celia J. Dodds RGN RCT RNT
Tutor, North Lothian College of Nursing and Midwifery

Isobel M. Gibson RGN SCM RCT
Clinical Teacher, North Lothian College of Nursing and Midwifery

Christina E. Gillies RGN RCT RNT DN (London)
Senior Tutor, Post-basic Courses, North Lothian College of Nursing and Midwifery

Mary K. Gillon BA RGN RMN RNT
Professional Adviser (Post-basic Nursing), National Board for Nursing, Midwifery
and Health Visiting for Scotland

Margaret C. Grubb RGN RCT RNT
Senior Tutor, Glasgow Northern College of Nursing

Jane E. Innes RGN SCM RNT
Assistant Director of Nurse Education, North Lothian College of Nursing and
Midwifery

The late **George J. McKenzie** BA RGN RMN RNT Cert. Neurosurg. Nursing
Lecturer in Nursing Studies, Dundee College of Technology

Robert G. Mitchell RGN RMN RNT
Tutor, South Lothian College of Nursing and Midwifery

Stephen J. Rigby RGN RMN RCT DN (London)
Former Tutor, North Lothian College of Nursing and Midwifery

Sister Eleanor E. Rodgers RGN RNMD RNT DN (London)
Tutor, St Joseph's Hospital, Rosewell, Midlothian

Elizabeth Ross RGN RCT
Clinical Teacher, North Lothian College of Nursing and Midwifery

Phyllis J. Runciman MPhil MSc BSc RGN SCM HV
Lecturer, Queen Margaret College, Edinburgh

Christine M. Slater RGN RNT
Tutor, North Lothian College of Nursing and Midwifery

Norah J. Stephen RGN RSCN SCM MTD
Former Divisional Nursing Officer (Midwifery), North Lothian District

Williamina W. Thomson BSc RGN SCM ONC RNT Dip.Nurs.Admin.
Nursing Officer (Education), Scottish Home and Health Department

James Wiley BA MSc RGN RMN RNT
Senior Tutor, North Lothian College of Nursing and Midwifery

Contents

CONTENTS

Section A
Physical and mental disorders

Chapter One
The nature of infection

This chapter is a selection of those aspects of infection which are most relevant to nurses. The subject is not as mysterious as it may appear, nor is it a daunting task to discover the principles of nursing which have been derived from the science of medical microbiology. For those who wish to pursue the subject further after reading this chapter, a reading list is given at the end which offers a wider perspective for increasing understanding.

INFECTION

Babies are normally born free of micro-organisms. However, they quickly acquire a population of various types, which they retain for the rest of their lives and to which others may be added. It might be expected, then, that infection would be extremely common, caused either by one's own micro-organisms or those from someone else. Indeed, everyone at some time or another has an infection, such as German measles or the common cold, although fortunately it is mild in most cases. Serious infections do occur, but they are surprisingly uncommon. The reason we do not all die from infections is the ability of the human body to protect itself. This ability is known as **resistance.** Some of its many aspects will be discussed in this chapter.

All micro-organisms have a point of origin. This is known as the **source of infection.** In order to infect others they must spread in one of several well-known ways. Further, they must invade the body of another person, again in one of a number of ways. Of course, they must not be overcome by this person's resistance. The newly infected person is known as the **host,** and now acts also as a source. Knowledge about sources, methods of spread and ways of invasion of the host is gained from scientific study of the biological characteristics and the natural history of micro-organisms. Tried and tested ways of prevention and treatment of infection are based on this study.

In the community the nurse is especially involved with the protection of individuals through immunization. In hospital, she is very much concerned with prevention of spread between patients, a process known as cross-infection. She is the guardian of her patients and must ensure, through her awareness and the intelligent application of knowledge, that no patient is exposed unnecessarily to infection either from her own actions or the behaviour of others. The community nurse is in the unique position of being able to educate the public about the dangers of infection and the ways to prevent it, particularly through elementary hygiene.

The meticulous application of sound principles is largely a matter for the conscience of the individual. Nurses must therefore embody a positive attitude towards preventing infection in their philosophy of nursing. Further, knowledge never stands still and the problems that have to be solved vary with the times. The profile of infection has altered considerably over a relatively short period. Old enemies such as tuberculosis and diphtheria are under control, as can be seen from the figures given in Table 1.1 of cases occurring in Great Britain since 1951. But new problems are always appearing, such as increasing numbers of wound, urinary and respiratory tract infections with Gram-negative bacilli. These are currently causing concern, as is the increasing resistance of many bacteria to antibiotics. And there is evidence that the old enemies spoken of are not dead but merely sleeping, waiting for the unguarded moment.

Table 1.1
The changing incidence of infectious diseases

Disease	Cases by year notified in Great Britain			
	1951	1961	1971	1981
(thousands)				
Pulmonary tuberculosis	50.3	22.2	10.5	6.6
Whooping cough	192.3	26.9	18.5	20.7
Measles	628.6	776.4	150.6	57.6
(numbers)				
Diphtheria	826	51	17	2
Poliomyelitis	2925	904	8	2

THE NATURE OF MICRO-ORGANISMS

Micro-organisms, as the name proclaims, are microscopic living things. Although widely dispersed in nature, fortunately only a small fraction of the total number of species causes disease in humans. Included among those that do are bacteria, viruses and fungi.

Bacteria

These are unicellular organisms, that is, they are each composed of one cell only. They vary in size, but are larger than viruses and can be seen through the ordinary light microscope. Reproduction occurs by simple binary fission. This means that each cell divides to form two, which divide in turn. Rates of reproduction vary considerably, one factor influencing the rate being the suitability of the environment. Even under optimum conditions different species vary considerably, for instance *Escherichia coli* divides about every 20 minutes, while *Mycobacterium tuberculosis* may take several days to reproduce itself.

In order to multiply, bacteria require a favourable environment. In fact, measures to kill bacteria or prevent growth depend on rendering their surroundings as unfavourable as possible. Broadly speaking, pathogenic bacteria survive best in the sort of environment that the human body provides. This includes a temperature of around 37°C, moisture, a supply of food and slight alkalinity. Some bacteria are absolutely dependent on a supply of oxygen (obligatory aerobes). Others can survive but not thrive in its absence (facultative anaerobes). Still others (obligatory anaerobes) require oxygen to be absent. Clearly, then, an anaerobic bacillus such as *Clostridium tetani* will be more likely to cause infection if it enters the body in a deep wound, say, a puncture wound contaminated with dirt or soil.

Bacteria require moisture; most types will be killed by drying. The gonococcus, which causes a form of sexually transmitted disease, is especially sensitive to lack of moisture. Stories of having 'caught it from a lavatory seat', while not impossible, are regarded with some scepticism since the bacteria are unlikely to survive there for long. On the other hand, certain bacilli have the ability to change into a form which is extremely resistant to adverse conditions. This resistant form is known as a **spore**. Shown in Figure 1.1 as clear areas, the spores, which house the materials

Figure 1.1
Bacilli showing sites of spore formation

necessary for reproduction, shed the rest of the bacterial cell. When conditions become favourable, the organism can return to its original form and begin to reproduce again. Two of the most important bacilli to have this ability are *Cl. tetani* and *Cl. welchii*, which cause tetanus and gas gangrene respectively.

Much of the effect of bacterial infection on the body is caused by products of the bacteria. These harmful substances are called **toxins**; when released they circulate in the bloodstream. In a severe infection they cause serious symptoms, collectively referred to as toxaemia. There are two types of toxins: *endotoxins*, released only when the bacterial cell dies and disintegrates, and *exotoxins*, released continually by the bacteria. Endotoxins are not likely to cause damage unless present in large quantities, when local tissue destruction may occur. A small number of bacteria, including *Cl. tetani*, *Cl. welchii* and diphtheria bacillus produce exotoxins. These travel in the bloodstream to distant parts and exert their effects there. Thus, the characteristic muscle spasm of tetanus is due to the effect of the exotoxin on the nervous system.

Enzymes play a large part in the life processes of bacteria, as in other living things. Some bacteria produce enzymes which can influence the course of an infection. *Staphylococcus aureus*, for example, produces an enzyme called coagulase. This protects the bacteria by creating a fibrin barrier around them. Another enzyme produced by *Staph. aureus* is penicillinase, which destroys penicillin thus rendering the bacteria resistant to it. *Streptococcus pyogenes* produces streptokinase, which helps it to spread through tissues.

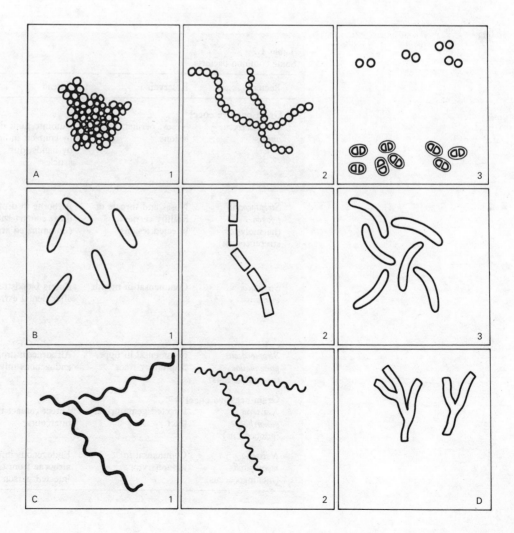

Figure 1.2
Classification of bacteria by shape
(A) Cocci (spherical bacteria)
　1. Staphylococci
　2. Streptococci
　3. Diplococci
(B) 1, 2 and 3 Bacilli
(C) 1 and 2 Spirochaetes
(D) Actinomyces

Classification of bacteria

The importance of classification lies in the need to be able to identify bacteria so that the most effective methods can be used to prevent spread and to treat infections.

Shape is the most elementary method of classification. Figure 1.2 shows the various shapes of bacteria.

Cocci are spherical bacteria. The various types are (1) staphylococci, which are found arranged in clusters; (2) streptococci, which grow in chains; and (3) diplococci, which grow in pairs and may be encapsulated.

Bacilli are bacteria which are rod-shaped, or nearly rod-shaped. Some of these are capable of producing spores.

Corkscrew-shaped or spiral bacteria are known as **spirochaetes**. In different spirochaetes, the coils of the spiral may be either tight or loose.

Actinomyces are branching micro-organisms, sometimes regarded as fungi, although they have some characteristics in common with bacteria.

Another simple method of classifying bacteria, which divides them into two categories only is Gram-staining. This technique involves a number of steps, but briefly it means that a prepared slide of bacteria is stained with a violet dye, washed, then stained with a red dye and washed again. Some bacteria will retain the violet dye and are referred to as Gram-positive. Others lose it but retain the red dye and are called Gram-negative.

Microbiologists use other more sophisticated methods which identify bacteria according to their characteristics. These include the appearance of colonies when grown on nutrient media, biochemical activities such as carbohydrate fermentation, and phage-typing (see p. 8). Some common bacteria, how they spread and the infections they cause are listed in Table 1.2

Table 1.2
Some common bacteria

Bacteria	Reservoir	Spread	Infections caused
Gram-positive cocci			
Staphylococcus aureus	Noses; perinei; infected lesions	Autoinfection; directly by contact; indirectly by hands, dust, other articles	Boils, styes, wound infections, osteomyelitis, pneumonia, septicaemia, food poisoning
Streptococcus pyogenes (haemolytic streptococcus)	Noses and throats of healthy carriers; infected lesions	Airborne in droplets; dust; contact with contaminated articles	Tonsillitis, otitis media, impetigo, scarlet fever, wound infections, associated with acute nephritis, rheumatic fever
Streptococcus viridans	Commensal in mouth	Enters bloodstream after dental extraction	Dental abscess; subacute bacterial endocarditis where heart valves have been previously damaged
Streptococcus pneumoniae (pneumococcus)	Commensal in upper respiratory tract	Airborne in droplets; endogenous infection	Pneumonia, otitis media, meningitis, conjunctivitis
Gram-negative cocci			
Neisseria gonorrhoeae (gonococcus)	Infected genitourinary tract	Direct contact in sexual intercourse	Gonorrhoea
Neisseria meningitidis (meningococcus)	Commensal in nasopharynx	Endogenous infection; airborne from carrier or infected person	Meningococcal meningitis, septicaemia

Table 1.2
Some common bacteria (*contd*)

Bacteria	Reservoir	Spread	Infections caused
Gram-positive bacilli			
Bacillus anthracis	Cattle; sheep; animal hides	Direct contact	Anthrax
Clostridium tetani	Faeces of humans and animals; soil and dust	Direct contact of wounds with soil or dust	Tetanus
Clostridium perfringens (*Cl. welchii*)	Animal faeces: soil and dust	Direct contact, ingestion	Gas gangrene, food poisoning
Mycobacterium tuberculosis	Infected cattle; respiratory tract of infected person	Airborne by droplets or contaminated dust; infected milk	Tuberculosis
Gram-negative bacilli			
Haemophilus influenzae	Commensal of upper respiratory tract	Endogenous opportunist infection	Chronic bronchitis, pneumonia, meningitis in children
Bordetella pertussis	Nasopharynx of infected child	Droplet spread	Whooping cough
Salmonella typhi (*and paratyphi* A & B)	Faeces of infected persons and carriers	Contaminated food, water or milk	Typhoid, paratyphoid A or B
Salmonella typhimurium (and many others)	Faeces of infected persons, infected cattle, pigs, poultry, mice	Contaminated food including meat products, poultry, milk and duck eggs	Food poisoning
Shigella sonnei	Faeces of infected humans	Direct or indirect contamination of food or feeding bottles; hand-to-mouth routes	Bacillary dysentery
Escherichia coli	Commensal in large intestine	Endogenous infection; direct or indirect spread	Wound infections, urinary tract infections, peritonitis, septicaemia, infant gastroenteritis
Proteus mirabilis *Proteus vulgaris*	Commensal in large intestine; soil	Endogenous infection; hands, dust or other articles	Wound and burn infections, urinary tract infections, septicaemia (resistant to many antibiotics)
Pseudomonas pyocyanea	Human intestines; soil, water; survives in disinfectant bottles, respirators and humidifiers	Endogenous infections; direct or indirect spread	Wound and burn infections; urinary tract infections; septicaemia (also resistant to many antibiotics)
Spirochaetes			
Borrelia vincenti	Commensal in mouth	Endogenous infection; direct contact	Vincent's angina
Treponema pallidum	Infected genital tract	Direct contact in sexual intercourse; intrauterine infection of fetus	Syphilis
Leptospira icterohaemorrhagiae	Infected rats	Contact with water contaminated by rat's urine, e.g. sewers	Weil's disease (haemolytic jaundice)

Viruses

Viruses are so much smaller than bacteria that a special type of microscope, the electron microscope, must be used in order to see them. They have been known for many years to be the causes of numerous communicable diseases. They are now also recognised as causes of other important infections. Most respiratory infections are now considered to be viral in origin, though frequently a bacterial infection occurs secondarily. The two most important viruses in this respect are the influenza virus and the *respiratory syncytial virus*. Diarrhoeal infections are also caused by some viruses, ingested perhaps with shellfish. In infants and young children the rotaviruses are well known to be responsible for diarrhoea. In addition there are infections rarely seen in this country, caused by viruses such as the *Lassa fever* virus and the *Marburg* virus. There is, too, a growing body of evidence which suggests that viruses play a part in causing some types of cancer and leukaemia.

Viruses differ from bacteria in the way they reproduce. Reproduction can only take place inside a living cell, which the virus has invaded. Bacteria are, of course, living cells and can be invaded by certain viruses called bacteriophages. Indeed, bacteria can be labelled according to the viruses which are capable of invading them. Another method of identification of different strains of bacteria has, consequently, evolved.

Bacteria are to a greater or lesser degree sensitive to antibiotics, while viruses are very little affected by them. There are only a few antiviral drugs at present, but others are being developed. Viruses themselves cause cells to produce a substance called interferon. This passes to neighbouring cells, providing a temporary resistance and probably limiting the course of the infection. Interferon has not yet been used therapeutically to any significant extent although its potential as an anti-cancer agent is currently being evaluated.

Viruses consist of either *DNA* or *RNA* inside a protein covering. When a cell is invaded, its nucleic acids are diverted from normal activities to make the nucleic acid and protein of the virus. These are assembled into new viruses, which are released to invade new cells (Fig. 1.3).

Within the body, viruses spread in various ways. A wart is an example of local spread from cell to cell. More extensive spread may occur in the respiratory tract, for instance in influenza. Spread by lymphatics and bloodstream (viraemia) causes symptoms of a generalized infection. Viruses often attack particular target organs,

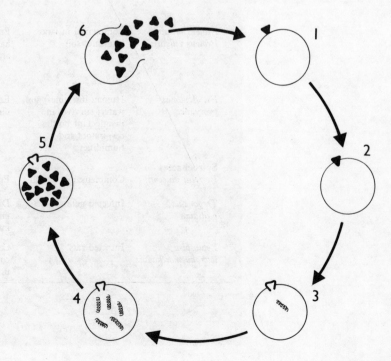

Figure 1.3
Replication of viruses

for example the spinal cord in poliomyelitis with resultant paralysis. Great advances have been made in the study of viruses and the continuing effort being put into this research reflects a growing awareness of their importance as infecting agents.

Fungi

From the nurse's point of view, fungal infections are less important than those caused by bacteria or viruses. The common fungal infections are of the hair, skin and mucous membranes. Occasionally some infections are of a serious and generalized nature.

Actinomycosis

Actinomyces israeli is an anaerobic branching organism. In pus it gives the appearance of gold-coloured granules. It can cause an infection of the jaw, often after injury. Infections of lungs and abdominal organs may also occur.

Moniliasis

Candida albicans, the causative micro-organism, is a *commensal* of the mouth, and often of the skin. The predisposing conditions which must exist before this infection occurs include:

1. Antibiotic therapy which suppresses normal flora.
2. Corticosteroid therapy given over a long period.
3. Diabetes mellitus.
4. General debility such as is found in subnutrition.

The common sites of moniliasis are the mouth (thrush), the vagina (vulvovaginitis) and skin folds.

Ringworm

Fungi causing ringworm are known as dermatophytes. They infect tissue which is keratinized, that is, hair, nails and skin. Animals such as cats, dogs, cattle and horses may act as sources, though the infection can be spread from person to person.

Athlete's foot *(Tinea pedis)*

This is a fungus infection of the skin, commonly spread during communal bathing. It is a particularly difficult infection to cure, and so measures are necessary to prevent spread, for instance in a household, by using separate bath towels and sponges.

SPREAD OF INFECTION

As already stated, the control of infection depends on an understanding of the ways in which spread occurs (Fig. 1.4). All pathogenic micro-organisms have a source. They must have a way of leaving that source, a way of travelling to a new host and a way of entering his body. The new host then becomes a source as well.

Sources of infection

Most infections originate with people who are either suffering from the infection or are carriers. Carriers are persons who harbour and disseminate micro-organisms without themselves showing any signs of the infection. Four categories are described:

1. Those who are incubating an infection and in whom features of the illness have not yet appeared.
2. Those who are recovering from the infection (convalescent carriers).
3. Permanent carriers (as distinct from types 1 and 2, who are temporary carriers)
4. Those with a subclinical, and therefore unrecognised infection.

Figure 1.4
Methods of spread of infection
and some preventive measures

Animals provide another, though less common, source of infection. Hens, mice and ducks may be sources of Salmonella, cattle of tuberculosis and brucellosis, dogs of rabies and parrots and budgerigars of psittacosis.

The route of exit

The way in which micro-organisms leave the body of an infected person depends on the part of the body which is the seat of the infection. Skin infections leave directly from the lesions. In respiratory infections micro-organisms leave in discharges from that tract, that is, in droplets (see p. 11) and in sputum. Bacteria from infected wounds leave in pus, from urinary tract infections in urine. Micro-organisms causing a number of infections leave in faeces — food poisoning, dysentery, enteric fevers, poliomyelitis and infectious hepatitis. The virus of serum hepatitis leaves in blood or blood products.

Modes of spread

Infection is spread from one person to another either directly or indirectly. Direct spread is relatively uncommon and requires direct contact of the appropriate nature, say, kissing in the case of herpes simplex and sexual intercourse in gonorrhoea or syphilis. Spread by indirect means accounts for most cases of transmission of infection. This includes indirect contact, that is, another person such as a nurse acts as an intermediary. Indirect methods of spread include the following also:

Fomites

These are any articles which have been used by or in contact with an infected person. If these are shared or passed on to another person without being disinfected, they may act as vehicles for transfer of pathogenic micro-organisms.

Food and drink

These can be instrumental in the spread of faecal-borne diseases if they have been contaminated by some person engaged in food preparation or cooking. Some infections originating in animals, such as tuberculosis, brucellosis and Salmonella food poisoning, are also transmitted in this way.

Air

Micro-organisms are being constantly discharged into the air from individuals' respiratory tracts. Coughing and sneezing are responsible for the spread of more micro-organisms than talking. They are expelled into the air in minute water droplets of varying size. The smallest dry up, remain suspended for long periods and may be inhaled. Larger droplets fall to the floor and dry up, leaving the dust contaminated. The dust can then be dispersed during cleaning. Airborne infections include tuberculosis, pneumonia, influenza, measles, the common cold and diphtheria.

Dust

As well as being contaminated in the way described, dust acquires micro-organisms from clothing, bed clothes, skin, hair and faecal matter.

Soil

Soil is a reservoir for micro-organisms deposited in it from animal faeces, including *Cl. tetani* and *Cl. welchii*.

Portals of entry

Infection may enter the body by inhalation, ingestion or through abrasions in skin or mucous membrane. Each of these portals of entry possesses protective mechanisms which help to prevent infection or to contain it locally if it occurs.

The fetus can acquire infections from which the mother is suffering. They enter the bloodstream of the fetus by means of the placenta. Examples are rubella and congenital syphilis.

RESISTANCE TO INFECTION

Resistance means the body's ability to defend itself against infection. It depends on a number of factors, some non-specific and others specific to a particular micro-organism. There are three principal lines of defence: outer defences (mainly mechanical barriers), inflammatory responses and immunity.

Outer defences

Skin provides a mechanical barrier to most micro-organisms but bacteria are found in hair follicles where they may set up infections. The resident population of skin bacteria prevents other pathogenic ones from living on it by competing with them for food.

Mucous membrane lines all body passages which open on to the surface. The mucus produced is a trap for micro-organisms. In the respiratory tract, cilia move this mucus to the outside. In the stomach, strong hydrochloric acid is produced, lethal to many bacteria. The outward flow of urine protects the urinary tract, while the acidity of the adult vagina renders it unsuitable for bacterial growth. Eyes are protected by the flow of tears which contain an antibacterial substance called lysozyme.

Despite these defences, pathogenic micro-organisms do gain access to the tissues. Then the second line of defence comes into action.

Inflammatory responses

Although most often associated with infection, inflammation is the body's response to any form of injury. The result of this process is that large numbers of phagocytic cells, i.e., polymorphonuclear leucocytes, and antibacterial substances are concentrated at the site of the infection or injury. First a dilatation of small blood vessels occurs in the affected area. The flow of blood is slowed down and the area becomes hot and red. Capillary walls become more permeable, and an exudate composed of fluid and polymorphonuclear leucocytes leaves the bloodstream. This results in swelling, which in turn causes pain by pressure on nerve endings. The exudate provides several defence mechanisms. The fluid helps to dilute toxins. Fibrinogen becomes converted to fibrin, creating a barrier to the local spread of the micro-organisms. Antibodies may also be present. The polymorphonuclear leucocytes destroy bacteria by ingesting them.

Immunity

When the body is invaded by pathogenic micro-organisms, it reacts by producing either antibodies or immune cells. **Antibodies** are protein substances — gamma globulins, fractions of one of the plasma proteins. **Immune cells** are lymphocytes with antibodies attached. The production of antibodies is known as the humoral response, that of immune cells the cellular response. In both cases the protection provided is effective only against the specific micro-organism provoking the response, which is referred to as the **antigen**.

Antigens are recognized by the body as 'not-self' and thus they must be rejected. About 7 days after invasion by the antigen, antibodies appear in the bloodstream. At the site of local infections they leave the bloodstream through capillary walls. The way in which antibodies work depends on the nature of the antigen. If it is a bacterial toxin, it is neutralized. If the bacterial capsule is the antigenic substance, it is removed, exposing the bacteria to phagocytosis. Where the bacterial cell wall is the antigen, the bacteria are caused to clump together facilitating phagocytosis. Immune cells carry a chemical which attracts phagocytes to the antigen.

When this process has occurred in response to a particular antigen, the individual is said to have developed immunity to it. A second exposure to the micro-organism results in rapid production of specific antibodies and an abortive or very mild attack of the disease.

Thus one way of developing immunity is to have the infection. The immunity produced in this way is usually long-lasting and may even be life-long. Subclinical infections produce a similar immunity. Because the process of disease is a natural one, immunity gained in this way is said to have been acquired naturally. And since the individual's own body has been active in producing the antibodies, the immunity is called **active immunity**. Active immunity may also be acquired artificially. This is what happens when we are vaccinated. A harmless form of the antigen is introduced into the body to provoke the immune response. These antigens may be toxoids, that is toxins treated with formalin, or vaccines made up of micro-organisms that have been either killed or weakened (attenuated).

Sometimes an individual may acquire antibodies from another source. In this case, the individual's body has not been active in the antibody production and the immunity is thus known as **passive immunity**. It is usually very short-lived because

Table 1.3
Acquired immunity

Acquired by	Nature	Duration
Infection	Natural active immunity	Long-lasting
Vaccination	Artificial active immunity	Long-lasting
Transplacental transfer	Natural passive immunity	Short-lasting
Injection of gamma globulin	Artificial passive immunity	Short-lasting

such donated antibodies are themselves foreign, and are consequently destroyed by the body. Like active immunity, passive immunity can be acquired naturally or artificially. Passive immunity is acquired naturally by the fetus, which is supplied with the antibodies possessed by the mother and is thus, at birth, temporarily immune to the same infections to which the mother is immune. When a person requires immediate protection from infection for a short period, antibodies (in the form of gamma globulin) are injected — an example of artificially acquired, passive immunity. The types of acquired immunity are summarized in Table 1.3.

Other factors

Other factors influence the body's ability to resist infection.

Age. The very young and the very old are more susceptible to infections than other age groups.

Hormones. Patients having corticosteroid therapy are more prone to infection, as are diabetics. In women, the protective acidity of the vagina is maintained by normal levels of oestrogen.

Malnutrition. Although often quoted as a reason for increased susceptibility to infection, there is no direct evidence to substantiate this. However, subnutrition is often found in conjunction with other factors which do predispose to spread of infection, such as overcrowding.

HOSPITAL-ACQUIRED INFECTION

Hospitals provide unparalleled opportunities for infection to occur. A large number of people are brought together, each with his own population of micro-organisms. The pathogenic micro-organisms which are commonly found in hospitals are both virulent and resistant to many antibiotics, and are therefore extremely dangerous. In addition, patients in hospitals are usually more susceptible to infection. They include the very young and the very old, those whose defences have been weakened by illness, or whose skin has been breached by surgery. Some treatments increase the hazard — radiotherapy, cytotoxic agents and immuno-suppressive therapy all interfere with white cell production and the immune response, while antibiotics destroy the body's normal protective bacteria.

Broadly speaking, hospital-acquired infections fall into three categories:

Wound infections.

Chest infections.

Urinary tract infections.

But this list is not exclusive. Other types of infection also occur, including gastrointestinal infections and serum or viral type B hepatitis (a particular hazard to hospital staff).

Wound infections

Surgical wounds are normally uncontaminated and heal without infection. Some, such as incisions for abscesses, should be regarded as infected or potentially so. As such they are sources of infection for others and require special precautions to be taken. Most clean wounds which become infected, do so in the ward. Burns become infected in the same way, and the risk is even greater because of the loss of the mechanical barrier — skin — and the presence of an admirable nutrient medium, the exudate. The micro-organisms involved in wound and burn infections include staphylococcus, streptococcus, proteus, pseudomonas and, less frequently, E. coli. Sources are almost always other humans, though autoinfection can occur. An obvious source is another infected wound, dispersing bacteria on to bedding, or dust, which may be picked up on hands or uniforms and transported to a new host. Pyogenic infections among staff, such as boils, styes or hand infections, are also ready sources. The one source not readily recognizable is the nasal carrier — 60% of persons who work in hospital carry staphylococci in their noses, thus presenting a potential hazard. A significant number also carry the haemolytic streptococcus in their noses and throats.

Chest infections

Chest infections acquired in hospital are frequently preventable. They may be the result of lack of attention to detail in carrying out nursing procedures. Patients may have difficulty in breathing either because of their illness or from postoperative pain. The inadequate lung ventilation which results leads to a retention of secretions that provide an admirable breeding ground for bacteria. Patients who are especially prone to chest infections include the following:

Postoperative patients

Operations on the thorax or upper abdomen carry a particular risk of infection because pain prevents deep breathing. Reduced mobility, for any reason, also increases the danger.

Unconscious patients

Loss of the cough reflex and incorrect positioning of the patient in bed increase the risk of infection.

Patients on ventilators

These patients must be protected by the removal of bronchial secretions by suction. If a tracheostomy has been performed, natural defences in the upper respiratory tract are by-passed. It is worth noting that *Pseudomonas pyocyanea* can survive happily in water and may colonize humidifiers and respirators.

Very ill patients

The lowered resistance, the weakness which prevents proper lung ventilation and some specific features of severe illness, such as pulmonary oedema, all predispose to chest infection. The following bacteria are found, but the importance of viruses in causing respiratory infections (see p. 8) must be remembered.
Pneumoccoci. These are found in the throats of many healthy people. They can cause pneumonia following virus infections or following the inhalation of saliva or vomitus.
Staphylococcus aureus. The widespread distribution of this micro-organism in hospitals makes it likely to cause chest infections in any of the circumstances discussed above.
Klebsiella pneumoniae. This sometimes causes pneumonia secondary to other infections.
Spread of pathogens causing chest infections is by airborne means, though opportunist infection by the patient's own commensals may occur.

Urinary tract infections

Urine is normally sterile, but bacteria gaining access to it can grow successfully. These include *E. coli, Strep. faecalis, Bacillus proteus* and pseudomonas. Infection by blood or lymphatic spread can occur, but in most cases it is due to ascending infection. Many cases are caused by a patient's own intestinal bacteria, particularly those of a woman since she has a short urethra, the orifice of which is in close proximity to the anus. It is also more likely to occur in patients confined to bed because the bottom sheet may act as a vehicle for transfer of bacteria; in addition there may be stasis of urine. The passage of any instrument such as a catheter or cystoscope into the bladder can introduce bacteria. The longer a catheter is left in the bladder, the greater the possibility of infection. It is also believed that clamping of catheters is more likely to lead to infection than free drainage. Any form of contamination of the catheter, the drainage tubing interior, the collecting bags, or of irrigation equipment also constitutes a hazard.

PREVENTION OF HOSPITAL-ACQUIRED INFECTION

Since micro-organisms cannot be eliminated completely from the hospital environment, prevention of infection must depend on governing the behaviour of workers and manipulating the environment. In this way, sources of infection can be controlled, the channels of spread blocked and susceptible persons protected.

Wound infections

In preventing wound infections, the overall aim is to prevent contamination with pathogenic bacteria. Contamination can occur during dressing procedures, so a technique which prevents this is necessary. Most hospitals have evolved their own methods; they vary in detail, but all are based on the principles of asepsis. Control of nasal carriers among the staff is essential, and provision must be made for their detection and treatment. There is considerable advantage in having a dressing-room separate from the ward. It is easier to clean thoroughly, and will not house the same concentrations of bacteria as a ward. Protection of clean wounds from infected ones may require isolation of patients with septic lesions.

Principles of aseptic technique are most often applied when carrying out a surgical dressing, but they are of equal importance in any procedure which is likely to permit the entry of micro-organisms into the tissues, including catheterization, bladder irrigation, venesection, intravenous infusion, lumbar puncture and marrow puncture. The risk of introducing infection during any invasive technique cannot be over-emphasised. The most important principles of asepsis are:

1. Nurses with infected lesions of skin or throat should not participate.
2. Packs from central sterile supply departments or from commercial suppliers should be checked for damage and expiry dates.
3. Equipment must be collected in advance, as any interruption to the smooth flow of the procedure may create a hazard, for instance, by causing a wound to be exposed unnecessarily.
4. Prescribed methods of cleaning dressing trolleys and dressing-rooms must be followed. These may vary from hospital to hospital.
5. Controversy exists regarding the wearing of masks; however, hair must be covered and clean gowns worn.
6. Hands must be washed at the beginning of the procedure and at any time during it when an unsterile article is touched.
7. Different types of packs require different methods of opening. The correct method that will avoid contaminating the contents should be ascertained.
8. Soiled dressings must be removed carefully from the wound, to prevent scattering of micro-organisms into the air. In most units the outer covering is removed by an assistant and the inner covering by the dresser, using forceps which are then discarded.
9. Used dressings should be put straight into a paper or plastic bag provided for the purpose and later incinerated.
10. Neither the wound nor any sterile material may be touched by hand.
11. Opportunity for infection is minimized by:

    No unnecessary talking.
    No unnecessary movement.
    Minimum exposure of wounds.
    Minimum disturbance of clothing and linen.

Chest infections

The prevention of chest infections depends to a large extent on the exercise of good basic nursing principles for ill, postoperative and unconscious patients. Consideration must be given to the patient's position in bed, changes of position, physiotherapy, and the use of suction to keep the respiratory passages clear. Details of this aspect of nursing care will be found in Chapter 6.

A patient suffering from a chest infection is an obvious source of infection for others and may need to be nursed in a single room. Collection of sputum requires special precautions. Disposable cartons with lids should be used and changed frequently. They should be handled carefully, collected into waterproof sacks and incinerated. Paper tissues should be used in place of handkerchiefs and disposed of in a similar manner. Hands should be thoroughly washed after handling sputum containers, not only to protect other patients, but also to protect the nurse herself.

Urinary tract infections

One of the most important ways of preventing urinary tract infections is to avoid passing catheters if at all possible. When such a procedure is necessary, it should be carried out strictly in accordance with the principles of asepsis. Indwelling catheters present a greater risk of infection than those removed immediately after insertion. At the same time it must be recognized that each time a catheter is passed, another opportunity for infection is created. Some authorities recommend weekly changing of indwelling catheters. Others believe that they may safely be left in place longer if drainage bags capable of being emptied without disconnecting the catheter are used. If the system remains closed in this way, less opportunity for the entrance of micro-organisms is provided.

Obstruction to the flow of urine should be avoided, since urine which remains in the bladder will act as a culture medium for bacteria. Tubing must, therefore, be kept free of kinks and other interference which would occlude the lumen. At no time should spigots be used, as this will not only interfere with the closed drainage system, but may introduce micro-organisms. If it becomes necessary to interrupt the flow of urine temporarily, a gate-clip should be used. Changes of drainage bags, when this becomes necessary, should be carried out with due attention to asepsis. In particular, care must be taken not to contaminate the catheter lumen at this time.

Backward flow of urine into the bladder is undesirable, and is prevented by maintaining the position of the drainage tubing and bag below the level of the bladder.

Cleansing of the urethral meatus, and perineal toilet for women is necessary several times a day. Thorough cleansing of the perineum for women after defaecation is especially important, not only for those with catheters, but also those who are confined to bed. Frequent changing of bottom sheets on the bed will also help prevent the transfer of micro-organisms from anus to urethra.

Environmental control

Control of the environment and of activities of staff, with the object of reducing infection in hospital, is best carried out by a Control of Infection Committee headed by a bacteriologist and including a nurse. Rules can be laid down governing all practices which might constitute an infection hazard. Policies regarding the use of antiseptics and antibiotics can also be drawn up. Among its tasks should be the education of all grades of staff in preventive measures.

Several aspects of environmental control merit further discussion.

Cleaning

Dust is a reservoir of bacteria, so cleaning must ensure its removal not its redistribution. Domestic workers must be educated in the importance of their role in infection control and in the safest methods of cleaning. To prevent dust dispersal, floor cleaning must be carried out by vacuum cleaners fitted with filters. Mops, if not cleaned properly, can be dangerous breeding grounds for bacteria and can actually increase the number of bacteria on floors. Mops should be thoroughly washed in hot water, steeped in a strong solution of phenol disinfectant such as Sudol 1% and then rinsed and dried.

Dishes should only be washed in a dishwashing machine. The importance of very hot water cannot be overemphasized. Dish cloths and drying cloths should be prohibited.

Dirty linen

Careful handling of soiled linen is necessary to prevent the dissemination of bacteria into the air. On removal from a bed, linen must be put straight into a container before being carried out. Careful and quiet making of beds is necessary for the same reason. A colour-coding system for laundry bags is necessary, so that infected or contaminated linen is clearly recognizable by the laundry staff. Proper steps to protect laundry workers and to disinfect the linen can then be taken.

Bedpans and urinals

Problems can be avoided if disposable types are used. These, however, create the difficulty of finding space for storage. Stainless steel bedpans and glass urinals are adequately treated in normal circumstances by automatic washers. Where disinfection of bedpan contents is considered necessary, for example in typhoid, it is customary to fill the bedpan with a phenol disinfectant (Sudol 1%) and leave it for at least an hour. It can then be cleaned in the bedpan washer. Some authorities, however, question the value of this practice.

Waste disposal

Certain types of used materials are an infection risk and their disposal must be carefully controlled. These include used dressings, infusion sets, syringes and needles. Dressings must be put into a waterproof paper sack of distinctive colour, sealed and incinerated. Sharp objects such as glass ampoules, scalpel blades and needles must be placed in a rigid cardboard box before disposal to avoid accidental injury to handlers and the risk of serum hepatitis.

Sterilization

Much hospital equipment needs to be sterile, that is, free from all living micro-organisms. A good deal of this equipment is supplied commercially and is disposable, for instance syringes, needles, infusion sets, catheters and dressings. These items are generally sterilized by gamma radiation. Equipment which is reused is sterilized locally in hospital central sterile supply departments. This category includes surgical instruments, glassware, surgical gowns and towels.

Boiling as a means of sterilization is not effective and is seldom used in hospitals. Most materials requiring sterilization are suitable for treatment either by steam under pressure or dry heat.

The autoclave (Fig. 1.5) is used to sterilize by steam under pressure. It employs the same principle as the pressure cooker — the greater the pressure steam is subjected to, the higher the temperature that can be achieved. Articles must be held at a predetermined temperature for a given time; the higher the temperature, the shorter the time, thus:

Temperature	Holding time
121 °C	15 min
126 °C	10 min
135 °C	3 min

Dry heat is only suitable for sterilizing materials which will not burn, such as all-glass syringes, metal instruments, powders and oils. A variety of methods is employed ranging from a Bunsen burner flame, used in laboratories to sterilize platinum wire loops, to hot air ovens and infra-red heated conveyer ovens.

Whatever the method of sterilization, the articles must be thoroughly cleaned first, as bacteria protected by dirt or blood are likely to survive.

Disinfectants are extremely unreliable as a means of killing bacteria. They are therefore not normally used for articles which must be sterile. Disinfectants are also unsafe for the storage of sterile instruments and, as a rule, should only be used where no other treatment is suitable.

Figure 1.5
A fully automatic high vacuum autoclave

INFECTION IN THE COMMUNITY

Infectious or communicable diseases are no longer the threat to life that they once were. This is mainly due to the institution of immunization programmes against many of these diseases, particularly the more serious ones such as diphtheria and

Figure 1.6
Distribution of the rash —
chickenpox and smallpox (see
Table 1.4)

poliomyelitis. To some extent, the advent of antibiotics and the improvement in living standards have also contributed to this change.

The number of infections that come under the category of communicable disease is considerable and cannot be discussed at any great length in this chapter. Emphasis has been placed on those diseases which occur most commonly and those which by their nature are serious hazards. Although it is customary to discuss sexually transmitted diseases separately, they are communicable diseases and, as such, have been included here. A list of the main communicable diseases and their distinguishing features is given in Table 1.4.

Sexually transmitted diseases

Gonorrhoea

The incidence of gonorrhoea has risen steadily for the past 30 years. While Figure 1.7 shows an overall decline since 1977, this is small, and the figures continue to give rise to concern. The causative micro-organism is the *Neisseria gonorrhoeae* (gonococcus), most often transmitted during sexual intercourse. A form of non-sexual contact is the infection of a newborn baby by its mother, causing ophthalmia neonatorum. On rare occasions indirect spread may occur, for example by using communal towels. Among the reasons suggested for the increasing incidence of gonorrhoea are:

1. Decreasing use of the sheath as a means of contraception (a sheath is a useful mechanical barrier to infection).
2. Ease of availability of the contraceptive pill.
3. Increasing promiscuity among young women (who provide an often undetected reservoir of infection).
4. Lack of parental control.
5. Changing moral standards.

Gonorrhoea has a short incubation period of 3 to 6 days. In men, a purulent urethral discharge is the main feature, but if left untreated, more serious complications will develop including urethral stricture, arthritis and sterility. In women an ascending infection of the reproductive tract occurs which can involve the ovaries and the uterine tubes (Fallopian tubes). Treatment with penicillin is still effective, although the gonococcus is becoming increasingly resistant, necessitating the use of broad spectrum antibiotics. Education and contact tracing is an important part of the control of this infection.

Figure 1.7
(A) New cases of gonorrhoea in
Scotland, 1976–82. (B) New
cases of genital herpes in
Scotland, 1976–82.

A

B

Table 1.4
Summary of communicable diseases

Disease and cause	Spread	Incubation period	Rash	Other features	Treatment	Other remarks
Measles Measles virus	Droplet (Affects mainly young children).	8–11 days.	Rapidly spreading, blotchy rash about fourth day. Coalescent macular spots. Fades in few days, followed by desquamation.	Catarrhal symptoms during 3- or 4-day prodromal period, i.e., sneezing, coughing, watery eyes and nose. Photophobia, Koplik's spots. Temperature rises to 40°C by about 4 days. Falls when rash fades.	No specific treatment. Nurse in warm, well-ventilated room. Shade from bright light. Encourage fluids. Isolate until rash disappears.	Complications may include: stomatitis, laryngitis, bronchitis, otitis media, corneal ulceration, convulsions, encephalitis. Routine vaccination available. Gamma globulin given to protect very young or ill children who are contacts. Notifiable.
Rubella Rubella virus	Droplet.	About 17 days.	Appears on first day. Small pink spots which coalesce. Fades in about 48 hours.	Sudden onset, sneezing, coughing, watery eyes and sore throat. Temperature rises to about 38°C. Falls when rash fades. Often a very mild disease.	No specific treatment. None usually required.	Complications are rare. Rubella is known to be liable to cause congenital defects in the offspring if contracted by pregnant women in first 3 months of pregnancy. In this situation, passive immunity with gamma globulin may be tried but is not very successful. Active immunization is available and should be encouraged for girls of about 13.
Chickenpox Varicella virus	Direct contact or droplet.	14–21 days.	Mainly confined to the trunk (Fig. 1.6). Rash appears on first day. Progresses through papular, vesicular and pustular stages. Successive crops permit spots at all stages to be seen together. Crusting precedes healing.	Symptoms in children may be very mild, in adults more severe. Headache, malaise, sore throat, fever. In adults, this virus causes shingles.	No specific treatment. Isolation at home until rash heals. Itching and irritation is treated with calamine lotion: antibiotics only for secondary bacterial infection.	Probably advantageous for children to have chickenpox, since the resulting immunity is life-long. Secondary bacterial infection with haemolytic streptococci or with staphylococci may occur. Other complications are rare.

Table 1.4
Summary of communicable diseases (*contd*)

Disease and cause	Spread	Incubation period	Rash	Other features	Treatment	Other remarks
Mumps Mumps virus	Droplet, direct contact, food contaminated by saliva from infected person.	14–21 days.		Tender swelling of salivary glands, headache, difficulty in chewing. Temperature may reach 39°C.	No specific treatment. Rest in bed, with soft diet and plenty of fluids. Analgesics and frequent mouth washes. Observation for complications.	Complications include orchitis, oophoritis and pancreatitis.
Smallpox Variola virus	Droplet. Contact with discharges from skin lesions or respiratory discharges of infected person. Indirect contact with articles contaminated by above.	About 12 days	Rash appears on third day and is distributed mainly on face, scalp and limbs (Fig. 1.6). Progresses through papular, vesicular and pustular stages, taking about 24 hours. Pustules dry to scabs in 8 or 9 days. These leave pock marks.	Prodromal symptoms are malaise, shivering, headache, backache, sore throat. Ulcers of upper respiratory mucosa may occur. Temperature rises again in pustular stage of rash and toxaemia occurs. Pneumonia is common.	There is no specific treatment. Good nursing care by staff recently vaccinated. Isolation in infectious diseases unit is essential. Antibiotics may be given to prevent secondary bacterial infection. Correction of water and electrolyte balance may be necessary. Care of skin and mouth is essential.	Complications include heart failure, secondary bacterial infection of respiratory tract leading to broncho-pneumonia, delirium, convulsions, corneal ulcers. Routine vaccination has recently been discontinued. A notifiable disease.
Infectious mononucleosis (Glandular fever) Probably caused by a virus.	Affects many young people. Spread occurs probably as the result of exchange of saliva such as occurs in kissing or sharing drinking utensils.	5–10 days.	Some cases present with a macular rash.	A variety of types occurs. Fever may be accompanied by a sore throat, by malaise, anorexia, headache and rash, or by enlargement of superficial lymph glands and the spleen. In some instances jaundice appears.	No specific treatment. Rest in bed is advisable during the febrile period. A soft diet may be helpful and adequate hydration is essential. In very severe cases corticosteroids may be used. Antibiotics are only useful in secondary bacterial infection.	Recovery always occurs, though the illness can persist for weeks or months. Complications are rare, the most serious being accidental injury to an enlarged spleen.
Diphtheria *Corynebacterium diphtheriae*	Droplet from infected persons or carriers.	2–5 days.		Usually begins with malaise, headache and sore throat. Infection is local and general symptoms are due to exotoxins. Grey membrane forms across pharynx and may cause respiratory obstruction. Tachycardia with	Immediate antitoxin, intravenously in severe or moderate cases, intramuscularly in mild. A trial dose may be used to detect sensitivity to horse serum. Patients and carriers should be isolated until 3	Active immunization, begun in 1942, has reduced the incidence dramatically. This should be carried out for all young children. Complications are involvement of the

Table 1.4
Summary of communicable diseases (*contd*)

Disease and cause	Spread	Incubation period	Rash	Other features	Treatment	Other remarks
				fall in blood pressure occurs due to effect of toxin on myocardium. Effects on nervous system may show as swallowing difficulties and disturbance of visual accommodation. Only a slight elevation of temperature occurs.	consecutive negative swabs are taken. The bacillus, but not the toxin, is sensitive to penicillin, which is given intramuscularly for 5–7 days. Respiratory obstruction due to membrane requires immediate tracheostomy.	myocardium, nervous system, respiratory obstruction and pneumonia. Notifiable.
Scarlet fever Haemolytic streptococcus	Droplet. Ocassionally by contaminated milk or ice cream.	2–4 days.	The rash appears in 24–36 hours. The face is flushed with pale area round the mouth. The erythema, which spreads over the body, has dark red points. Fades in about 3 days. After first week, skin peels.	Sudden onset. Temperature rises, throat becomes sore. There may be vomiting. Tonsils are red and swollen, covered with 'exudate.' The tongue, furred in beginning, peels, leaving strawberry appearance. Condition improves when rash fades. In some children, disease is very mild.	Penicillin is effective against the streptococcus. Most cases can be cared for at home. Rest, with plenty of fluids and analgesia, is generally all the care required.	Complications are less common nowadays. These include otitis media and skin infections. Acute glomerulo nephritis and rheumatic fever are due to sensitivity to the streptococcus. Notifiable.
Whooping cough *Bordetella pertussis*	Droplet. Direct contact.	7–14 days.		Onset is gradual. Two steps occur: 1. Catarrhal stage with cough, vomiting, slight elevation of temperature and possible convulsions. This lasts about 10 days. 2. The second stage is characterized by paroxysms of coughing, each series of coughs followed by inspiratory 'whoop'. The child is usually better after 4–6 weeks.	No specific treatment. Antibiotics to control secondary infection is necessary. Mild disease in children best cared for at home. Light sedation may be helpful. In severe illness, admission to hospital may be necessary in case of pneumonia.	Complications such as hernia, rectal prolapse and sub-conjunctival haemorrhage are due to increased intra-abdominal or intrathoracic pressure. Laryngitis, bronchitis and bronchopneumonia may occur. Active immunization is given to children as part of triple vaccine. Notifiable.

Table 1.4
Summary of communicable diseases (*contd*)

Disease and cause	Spread	Incubation period	Rash	Other features	Treatment	Other remarks
Bacillary dysentery *Shigella sonnei* *Shigella flexneri*	Food contaminated by carriers or cases.	3–7 days (may be less).		Sudden onset with abdominal pain, diarrhoea. Vomiting not common. The temperature may be elevated. In about a third of patients blood and mucus appear in stools.	Antibiotics are usually better reserved for seriously ill patients. Most people recover in a few days. Adequate hydration is important, and in young infants and those very ill, intravenous correction of electrolyte balance may be necessary.	Control of spread includes notification. Prevention of spread depends on strict hygiene, especially after defaecation. Only the very ill need be admitted to hospital, where isolation techniques should be practised. Children with dysentery should be kept from school.
Typhoid *Salmonella typhi*	Water, milk and food which have been contaminated by cases or carriers. Occurs in U.K. usually only if imported.	7–21 days.	Scattered rose pink spots appear about seventh day and last for 3 or 4 days.	Insidious onset, with anorexia, headache, malaise, gastrointestinal upset. Temperature rises over a week to about 40°C (step-ladder phenomenon). Remains high for a week then falls during third and fourth week. The pulse is slow. Spleen is enlarged. Haemorrhage or perforation of the intestine is a danger.	Chloramphenicol is effective, as may be Ampicillin. Corticosteroids, e.g. prednisone, may be used. Admission to infectious diseases unit is essential. Nursing is mainly basic care, with particular attention paid to fluid balance and oral hygiene. Measures to prevent spread are essential.	A carrier state develops in about 5% of cases, 2% being chronic. Measures to prevent spread by carriers are essential, notification is obligatory. It enables investigation into the source and institution of measures to control spread of the disease. Prophylactic vaccine is given to those entering areas where typhoid is endemic.

Genital herpes

Although the actual numbers that occur are much less than gonorrhoea, the disturbing fact about this condition is the dramatic increase in its incidence. Figure 1.7 shows that in Scotland since 1976 the increase has been in excess of 50%. Genital herpes is caused by a type of the herpes simplex virus, spread by direct sexual contact. The virus enters through an abrasion or break in mucous membrane. It causes an initial outbreak, characterised by the appearance of fluid-filled vesicles on the genitalia. These break down and ulcers form, taking perhaps weeks to heal. The main problem for the sufferer at this time is the very severe pain and discomfort experienced. The virus remains dormant between attacks, lodging in nerve ganglia. Subsequent infections are not usually as severe as the first.

While a considerable increase in cervical cancer is associated with genital herpes, it is considered that the increased risk to any individual is small. Another problem is the risk of a newborn infant becoming infected during delivery if the mother has active vaginal lesions. In this situation, delivery by caesarian section may be carried out.

So far, treatment is limited in its effectiveness. Local application of idoxuridane is helpful. Intravenous administration of acyclovir, an antiviral agent, leads to more rapid healing of the ulcers and shortens the attacks. Work is currently in progress at Birmingham University on the development of a vaccine. This could well be effective in helping sufferers as well as giving immunity to those at risk.

Syphilis

Syphilis is caused by the *Treponema pallidum*. The incidence is less than that of gonorrhoea but it is a much more serious disease. There is an increasing incidence of syphilis on a world-wide basis, although in Great Britain the number of new cases each year remains fairly constant. Spread is again mainly by sexual intercourse; however, the spirochaete can enter through an abrasion in the skin and may infect a nurse or doctor caring for infected persons. Fortunately this is a very rare occurrence, but it nevertheless dictates extreme caution.

Congenital syphilis occurs in babies born of infected mothers who have been untreated. Screening by means of blood tests is now carried out to detect such women and give them early treatment. The incubation period of syphilis varies from 10 days to 3 months, after which the primary sore or chancre, appears at the site of infection, which may be the penis, labia or lips. In the secondary stage, skin manifestations such as an erythematous rash, condylomata and snail-track ulcers of the buccal mucosa appear. The third stage may occur from 2 to 20 years later and be manifested in lesions anywhere, but particularly in the cardiovascular and central nervous systems. Treatment over a period of 12 days by penicillin is still effective, though other drugs may be necessary.

Nursing care

Nursing the patient with a sexually transmitted disease requires a very special type of person. Much of the contact with these patients is in out-patient departments, which are usually open in the evenings. The extent to which patients will be willing to come forward for treatment depends very much on the reception they meet in these treatment centres. Nurses should be very careful not to let their own personal feelings affect their attitudes to their patients. No moral judgements must be made or expressed. Further, all confidences must be respected and information divulged only for the purpose of treatment. This applies especially to employers, relatives and also to the patient's husband or wife, though usually the spouse will be involved in the same course of investigation or treatment.

The nurse must be particularly careful not to risk becoming accidentally infected herself. She must avoid contact with any discharges, observe scrupulous hygiene of her hands and wear gloves when attending patients if she has any cuts or abrasions. She should also be careful when handling syringes, needles and specimens. Nurses may be asked for advice by members of the public. They therefore must have an understanding of the subject and a knowledge of the facilities available for treatment.

Contact tracing is an important part of controlling sexually transmitted disease. This is usually carried out by trained personnel, including social workers and health visitors who have had specific preparation for this work. A social worker should be employed in clinics where these diseases are treated, since they are often only one aspect of a social problem which may include marital difficulties and separation.

Acquired immune deficiency syndrome (AIDS)

Although this is discussed in the context of sexually transmitted diseases, this is not the exclusive means of spread. AIDS is a disorder characterized by severe immune deficiency, as a result of which there occurs opportunistic infection often by normally harmless micro-organisms. A rare form of cancer, *Kaposi's sarcoma*, also occurs in a very large proportion of cases. The mortality rate is also very high.

The cause of AIDS is not known, though it has been suggested that a virus may be responsible. Symptoms include persistent high temperature, a persistent cough, diarrhoea, loss of weight and lymph node enlargement.

Most of those affected are male homosexuals; a much smaller proportion are haemophiliacs, heroin addicts or Haitians. A common factor among the first three groups is the possibility of transmission in body fluids and infection by inoculation. The connection with Haitians is not known.

As a result of the mystery surrounding the disorder and its serious consequences there is much concern among homosexual males, to the point where promiscuity has decreased. Suggestions that AIDS may be occurring as a result of heterosexual activity lends urgency to the search for the cause.

Controlling infection in the community

Broadly speaking, control consists of dealing with two aspects: the prevention of importation of diseases from abroad, and the prevention of spread of those diseases endemic to a country.

Imported infections

Travellers going abroad

The speed of modern travel means that a person may go abroad, acquire an infection and return home before the incubation period is over. The most effective way of dealing with this is to ensure that travellers are vaccinated against diseases endemic in those regions they propose to visit. International health regulations provide for requirements to be made for travellers to such areas to be in possession of a valid international certificate of vaccination against appropriate infections.

A number of countries still insist on vaccination against yellow fever. These include Cameroon, Central African Republic, Gambia, Nigeria, Uganda and Senegal. Vaccination against cholera is required for Swaziland. Visitors to central Africa, central and south America, Asia and parts of the Middle East are recommended to take precautions regarding malaria. Vaccination against typhoid, and poliomyelitis is also advised for travellers to areas other than Canada, the United States, Australia, New Zealand and northern Europe.

Much responsibility rests with port and airport medical officers to ensure that no person with a serious infection is allowed to land undetected in the country. They will have advance information available regarding any outbreaks or epidemics of infections in areas from which ships or planes are arriving, and so will be on the alert. Captains of ships and planes are required to make a declaration of the health of passengers and crew on arrival, and nobody may land until the medical officer is satisfied.

Immigrants

As well as the infections discussed above, immigrants may be suffering from other infections, particularly tuberculosis. This may be detected by screening on arrival, and treatment is provided.

Imported food

Medical officers at disembarkation points are responsible for inspecting and taking samples of all food imported into the country. Many people in Britain will recall the 1964 outbreak of typhoid in Aberdeen, where more than 300 people were infected by one can of corned beef containing *Salmonella typhi*. This sort of outbreak is rare but it shows what could happen if vigilance was relaxed.

Imported livestock

Importation of live animals is rarely a cause of infection in Great Britain. Hides, wool and bone meal are frequently infected with *Bacillus anthracis*. This is a risk for handlers, though infections are surprisingly uncommon. Parrots and budgerigars can bring with them psittacosis and dogs can carry rabies. The increasing illegal importation into Great Britain of pets such as dogs has caused considerable anxiety because of the danger of rabies being introduced into the country.

Endemic infections

Prevention of these can be considered under the following headings: immunization; notification; source and contact tracing; food hygiene; health education.

Immunization

As already pointed out, immunization has been greatly responsible for the decline of communicable disease in the U.K. and many other countries. Infant immunization for diphtheria, whooping cough, tetanus and poliomyelitis is routine. To this may be added BCG vaccination for tuberculosis. A typical schedule is given in Chapter 18.

Notification

This is required by law for certain specified infections. There are a number of reasons for its importance. By means of notification, the effectiveness of immunization, medical policies and services can be assessed. Also, the relationship of infections to factors such as occupation and social grouping can be judged and the geographical distribution of cases seen. Notification is made to the area's chief medical officer by the doctor who diagnoses the condition. Included in the list of notifiable diseases are:

Acute poliomyelitis	Measles
Anthrax	Ophthalmia neonatorum
Cholera	Puerperal fever
Diphtheria	Rubella
Dysentery	Scarlet fever
Enteric fever	Smallpox
Erysipelas	Tuberculosis
Infective jaundice	Whooping cough
Malaria	

Source and contact tracing

Until the source of an infection is identified, spread can still occur. Contact tracing is especially important in food poisoning and in serious infections such as typhoid, since it identifies further possible sources of the infection. In tuberculosis, known contacts must be screened by X-ray. Contacts of persons who develop poliomyelitis must be immunized, and a booster immunization is given to diphtheria contacts, who must also be screened to detect whether they are carriers of the micro-organisms.

Food hygiene

Infections spread by food are mainly preventable and common sense hygiene is all that is required. Water-borne diseases are virtually unknown in most Western countries due to the reliability of water supplies and the efficiency of methods of sewage disposal. Most food-borne infections are the result of contamination either by a carrier or an infected person during the cooking or the preparation of food. Contamination at source also occurs, for example duck eggs may be infected with Salmonella, as may be poultry. Carriers and those with infected skin lesions must not be permitted to work in any food trade. Simple hygiene measures which will prevent food poisoning include:

Preparing food under clean conditions.
Frequent handwashing, especially after defaecation.

Eating cooked food immediately, or storing it under refrigerated conditions.
Avoiding precooking meat for heating later.
Thorough cooking of food and, if frozen, thorough defrosting before cooking.

Health education

Awareness is increasing of the importance of health education as a means of preventing many forms of illness, including communicable diseases. Its purpose is to convince people of the need for measures to promote health and to persuade them to change their style of living if it is likely to lead to ill health. Health education is carried out by many workers, including local authority health education officers, health visitors, general practitioners, teachers and social workers. Much teaching is also carried out informally by nurses in contact with their patients. A wide variety of methods is used in health education, each designed to meet a particular situation. A back-up service of posters, films and tape recordings is often provided by resource centres. Most of us are familiar with mass media techniques that use radio and television extensively for informing the public on topics such as immunization and sexually transmitted disease. Where a special need exists, say, to encourage immunization in a particular area, a concentrated campaign using a number of techniques may be mounted.

PRINCIPLES OF NURSING IN COMMUNICABLE DISEASE

Many of the minor communicable diseases do not require admission to hospital, and such has been the decline in serious infections that fever hospitals, once busy, have now been converted to other types of work, leaving perhaps one or two wards to be used for the original purpose.

The basic principles of nursing care are the same for these diseases as for all forms of illness. However, they have a special importance in serious infections where, apart from treatment with antibiotics, the patient's progress depends to a large extent on good nursing.

Rest

This is an important part of the treatment of any illness. In serious infections the need for rest is even greater because, as a result of the disease, the respiratory rate, pulse rate and temperature are increased. In order to prevent further strain on the heart, rest is essential. A quiet, non-stimulating atmosphere is necessary because of the heightened irritability which often accompanies fevers. It is necessary to encourage sleep by all means at the nurse's disposal, avoiding the use of drugs if possible.

Hygiene

High temperatures are accompanied by profuse sweating, which leads to much discomfort. The daily bed-bath is therefore of considerable importance. A wash at intervals during the day is also helpful. While an increased temperature is the body's way of combating the infecting micro-organisms, a temperature of over 40°C can be harmful to its own cells. Tepid sponging and other temperature-reducing treatments must therefore be employed to prevent body temperature from exceeding this level. Clothing should be light and loose, cotton being more comfortable than other materials. It will be necessary to change bed linen frequently.

Oral hygiene

Sweating, increased respiratory rates and high temperature cause water to be lost from the body, and the mouth will become dry and uncomfortable. Since the patient is unlikely to be eating much, salivation will also be diminished. Some infections may be accompanied by lesions in the mouth or lips. Frequent and careful oral hygiene is therefore necessary, and a mouth wash should be available at all times.

Fluid balance

The loss of water by seriously ill patients (noted above) is greatly increased if vomiting or diarrhoea are features of the disease, and these features may also cause severe electrolyte deficiency. At least 3 litres of fluids should be taken daily, and in cases of severe loss, replacement by intravenous means may be necessary with additives such as potassium chloride to correct the electrolyte imbalance. Oral fluids should include glucose drinks and fruit juices, which provide vitamin C and potassium.

Diet

Various proprietary protein supplements are available to be added to milk; these should be given when the patient is disinclined to eat. Once the patient's temperature has begun to fall and his appetite returns, a light diet, attractively presented, can be given, supplemented as described.

Skin care

The essentials of skin care are fully discussed in Chapter 14. It is worth remembering that cleanliness and change of position are two of the most important principles. Itching, such as occurs in chickenpox, leads to scratching and consequent secondary infection. To minimize irritation soothing lotions should be freely used. Anal tenderness will accompany diarrhoeal diseases, and a suitable barrier cream should be provided.

Observation and records

Pulse, temperature and respiratory rates must be recorded at intervals as requested by the doctor. This may be hourly or less frequently. In serious infections, blood pressure readings may be needed, and daily urine testing may be required. A fluid balance record is a useful guide in preventing dehydration. In diarrhoeal diseases, a record should be kept of the frequency and nature of stools.

Prevention of spread

The protection of other patients and of the staff is an important part of nursing infected patients. All staff should be recently vaccinated against any serious infection that is being nursed. These patients also require isolation in an infectious diseases unit. Ideally, this should be carried out in a single room, the door of which is kept closed. Rooms specially designed for this purpose may have vestibules as air-locks, so that air from the room which may be carrying micro-organisms does not enter the rest of the ward. Air must not be recycled by air conditioning systems, but should be expelled to the outside.

All persons entering the room should wear protective gowns, and masks are necessary when the micro-organism is spread by air. For infections spread by the faecal route, urine or blood, gowns need only be worn when in actual contact with the patient, his bed or excreta. Gloves should also be worn for highly infectious and serious infections such as diphtheria, as well as when removing sanitary utensils containing infected faeces or urine. Hands should be washed immediately before and after removing gowns and masks. Gowns should be hung on hooks inside the room or in the vestibule, spaced in such a way that they do not touch each other.

Cleaning of the rooms should be carried out in the usual way, but separate utensils must be kept stored in a cupboard in each room. Terminal cleaning must include washing floors and walls with hot water and soap, and fumigation may be necessary. Linen should be disposed of as indicated on page 16, in appropriately identified plastic bags. The advice of the central sterile supply superintendent should be sought when it is necessary to use any equipment from that department, as, even though expensive, it may be desirable to use disposable equipment. Disposable items must also be collected in colour-coded plastic bags in the room, put into another bag when being removed and incinerated.

Disposal of excreta can be a problem in the enteric fevers. Separate bedpans and urinals are essential. The conventional method of disinfection is described on page 17.

Prevention of spread of infection depends ultimately on knowing the methods by which micro-organisms are transmitted and adjusting behaviour accordingly. If the rules that are laid down are observed, then prevention of spread is a simple matter and can be accomplished even in the most unsatisfactory conditions.

SUGGESTED ASSIGNMENTS

1. Imagine that you have been invited to talk to a young wives group at your local church. Outline how you would explain to them the purpose and advantages of infant immunization.

2. Read the prescribed procedure for carrying out a simple surgical dressing in your own hospital. Demonstrate how it complies with the principles set out on page 15 for practising aseptic technique. (A simple method is to label each stage of the procedure with code letters or numbers representing the appropriate principle or principles.)

3. The protection of hospital staff from infection is very important. How are staff in your hospital protected in regard to:

Collection and transport to the laboratories of specimens of sputum, blood and pus?

Arrangements for disposal of used intravenous infusion sets, hypodermic syringes and needles and scalpel blades?

Removal of used linen from wards?

4. Nurses play a vital part in the prevention of infection in hospital wards and in the community. Could their preparation for this responsibility be improved? If *yes*, how?

FURTHER READING

Catterall R D 1979 Venereology and genitourinary medicine, 2nd edn. Hodder & Stoughton, London
Collee J G 1981 Applied medical microbiology, 2nd edn. Blackwell Scientific, London
Gibson G L (ed) 1974 Infection in hospital. A code of practice, 2nd edn. (3rd edn in preparation) Churchill Livingstone, Edinburgh
Lowburg E J L (ed) 1981 Control of hospital infection, 2nd edn. Chapman & Hall, London
Parker M J, Stucke V A 1982 Microbiology for nurses, 6th edn. Bailliere Tindall, London

Chapter Two
The locomotor system

In health a person must be able to stand upright, sit, walk, run, jump and perform the many complex movements necessary in everyday life. To do this it is vital that the bones, joints, voluntary muscles, sensory and motor nerves are all healthy and in perfect working order. Distortions and malfunctioning of any part of these systems will cause a proportionate reduction in locomotor efficiency.

Orthopaedic conditions, their prevention, treatment and nursing, is a speciality in its own right, and there are many excellent textbooks on the subject from which a detailed knowledge of such disorders can be gained. The purpose of this chapter is to provide some basic information about the working of the locomotor system which can be applied in general nursing care and some guidelines to the treatment of a limited number of orthopaedic conditions which the nurse may meet in a general hospital.

ANATOMY AND PHYSIOLOGY

Maintenance of body shape and the protection of vital organs are two of the functions of the skeleton. A third function is that it forms a system of levers and joints so that the action of voluntary muscles, stimulated by motor nerve fibres, will cause movement of a part of the body.

How joints and muscles work

A joint is any place in the body where two or more bones touch (or articulate). Some joints are fixed, such as the joints between the bones of the adult skull. These sutures, as they are called, ossify early in childhood and, of course, movement is not possible at such joints.

A second type of articulation is the slightly movable joint; here the union between the bones is formed by cartilage. Examples of such joints can be seen at the symphysis pubis of the pelvis, or the union between the bodies of the vertebrae. Cartilaginous joints allow very slight movement to occur between the bones; for example, the movement between any two vertebral bodies is very limited and in some cases non-existent, though the composite range of movement of the whole spinal column is fairly wide.

It is the third type of joint, however, which is of major importance in locomotion, namely the freely movable joint.

Characteristics of a freely movable joint

The articulating surfaces are smooth and complementary to each other — as in the shoulder, hip and knee joints on the skeleton. These surfaces are made even smoother by a covering of tough resilient cartilage which also acts to some extent as a shock-absorber. The bones which form a joint are held together by bands of fibrous tissue called ligaments. All freely movable joints are enclosed in a sleeve of this fibrous tissue. This is called the joint capsule, or capsular ligament, because it encapsulates the joint and holds the bones in place without unduly restricting movement.

Some freely movable joints have additional ligaments situated within the capsule (intracapsular ligaments) and others which lie outside the capsule (extracapsular ligaments). These ligaments lend extra stability to the joint and prevent undesirable movement. Intracapsular ligaments hold the bones together without limitation of movement. An example of this can be seen in the hip joint, where a ligament passes from a small depression on the head of femur to an attachment in the cup-shaped part of the innominate bone of the pelvis which is called the acetabulum. This ligament effectively tethers the ball-like head of the femur to the socket-shaped acetabulum (Fig. 2.1).

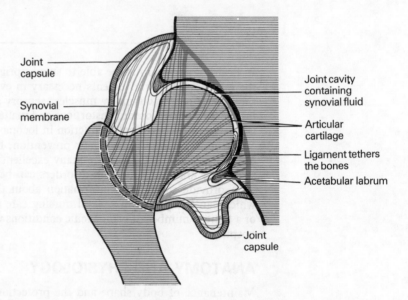

Joint capsule
Synovial membrane
Joint cavity containing synovial fluid
Articular cartilage
Ligament tethers the bones
Acetabular labrum
Joint capsule

Figure 2.1
A freely movable joint

Though freedom of movement is essential, excessive movement or movement in undesirable directions must be prevented. For instance it would be difficult to walk if the leg bowed or went into a knock-kneed position at every step. This is where the extracapsular ligaments come into play. Strong bands of fibrous tissue called collateral ligaments on the inner (medial) and outer (lateral) aspect of the knee prevent this undesirable movement. The patellar ligament (though technically a tendon) performs a similar function anteriorly.

Sometimes, in addition to the stability conferred on a joint by the shape of the articulating surfaces and the supportive ligaments, joints are further stabilized by structures within the capsule. These are commonly wedges or pads of cartilage which deepen a socket or build up an area deficient in bone. Examples of these intracapsular structures are found in the shoulder and hip joint where the glenoid and acetabular labra deepen the respective sockets. Similarly in the knee joint, the half-moon shaped (semilunar) cartilages known as menisci build up the medial and lateral aspects of the table-like head of the tibia, thus increasing the stability of the joint.

All joints, mechanical or biological, require lubrication to cut down friction and wear and to permit free action. In mechanical joints lubricants such as oil, grease, silicone or graphite have to be regularly maintained and replaced, as motorists know to their cost. Freely movable joints are lubricated by a clear, viscid fluid called synovial fluid. It is secreted by a specialized tissue, the synovial membrane, which lines and covers all nonarticular surfaces within a joint capsule. In health the secretion of synovial fluid by this tissue is sufficient to provide a small lubricant cushion between joint surfaces. As with other secretory membranes, like the pleura for example, irritation — mechanical, chemical or bacteriological — will stimulate an increase in production of the exudate. Thus, as pleural effusion is associated with pleurisy, so joint effusion may be associated with infection or injury.

Bursae

Some joints, due to the type of load they are required to bear, are subject to excessive friction or pressure, for example the knee in the kneeling position. In such cases small, fluid-filled sacs or bursae of synovial tissue act as cushions to buffer the joint from a jarring shock.

The action of muscles of locomotion

The groups of muscles which produce movement act synchronously — when the flexor muscles in the upper arm contract to bend the elbow, the extensor muscles relax to permit the action. The jerky movements of the child suffering from cerebral palsy are due to malfunctioning of the neural control, the system that allows this synchronous action to occur.

Terminology

Muscle contraction

Increased stimulation by motor nerve fibres causes muscle fibres either:
    1. To shorten the muscle, the tension remaining the same (isotonic contraction), or
    2. To increase the tension, the length of the muscle remaining the same (isometric contraction).

Muscle relaxation

Decreased stimulation by the motor nerve results in either lengthening of the muscle or decrease in the tone.

Muscle tone

In health all muscle fibres are held in a state midway between contraction and relaxation and are ready for instant action to produce a smooth movement. This state is referred to as muscle tone (Fig. 2.2).

Maximum muscle contraction potential does not occur during activity in normal body states.

Spasm   Contraction   Tone   Relaxation   Flaccidity

MUSCLE ACTION

Figure 2.2
Muscle action

Abnormal muscle action

Muscle spasm

Excessive muscle contraction is referred to as muscle spasm. In this state the affected muscles are rigid and stone-like in quality. Muscle spasm can also occur in conditions other than orthopaedic disorders. The board-like abdomen of the patient with a perforated peptic ulcer or the painful and disabling leg cramp sometimes experienced by swimmers are other examples of muscle spasm.

Sudden dramatic muscle contraction, say, when a mother lifts a very heavy object to free her trapped child, can be sufficiently violent to fracture bones or to tear muscle tendons from their bony attachments. One reason patients undergoing electroconvulsive therapy in psychiatric hospitals are given relaxant drugs as part of their anaesthetic is to prevent the violent muscle contractions which would otherwise be produced by the passage of the electric current through the body.

Muscle spasm is always acutely painful. It immobilizes the affected joint and can spread to adjacent muscles causing further pain and immobility.

Flaccidity

Just as muscles do not normally fully contract, similarly muscles do not normally fully relax. When a muscle cannot contract due to a disorder of its nerve supply, the muscle is said to be flaccid or paralysed. When a patient is unable to contract any of the muscle groups around a joint, that joint is said to be flail. Such a situation can arise in patients suffering from poliomyelitis. In this case the joint must be protected, because without support the limb will fall into abnormal positions causing stretching of ligaments and tendons.

Simple measures to relieve muscle spasm

Muscle spasm caused by inflammatory or other painful lesions can often be relieved by the application of local heat.

Local heat

Local heat applications all aim to increase the circulation to the affected muscle thus raising the temperature locally. The nurse should realize that there is always the danger that skin may be burnt in the process and take care to prevent this. The following are some methods of applying local heat:

1. A carefully protected hot water bottle or electric heat pad.
2. Hot baths — total immersion or immersion of the affected part only.
3. Wax baths — similar to item 2 but the heat is retained for longer by the wax and only the affected part is immersed.
4. Poultices — preparations such as Kaolin contain a counter-irritant, thus the action is two-fold; these need frequent reapplication.
5. Hot fomentations ⎫
6. Warm wool   ⎬ largely superseded by other methods.
7. Counter-irritants ⎭
8. Infra-red rays from a special lamp — superficial heat.
9. Ultrasonic massage: very high frequency sound waves penetrate tissue to the required depth and increase blood flow to the affected part.

Correcting posture

It is useful to remember that the patient having bed rest and skin traction may complain of acute lumbar or groin pain due to abnormal positioning of the pelvis. By gently altering the patient's position in bed so that the anterior iliac spines are level and the hips abducted, the muscle spasm can often be relieved. The importance of correct posture in bed or in a chair is discussed later in this chapter.

Movement

A muscle or group of muscles producing movement must, obviously, be attached on either side of the joint so that when the muscle length is decreased the effect is to pull the two bones into a position where the angle between them is decreased.

The muscle passes from a fixed point, across a joint to its attachment on the other bone(s), and when it contracts and the opposing set of muscles relax, movement is produced.

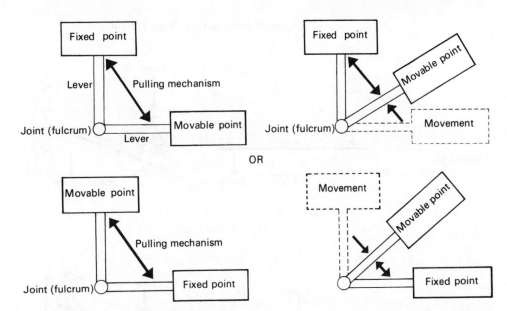

Figure 2.3A
Movement

Figure 2.3B
Fixed and movable points

The upper bone will be pulled towards the lower, or the lower towards the upper depending on whether the upper or lower end of the muscle is used as the fixed point. Thus muscles and joints are versatile in the movement they can produce (Fig. 2.3).

Figure 2.3C
Lever and fulcrum principle

A fulcrum is a specific point against which a lever may be placed to exert pressure. Pressure of the lever against the fulcrum causes increased force at the tip of the lever. The longer the lever and the closer the fulcrum to the point to be moved, the greater the force which is exerted. This principle has been used to move great weights throughout man's history. It is still used today in engineering achievements. A simple example from daily life is the use of a metal bar as a lever against a wheel rim to remove a tyre for puncture repair. Using a lever against a fulcrum allows great force to be exerted with minimum expenditure of effort.

Movement at a joint also uses this principle. This allows for maximum efficiency in that normal movements are achieved by the use of minimal amounts of muscle effort. The general state of 'readiness' of muscles in good tone and the co-ordinated action of the nervous system are also essential to locomotor efficiency.

Types of lever action

The anatomical shape of the bones involved and the siting of the muscle attachment cause different types of lever action.

The longer the lever, the greater is the force applied at the fulcrum.

Greater force is needed to raise the whole body weight when standing on tiptoe than is needed to nod the head. The relative position of the fulcrum in each case reflects this (Fig. 2.4A–C).

Types of lever action (Figs 2.4A–C)

Figure 2.4A

Figure 2.4B

Figure 2.4C

It is important for the nurse to know the full range of normal movement for each joint (Fig. 2.5A–H). This knowledge is required when joint mobility has to be retained in a paralysed limb and the nurse must assist with passive movement of the joint.

Joint movements (Figs 2.5A–H)

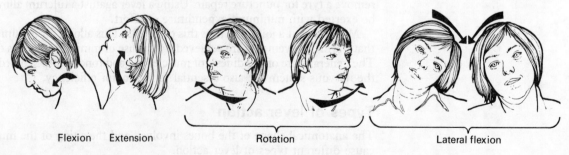

Flexion   Extension   Rotation   Lateral flexion

Figure 2.5A
Head and neck movements

Gently helping a patient to move the neck through its full range of movements may sometimes alleviate neck pain or headache.

Figure 2.5B
Shoulder movements

A combination of these six movements, shown in Figure 2.5B, is used when children swing their arms in a wide circle while playing at 'being a windmill'. This complex movement is called circumduction. Circumduction is also possible at the hip joint and is a movement commonly used in ballet (Fig. 2.5A–H).

Figure 2.5C
Elbow and forearm movements

Figure 2.5D
Wrist movements.

Wrist mobility makes a very important contribution to very fine movements of the hand.

Figure 2.5E
Hip movements

Figure 2.5F
Knee movement

Figure 2.5G
Ankle movements

Figure 2.5H
Forefoot movements

Position of rest

Excessive muscle contraction can be caused solely by abnormal joint position. It is, therefore, important that the nurse should know the position of rest for each of the major joints. In this position no undue tension is put on the muscles or strain on the ligaments or the joint. By gently moving a joint into the correct position, muscle spasm can often be relieved or minimized. It is also important when the patient has a paralysed limb. The muscles are unable to contract, so they are unable to support the limb. Thus it will tend to flop into abnormal positions which will strain the joint and can cause deformity. The nurse must ensure that when she is working with such a patient she holds the limb in a normal position at all times, and that when she leaves the patient the limb is gently but firmly supported by pillows and pads so that the desired position will be maintained.

Position of rest for important joints (Figs 2.6A–I)

Even if not paralysed, a person sitting in bed or in a chair will be more comfortable if the shoulder joint is supported in the position of rest.

There are circumstances which dictate that a special position should be adopted, other than the position of rest. For example, the straighter positioning of the fingers of the stroke patient to prevent contractures of the small joints.

Sometimes the pathology indicates that full recovery of joint function is unlikely. Here it is important that the joint is held in the best position for function. The positions of function and of rest are often similar, but occasionally the position must be modified in the knowledge of the occupation the patient wishes to follow after discharge.

Figures 2.6A–I
Positions of rest

Figure 2.6A
Shoulder
60 degrees abduction
30 degrees forward flexion
45 degrees rotation

Figure 2.6B
Elbow
90 degrees flexion
Forearm midway between
pronation and supination

Figure 2.6C
Wrist
30 degrees dorsiflexion
Slight ulnar deviation

Figure 2.6D
Thumb
45 degrees abduction
Thumb opposed to fingers

Figure 2.6E
Fingers
Lightly curled

Figure 2.6F
Hip
5–15 degrees abduction
30 degrees forward flexion
No rotation (toes point to ceiling)

Figure 2.6G
Knee
5–15 degrees flexion
Patella points to ceiling

Figure 2.6H
Ankle
Neutral — 90 degrees
angle (No inversion or eversion)

Figure 2.6 I
Spinal column
Shoulders level:
pelvis level: no rotation
Support lumbar and cervical
curves

The positon of rest and the position of function are identical in the case of the ankle joint (Fig. 2.6H). It is essential that this positon is maintained, with support if necessary, if a person is going to be unable to walk for some time.

LOCOMOTOR EFFICIENCY

The information in the preceding section gives guidance about the positions of rest and positions of function for the major joints in the body. The importance of knowledge in this area cannot be overemphasized. The nurse who uses this information to observe the patient, in bed or in a chair, to ensure that all joints are maintained in the best possible (optimum) position not only contributes to therapy, but does much to ensure the patient's comfort and sense of well-being.

The ability to ensure correct body alignment and joint position is a skill which the nurse may undervalue. There are some who may regard the ability to position supports and pillows as trivial. This is not the case, as is evident when one compares the efforts of the junior trainee with the deft movements of the experienced nurse, and the evident comfort of the patient after such expert attentions.

POSTURE AND BODY MECHANICS

In order to maintain the upright position with minimum effort, it is vital that weight transmission and balance are efficient. If the head, thorax and pelvis are thought of as loads which have to be carried by the legs, it is obvious that if the weights are piled in a straight column and balanced on straight legs, the amount of muscular effort needed to maintain this position will be minimal. The load is further stabilized when the feet are apart, as this gives a broader base for weight transmission (Fig. 2.7).

The same is true of sitting positions. Strange as it may seem the slouching position is more tiring as it causes strain and muscle tension (Fig. 2.8).

STABLE COLUMN
Body alignment allows gravitational pull
to pass straight down weight-bearing line

UNSTABLE COLUMN
Poor alignment causes fatigue due
to muscle and ligamentous strain

Figure 2.7
Posture — standing

Muscle tension

Decreased
lung expansion

Ligamentous strain

Figure 2.8
Posture — sitting

Posture during normal activity

Good postural habits are vital to nurses since, by minimizing the amount of muscular effort needed for work, they help the nurse not only to complete the task with less fatigue, but also to avoid the possibility of joint strain. The major points of good posture are:

1. Head held high.
2. Chin tucked in.
3. Shoulders level.
4. Lower abdomen flat.
5. Curves of the spine maintained without exaggeration.
6. Pelvis level.
7. Knees relaxed.
8. Feet pointing straight ahead.

Good posture and body alignment must, however, be maintained not only when standing and sitting but during activity.

Lifting patients is achieved by a series of dynamic movements. Not only has a load to be lifted, but it has also to be moved to a different relative position. Good postural habits and lifting techniques all aim to ensure that whether standing still or moving, the nurse maintains balance and equilibrium. Smoothness of action and easy transmission of weight during movement are emphasized in training for many sports. Correct ratios of balance to speed and to direction of movement all contribute to a magnificent throw of the javelin. The same application and thought and practice which must be applied to the 'weight lifting training' nurses must do if they are to perfect their skills to the level that professional competence and patient safety demands.

The following summary may help the student to learn postural habits which will use efficiently the body's system of levers and joints.

1. When carrying or lifting, the load should be held close to the body. This simplifies weight transmission and thus minimizes effort.

2. When carrying a load, the elbows should be flexed and held close to the side of the body. This utilizes the stronger muscles of the upper arm, rather than demanding a combined effort from arm and shoulder muscles.

3. When lifting, the load should be faced, thus avoiding rotary strains of the spine.

4. Shoulders and pelvis should be held on the same plane and never twisted.

5. A broader base of support increases stability. By placing one foot in front of the other, the base of support is increased towards the object to be lifted.

6. To lift objects from a lower work level, the knees should be bent and the spine kept straight. This allows the load to be carried by the stronger thigh and buttock muscles rather than the weaker spinal muscles.

7. Stand close to the object to be moved. This helps to maintain the body's centre of gravity over the base of support and so increases stability.

8. The flexor muscles of the arm are usually stronger than the extensors, so always lift or turn objects towards oneself.

9. Whenever possible, turn or slide the object to be moved. Extra effort is needed to lift a load against the force of gravity.

10. Always use smooth, continuous movements as opposed to jerky, stop-start manoeuvres. Less effort is required to keep an object moving than to start the movement.

11. Try to move a patient on a level surface. Unless contra-indicated, lower the backrest before moving a patient towards the head of the bed.

12. A lifting or turning sheet is often helpful as it reduces the amount of contact surface and therefore friction. When using a lifting sheet, it is helpful if the patient is able to flex knees, hips and neck.

13. Never attempt to lift a heavy load without help. To do so is to put both your own and the patient's safety at risk.

14. When lifting a heavy static weight, if the nurse is not required to move from A to B with the object, it is sometimes useful to prepare for the lift by 'fixing' or contracting pelvic and gluteal muscles. A knee braced against a solid support can also help to prepare for such a lift.

Posture in bed or in chair

It is just as important for the patient to maintain good posture and body alignment in bed or when sitting in a chair. A sagging mattress can cause flexion contractures of the hip in an amazingly short time. Improperly placed pillows at head and neck can lead to round shoulders and decreased chest expansion. Knees permanently flexed will cause shortening of the hamstring tendons and therefore knee flexion contractures. These deformities do not take long to develop so the vigilant nurse must be aware of the hazards and take steps to prevent them. This means constant intelligent observation of the patient in bed or in a chair. Untrained observation is of little use to the nurse. Knowledge of normal body function must be applied to each observation. Only by constant awareness of potential malfunctioning or dangers can the warning signs be detected soon enough.

Observation and maintenance of the best possible position for the patient is, of course, not only applicable to orthopaedic care. The nurse's knowledge of physiology and body mechanics must be interrelated. It should be obvious that a patient having oxygen therapy who is allowed to slip from the upright sitting position into a slumped position is no longer able to gain the full benefit of the therapy.

Complications of enforced inactivity

Problems associated with inactivity and bed rest are many and varied, and it is perhaps appropriate at this point to summarize the major problems which the observant nurse can prevent or minimize.

Muscle atrophy

Inactivity results in muscle atrophy. The muscle becomes smaller and its circulation diminishes, resulting in decreased endurance and rapid fatigue. The individual becomes less active and further atrophy occurs. A dramatic example of this can be seen in the patient who has had a plaster cast removed after several weeks of immobilization; the same process of atrophy begins in the bed-fast patient after only a few days. It is therefore important to encourage the bed-fast or chair-fast patient to do active exercising of thigh, lower leg and foot muscles to minimize this atrophy. Patients wearing a plaster cast should also engage in an active exercise regime at least once hourly unless contra-indicated.

Joint contractures

Joints which are held immobile will soon become stiff. This may result from shortening of muscle tendons, capsular ligaments or the muscles themselves. In terms of the patient's well-being, the consequences may mean longer convalescence, discomfort or pain during rehabilitation, and possibly a persistent deformity. It is, therefore, an important nursing responsibility to prevent joint contractures, whenever possible, by good positioning and regular exercise.

Drop foot deformity

The nurse should note that if the foot is not supported, tendons of the calf muscles tend to shorten while the muscles of the anterior portion of the leg lengthen. Even a mild degree of drop foot can cause many weeks of painful rehabilitation. If severe, it will mean that the patient cannot put the heel to the ground when attempting to stand. Maintenance of the foot in a functional position at all times should be ensured, and special appliances should be used to maintain this position if the bed rest is prolonged. Again, instruction and encouragement with active exercise, if the patient is able, will be essential.

Hypostatic pneumonia

A slouched or horizontal position in bed, lack of mobility, tight bandages around the chest and upper abdomen all cause a decrease in chest expansion. Severe pain and the administration of analgesics which depress the respiratory centre in the medulla can contribute to lung congestion. Inactivity lowers the basal metabolic rate, therefore CO_2 production is less, resulting in a further reduction in respiratory stimulus. The horizontal position allows pooling of secretions in the bronchial tree and if dehydration occurs, these secretions become tenacious and difficult to expectorate. This bronchial stasis provides an ideal medium for the growth of pathogenic organisms. Thus the stage is set for the development of hypostatic pneumonia and chest infections. Awareness of this potential hazard should make the nurse vigilant in ensuring that the patient's posture allows optimum lung ventilation. Instruction and assistance with deep breathing exercises and expectoration are also essential.

Pressure necrosis

The effect of prolonged pressure on vulnerable areas of tissue is well known and is fully discussed on page 517.

Disuse osteoporosis

The exact mechanism of calcium deposition and bone formation is not known. It is known that inactivity and lack of weight-bearing results in loss of calcium from the skeletal system. To minimize this loss, patients on prolonged bed rest, unless contra-indicated, have the head of the bed raised for several hours per day, as this simulates weight-bearing stress.

Renal calculi

The calcium lost from the skeletal system is excreted by the kidneys. Research has shown that increased calcium excretion begins as early as the third or fourth day of bed rest and reaches a peak by the fourth or fifth week. This increased calcium excretion may lead to the formation of kidney stones. Other precipitating factors are stasis of urine, decreased urinary output, urinary tract infection and an alkaline urine which is associated with decreased muscular activity. Raising the head of the bed will aid gravitational drainage and this, plus a high fluid intake, helps to minimize the problem.

Bladder and bowel problems

The patient confined to bed in the supine position has particular difficulty with elimination. Lack of privacy and attempting to use a bedpan or urinal in an unnatural position make it difficult for the patient to relax the perineal and sphincter muscles. The nurse must recognize that the patient who asks for frequent bedpans but passes only small amounts of urine, or the older patient who is frequently incontinent, may be suffering from retention of urine with overflow (p. 356).

Constipation and faecal impaction are also common problems with the immobilized patient. Neither lying supine nor sitting with the knees extended will promote the normal reflexes necessary for defaecation. The patient with faecal impaction may pass frequent small amounts of liquid faecal material which can be misinterpreted as diarrhoea. The nurse should always try to help the patient to achieve as natural a position as is compatible with the splintage being worn. Raising the head of the bed and/or judicious use of pads or supports may assist with the achievement of a more natural position for elimination.

Thrombosis

The problems of phlebothrombosis and thrombophlebitis associated with bed rest are fully discussed on page 290. Pulmonary embolism as a result of thrombosis formation can also occur (p. 291).

Fat embolus

When a major bone is fractured, fat globules from the bone marrow may enter the circulation and give rise to symptoms 24 to 48 hours after the fracture. The first sign may be a sudden or progressive pyrexia followed by restlessness, chest pain and dyspnoea. Tachycardia and cerebral symptoms develop and, if a large quantity of fat has been released into the circulation, the prognosis is poor. One sign which the nurse must report urgently is the appearance of a petechial rash especially over the chest, neck and shoulders. (Petechiae look like tiny bruised spots in the skin.) Sometimes symptoms are mild and fleeting and slight confusion or unexplained incontinence sometimes indicates that fat embolism has occurred.

Postural hypotension

Patients who have been confined to bed for long periods may experience vertigo on assuming the upright position. Sometimes fainting will occur. This is known as postural hypotension and is due to sudden pooling of blood in the abdominal viscera and legs. Before ambulation, therefore, the nurse should prepare the patient gradually by raising the head of the bed for short periods or allowing him to sit up if permitted. The application of support bandages or stockings may also help to minimize the pooling of blood in the peripheral circulation and to prevent oedema of the dependent extremities.

Body position as part of therapy

There are many occasions in which the nurse's knowledge of optimum joint position plays a vital part in treatment. Perhaps a few instances would start the learner thinking about the relationship between anatomy, types of therapy, the aims of the treatment, and the constraints imposed upon such treatment. For example, a patient may be suffering from osteoarthiritis of the left hip. If you look at the effect that the pain caused by this disease has had upon the patient's posture you will usually see that the hip is held in an unnatural position. It is often flexed, so that the patient has difficulty in placing the foot flat on the floor. Pain and muscle spasm often cause external rotation and adduction of the hip joint so that the knee-cap (patella) points away from the opposite leg instead of straight ahead. Flexion and external rotation of the hip will also cause tilting of the pelvis and alteration of the spinal curve in the lumbar region. This vicious circle of stiffness, due to distortion of joint surfaces, pain, spasm and shortening of ligaments and tendons, places the patient in a very unhappy situation. Attention paid to pillows which will support the joints in their most appropriate position will do much for the patient's comfort.

Selection of the appropriate position for a patient to adopt takes knowledge, judgement and skill. For the patient admitted for surgical correction by arthroplasty, the position of function is not possible at this stage. Therefore joints should be supported in the manner the patient prefers and must be prevented from falling into a strained position. If the hip is flexed and externally rotated, it should be supported in this position. Unsupported the weight of the leg will cause pulling on the short-ened ligaments and will cause further pain and resultant spasm. Whether the patient is up or in bed, dorsal or in a lateral position, the observant nurse should ensure that all joints are supported in the most comfortable position prior to surgery. In the early postoperative stages, the nature of the surgery required to relieve the condition means that there is a risk of joint dislocation. The patient must, therefore, be nursed with the hip supported in its most stable position, that of abduction and slight internal rotation, and this position must be maintained at all times and during all nursing procedures.

The art of placing pillows so that they give appropriate support without compro-mising vital structures is a skill which all nurses must develop. For example, a pillow to support the leg must not compress the back of the knee, which would increase the patient's risk of thrombosis of the deep leg veins. It should, however, support the head of the tibia and should also be able to hold the heel clear of the mattress without compressing the calf muscles. Knowledge of surface anatomy, proximity of nerves and blood vessels, normal joint positions and awareness of the outcome to be achieved by the support all contribute to the nurse's ability to use pillows and other supports judiciously and appropriately.

TRAUMA AND THE PROCESS OF REPAIR

The repair process for soft tissues and bone is fundamental to any consideration of the remote complications of injury or surgery. Tissues vary in their capacity for true repair. In connective tissue such as bone, repair is almost perfect. A year after a fracture it may be impossible to identify the site of the injury. Other tissues, however, are so highly specialized that it is impossible for them to regenerate — for instance the nerve cells of the brain. Notable exceptions to this rule are the cells of the liver and kidney, which are capable of dramatic proliferation, though the struc-ture may be disorganised.

The process of repair for all tissues is basically the same but is influenced by the degree of specialization of the cells, the vascularity of the part, the presence or absence of infection and the degree of tissue destruction. There are, of course, a number of other factors involved, many of which are as yet ill-understood and the subject of much experimental work.

Methods of repair

It is convenient to discuss tissue repair under two headings:

1. Healing by primary union.
2. Healing by granulation tissue.

Healing by primary union

This occurs in clean, incised wounds, such as a stitched, surgical incision, where there is little or no loss of tissue and the cut edges of the wound are in close opposition.

The space between the cut surfaces fills with plasma, which forms a sticky medium into which two types of cells grow: (1) fibroblasts and (2) vascular endothelial cells. This occurs very rapidly (within the first 24 hours or so). At the same time small blood vessels of the injured part enter a phase of great activity. The endothelial lining of the capillaries proliferates and these capillary buds join up with neighbouring buds to form a branching network. The buds quickly multiply and a lumen is established which communicates with the parent vessel. In the same way the lymphatic endothelial cells divide rapidly to establish a primitive lymphatic system.

The narrow gap on the skin surface is bridged by epithelial cells which grow in from the wound edges. Hair follicles and sweat glands (specialized cells) are not reproduced. Healing is complete and the resultant scar tissue gradually shrinks.

Healing by granulation tissue

Where there has been loss of tissue or infection the fibroblast are unable to 'sew' the wound surfaces together and repair starts at the base of the wound.

The wound defect is filled by a blood clot, plasma and inflammatory exudate. As in healing by primary union fibroblasts and vascular endothelial cells proliferate, but in addition wandering, scavenger cells play an important part in the process. The resulting granulation tissue is highly vascular and easily damaged. It is, therefore, very vulnerable to careless dressing technique or inappropriate dressings.

The scavenger cells at first are mainly polymorphonuclear leucocytes. They ingest bacteria and debris and keep the surface of the wound free from serious infection. A granulating surface has remarkable powers to resist serious bacterial infection, but if there are foreign bodies or dead tissue in the wound, suppuration occurs and the process of healing will not take place.

When the wound is 'clean' (though not necessarily bacteriologically sterile) epithelial cells begin to grow in from the wound edges to cover the granulation tissue. As healing proceeds the granulation tissue contracts (collagen formation) and becomes less vascular. Parts of the wound may fail to heal because of avascularity or the presence of a foreign body. Persistent infection will also delay healing. Ulcer formation is associated with the former and the development of a sinus with the latter.

Factors which influence repair

Nutrition

When suffering from a major injury, malnutrition or starvation, the body is in negative nitrogen balance (Ch. 4) and wound repair is slow. Thus, unless contraindicated due to another disease condition, a high protein diet is indicated following trauma or surgery. The part played by vitamins in tissue development and repair should not be ignored, and vitamins C and D may be prescribed as a nutritional supplement.

Hormonal control

Endocrine glands influence repair either by systemic effects on metabolism or by direct action on the affected tissue. Cortisone, for example, inhibits vascular changes and discourages collagen formation, therefore patients having cortisone therapy may show evidence of slow healing.

Local vascularity

Tissues which have a good blood supply heal well. If vascularity is normally poor or has become so because of disease, healing is slow. Wounds of face or scalp, therefore, heal quickly while those on ankle or shin are notoriously slow.

Lymphatic drainage

Obstruction to the lymphatic drainage will cause oedema which delays healing.

Mechanical factors

Excessive movement tears young granulation tissue. In soft tissue, this tends to produce a dense thickened scar. In bony tissue, movement at a fracture site may convert osteoid tissue into fibrous tissue, and a pseudarthrosis or false joint may be formed.

Anchorage to subjacent structures

Where layers of tissue are firmly bound to other tissue, healing is slow. Wounds over the 'shin', for example, heal badly.

Repair of specific tissues

Bone

Despite the specialized nature of the tissue, bone heals well. It is worth remembering that bone is not merely a rigid skeleton but is constantly changing in response to the physical or chemical demands of the body. An area of bone constantly subjected to extra stress will, over time, develop a buttress system to strengthen the area. The repair of bone consists of two processes:

1. The formation of osteoid tissue.
2. The deposition of calcium and phosphorus (ossification).

Granulation tissue forms in the haematoma which surrounds the broken bone ends. Very quickly the fibrous tissue so formed differentiates into fibrocartilage. Almost simultaneously, specialized cells called osteoblasts proliferate and a loosely woven osteoid tissue called callus forms a sleeve round the fractured bone ends. This tissue unites and helps to stabilize the fracture, but it is not strong enough to permit weightbearing or prevent movement without additional splintage. Gradually more calcium and phosphorus salts are laid down in the tissue so that true bone is reformed. Restructuring and remodelling occurs; eventually the bone is restored to its former shape.

Muscle

Voluntary muscle may regenerate to a very limited extent depending on the type of injury. When involuntary muscle is damaged, repair is by fibrous tissue replacement.

Tendons

Collagen fibres heal very well provided that the gap is not too great. Divided tendons are therefore sutured to facilitate repair. Tendon sheaths repair by fibrous tissue and if there is extensive destruction of the sheath adhesions tend to form.

Serous membrane

These tissues heal by fibrous tissue formation. The surface endothelium *may* cover the fibrous scar to restore the smooth membrane. Sometimes two or more adjacent surfaces are involved, and the fibrous tissues coalesce and become adherent. This is particularly likely if infection is present.

Articular cartilage

Repair is poor due to the relative avascularity of this tissue. The repair is usually by formation of fibrous tissue rather than articular cartilage.

Central nervous system

The brain and spinal cord have no power of regeneration.

Peripheral nerves

The repair process is complex and occurs after an extended period of time. If a peripheral nerve has been divided by an injury the nerve sheath must be sutured for regeneration to occur.

Skin

Small defects are quickly covered by epithelium, but the scar is thinner than normal skin and often unstable.

Fat

If fat cells have been destroyed they do not usually regenerate.

Solid organs

Specialized cells have little capacity for true healing. Repair is effected by connective tissue replacement.

DISORDERS OF THE LOCOMOTOR SYSTEM

As in other systems of the body, the locomotor system can become disordered by injury, disease or congenital malformation. In broad terms and excluding the neurological manifestations that affect locomotion, the system will be unable to function efficiently if its structure is altered. For example, if a long bone is fractured the muscles cannot pull upon it as a lever, therefore movement is impossible. Similarly if the smooth surface of a joint is destroyed due to osteoarthritis, movement is reduced. Pain and resultant muscle spasm lead to further limitation of function.

Inflammatory responses give rise to swelling and exudate, which again result in loss of movement. In a less direct way the same effect is produced by congenital deformities or deformity as a result of trauma. Distortion of the shape of, say, the femur can lead to alteration of the lines of weight transmission, muscle spasm, extra wear and tear on joints, arthritis, pain and limitation of movement.

The purposes of orthopaedic treatment

The aims of orthopaedic treatment are:

1. To restore or maintain function.
2. To increase movement.
3. To prevent deformity.
4. To restore stability.
5. To correct deformity, if present.
6. To relieve pain.
7. To aid diagnosis.
8. To excise dead or infected tissue.
9. To develop powers of adaptation or compensation if loss of function or disability is inevitable.

Multidisciplinary management

Care of the person suffering from an orthopaedic condition requires the involvement of a team of people with a wide range of skills (Fig. 2.9). If an operation is necessary it is only one step in a carefully planned campaign from conservative management right through to the patient's independence and rehabilitation. At all times, the nurse must encourage and give explanations to the orthopaedic patient, whose road to recovery may be prolonged, painful and sometimes discouraging.

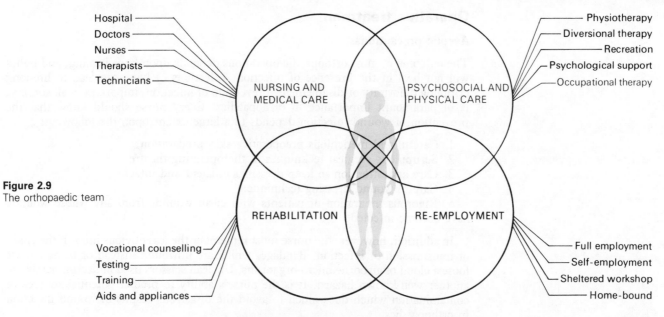

Hospital
Doctors
Nurses
Therapists
Technicians

NURSING AND MEDICAL CARE

PSYCHOSOCIAL AND PHYSICAL CARE

Physiotherapy
Diversional therapy
Recreation
Psychological support
Occupational therapy

REHABILITATION

RE-EMPLOYMENT

Vocational counselling
Testing
Training
Aids and appliances

Full employment
Self-employment
Sheltered workshop
Home-bound

Figure 2.9
The orthopaedic team

Orthopaedic treatment can be categorized as either conservative or operative, though often a combination of the two is required.

Conservative treatment

Active exercises

Normal joint function requires good muscle control. Specific exercises aimed at one muscle or group of muscles will be required if:

1. The muscles are weak and deformity is liable to occur due to the pull of the antagonist group of muscles. This can be caused by (a) nerve or muscle tissue damage; (b) brain or spinal cord lesions; (c) tendon injuries.
2. The joint has limited mobility following injury.

Passive movements

The therapist gently moves the joint through its full range of normal movement. Often this is combined with active exercise, when it is known as assisted movement. The manipulation is always gentle, never forced and can be used for the following reasons:

1. To prevent stiffening of the joints in a paralysed limb (hemiplegia following a cerebrovascular accident).
2. To correct deformity (club foot).
3. To restore joint movement (following immobilization).
4. To relieve muscle spasm (leg cramp).

Active exercise is encouraged whenever possible. It is only when the patient is unable to contract his muscles that passive movements would be carried out by the nurse or therapist in an attempt to maintain joint mobility. N.B. The term 'passive exercise' is a misnomer, as 'exercise' is always *active*.

Splinting

Sometimes it is necessary that certain joints or a limb should be held immobile in a prescribed position, using various appliances and materials. Splinting is used to:

1. Relieve pain.
2. Diminish muscle spasm.
3. Prevent undesirable movements.
4. Immobilize fractures in alignment until healed.
5. Maintain stable joint position after dislocation until the capsule is healed.

Operative treatment

Aseptic precautions

The outcome of most orthopaedic operations depends upon bone healing, and bones will not heal in the presence of infection. Infections of bone can lead to life-long crippling deformity or disablement. Prevention of infection, important in all surgery, is of paramount importance in orthopaedics. Every nurse should know that the prevention of wound infection depends to a large extent upon the following:

1. Careful and meticulous preoperative skin preparation.
2. Scrupulous surgical techniques in the operating theatre.
3. Care and attention to keep dressings efficient and intact.
4. Careful wound dressing technique.
5. Rigorous separation of patients with clean wounds from any whose wounds have become infected.

In addition, however, the nurse must remember the less obvious links in the chain of transmission of infection. Bandages which are unwound instead of being cut let loose a cloud of airborne micro-organisms. Unclean scissors used indiscriminately are another well-known hazard. It is the nurse's ability to predict potential sources of contamination which does much to avoid the disastrous results of wound infection in orthopaedics.

Orthopaedic operations can be classified under the following headings:

Operations on bones

1. Division of the bone (osteotomy) to alter its shape or correct deformity.
2. Internal fixation — metal plates, screws or special nails used to immobilize divided bone after fracture or osteotomy.
3. Bone graft. A piece of bone or bone chips used to support or encourage healing after fractures (especially if non-union occurs), osteotomy or removal of a bone tumour.
4. Removal of pieces of bone: for histological examination (biopsy) or because excess bone is pressing on adjacent structures and causing pain.
5. Operations for bone infections. It may be necessary to remove dead pieces of bone (sequestrectomy) which act as foreign bodies and delay healing, or to drain abscesses.

Operations on joints

1. Division of capsule or fascia to correct deformity (capsulotomy or fasciotomy).
2. Excision of synovial membrane for investigative reasons (biopsy) or therapeutic reasons (synovectomy).
3. Excision of joint surfaces to create a false joint and permit movement (pseudarthrosis).
4. Fixation of a badly damaged or painful joint (arthrodesis).
5. Refashioning of a joint by insertion of a prosthesis (arthroplasty).
6. Stabilization of a flail joint or one where there is recurrent dislocation.

Operation on muscles and tendons

1. Suturing where structures have been divided.
2. Division of a tendon to correct deformities (tenotomy).
3. Tendon transplant to restore function to a joint.

Operations on peripheral nerves

1. Suturing of a nerve sheath when a nerve has been divided.
2. Dissection to free a nerve from pressure due to ganglia, fascia, bone or tumour.
3. Division of nerve supply to overactive muscles.

Operations to repair skin defects and deficient blood supply

1. Skin grafts or tissue transplant.
2. Venous or arterial surgery.

Amputation

This may be necessary when a limb or part of a limb has become a useless encumbrance because of one of the following:

1. Death of tissue.
2. Gross and intractable sepsis.
3. Gross deformity.

Diseases affecting joints

The multidisciplinary nature of care and therapy required by people with disorders of the locomotor system is perhaps best illustrated in the management of patients with joint disorders. It is not possible here to describe and discuss all the diseases which may affect joints but as rheumatoid arthritis is one of the major crippling diseases, perhaps this condition could be used to illustrate some important points of nursing management of patients with joint disorders in general.

Throughout this section the reader will be referred back to general points which have been discussed more fully elsewhere.

The physician initiates the plan of treatment which involves the nurse, physiotherapist, occupational therapist and medical social worker in a team effort. All have an important job to do as they make their own specialist contribution but the nurse has a major role to play, as she contributes to every aspect of treatment.

Rheumatoid arthritis

Rheumatoid arthritis is a chronic form of polyarthritis characterized in the majority of patients by exacerbations and remissions. The cause is still unknown but research suggests that disorders of the immune system play an important part in the development and perpetuation of the joint inflammation as well as the extra-articular manifestations such as skin nodules. What initiates and maintains the disease process is not clear. What has been established is that rheumatoid arthritis is an inflammatory disease unlike osteoarthritis which also affects synovial joints but in which inflammation does not play a major role. In this section some important facets of the nursing care of adult patients with rheumatoid arthritis will be described. Most of the text reflects experience gained from nursing such patients in a specialized hospital unit but much of what is suggested would, with appropriate modification, be equally applicable to the care of patients at home.

The first thing that the nurse must appreciate is that the patient is suffering from a chronic disease and is worried and often very bitter. Questions spoken and unspoken fill the air. Will I become a helpless cripple? Am I going to lead a normal life again? What did the doctor mean? The nurse plays an important role in listening to the patient and identifying the hidden fears and misconception he may have. This requires a great deal of time, patience and understanding coupled with factual knowledge about the disease process and the prospects for individual patients. The nurse must inspire in the person confidence and belief that even if cure is not possible, the treatment will lead to improvement in his condition.

A regime of medical treatment will be prescribed and nurses must ensure that the total programme is tailored to suit the individual needs of the patient. The role of the nurse in this blending of treatment and care to form an integrated pattern cannot be overemphasized. In any situation where cure is not possible, good and skilful nursing is of supreme importance. Although it is the doctor who prescribes the appropriate therapeutic regime for each individual patient, it is the nurse who organizes the therapy, diet, environment, rest and other aspects of the patient's day so that the needs of the individual are met. The processes of assessment, planning, teaching, explanation, reassurance and encouragement all play an important part in the building up of the patient's confidence to face the future.

For convenience the usual treatment can be described in three stages and at each one the nurse's attention to detail and knowledge of the person play a major part. The three stages of management of a patient suffering from early active rheumatoid arthritis are:

1. Rest phase.
2. Remobilization.
3. Rehabilitative phase.

Patients with less active disease, for example the elderly and severely crippled, have a modified regime of treatment. The nursing care required may be classified under the following headings:

1. General care and comfort of the patient.
2. Alleviation of pain.
3. Prevention of deformity (in a specialist unit nurses would also participate in the correction of deformity).
4. Careful observation.
5. Support, teaching and encouragement of the patient and the maintenance of his morale.
6. Rehabilitation of the patient.
7. In a specialist unit nurses would also be involved in the maintenance of improvement and the provision of continuing support.

Phase 1 — Rest

General care

A bright, well-ventilated room with a good outlook is essential. The bed must have a firm mattress and fracture boards may be used to ensure this. A back rest with the necessary number of pillows is used to keep the patient in an upright postion. The minimum number of pillows required for comfort should be allowed. This position is maintained for most of the day except for rest and treatment periods. The limbs must be correctly positioned (see pp. 37–38). A large cage with a padded foot board should be placed over the legs and feet. This should be anchored in position by straps if possible (Fig. 2.10). The bedclothes should be light and a soft blanket next to the patient is warm and comforting. The patient's own clothing should be light and easy to put on.

Figure 2.10
1. As few pillows as necessary for comfort
2. Back rest
3. Upright position
4. Padded footboard
5. Foot and ankle in position of function
6. Bed cage
7. Anchoring straps.

The nurse must always remember that in the acute phase of the disease the joints are swollen, inflamed and painful. Movement will inevitably cause an increase in pain and muscle spasm, therefore the patient must be lifted and turned very carefully to avoid jarring of the joints. As this person is completely bedfast special care must

Figure 2.11
Skin tight POP splints (Courtesy
of Dr T. M. Chalmers,
Consultant Rheumatologist.
Northern General Hospital.
Edinburgh)

be exercised when assisting with elimination. Great care must be taken to ensure that bed pans are positioned accurately and comfortably and that they are removed as soon as the patient wishes this. The limbs should be placed as close to the position of function as possible (see pp. 37–38). Skintight plaster of Paris splints are used to ensure this (Fig. 2.11). During this phase, of rest and immobilization, the patient is totally dependent upon the nurse, therefore he will require assistance with most of the activities of daily living. Daily bed bathing, oral hygiene and hair care are all necessary but special attention must be paid to pressure areas (see p. 517). The patient is unable to move about the bed and often perspires excessively due to active disease or as a result of the administration of salicylates. The patient with subcutaneous nodules requires particularly good skin care as the area over the nodules is very prone to breakdown (Fig. 2.12). Nodules are frequently found at the elbows

Figure 2.12
Subcutaneous nodules (Courtesy
of Dr T. M. Chalmers)

but may occur over any bony prominence and they may become ulcerated following a minor knock or merely pressure. If skin breakdown does occur it often becomes infected and difficult to heal. The use of aids such as foam pads, air-rings, sheep-skins or polystyrene bead bags can be of great assistance in the plan for skin care.

A well-balanced diet is given. If the patient is underweight extra milk and protein are added. Often however the patient is obese and it is most important to restrict carbohydrate to reduce weight. This is necessary if weight-bearing joints are involved. An adequate fluid intake will help to prevent urinary tract infections and constipation (see p. 42). Assistance with feeding must be given in an unhurried fashion. The nurse should always sit by the bedside and give her full attention to the patient at mealtimes.

Alleviation of pain

1. Rest splints are used for the relief of pain.
2. Special procedures such as the aspiration of effusions and local injections into the joints are carried out by the doctor.
3. Many drugs have been used to alleviate the pain characteristic of rheumatoid arthiritis and one of the most useful is acetylsalicylic acid (Aspirin). No pharmacological agent has yet been found to cure the condition and nurses must have a wide knowledge of the uses and side effects of the drugs prescribed so that they can detect and report any undesirable signs at the earliest possible moment. Accurate timing of drug administration is important. This means a departure from the traditional medicine round of three times a day. The drug must be given with or immediately after a meal to reduce irritation of the gastric mucosa, the early morning and bedtime dose being given with a glass of milk or a small snack. If extra analgesia is required to supplement the antirheumatic medication it is best given between the usual medicine times and at bedtime. A mild sedative is often required in the initial stages but it is undesirable to use strong hypnotics or drugs of addiction.

Prevention of deformity

Good posture and position in bed are essential at all times (see p. 40). Skintight unpadded rest splints designed to hold the affected joint in the position of function without muscle strain, should be used to prevent further flexion deformities of the knees or wrists and to prevent ulnar deviation of the fingers (Fig. 2.13).

Figure 2.13
Ulnar deviation of the fingers
(Courtesy of Dr T. M. Chalmers)

Observation

As rheumatoid arthritis is an inflammatory disease temperature, pulse and respiration rate are normally recorded twice per day or four hourly if the patient is febrile. The nurse must note and report the duration of early morning stiffness, any increase in pain, tenderness or involvement of other joints (Fig. 2.14).

Figure 2.14
Deformities and stiffness of the feet (Courtesy of Dr T. M. Chalmers)

Any signs of the plaster being too tight (see p. 59) such as colour changes, swelling or pain, should be reported immediately; if the plaster is too tight it will need to be removed at once. Pressure or rubbing of the plaster on bony prominences or rubbing at the edges of the plaster must be avoided lest abrasion of the skin occurs (see p. 61). The nurse must be able to report on the effectiveness of the prescribed drugs or any untoward effect which they may produce. Urine testing is important. Albuminuria may be present if there is renal involvement. Certain drugs, for example gold or D-penicillamine, may also produce protein in the urine. Glycosuria may develop in patients receiving high doses of steroids. The nurse must always be on the alert for any of the other possible complications that can arise due to immobilization and bed rest (see pp. 41–42).

Maintenance of morale

During this period of rest and immobilization the patient requires support and encouragement and his mind must be kept occupied. In addition to listening, talking and conversation between nurse and patient simple measures such as changing the position of the bed so that there is a view from the window will help. Full use can be made of television, books from the library and other diversions which all help to pass the time. Some patients who are ambulant may be of the greatest assistance simply by sitting and chatting with the bedfast patients. Visitors can also be of help and they too need support and advice from nursing staff. At this stage anxiety about the family and about the home may dominate the patient's outlook. The nurse may seek the help of the medical social worker to relieve the patient's worries.

The duration of phase 1 is usually about three weeks and towards the end of this period rest splints will be removed for short intervals during the day but are firmly and carefully secured at night.

Phase 2 — Remobilization

After the period of immobilization the physiotherapist starts a programme of graduated, non weight-bearing exercises beginning with general exercises designed to regain muscle tone and progressing to exercises designed to build muscle strength and joint mobility. Some patients may be over enthusiastic and may therefore have to be carefully supervised as too much exercise can cause a recurrence of joint inflammation.

It is the physiotherapist who will regulate the progression from day to day. Some increase in pain and stiffness is usual following unaccustomed exercise but if it is confined to the muscles it is not a contra-indication to further treatment. Once again reassurance, support and encouragement from the nurse is essential. The patient is still very dependent at this stage but is now able to be taken in a chair to the bath and toilet. Less assistance will be required with feeding each day and the person must be encouraged towards greater independence. He is now able to sit out of bed and weight-bearing is permitted when adequate muscle strength has been developed.

Each day activities are slowly increased, and when the physician is satisfied that disease activity has been controlled, the last phase of the treatment begins.

Phase 3 — Rehabilitation

At this stage patients are up for much of the day. They dress in their own clothes, wear shoes and go to the day room for meals and recreation. Physiotherapy is still carried out in the ward but in addition the patient now attends the physiotherapy department for further treatment and training in the performance of essential activities such as climbing stairs and rising from a chair. A simple series of exercises, free and against resistance, must be learned by the patient. These will need to be performed daily at home to maintain movement, joint stability and to prevent contractures. The occupational therapist is also concerned in the rehabilitation programme. The patient is assessed in the activities of daily living by nursing staff. Where there are problems with personal and domestic activities, special retraining may be necessary. The occupational therapist's contribution to this aspect of rehabilitation is when the patient needs to use special aids and equipment such as modified cutlery or tools. Modification of the home may also be required, for example rails to help rising from the lavatory or bath or to negotiate stairs.

Both physiotherapist and occupational therapist have an important role in the final assessment of the functional level obtained, and translating this in terms of capacity for employment or work in the home. They collaborate with the nurse and medical social worker who will by now have a thorough knowledge of the patient's social background and the difficulties likely to be encountered in the process of resettlement. When the patient has reached the maximum degree of improvement the nurse as part of the team must help prepare him to face the future. By the time of discharge from the ward careful instructions should have been given about exercise and the wearing of splints at night, the limits of physical activity, the continuation of regular doses of anti-inflammatory drugs and the importance of returning to the follow-up clinic so that the physician can adjust the regime of treatment as required. Hospital admission as well as establishing reasonable control over the manifestations of the disease provides an opportunity for educating the patient to take a realistic view of the limitations within which he or she may have to live.

Joint injuries

In order to function efficiently the articular surfaces of a joint must be smooth, held in the correct position and able to slide one upon the other. Congenital abnormalities may be responsible for joint disorders, but the commonest cause is trauma.

Strains

If a joint is forced beyond its normal position but there is no tissue damage, the joint has been strained. The sufferer will complain of pain when he attempts specific actions, but there will be no evidence of swelling, deformity or loss of function. Local heat may give comfort by relieving muscle spasm and mild analgesics help the patient to persist with gentle exercise of the part.

Sprains

When a joint is forced into an abnormal position and some fibres of muscle, tendon or ligament are torn, the body response is pain, local swelling, limitation of movement and often local bruising. But there is no deformity or loss of function. This injury is referred to as a sprain. X-ray investigation will rule out the possibility of fracture. Though any joint can technically, be sprained the commonest site is the ankle joint. Treatment is usually the application of a support bandage with the joint in the position of rest. The amount of exercise allowed during the process of healing depends upon the severity of the sprain.

Torn ligaments

This term is used when the traumatic force has been severe enough to tear ligaments or dislodge them from their bony attachments. Such an injury is much more serious as the joint is now unstable. If the ligament has been wrenched from its bony attachment and has taken with it a flake of bone, immobilization of the joint may allow bone healing to occur, thus reattaching the ligament. If, on the other hand, the ligament has been divided at some point along its length and that ligament is a vital factor in the affected joint's stability, surgery may be necessary so that the ligament can be sutured. Common sites for this injury are the knee and ankle joint. Treatment involves splintage in the rest position, then remobilization of the joint when sound healing has occurred.

Subluxation and dislocation

When the ligaments which support the joint are torn or cut the joint is unstable. In consequence the bones are able to slip from their normal position of close alignment of articular surfaces into an abnormal position. When the articular surfaces are completely out of alignment the term dislocation is used. If the disarticulation is only partial, the term subluxation is used.

The degree of damage to the ligaments is an important consideration in this type of trauma, whether due to surgery or accidental injury. The young man who sustains a dislocated hip in a road traffic accident may require similar nursing care in the early stages to the elderly lady who has undergone surgery to replace the head of the femur by a prosthesis. The accident may, and the operation certainly will, have divided the ligament which tethers the femoral head to the acetabulum. In either event the joint is potentially unstable, that is, liable to dislocate.

Most often the head of the bone is forced out through the capsule like a button through a button-hole. When the bone is relocated, healing of the capsule by fibrous tissue can occur and the joint is once more stable. Sometimes, however, the damage to the supporting ligaments is extensive and spontaneous repair is impossible. The joint never regains its stability and the patient has recurrent dislocations which occur during the performance of simple, everyday movements. The commonest site for this unusual injury is the shoulder joint and the sufferer may find that as he tries to put on his coat the joint slips out of position. In this situation surgical repair of the joint supports will be required.

When a joint is dislocated the features are pain, deformity and loss of function. Obvious swelling and bruising vary with the affected part. The treatment is to realign the articular surfaces as soon as possible (before oedema of the injured tissue makes this more difficult) and to support the limb in its most stable position. The stable positions of joints such as the fingers, thumb, wrist, elbow, ankle and knee are often similar to their positions of rest. Sometimes, however, due to the shape of the bones involved, exaggeration of certain planes of movement will make the joint less likely to dislocate.

When healing has occurred, either spontaneously or following surgical repair, intensive physiotherapy will be required to mobilize the joint fully so that the former range of movement is restored.

Complications of joint injuries

Synovial effusions

Response to injury causes increased secretion of synovial fluid. This can be felt as a fluctuant swelling around the joint. A common site is the knee, especially when the injury has torn part of the meniscus from its attachment. If effusion persists, it may require aspiration.

Haemarthrosis

In severe joint injuries, particularly where a fracture line involves the joint, bleeding may occur. This usually requires aspiration.

Damage to adjacent nerves

This is particularly liable to happen in shoulder injuries where damage to the circumflex nerve leads to paralysis of the deltoid muscle.

Osteoarthritis

This can be a late complication when a fracture has disrupted the smooth articular surface.

Fractures

A fracture is an interruption in the continuity of a bone. Fractures are most commonly caused by injury but can also occur due to a pathological defect in the bone, for example, a cyst or certain metabolic disorders which cause the bones to be weak and brittle. In fractures due to injury, the violence can be direct or indirect (Fig. 2.15 A–D).

Figure 2.15
Causes of fractures
(A) Direct violence
(B) Indirect violence
(C) Indirect violence: muscular
    effort
(D) Pathological defect of bone

Types of fracture

Fractures may be described as 'closed' (where the skin over the fracture site remains intact) or 'open' (where a wound over the fracture site allows communication between the bone and the air). An open fracture is sometimes referred to as a compound fracture.

Fractures may also be described as 'simple' or 'complicated'. A simple fracture, as its name implies, is a break in the continuity of the bone which does not involve any other structure. A complicated fracture, however, involves injury to adjacent structures. Thus, a compound fracture is by definition a complicated fracture as it

Figure 2.16
Types of fracture

Oblique Transverse Comminuted Greenstick Impacted Complicated Muscle tissue

involves damage to surrounding muscle and tissue. A closed fracture, on the other hand may or may not involve injury to adjacent structures and, therefore may be either simple or complicated.

Sometimes the terms used to describe fractures refer to the way in which the bone has broken. The terms transverse, oblique, spiral, hairline or crack fractures are self-explanatory. If the injury has caused the bone to splinter, the term comminuted fracture is used. On other occasions, the nature of the injury causes the bone ends to be driven into one another and here the terms impacted or compressed fracture would be used. In children, injury may cause the bone to bend rather than snap and the term greenstick fracture is used (Fig. 2.16).

Finally, words may be used to describe the exact anatomical position of certain commonly occurring fractures. The cervical fracture of the femur indicates that the site of injury is the femoral neck. The pertrochanteric or intertrochanteric fracture of the same bone indicates that the fracture line runs between the trochanters of the femur. The supracondylar fracture of the humerus indicates that the site is just above the lower condyles of the humerus. On other occasions a particular fracture bears the name of the doctor who first described it, such as Pott's fracture or Colles' fracture. These doctors' names are only used to identify specific types of fracture of the ankle and wrist respectively.

Signs and symptoms of a fracture

1. Loss of function.
2. Deformity.
3. Shortening of the affected limb.
4. Abnormal mobility.
5. Local tenderness.
6. Swelling and bruising.

Complications of fractures

1. Early: injury to blood vessels, joints, nerves, viscera.
2. Late: infection, mal-union, non-union.

Sequelae of fractures

Shock (first 24 hours).
Fat emboli (first 48 hours) (p. 42).
Pulmonary infarction (2 to 3 weeks after injury) (p. 291).
Hypostatic pneumonia
Pressure necrosis (p. 517) } any time during bed rest.
Renal calculi (p. 347)

Principles of treatment of fractures

Figure 2.17 (p. 58) illustrates the deformity that can result when a fracture occurs.
There are three basic principles to be observed in the treatment of this type of injury:

Figure 2.17
Fracture deformity

1. Reduction of the fracture. The surgeon, by the application of traction and gentle manipulation, counteracts the muscle pull and restores normal alignment to the bone.
2. Immobilization of the fracture site until healing (bony union) occurs.
3. Restoration of full physical function.

Methods of immobilizing a fracture

Some form of fixation or splintage is required to hold the bone ends in alignment until healing occurs. This may be achieved by internal fixation involving surgical intervention or by external splinting.

Internal fixation

Various devices have been invented to hold a fracture securely. They are usually made of special metals which do not cause an inflammatory response in the body. Figure 2.18 shows some of the more common types of internal fixation.

A. Bone plate   B. Bone screw   C. Tri-flange nail   D. Tri-flange nail and plate   E. Intramedullary bone nail

Figure 2.18
Common types of internal fixation

External splinting

There are many splints which can be applied to immobilize a fracture, but the commonest is plaster of Paris. Therefore special attention is given here to the care of patients wearing plaster casts.

Care of patients in plaster

The diagnosis, reduction and immobilization of fractures is the province of the medical practitioner. The decision about whether to use internal fixation by screws, pins, plates or nails is his, and he will perform the necessary operation. Similarly, if external splintage of the fracture is the chosen method of immobilization, the doctor will be closely involved with its application. Diagnosis, reduction and immobilization all take place in a matter of a few hours or, at most, a day or two. The period of immobilization necessary to allow healing to occur extends for many weeks (6 to 8 weeks for an upper limb; 3 months and longer for a major weight-bearing bone). It is this period of healing which is the prime concern of the nurse.

The commonest method of immobilization is the application of a plaster of Paris cast to the affected part. These casts are often extensive and may encase the whole lower limb (above knee plaster) the limb and torso (hip spica, which can be single- or double-legged), the torso alone (plaster jacket), the torso and shoulder (shoulder spica) or the torso and head (Minerva jacket). Preserving the efficiency of the cast and at the same time keeping the patient clean and comfortable can tax the ingenuity of the most skilful nurse. No single 'best' method can be defined — nurses working in orthopaedic centres are continually devising better ways of solving recurrent problems. What follows is merely an outline of some points which may help the inexperienced nurse who finds herself working for a short period in an orthopaedic unit.

The first thing to remember is that, although we shall be talking in terms of the plaster's efficiency and well-being, it is really the patient inside the cast who is our prime concern. Every complaint of pain or discomfort made by the patient must have prompt attention. It may be that the discomfort is only fleeting and insignificant, but on the other hand it could be a warning of imminent danger. A patient in a newly applied cast may complain of all manner of sensations at first — sharp pain, dull ache, throbbing sensation, sensations of heat, cold, itch or swelling. These impressions may be merely the brain trying to identify just exactly what the leg is feeling at the time. However, amongst all these sensations there may be one which is significant; therefore all must be heeded, lest the one important complaint be missed. If pressure is present under a plaster the patient will only experience discomfort for a few hours. After this time the part becomes numb, and although the patient says he is now comfortable, the pressure persists and the damage continues. Warning signs are **numbness and tingling**, a **burning sensation** or **persistent pain** over one part of the plaster. Remember it is not only the bony eminences which are vulnerable now. Any part of a plaster may have a ridge or dent in its inner surface that can cause pressure.

Observation of the circulation

The need for close observation of the circulation to the extremity when a plaster has been newly applied cannot be overstressed. It may be difficult for the inexperienced nurse to comprehend the speed with which the situation can deteriorate from impaired circulation to permanent damage. A paralysis of such severity that the patient may never regain the use of his hand or foot can occur within 24 hours. Inspecting the fingers or toes after application of a plaster is as important as checking the pulse after surgery. They should be warm and of good colour. Nurses should be familiar with the blanching test (capillary flush). The nails of the fingers or toes are each compressed in turn. When the pressure is released, blood should rush back into the nail bed, that is the nail should turn from white to pink **at once**. If the return of colour to the nail is sluggish, then the circulation is for some reason impaired. This state must be reported immediately. Inspection and the blanching test should be carried out ½ to 1 hourly for 24 hours and should be observed regularly for several days. If there is any sign of circulatory impairment, the observations must be done every 10 to 15 minutes.

Cardinal signs of circulatory impairment

These are:

Coldness.
Blueness or pallor.
Oedema.
Loss of movement or stiffness.
Numbness or pain.
Sluggish return of blood after blanching test.

If several of these signs are present together, the situation is urgent and the doctor must take steps to relieve the pressure immediately.

Care of the cast

Plaster of Paris bandages are made by impregnating an open weave material with anhydrous gypsum, which we call plaster of Paris (calcium sulphate from which the water of crystallization has been removed). Plaster casts are made by wetting the bandages and applying them smoothly and evenly to the area to be encased. Great care is taken to mould the plaster to the contours of the patient so that pressure is avoided. The addition of water to anhydrous gypsum allows a chemical reaction to occur which reconverts the plaster of Paris to the rock-like gypsum. Setting occurs quite rapidly, but the full potential strength of the cast is not achieved until all the excess water has been removed by evaporation. At this stage, when the plaster is set but not yet dry, it is very susceptible to damage by cracking or denting. This vulnerable period may last for as long as 48 hours for an extensive cast.

Supporting the wet cast

Care of the cast begins before the patient returns from the plaster room. It begins with the preparation of the bed. A firm mattress, bed cradle and fracture boards are vital. Pillows to support the cast will also be needed. Mattress and pillows will need waterproof protection to prevent dampness and mustiness caused by the wet plaster. For a plaster jacket, three pillows laid across the bed should be sufficient. For a hip spica, one pillow at waist level and two pillows laid lengthwise to support the leg are required. If both legs are encased in plaster, two or more pillows will be needed for the second leg. A pillow for head and shoulders will be needed for the patient who has not had an anaesthetic.

The nurse should never lay a damp plaster cast directly on to a mattress. If she does, the cast will become flattened over bony prominences such as the sacrum or the heel and damage to the underlying tissue will be unavoidable. It is essential that the pillows are positioned to support the contours of the plaster. Any sharp break in pillow alignment and support might cause the plaster to sag and crack at some strategic point. This is particularly likely to happen at the leg and body junction of the hip spica but may also occur at the knee.

When lifting the patient on to the bed, care must be taken to support the cast with the palms of the hand and not the fingers. Fingers can make indentations in a recently set plaster.

Drying the cast

Natural evaporation of moisture by exposing the cast to the air is preferred by many surgeons, as this gives the cast a chance to develop its full potential strength. Accelerated drying using heat lamps or a heat cradle is not usually recommended but is sometimes used in out-patient work. Though slow drying by exposure to the air is desirable for the cast, from the patient's point of view it is a lengthy, tedious and uncomfortable time. There is not a great deal that can be done about his enforced lack of mobility at this stage, but the nurse should give him reassurance and company as well as access to any diversion or entertainment the ward can provide.

The physical discomfort may be due to unaccustomed immobility, and ease can sometimes be gained by helping or encouraging the patient to move the parts of the body that are not encased in plaster into different positions. Much discomfort is caused by the fact that the patient has a large, wet, cold object in bed with him — namely the plaster. During application, due to the chemical reaction which is taking place, heat is generated and the plaster feels nice and warm. The patient may even feel that it is too hot and sometimes needs reassurance that he is not being burnt. Very soon, however, as the water evaporates, the plaster becomes profoundly cold. As water evaporates from the plaster heat is lost from the whole body. It should not be surprising, therefore, that the patient soon feels cold and shivery. Even with a relatively small cast such as an above-the-knee plaster, both legs will feel the chill badly. Make sure that all areas of the body not encased in plaster are warmly wrapped up. Use of small blankets next to the skin and a warm sock will not only help to prevent draughts but will stop the patient placing his 'good leg' on a sodden area of bed linen.

Turning the patient

The patient with an extensive cast in position must be turned from dorsal to prone position to allow drying of the back of the plaster and care of the pressure areas. Timing of the first turn requires professional judgement. During this first turn, more help will be needed than with subsequent turns, as the plaster must be fully supported to prevent cracking. Turning should always be done on the leg which is **not** encased or, in the case of a double hip spica, over the side which has **not** been operated on. Pillows to support the entire length of the cast must be positioned in readiness so that lifting the patient once he is turned is avoided. Lifting at this stage is uncomfortable for the patient, endangers the soft cast and places an unnecessary strain on the nurses' backs.

As soon as the turn is completed, the nurses should check the patient's position to see that the toes are not pressing against the mattress. Note should also be made of the body position. Too many pillows at head and shoulders will cause the cast to dig into the chest. If the pillow under the lumbar curve is not positioned correctly, the plaster edge may cut into the soft tissue of the buttocks.

When the cast has hardened regular turning can be managed by two or even one nurse. The patient soon becomes skilled at helping, and some manage to turn themselves without assistance. Pillows are no longer necessary for plaster protection but are used for the comfort of the patient. Support at the upper edge of a body plaster lifts the pressure from the patient's chest and makes breathing easier. Pillow support at buttock level prevents the plaster cutting into soft tissues. Lumbar support prevents pressure which would otherwise occur in this area if the patient was left with only the top and bottom of the plaster supported. Similarly with leg plasters, the heel must be supported clear of the bed, but the wearer of the plaster will be more comfortable if the plaster is supported along its length. If allowed to hang with only the foot supported, the top edge will cut into the front of the thigh. A pillow between the legs is also useful as it prevents the sound leg banging against the plaster.

Placing the patient on a bedpan

The plaster will be carefully trimmed and bound to allow the patient to use a bedpan or urinal and to leave access for perineal and anal toilet. To prevent soiling or wetting of the plaster, however, the nurse must develop some skill in the positioning of sanitary utensils. The following points will help to prevent accidents:

1. Elevate the head of the bed or place extra pillows under the shoulders to prevent urine or faeces running back under the plaster.
2. Place an absorbent pad at the cast edge as an additional safeguard — this pad must be removed with the bedpan.
3. Position the bedpan by rolling the patient to the unaffected side and placing the pan so that the buttocks contact the rim of the utensil. Position pillows to support the back and limbs and roll the patient on to his back.

Care of the patient's skin

Good powers of observation are vital when caring for patients in plaster. All visible skin must be inspected daily for signs of abrasion or irritation. Immediately after plaster application, the nurse should ensure that the patient's fingers or toes are thoroughly washed so that this inspection can be carried out.

Chafing and irritation are particularly likely at cast edges. In cases where there are no wounds in the vicinity of the plaster edges, the fingers, lightly dusted with talcum powder, should be used to explore the skin as far as it is possible to reach. The exploration can reveal skin eruptions and is also useful in removing plaster crumbs and debris from the cast.

Other areas which are commonly vulnerable to pressure are the heel of the 'good' foot, which is used by the patient to heave himself about in bed. The elbows receive a lot of friction as the patient tries to see what is going on around him. These places can be easily cared for and therefore should never be allowed to get to the stage of skin breakdown.

Inspecting the plaster involves more than merely looking at it. The experienced nurse uses her sense of smell as well as her senses of sight or touch. Learning to use the sense of smell discerningly takes time, but occasionally even an inexperienced nurse can locate the exact position of the musty odour which may be the only sign of a plaster sore. It is sometimes possible to detect the postion of an area of necrosis by the temperature of the cast, as the plaster tends to become much hotter over an area that is beginning to discharge.

Arm and leg plasters

The previous section was mainly concerned with the problems associated with care of patients in large casts. There are also some important points to note about the patient wearing an arm or leg plaster.

To prevent oedema following the application of an arm or leg plaster, it is usually necessary to support the extremity in an elevated position. If oedema occurs, the doctor may require the limb to be supported in a position equal to or higher than the level of the heart.

Full arm plasters should be supported in a sling when the patient is out of bed. The weight of an unsupported cast on the shoulder is considerable and will cause the patient discomfort. The patient in an arm plaster should also be reminded to exercise the shoulder joint several times daily to avoid unnecessary stiffness.

Long leg plasters must be supported on pillows when the patient is using a bedpan; otherwise, the patient will feel insecure and uncomfortable,

Care of the patient when the plaster is removed

Although a plaster cast looks clumsy and awkward, it is in fact a highly efficient fixation apparatus. The patient himself may not realize until the cast is removed just how efficient it was. This is a difficult time for the patient. He has tolerated the long weeks needed for healing to take place and at last the day he has been waiting for arrives. The bone has healed and the plaster can be removed. Now to his consternation he is suddenly aware of many aches and pains; even minute changes of joint position will cause acute discomfort. Joint structures and muscles that have become contracted are suddenly stretched. Circulation has become sluggish, and coldness, mottling and swelling often occur. The patient is frightened to discover that, although the primary problem was the hip, it is now the knee which gives rise to pain, and he will need physical and emotional help. Joints should be supported in a relaxed position and assurance given that with time and exercise function will improve.

When a plaster has been worn for a considerable time, the skin may become covered with a dense yellow scale. This is partly dead skin and partly skin exudates. It is usually considered unwise to try to soften this loosely adherent scale or to remove it forcibly, as this will cause rawness and bleeding. The scale can be cleaned away gently and gradually over a period of several days.

Traction

Traction literally means the drawing of a body along a surface. In other words traction involves pulling. When two opposing pulling forces are applied to an object, as shown in Figure 2.19A, an area of tension is created between them.

Figure 2.19B shows two examples of pulling forces in everyday life. When the opposing forces are equal, the pulling is balanced and neither side can win.

Figure 2.19A
Traction

Figure 2.19B
Examples of balanced traction

Figure 2.20
Traction (A) Equal weights
(B) Equal pull

This is the principle used when traction is applied in the treatment of certain orthopaedic disorders. The pull in one direction is the patient's body weight; in the other, it is a weight or force which exactly matches or counterbalances the patient's weight.

Neither of the methods of applying traction shown in Figure 2.20 would be practical, of course. Various pieces of apparatus are therefore used so that the pulling force can be exerted on the appropriate bone or joint. These devices commonly consist of:

1. A mechanism for attaching the patient to a length of cord.
2. A pulley or series of pulleys over which the cord can run.
3. A weight or several weights to counterbalance the patient's body weight.

or

1. A mechanism for attaching the patient to a length of cord.
2. A splinting device which will create a fixed point against which traction can be exerted.

Common methods of achieving traction

Skin traction

Traction is applied to the skin and thus indirectly to the skeletal system. Various tapes or bandages can be used to provide adhesion. When these skin extensions, as they are called, are attached to a weight or splint they allow a pull to be exerted on the skin and skeletal system.

Figure 2.21
Thomas splint

Leather covered ring

Angle to accommodate greater trochanter of femur

Extension bow

Skeletal traction

Traction is applied directly to the skeletal system using special appliances such as a Steinmann pin, Kirschner wire, or skull calipers of various makes.

Traction may be of short or long duration. It will be of short duration, for instance, when the surgeon manipulates a fractured limb — this procedure is known as reduction of the fracture. It will be of long duration if the surgeon chooses to immobilise a fractured shaft of femur by traction until the fracture has healed. For this long-term immobilization and traction a Thomas splint is commonly used (Fig. 2.21). The ring of the splint is gently pushed over the patient's leg until the ring impinges on the patient's ischial tuberosity. Then when the patient's leg is attached to the cords and cords are secured to the W shaped bow at the lower end of the splint, the pull against the fixed point can be exerted.

Traction is used for a variety of purposes in orthopaedic work:

1. To realign fractured bone ends.
2. To realign joint surfaces which have become dislocated.
3. To overcome muscle spasm.
4. To correct deformity caused by shortened tendons or ligaments.
5. To immobilize joints.
6. To immobilize fractures.
7. To relieve weight-bearing stress on a joint.
8. To relieve pressure on a nerve or nerve root.

Balanced traction

Balanced traction, as its name implies, is an exact counterbalancing of body weight to the pull of traction weights. Some systems increase the pull exerted by the weights by running the traction cords over a zig-zag arrangement of pulleys. Thus when the bed is tilted the pulley becomes the pivotal point. Gravity pulls the patient's weight in one direction but also acts upon the weight to exert the counter-pull (Fig. 2.22).

Once the essential nature of traction as a system of counterbalancing forces has been grasped, it is easier to appreciate the several variations on a theme which can be seen in orthopaedic practice.

Figure 2.22
Traction (A) Leg traction
(B) Head traction

Body weight *Counter-weight* *Counter-weight* *Body weight*

A   B

Figure 2.23
Fixed traction

Fixed point

Area of tension

Force

Fixed traction

An alternative method of applying traction to a body is by exerting a pull against a fixed point (fixed traction), as if a dog were pulling a lead attached to a post (Fig. 2.23). This situation can be imitated when applying traction to the upper or lower limb (Fig. 2.24).

Nursing care of patients on traction

Skill in the nursing care of patients on traction develops with knowledge and experience. Patients in plaster casts have their problems, but these are usually simpler than those of the patient on traction. The patient in a cast can be moved as often as required or desired for comfort or skin care without endangering the immobilised part. Patients on traction, on the other hand, usually have to be nursed in one

Figure 2.24
Traction against a fixed point

Figure 2.25
Slipper bedpan

position, commonly supine. The aim of good nursing is to keep the patient clean, comfortable and free from pressure sores or other complications of his enforced and prolonged recumbency, not the least of which may be boredom and depression.

Special thought must be given to make feeding and elimination as easy as possible. At first the patient will require assistance with feeding when lying flat. Later he will learn to feed himself if food is presented in a readily 'forkable' manner.

Certain appliances are of value in helping to overcome some of these problems. An overhead trapeze is an invaluable aid to mobility, and a sheepskin pad may help to protect sacral skin from pressure. A fracture bedpan, sometimes called a 'slipper bedpan' because of its shape (Fig. 2.25), is easier for the recumbent patient to use. Female patients often find a female urinal easier to use than a bedpan for micturition.

Ensuring the warmth and comfort of the patient on traction also requires some thought. The bed linen must often be put on in a special manner to allow the traction ropes to run freely or to accommodate a splint. This results in a series of very uncomfortable draughts for the patient. Use of warm socks and small extra blankets will help to prevent this discomfort. The patient feels exposed and vulnerable in the 'divided bed' that is necessary to accommodate traction. Normal briefs cannot be worn as they cannot be put on and removed due to the traction equipment. A special garment with side ties should therefore be provided for the patient's peace of mind. Prism spectacles (Fig. 2.26) can be used to make reading less fatiguing, and strategically positioned mirrors will help him to keep in touch with the activity around him.

Figure 2.26
Patient using prism spectacles
for reading

Figure 2.27
Balanced traction

A

B

Points to note in the care of patients being nursed in different types of traction

Balanced traction

A state of traction is achieved by using metal weights as the traction force and the patient's body weight as the counter-traction (Fig. 2.27). The degree to which the bed is elevated and the amount of weight applied will depend upon the weight of the patient, but both must be sufficient to maintain a balanced pull. The patient must not slide up or be pulled down the bed by excessive weight in either direction. There are certain points to note with balanced traction:

1. The patient is nursed in a supine position.
2. Bed elevation is maintained continuously.
3. Friction is reduced by ensuring that ropes run freely over pulleys.
4. Weights must hang free at all times.
5. No extra pillows are allowed as this increases friction and reduces traction.
6. Correct body alignment must be maintained at all times.
7. The patient must not be allowed to slip towards the head or foot of the bed.
8. The patient should be taught to move himself up the bed as and when required.

Fixed traction

An alternative method of achieving traction is to exert a pull against a fixed point. The axilla and ischial tuberosity are anatomical fixed points against which a pull may be exerted via a splint such as the Thomas leg splint (Fig. 2.28). Slings are used to support the leg in the splint, and pads are positioned to maintain the optimum position of the knee. As this splint is heavy, it is usual to arrange a system of pulleys and weights to counterbalance the weight of the splinted leg. This time the weights act as a device to aid the patient's mobility in bed and are not involved in the maintenance of traction.

There are certain points to note with fixed traction:

1. The ring of the splint must fit snugly against the ischium in order to maintain the traction. This will be achieved if the traction tapes are kept firmly tied over the extension bow at the lower end of the splint. Check twice daily.
2. The ring of the splint can exert pressure on the groin and cause tissue necrosis. To avoid this the nurse must: (a) keep the area clean and dry by 2-hourly attention, and (b) teach the patient to ease the tissue gently under the ring to a different position every hour or each time he feels discomfort, whichever is the more frequent.
3. The patient can be nursed in the sitting position with this type of traction, but he should lie flat for several hours each day to prevent hip contractures.
4. The patient should be taught how to use his arms and sound leg to increase his mobility in bed and to allow inspection of the vulnerable sacral area.

Fixed point
(ring of splint
against groin)

Skin extensions

Traction force

Extension
tapes or cords
tied securely
over
extension bow

Figure 2.28
Fixed traction (Note: the ring fits
snugly into the groin, but the
point of pressure (not shown) is
the ischial tuberosity)

General observation of the patient on traction

1. Circulation — skin colour and joint mobility must be checked. Note any complaints of numbness, coldness or swelling of the extremity. Avoid pressure in the popliteal space.

2. Skin condition — check areas over Achilles tendon, heel, dorsum of the foot and sacral area. (Check groin and buttocks if fixed traction is being used.)

3. Body alignment and position of the extremity — is traction being achieved and maintained?

4. Counter-traction — is this efficient, or does the patient have to be regularly moved up the bed? If he does, increasing the tilt of the bed may improve matters.

5. Outer bandages and securing tapes — are these neatly and securely in position? Remove and reapply as required. (Note: The traction tapes and rubber foam bandages, should not be reapplied without specific instruction.)

6. Supporting pads and slings — are they correctly positioned to do the required job?

7. Prevention of deformity — have measures been taken to prevent foot drop, or hip flexion in the sitting patient?

8. Pressure — is there any pressure on the lateral aspect of the leg over the head of the fibula? Pressure here can damage the lateral popliteal nerve and so cause foot drop.

9. Comfort — traction should never be a source of discomfort for the patient. Listen carefully and investigate promptly every complaint.

10. Complications — hypostatic pneumonia is a constant threat to the patient, especially if he is elderly. Encourage deep breathing and regular coughing. Ensure adequate fluid intake.

General exercise of the joints and muscles not immobilized by traction is vitally important and the nurse plays a large part in this task by her teaching, encouragement and frequent reminders. Diversional therapy cannot be overemphasized since the orthopaedic patient, being closely confined to bed for an extended period, quickly becomes bored and depressed.

Application of principles

Throughout this chapter an attempt has been made to give broad outlines of some of the more important aspects of body mechanics related to function. It is to be hoped that the thinking nurse can apply these principles to a variety of situations and patients other than those with disorders of the locomotor system. Specific details of particular diseases and conditions have been deliberately avoided as the nurse needing a deeper knowledge would be advised to study a more specialized text in order to develop the art of orthopaedic nursing.

A knowledge and appreciation of the principles of orthopaedic care can serve the nurse well in her own life as well as in the treatment of her patients. Maintenance of a healthy musculoskeletal system is vital for everyone, not only those who have suffered injury or disease to bones or joints.

SUGGESTED ASSIGNMENTS

1. How would you help a bed-fast or chair-fast person to maintain good muscle tone? How would you teach the patient and his relatives the required measures when he is being looked after at home?

2. Observe the nursing staff with whom you work for two spans of duty. List the occasions and circumstances in which there was particular risk of back strain. Devise a programme which would help junior staff to develop good postural and lifting habits.

3. For each patient in your care, list the most likely complications which could be prevented or minimized by nursing action. Design a plan for care which highlights these preventive actions.

4. Examine the various types of chair (upright, wheel, easy) in the unit in which you work. List the good points and bad points for each type. Which chair would you select for each of the patients in your care? How would you make the most of the chair's good features and how would you minimise the effect of its bad points?

5. What housing alterations or aids would help an active young married woman who has suffered permanent loss of power in her left arm, to achieve maximum independence in the activities of daily living?

6. Prepare a list of conditions (other than bone or joint disorders) which have an adverse effect on the mobility of patients you have nursed. Describe the nursing actions which were aimed at re-mobilization.

7. Small boys, when wearing a plaster cast, are not noted for keeping the plaster clean, dry and intact. What advice would you give the mother of a 7-year-old who has to wear a below-knee plaster for the next 4 weeks? How would you instruct her about observations of circulation?

FURTHER READING

Apley A G 1982 A system of orthopaedics and fractures, 6th edn. Butterworths, London
Brunner L S, Sudarth D F 1980 Textbook of medical surgical nursing. Lippincott, Philadelphia
Farrell J 1983 Illustrated guide to orthopaedic nursing, 2nd edn. Blackwell Scientific, Oxford
Larson C B, Gould M 1978 Orthopaedic nursing, 9th edn. Mosby, St Louis
Mourad L 1980 Nursing care of adults with orthopaedic conditions. Wiley, New York
Powell M 1982 Orthopaedic nursing and rehabilitation, 8th edn. Churchill Livingstone, Edinburgh
Roaf R, Hodkinson L J 1980 Textbook of orthopaedic nursing, 3rd edn. Blackwell Scientific, Oxford
Rowe J W, Dyer L (eds) 1977 Care of the orthopaedic patient. Blackwell Scientific, Oxford
Webb J T 1977 Notes on orthopaedic nursing. Churchill Livingstone, Edinburgh

Chapter Three

The nervous system

In order to give nursing care to patients suffering from the effects of injury to, or disease of, the nervous system and, equally important, to appreciate the significance of observations which the nurse will be asked to make, an understanding of the structures involved and how they function is essential.

ANATOMY AND PHYSIOLOGY

Nerve tissue is made up of millions of nerve cells and their processes. These are the functional units of the nervous system and they are supported by a connective tissue called glia.

1. **Neurones.** These nerve cells vary in size and shape, each consisting of a cell body containing a nucleus embedded in protoplasm. Processes arise from the cell, a number of short ones called dendrites and a long one called the axon or nerve fibre.

Impulses are received by the dendrites, transmitted to the cell body and conducted from the cell body by the axon.

The dendrites and axon have similar structures:

a. A delicate central fibre called the axis cylinder.

b. The myelin sheath composed of adipose tissue. A number of nerve fibres do not have a myelin sheath and are described as non-myelinated. In order that impulses may be transmitted along myelinated fibres the myelin sheath is absent at intervals and these spaces are known as the Nodes of Ranvier.

c. The neurilemma is a delicate membrane surrounding the myelin sheath of the peripheral nerves only i.e. those found outwith the skull and vertebral column.

The myelin sheath has several functions:

  i. to protect the axis cylinder.
  ii. to act as an insulator.
  iii. to stimulate transmission of impulse through the nerve fibre (Fig. 3.1).

Figure 3.1
A neurone

2. **The Glia.** This is a tissue, consisting of cells and fibres, found in the brain and spinal cord. There are three types of glial cells, astrocytes, oligodendrocytes and microglia. Their collective functions are to protect, support and nourish the neurones.

Nerve tissue has two properties.

Irritability. The ability to respond to stimulation which is partly electrical and partly chemical.

Conductivity. The ability to transmit an impulse.

Generation of a nerve impulse. The propagation of a nerve impulse is an electrochemical process. The nerve cell has a 'resting potential' of — 70 millivolts (mV). The axon membrane separates the extracellular fluid (rich in sodium ions Na^+) from the intracellular fluid (rich in potassium ions K^+). In the resting state the axon membrane is relatively impermeable to sodium, and the 'sodium pump', a metabolic process, excretes any sodium entering the nerve cell. An impulse begins with the axon membrane becoming permeable to sodium ions, which then pass in. They take with them positive charges which alter the cell potential from — 70 mV to +40 mV, and this change is termed an 'action potential'. Immediately following this an equal number of potassium ions leave the cell and the potential returns to — 70 mV thus restoring the electrical status quo. When the impulse passes, sodium is pumped out and potassium returns to the cell thus restoring the chemical status quo. These alterations in the state of the axon membrane are propagated along the nerve. A nerve impulse lasts about 1 millisecond during which the complete process occurs (Figs 3.2 and 3.3).

Chemical transmitters and the synapse. There is no anatomical continuity between neurones. The axon of one neurone divides into small branches that terminate in small swellings called the terminal buttons or end feet. These lie in close proximity to the dendrites of the next neurone. The action potential of the cell i.e. +40 mV is not strong enough to permit passage of impulse over this synapse and a chemical bridge is necessary. The terminal button manufactures and stores a chemical transmitter. There are a number of chemicals known to act as transmitters such as acetylcholine, noradrenaline and dopamine.

When an impulse arrives at the terminal button the chemical transmitter is released which excites the next neurone and initiates another impulse. The released

Figure 3.2
Generation of a nerve impulse

Figure 3.3
Transmission of a nerve impulse

Figure 3.4
Chemical transmitter and a synapse

chemical is then neutralized by enzymes which ensure that the synapse remains inactive prior to the arrival of another impulse. The synapses between neurones, and those between neurones and structures they supply, function in the same manner (Fig. 3.4).

Functionally, the nervous system can be divided into two parts:

1. **Somatic system** — this part is under voluntary control.
2. **Autonomic system** — controls smooth muscle, cardiac muscle and the secretory glands of the body.

For descriptive purposes however the nervous system is divided into:

1. The central nervous system.
2. The peripheral nervous system.

The central nervous system
The brain

The brain can be anatomically divided into three parts: the **cerebrum**, the **cerebellum** and the **brain stem**.

The cerebrum

This forms the largest part of the brain and is divided by the falx into two hemispheres, the **left** and **right cerebral hemispheres.** The hemispheres are connected by a group of nerve fibres called the **corpus callosum** situated deep within the cerebrum. The cerebral hemispheres are divided into lobes — the **frontal, parietal, temporal** and **occipital lobes.** The lines of demarcation of these lobes are not exact.

The outer part is composed mainly of nerve cells (grey matter) and is called the **cerebral cortex.** The lobes are connected by **nerve fibres** or tracts (white matter). An important area situated within the cerebrum is the **internal capsule.** This consists of nerve fibres which either transmit nerve impulses from the body to the cerebral cortex (sensory) or from the cerebral cortex to the body (motor) (Fig. 3.5). A haemorrhage within the internal capsule may interrupt the pathway of nerve impulses controlling voluntary movement, resulting in paralysis of muscles. Most cerebrovascular accidents (strokes) result from bleeding within the internal capsule.

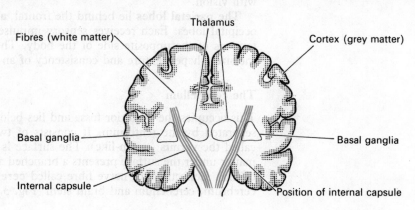

Figure 3.5
Coronal section of brain

Figure 3.6
Cerebrum: right lateral view

Figure 3.7
Lobes of the cerebrum

The outer surface of the cerebrum consists of elevations called **gyri** (singular: gyrus) and of depressions called **sulci** (singular: sulcus). A well-defined sulcus, the **central sulcus**, separates the frontal from the parietal lobe. Immediately posterior to the central sulcus lies the **postcentral gyrus,** which is the site of the sensory cortex. Anterior to the central sulcus is the **precentral** gyrus, which is the site of the motor cortex (Fig. 3.6).

One cerebral hemisphere tends to be dominant, and in the right-handed person this is the left hemisphere. The left hemisphere controls movement on the right side of the body and the right hemisphere controls movement on the left.

The functions of the cerebrum can be subdivided according to the lobular divisions (Fig. 3.7).

The frontal lobes occupy the anterior fossa. The anterior portions are concerned with behaviour, learning, creative thinking, personality, emotional responses, memory and ethical values. The posterior portions initiate the motor function by which movement occurs in the opposite side of the body. The dominant hemisphere is responsible for speech.

The temporal lobes occupy the front portion of the middle fossa and receive impulses from the special senses of smell, taste and hearing. The temporal lobe of the dominant hemisphere is important for understanding the spoken word.

The occipital lobes occupy the rear portion of the middle fossa and are concerned with vision.

The parietal lobes lie behind the frontal, above the temporal and in front of the occipital lobes. Each receives sensory impulses from the skin, muscles, joints and tendons of the opposite side of the body. The cortex of these lobes can recognize the size, shape, texture and consistency of an object.

The cerebellum

This occupies the posterior fossa and lies below the occipital lobes from which it is separated by the tentorium. It consists of two hemispheres and a central section called the **vermis** (worm-like). The surface is composed of grey matter. The white matter under the surface presents a branched appearance called the **arbor vitae** (tree of life). Collections of nerve fibre called **cerebellar peduncles** (tracts) connect the cerebrum, cerebellum and brain stem (Fig. 3.8).

Figure 3.8
Cerebrum, cerebellum and brain stem: relationships

The cerebellum controls balance and co-ordination of voluntary muscle movements. Impulses are received from muscles and joints indicating their position in relation to the body, and impulses from the semicircular canals in the ears indicate the position of the head in space.

By influencing the contractions of skeletal muscles the cerebellum maintains balance and ensures smooth and precise actions.

The brain stem

This lies deep in the midline. It is an elongated structure which passes from the cerebrum through an opening in the tentorium called the tentorial hiatus and enters the posterior fossa where it connects with the cerebellum. Anatomically it can be divided into three parts (Fig. 3.8):

1. **The midbrain** lies below the cerebrum and is composed of two groups of nerve cells and nerve fibres called the **cerebral penduncles**. It is by means of these peduncles that nerve impulses pass from the cerebrum to the cerebellum and spinal cord, and from the cerebellum and spinal cord to the cerebrum.

2. **The pons varolii** lies below the midbrain and anterior to the cerebellum. It is composed mainly of nerve fibres which connect the two hemispheres of the cerebellum and allows communication between the cerebral cortex and the spinal cord.

3. **The medulla oblongata** lies below the pons varolii and is continuous with the spinal cord. The outer part consists of nerve fibres which run to and from the higher areas of the brain and the spinal cord. The inner part consists of nerve cells some of which act as relay stations for sensory nerves travelling to the cerebrum.

Deep within the medulla are groups of cells associated with involuntary reflex activities called the **vital centres**. These are:

The **respiratory centre** which controls the depth and rate of respirations.
The **cardiac centre** which controls the force and rate of contractions of the heart.
The **vasomotor centre** which controls the calibre of blood vessels, particularly arterioles.

This area also contains the reflex centres of coughing, sneezing, swallowing and vomiting.

Travelling from the medulla through the brain stem and up to the cerebral cortex is a network of nerve cells and their fibres. This network is called the reticular formation. If all sensory impulses reaching the body were sent to the brain it would be, literally, swamped. The function of the reticular formation is to determine which sensory impulses will be allowed to reach the cerebral cortex. A state of arousal within the cerebral cortex is activated by the reticular formation. Any factor which impairs the function of this network (for example, head injury) will prevent sensory information reaching the cerebral cortex and an alteration in conscious level will result.

Figure 3.9
(A) Vertebral column (lateral view)
(B) A typical vertebra

Cervical
(7)

Intervertebral
foramina

Thoracic
(12)

Lumbar
(5)

Sacral
(5)

Coccygeal
(4-5)

A

Central canal

Posterior horn

White matter

Anterior horn

Grey matter

Figure 3.10
Section through spinal cord

The spinal cord

The spinal cord, a direct continuation of the medulla oblongata, lies within the vertebral canal of the vertebral column (Fig. 3.9) and, like the brain, is surrounded by the meninges (p. 81). The spinal cord extends from the first cervical to the first or second lumbar vertebra. The cord is divided into segments, 8 cervical, 12 thoracic, 5 lumbar, 5 sacral and 1 coccygeal. The centre of the spinal cord contains **grey matter,** composed of nerve cells, grouped in the shape of an H, surrounded by **white matter** (nerve fibres) arranged in tracts. In the centre of the spinal cord is the **central canal,** a continuation of the fourth ventricle. This canal is normally obliterated in whole or in part. The posterior limbs of the H are known as the **posterior horns** and the anterior limbs as the **anterior horns** of grey matter (Fig. 3.10).

The anterior horns contain the cell bodies of the lower motor neurones. They receive voluntary motor impulses from the motor cortex of the brain via the upper motor neurones, which descend in the lateral columns of the spinal cord as the **pyramidal or corticospinal tracts** (Fig. 3.11). The axons of the lower motor neurones leave the spinal cord by the anterior nerve roots and reach the organ innervated by the peripheral nerves. The transmitted substance released at nerve endings is acetylcholine. The posterior horn cells receive sensory impulses from the periphery via the peripheral nerves and the posterior nerve root. Thus the spinal cord conveys motor impulses from the brain and sensory impulses to the brain via tracts of white matter. Thirty-one pairs of spinal nerves arise from the spinal cord and emerge from the vertebral canal through the intervertebral foramina (Fig. 3.12).

A motor response to a sensory stimulus, which occurs without reference to the brain is called a reflex response; the withdrawal of a limb from a painful stimulus, coughing and the tendon reflexes are examples. If the tendon of the quadriceps muscle is stretched by tapping with a tendon hammer, the sensory stimulus passes centrally in the peripheral nerve and posterior nerve root and activates the anterior horn cells. They respond by passing motor impulses to the quadriceps muscle via the anterior roots and peripheral nerve causing the muscle to contract. This is an example of a simple segmental reflex arc (Fig. 3.13). More elaborate reflex actions may involve many segments of the cord at many different levels.

Although the spinal cord ends at the level of the first lumbar vertebra, the spinal meninges extend as low as the second sacral vertebra. The spinal nerves arising from the lower end of the cord hang down within the theca until they leave at their appropriate levels (theca, space containing CSF formed by the meninges). These nerve fibres form the **cauda equina,** so called because they resemble a horse's tail.

MOTOR CORTEX

Motor fibres crossing in medulla —   — Medulla   UPPER MOTOR NEURONE

Spinal cord

Peripheral nerve   Spinal cord

LOWER MOTOR NEURONE

Muscle

Figure 3.11
Pyramidal tract

Vertebral disc

Intervertebral foramen   — Spinous process

Vertebral body

Anterior nerve root emerging from spinal cord

Figure 3.12
Spinal nerves emerging through intervertebral foramina

Influence from brain   Sensory pathways

Posterior horn

Figure 3.13
Simple segmental reflex arc
(knee jerk)   Anterior horn of spinal cord   Motor pathway

Posterior spinal artery

Coronal artery

Sulcal artery
(one on each side)

Supplementary vessel from aorta

Anterior spinal artery

Figure 3.14
Segment of spinal cord: blood
supply

An anterior and two posterior spinal arteries extend the length of the cord getting additional supply from branches of the aorta (Fig. 3.14). The anterior artery gives off branches which encircle the cord anastomosing with the posterior spinal arteries. At various intervals another branch leaves the anterior spinal artery and supplies the substance of the cord.

Motor pathways

Although the motor pathways should be considered as an integrated system, it can best be understood if considered in two parts working in co-ordination:

1. The corticobulbar and corticospinal tracts collectively known as the *pyramidal tract*.
2. Other pathways involved in motor activity are described as *the extrapyramidal tract*.

1. *The pyramidal tract*

This pathway probably arises in many parts of the cerebral cortex, but predominantly within the motor area of the cerebral cortex of the precentral gyrus. Present are large pyramidal shaped cells — Betz cells — which are considered to give rise to the axons of the pathway. The fibres pass through the internal capsule to the mid brain. It is within the internal capsule that fibres pass through the pons varolii to the medulla. Within the medulla on each side of the midline is a ridge called the pyramids. It was the presence of fibres in this area which gave rise to the name of pyramidal tract. During the passage through the brain stem, fibres are given off to the motor nuclei of cranial nerves. While all fibres will cross in the medulla to innervate motor nuclei on opposite side, there are instances where the fibre sends a branch to innervate the motor nuclei on same side as in the motor nucleus of the branch of the facial nerve controlling the upper part of the face. An appreciation of this will explain the following feature. If, for example, there is interference to the pathway from the left hemisphere affecting fibres to facial nerves, then paralysis of the right side of the face occurs. However, as the branch to the upper part of the face is also innervated by fibres from the pathway from the right hemisphere, i.e. the same side, the muscles of the upper part of the face are not affected.

The components of tracks innervating the cranial nerve nuclei are called the corticobulbar tracts to distinguish them from fibres going to the spinal cord — the corticospinal tracts — but otherwise there is little else to distinguish them (Fig. 3.15).

Approximately 85% of fibres of the corticospinal tracts cross within the medulla in the decussation of the pyramids to the opposite side then descend in the white matter of the spinal cord between the anterior and posterior columns of grey matter.

Figure 3.15
The corticobulbar tracts

Figure 3.16
The corticospinal tracts

Remaining fibres do not cross
in decussation of pyramids
but at level of termination
descend in white matter in front

85% of fibres cross
in decussation of pyramids in medulla
and descend in white matter between
anterior columns of grey matter

The remaining fibres descend in the white matter between the anterior columns of grey matter and cross to the opposite side at the level of termination (Fig 3.16). The corticospinal tracts terminate either

    a. Around Alpha cells in the anterior column of grey matter.

or

    b. Around an internuncial neurone which synapses with Alpha cells. Alpha cells innervate muscle fibres of voluntary muscles.

2. The extrapyramidal tract

In the past the extrapyramidal tract was thought to consist of all pathways excluding those of the pyramidal tract. However both anatomical and physiological separation are becoming increasingly more difficult and the tract has come to be considered as a functional rather than an anatomical unit. The tract is composed of fibres arising from:

  i.   wide spread areas of the cortex but especially frontal and parietal lobes.
  ii. the cerebellum.
  iii. the basal ganglia.

The **basal ganglia** consists of several masses of grey matter embedded in the white matter of the cerebral hemispheres. The term 'basal ganglia' is used most frequently to denote motor nuclei that are closely related functionally.

The **corpus striatum** is the major centre in the extrapyramidal tract and is divided into the lenticular nucleus and the caudate nucleus. While the division is of secondary importance in respect of function an understanding of anatomical relationship is of value. The lenticular nucleus is wedge-shaped and about the size of a Brazil nut. The narrow part is called the globus pallidus (pale globe) and the lateral portion is called the putamen (Fig. 3.17).

The caudate nucleus consists of a head which tapers into a slender tail. The head bulges into the anterior horn of lateral ventricle and the first part of the tail lies along the floor of the lateral, the ventricle and then extends forward to the temporal lobe terminating at the amygdaloid nucleus. The caudate nucleus and amygdaloid nucleus have no functional relationship (Fig. 3.18).

There are many afferent and efferent intranuclear connections within the corpus striatum.

The particular contribution of the corpus striatum to motor function is poorly understood, but it is seen to participate in three ways:

a. it may provide for motor activity of an autonomic type including response to emotion.
b. to relay influence of cerebral cortex on voluntary muscles.
c. to exercise an influence on fibres of the pyramidal and extrapyramidal tracts.

Figure 3.17
The lenticlear nucleus of the corpus striatum

Figure 3.18
The caudate nucleus

Figure 3.19
Interconnections between
structures involved in extra
pyramidal tracts

Figure 3.20
The final common pathway

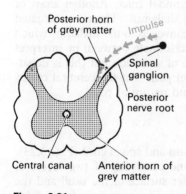

Figure 3.21
Cross section of spinal cord

Fibres arising from the cortex, cerebellum and basal ganglia form tracts which descend in the white matter of the spinal cord. The tracts terminate around Gamma cells in the anterior column of grey matter (Fig. 3.19).

The extrapyramidal tract exerts its influence by modifying the muscle fibres in the muscle spindle thereby modifying response to change in tension. Without such influence, normal smooth movements would be impossible and maintenance of posture and balance would be severely affected.

The final common pathway

The pyramidal pathways convey impulses to the large Alpha cells whose axons are distributed to muscle fibres of motor units. The extrapyramidal pathways convey impulses to the smaller Gamma cells whose axons are distributed to the muscle spindle in muscle fibres.

The alpha neurone is called the final common pathway.

Influences descending in pyramidal and extrapyramidal tracts constitute the *upper motor neurone*.

The alpha neurone or final common pathway constitutes the *lower motor neurone* (Fig. 3.20).

The sensory pathways

In order that we may be made aware of our internal and external environment, sensations must reach the sensory area of the brain. Sensory nerves bring such information from the skin and deeper structures.

Within the skin are four types of receptors which are sensitive to touch, pain, cold and heat. From the joint capsules, receptors convey information about position of joints in space, and from the muscle spindles information concerning degree of contraction of muscles. These nerves are called proprioceptors. The deeper structures also contain nerves transmitting sensations of pain.

The stimuli will either travel via the sensory cranial nerves (from the head) or the peripheral spinal nerves (from remainder of body).

Sensory nerve cells arise in the spinal ganglia which lie outside the spinal cord and the nerve fibres travel to the posterior horn of grey matter in the spinal cord. The sensory fibres outside the spinal cord form the posterior nerve root and are separate from the motor fibres. When receptors are stimulated impulses are transmitted to the posterior nerve root and from there conveyed to the posterior horn of grey matter (Fig. 3.21).

The nature of the sensation being transmitted to the brain will determine the pathway taken.

Figure 3.22
The sensory pathways

The posterior tracts

Nerves conveying sensations of touch or proprioception (i.e. sense of position of joints and muscles) enter the posterior horn cells of grey matter. They ascend the spinal cord in the posterior column of white matter to the medulla. In the medulla they synapse with a second group of nerves which cross to the opposite side — sensory decussation — and travel to the thalamus. In the thalamus a synapse occurs with a third group of nerves which travel to the sensory area of the cortex (Fig. 3.22).

The anterior tracts

Nerves conveying sensations of pressure, pain and temperature enter the posterior horn cells of grey matter. They synapse with a second group of nerves which cross to the opposite side and ascend in the anterolateral columns of white matter to the thalamus. These fibres have already crossed and there is no decussation in the medulla. In the thalamus, a synapse occurs with a third group of nerves which travel to the sensory area of the cortex (Fig. 3.22).

Tracts which travel from spinal cord to thalamus are called the spinothalamic tracts, and those from thalamus to sensory cortex, the thalamocortical tracts.

The thalamus. As already stated the term 'basal ganglia' is used most frequently to denote motor nuclei that are closely related functionally, and some of these nuclei have been mentioned when discussing the extrapyramidal tract. Another mass of nerve cells forming part of the basal ganglia is the thalamus. These are situated below the corpus callosum. All sensory impulses are conveyed to the thalamus which is thought to perceive sensation but is unable to discriminate between or interpret these stimuli. There may be some crude appreciation of sensation but this is debatable. If pain occurs, the thalamus has a 'perception of pain' but the cerebral cortex analyses information in terms of locality, intensity and nature of pain.

The meninges

These consist of three membranes which cover the brain and spinal cord (Fig. 3.23).
1. **The dura** (hard) is a white, inelastic membrane consisting of two layers of fibrous tissue. The outer layer is attached to the under surface of the skull and the inner layer covers and protects the brain and spinal cord. The inner layer forms folds notably the tentorium cerebelli which separates the anterior and middle fossae of the

Figure 3.23
The meninges

skull from the posterior fossa, and the falx cerebri (falx *L*. a sickle.) which incompletely separates the anterior and middle fossae (Fig. 3.24).

Between the two layers are sinuses which allow drainage of venous blood from the brain. These are called the *venous sinuses*.

2. The arachnoid (spider-like) lies immediately under the dura and is a serous membrane. Web-like processes extend from the arachnoid to the third membrane, the pia. Separating the dura from the arachnoid is a potential space called the **subdural space.**

3. The pia (tender) is a delicate membrane which is firmly attached to the brain and consists mainly of small blood vessels.

Between the arachnoid and pia is a space called the **subarachnoid space,** which is filled with **cerebrospinal fluid (CSF).**

Figure 3.24
Horizontal section of skull
showing cranial fossae

The ventricles

At the centre of the cerebrum are two irregular-shaped cavities, one in each hemisphere. These are the **left** and **right lateral ventricles.** Each lateral ventricle communicates with the third ventricle via an opening called the **interventricular foramen.** The third ventricle communicates with the fourth ventricle via a canal called the **aqueduct of the midbrain,** which lies between the medulla and cerebellum. The fourth ventricle is continuous with the central canal of the spinal cord.

Formation, circulation and absorption of CSF

Cerebrospinal fluid is formed from the blood by the action of vascular processes called choroid plexuses which are found in the lateral, third and fourth ventricles. It is a modified form of plasma consisting of water, protein, glucose, minerals and a few lymphocytes.

The circulation of CSF commences in the lateral ventricles from where it flows into the third ventricle, through the interventricular foramen and then into the fourth ventricle via the aqueduct of the midbrain. It leaves the roof of the fourth ventricle by two openings called the **medial and lateral foramina** and enters the subarachnoid space. As the fourth ventricle is continuous with the central canal of the spinal cord, cerebrospinal fluid also flows into the central canal (Fig. 3.25). It is absorbed back into the venous circulation through projections in the arachnoid called arachnoid villi to the jugular veins and back to the heart. Any obstruction within the ventricular system will result in impairment in flow of CSF, the ventricles will dilate and intracranial pressure will increase.

The composition of CSF is standard but changes occur in disease.

The pressure range is 60 to 180 mm of water, the specific gravity of water being identical to that of CSF. Examination of this fluid can therefore be an important aid in diagnosis.

Figure 3.25
Flow of cerebrospinal fluid (CSF)

Lateral ventricles

Interventricular foramen

Third ventricle

Aqueduct of midbrain

Foramen of fourth ventricle

Fourth ventricle continuous with spinal canal

Pia mater adherent to cerebrum

Arachnoid mater

Subarachnoid space

Cerebellum

The peripheral nervous system

The peripheral nervous system consists of:

1. The cerebro-spinal system
2. The autonomic system.

The cerebro-spinal system

The cranial nerves

There are 12 pairs of cranial nerves arising mainly in the brain stem. They are composed of either sensory or motor fibres or both. While certain cranial nerves carry fibres from the autonomic system it is important to appreciate that the cranial nerves, in themselves, form part of the somatic system (Table 3.1).

Table 3.1
The cranial nerves

Number	Name	Type	Function
1	Olfactory	Sensory	Convey sense of smell
2	Optic	Sensory	Convey sense of vision
3	Oculomotor	Motor	Control muscles which move eye up, in and down Carry **parasympathetic** fibres which constrict circular muscles of iris
4	Trochlear	Motor	Control muscles which move eye downwards and outwards
5	Trigeminal	Mixed	Sensory: convey sensations of pain, temperature and pressure from head and face Motor: innervate muscles of mastication
6	Abducent	Motor	Control muscles which move eye outward
7	Facial	Mixed	Sensory: convey perception of taste from anterior two-thirds of tongue Motor: control muscles of face Carry **parasympathetic** fibres which stimulate salivary and lacrimal glands
8	Acoustic (2 parts): — Cochlear — Vestibular	Sensory	Cochlear: convey perception of sound Vestibular: fibres from semicircular canal of ear convey impulses to cerebellum and assist in maintaining body equilibrium
9	Glossopharyngeal	Mixed	Sensory: convey perception of taste from posterior third of tongue and sensation from soft palate and tonsils Motor: innervate muscles of pharynx and control swallowing Carry **parasympathetic** fibres to parotid glands
10	Vagus	Mixed	Sensory: convey impulses from respiratory and digestive structures and back of ear. Motor: control voluntary muscles of pharynx and larynx. Individual groups of **parasympathetic** fibres: 1. stimulate peristalsis and control secretions from digestive tract, liver, gall-bladder, pancreas and kidneys 2. control constriction of bronchi and bronchioles 3. decrease rate and force of heart beat.
11	Accessory	Motor	Control sternomastoid and trapezius muscles Fibres travel with vagus nerve to supply muscles of pharynx and larynx
12	Hypoglossal	Motor	Control muscles of tongue

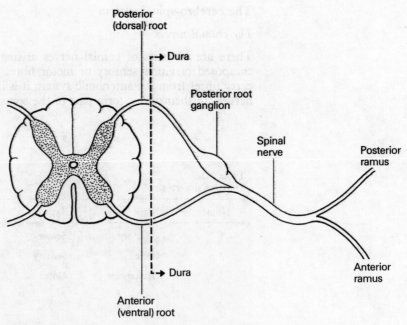

Figure 3.26
A typical nerve

The spinal nerves

There are 31 pairs of spinal nerves:

8 cervical
12 thoracic or dorsal
5 lumbar
5 sacral
1 coccygeal

The spinal nerves emerge in pairs from each side of the spinal cord. A typical nerve is shown in Figure 3.26; it consists of a mixture of sensory and motor fibres derived from the posterior and anterior nerve roots.

The autonomic system

The autonomic nervous system comprises:

1. A sympathetic component
2. A parasympathetic component.

Sympathetic nerve fibres

These leave the cord with the motor fibres between the first thoracic and second lumbar segments. They soon leave the motor fibres and join the sympathetic chain, branches of which go to the blood vessels, air passages, digestive tract, bladder and bowel. The sympathetic system is particularly active in states of stress and fear. A chemical transmitter substance, noradrenaline, is released at sympathetic nerve endings causing the pupils to dilate, the heart to accelerate, skin and blood vessels to constrict thus increasing blood pressure.

Parasympathetic nerve fibres

These leave the central nervous system with some of the cranial and sacral nerves. The cranial outflow includes the vagus nerve, which supplies most of the internal organs. This system is sometimes called the 'emptying system' as it speeds up digestion of foodstuffs and plays an important part in defaecation and micturition. The parasympathetic activating substance is acetylcholine.

In most cases the actions of the sympathetic and parasympathetic nerve fibres are mutually antagonistic, circumstances determining which action will predominate at any given time.

DISORDERS OF THE NERVOUS SYSTEM

Head injuries

Head injuries are usually caused by either the head coming to a sudden stop after travelling at a considerable speed (someone falling from a height and coming to an abrupt halt on reaching the ground) or an object travelling at speed striking the head (a metal fragment from a bomb explosion).

A series of events can then occur.

There can be a fracture of the skull either at the point of impact or at a point distant from it. If a blood vessel is ruptured blood will escape and result in the formation of a blood clot between the skull and the dura. Movement of the skull may separate the dura from the brain and cause rupture of blood vessels passing between them. This is an **extradural haemorrhage** (Fig. 3.27A).

Although the skull comes to a halt, the brain continues to travel within it. The brain strikes one side of the skull then moves in the opposite direction to strike the other side. This is known as the **contra coup** (opposite to blow) injury and as a result both sides of the brain suffer.

Several injuries can result from this movement of the brain:

1. Blood vessels passing from the cerebral cortex to the dura may rupture resulting in a **subdural haemorrhage** (Fig. 3.27B).

2. Any ruptured blood vessel on the surface of the brain or passing through the subarachnoid space may bleed into the subarachnoid space resulting in a **subarachnoid haemorrhage** (Fig. 3.27C).

3. The force may be sufficient to cause tearing of blood vessels within the brain resulting in an **intracerebral haemorrhage** (Fig. 3.27D).

4. The brain may be bruised; this is called **contusion**. If the brain is bruised, swelling can occur resulting in an increase in intracranial pressure.

5. Movement of the cerebrum can cause a transient distortion of the brain stem which results in loss of consciousness. This is known as **concussion**. If damage is slight then loss of consciousness will be temporary; if severe then a state of prolonged loss of consciousness will result.

As the maximum damage to the brain always occurs at the time of the accident, an improvement in the patient's condition will normally follow unless recovery is complicated by a rise in intracranial pressure.

A Extradural haemorrhage

B Subdural haemorrhage

C Subarachnoid haemorrhage

D Intracerebral haemorrhage

Figure 3.27A–D
Types of intracranial haemorrhage

Investigations

The following techniques may be employed as an aid to assessing the degree of damage sustained following a head injury:

Computerised axial tomography (CAT) scan

This is a non-invasive X-ray procedure which allows the densities of a transverse slice of the brain to be seen by producing an image at any given level. Any abnormalities such as an extradural haematoma (Fig. 3.28) will be demonstrated. The scanner (Fig. 3.37) employs conventional X-rays but instead of using a film, a computer produces a picture.

Figure 3.28
Extradural haematoma
demonstrated by CAT scan.

Echoencephalography

This utilizes sound as a basis. Ultrasonic impulses from a machine called an ultrasonic diasonoscope are directed through the patient's skull. The bones of the skull and the midline structures of the brain act as reflectors and will reflect a number of these impulses back to their initial source. These reflected impulses are seen on a screen and can be photographed. Any shift in the midline structures of the brain from, say, the pressure of a blood clot, will be demonstrated (Fig. 3.29).

The advantages of this procedure are that no special preparation of the patient is necessary and it is rapid and safe.

Angiography

This entails the injection of a radio-opaque contrast medium into the carotid artery or the vertebral artery during which radiographs are taken. The films will demonstrate the cerebral arteries and returning venous circulation. Any abnormalities can then be localized.

If the patient's condition allows, the procedure is explained and written permission is obtained. If it does not, written consent of the next of kin is obtained.

A sedative may be given on the evening prior to the angiography and, if a general anaesthetic is to be used, no fluid or food is given during the 6 hours prior to the procedure.

On return from the X-ray department the patient is placed in the recumbent position for 24 hours. If a general anaesthetic has been given, the patient is placed in the lateral position until fully conscious. The routine observations following general anaesthesia are maintained.

Rarely do complications arise, but the nurse must be aware of two possible major problems.

Figure 3.29
Echoencephalogram (A) Normal
(B) Midline shift to left

A   B

A haematoma may occur at the site of the injection and, if sufficiently large, will compress the oesophagus and trachea. The nurse must observe the patient's neck for evidence of swelling; this, and any difficulty experienced in breathing or swallowing, must be reported.

Spasm of the cerebral arteries or oedema may occur giving rise to an increase in intracranial pressure. The clinical features of this condition are described under observations (p. 92). Fortunately these complications are very unusual.

Types of head injury

The severity of a head injury is greatly influenced by age. A small child can have a serious fall with little or no effects, while in the elderly a slight bump can lead to severe intracranial damage.

Head injuries may be divided into two main groups:

Closed — the skull may be fractured but the meninges remain intact.
Open — the skull is fractured and the meninges and brain are exposed.

The types of fracture are:

Simple — no break in the skin (Fig. 3.30A).
Compound — the scalp is breached (Fig. 3.30B).
Comminuted — the bone is broken in several places (Fig. 3.30C).
Depressed — a piece of bone is driven inwards (Fig. 3.30D).

Figure 3.30
Fractures of the skull

The X-ray appearance of a fracture of the vault of the skull is shown in Figure 3.31.

It is the site of the fracture which is important rather than the fracture itself. Two areas are of particular importance:

If the frontal bone is damaged and there is a breach in the dura, CSF can escape via the frontal sinus from the nose. This is called **rhinorrhoea**.

If the fracture occurs at the base of the skull and the petrous bone, which contains the middle ear, is damaged, a breach in the dura will result in an escape of CSF from the ear. This is called **otorrhoea**.

Figure 3.31
X-ray of fracture of the vault of the skull

The nurse must remember to observe the nose and ears and report any discharge immediately. If such a discharge is observed, under no circumstances should the nurse attempt to stop the flow by plugging either the nostrils or ears as this may result in infection from the back flow of CSF being introduced into the subarachnoid space. The orifice should be covered with a sterile dressing until the patient is seen by a doctor.

Intracranial bleeding

Bleeding may occur outside the dura, extradural haemorrhage; under the dura, subdural haemorrhage; or into the cortex of the brain, intracerebral or subarachnoid haemorrhages.

Extradural haemorrhage

Haemorrhage may result from injury or, in some instances, from disease (p. 85). This occurs most commonly following injury to the temperoparietal region of the skull because of the large number of blood vessels in that area, but it can also occur following injury to any area. The onset of clinical features will depend on the site of impact and the degree of haemorrhage.

If haemorrhage is mild to moderate, the patient may or may not become unconscious at the time of injury, but as the clot formation increases in size an impairment in the conscious level will occur. If the middle meningeal artery is ruptured the result is the very rapid formation of a blood clot with a correspondingly rapid impairment in the conscious level.

Other features that may occur depend on the site of injury; they include headaches, neck stiffness, vomiting, paralysis of one side of the body and an increase in the size of the pupil of the eye on the side of bleeding.

The urgency of immediate surgical treatment is dependent on the clinical findings made on admission. X-ray of the skull and echoencephalography may be carried out, but the surgeon would not allow these diagnostic procedures to delay operation in a case of urgency. The patient is taken to the operating theatre where hair is shaved from the area considered appropriate. The scalp is incised and a hole made in the skull and widened by means of a burr. When the clot formation has been confirmed the exposed piece of bone can be removed. The clot is evacuated by suction and the bleeding vessel controlled by diathermy. The dura can then be opened to ensure there is no bleeding below this level. A drain is placed in position and the scalp incision closed with silk sutures.

Ideally, the patient should be transferred from the operating table to his bed as this will avoid unnecessary movement on his arrival back in the ward.

Following the removal of the clot and relief of pressure on the brain there may be a rapid improvement in the level of consciousness.

Subdural haemorrhage

This can range from an acute type, which usually occurs following a blow of considerable violence when bleeding is severe, to a chronic type, which follows an injury of milder degree when bleeding occurs slowly. Clinical features may be evident within the first few days or may not appear until weeks after the injury. These features include headaches increasing in intensity, drowsiness, changes in normal pattern of behaviour and confusion. If the motor cortex is involved then paralysis of one side of the body will occur. Pressure on the cerebral cortex will lead to fits. There is one classic feature — namely, the variations which occur in the levels of consciousness. The patient may be alert and talking but within a short time may become drowsy and uncommunicative. He is, however, easily aroused and will then appear as alert as before.

As this condition does not demand the same degree of urgency as an extradural haemorrhage, an X-ray of the skull will be taken to determine the site of any fracture. An echoencephalography and angiography are also carried out.

The operative measure is to evacuate the clot and control any bleeding vessels. The technique is similar to that described for extradural haemorrhage.

Intracerebral and subarachnoid haemorrhages

As most haemorrhages occurring in the cortex result in bleeding into the subarachnoid space producing a subarachnoid haemorrhage, the two conditions can be discussed together. The amount of blood found in the subarachnoid space is determined by the degree of injury to the cortex or the size of the torn blood vessel passing through the subarachnoid space itself.

The clinical features will depend on the severity of damage and the resulting haemorrhage. These range from headaches, neck stiffness, rise in temperature, irritability and photophobia (dislike of bright light) to progressive impairment of the conscious level.

Examination of CSF for evidence of blood is the diagnostic aid used in this condition. The procedure is called a **lumbar puncture** (p. 127).

In most cases, apart from a period of rest in bed, no specific treatment is necessary. There is no procedure which will hasten the reabsorption of blood from the subarachnoid space. The patient's recovery is spontaneous.

In the remainder of cases where there is delay in recovery and definite clinical features are present such as weakness of voluntary muscles of one side of the body (hemiparesis) and impairment of conscious level, surgery will be contemplated. An angiography will be carried out to determine the site of the haemorrhage.

If only a small area of the cortex is involved the clot can be aspirated through a burr hole in the skull. If, however, an extensive area of the cortex is involved then the skull will be exposed, a piece of bone removed and the clot evacuated. Any bleeding vessels will be controlled and the bone opening will be closed.

Nursing observations

The following are the observations the nurse must make and record as part of her total care of the patient.

Assessment of neurological status

There is no doubt that an assessment of the conscious level is the most important indicator of an improvement or a deterioration in the condition of a patient who has sustained a head injury. In assessing the conscious level of a patient it is important that the nurse realises that this is an assessment of brain function as a whole, and is not confined to any specific area of the brain. The problem in making an assessment of conscious level is that the degrees of impairment cannot be defined accurately. The use of terms such as stupor, semi-conscious, semi-comatosed, are ambiguous and should be discouraged.

A system which was devised in Glasgow, has proved to be an accurate formula for recording any impairment of the conscious level. Using this *Glasgow Coma Scale* (Fig. 3.32) the nurse assesses and records the patient's neurological status in relation to three aspects of his behaviour:

Figure 3.32
Glasgow Coma Scale
(reproduced by kind permission
of Mr G. Teasdale, Southern
General Hospital, Glasgow)

1. **Opening the eyes**
   a. *Spontaneous opening*. The patient will open his eyes when awake and close them when asleep; this suggests that the reticular formation of cells in the medulla are functioning. It is important for the nurse to realise that certain patients with damage to the brain will have a reversed diurnal rhythm and, as a result, will be awake during the night and asleep during the day.
   b. *Opening to speech*. The nurse addresses the patient by name and asks him to open his eyes. The loudness of sound necessary will indicate the patient's ability to respond.
   c. *Opening to pain*. The acceptable method of applying a painful stimulus is pressure to the finger nail bed; it is used only if the patient is unable to respond to speech.
   d. *No eye opening*. The patient does not respond to a painful stimulus. This lack of response suggests a marked degree of damage to the reticular formation of the medulla.

2. **Verbal response**
   Here the nurse is assessing the degree of orientation that the patient possesses in relation to self, time and place. It is however important that the questions asked are those which the patient could reasonably be expected to answer and must not be too specific. The nurse herself might, if suddenly asked the date, have difficulty in answering!

3. **Motor response**
   The nurse must assess the patient's motor response in relation to the following:
   a. The patient's ability to obey commands. Initially he should be requested to perform simple movements, for instance, 'lift your right arm'. If he is able to perform simple movements, then he can be asked to perform movements of a more complex nature, such as 'touch the middle finger of your left hand with the thumb of your left hand'.
   b. The patient's response to painful stimuli. The nurse can assess the patient's ability to move a limb to remove a painful stimulus, for instance if pressure is applied over the supra orbital region does the patient attempt to move his hand and arm in the direction of pressure.?

When assessing the patient's motor responses the nurse must consider two important points:

1. The strength of limbs on both sides of the body.
2. The power of limb movement. While it is appreciated that making a specific distinction regarding degrees of power is not possible, the nurse should observe the following criteria:

if limb movements are considered appropriate to those in health they are recorded as normal power;
if one limb shows normal power but its opposite appears less strong this is recorded as mild weakness;
if one limb shows normal power but its opposite is markedly weaker this is recorded as severe weakness.

The clinical significance lies not so much in the degree of weakness of a specific limb but in the comparison between opposite limbs.

Pupillary reaction

The reaction of the iris of the eye to light can indicate displacement of the brain due to pressure. It should be remembered that all smooth muscle is normally in a state of partial constriction. If the eye is exposed to the bright light from a torch, the parasympathetic fibres travelling within the third cranial nerve will cause further constriction of the iris and the pupil will become smaller.

If the brain is displaced the only escape valve is through the tentorial hiatus. The brain squeezes through and displaces the third cranial nerve, which ceases to function (Fig. 3.33). As parasympathetic control is lost the iris will relax and the pupil will dilate.

Figure 3.33
Displacement of brain

The significance of this observation is that the greater the amount of brain squeezed through the tentorial hiatus, the greater the pressure brought to bear on the reticular formation of the brain stem. It will be remembered that the reticular formation activates a state of arousal in the cerebral cortex which affects the level of consciousness.

The nurse should make the following observations regarding iris reaction of both eyes:

Are both reacting briskly to light?
Is one reacting more sluggishly than the other?
Is one pupil larger than the other?
If so, is it still reacting to light or has reaction ceased?

The nurse must always remember to ascertain if the patient has a glass eye or contact lens: failure to do so has led to unnecessary anxiety in the past!

Features of increased intracranial pressure

In a rigid container such as the skull, an increase in volume will result in an increase in pressure. If the contents are semisolid (as is the brain) and an increase in pressure arises, the contents will flow out.

If for any reason there is an increase in volume within one of the fossae of the skull, such as a clot of blood or a tumour, the pressure within the fossae will rise and the semisolid brain will flow out. This will eventually result in compression of the brain stem with a resulting disturbance in function.

Irrespective of the cause of increased intracranial pressure the nurse should be able to recognize certain features:

Headache, particularly on waking in the morning.
Blurring of vision.
Nausea accompanied by vomiting.
A slowing of the pulse rate.
A rise in the systolic blood pressure.
Slowing and irregularities of respiration. If the brain stem is damaged the respirations become periodic. The patient will take a few rapid breaths and then stop breathing completely. After a few seconds he will begin breathing again.
An impairment of the conscious level.

The vital signs

The frequency of observation of temperature, pulse, respirations and blood pressure will depend on the individual patient and his injury. In the initial acute stage or immediately after surgery, observations are made every 15 to 30 minutes. As the patient's condition improves these observations can be made at less frequent intervals. Any change, sudden or gradual, must be reported as complications may be averted or treated by prompt intervention.

Nursing care

The principles of nursing care are basically the same in all classifications of head injuries.

Respiratory function

Maintenance of a clear airway is of prime importance and takes precedence over all other care. Depression of respiratory function is the commonest cause of deterioration in the unconscious patient. It can be the result of several factors. The jaw tends to fall downwards and the tongue backwards, thus blocking the upper part of the respiratory tract. As the cough and swallowing reflexes are not functioning, secretions from the mouth and pharynx trickle down into the trachea. These secretions, and secretions formed in the bronchi, which are not cleared can block the lower respiratory tract. Another hazard facing the patient is that blood from the mouth and any vomitus can be inhaled into the respiratory tract. If the nurse observes the following rules the risk of respiratory difficulties for the patient will be greatly diminished.

Dentures should be removed and placed in the appropriate receptacle. The patient should be placed in the semiprone position, which can be maintained by placing a pillow under the lower part of the chest to prevent him falling forward; if the upper leg is flexed and a pillow placed between the legs he will not fall backwards (Fig. 3.34). A waterproof square covered by a disposable towel should be placed under the patient's head. This will protect bedding should vomiting occur. The lateral positions can be used as an alternative. The patient's position should be altered every 2 hours to help ventilation of both lungs. The changing of position requires at least two nurses — an individual nurse should never attempt it on her own.

Observation should be made of the skin for evidence of cyanosis which might indicate blockage within the respiratory tract. The respirations should be observed for any change which might suggest difficulty in breathing.

Although correct positioning will do much to ensure drainage of secretions, it is often insufficient. Excessive secretions can be aspirated by using a suction machine and catheter. The catheter is connected to the tubing from the suction machine, inserted gently into the mouth and directed to the pharynx. Suction is then applied and the secretions aspirated. A fresh catheter is then connected to the suction machine and gently inserted into each nostril to allow for aspiration of secretions. While a soft rubber catheter is ideal in that it lessens the risk of injury to the mouth, it does tend to curl before reaching the pharynx and a polythene catheter is more

Figure 3.34
Unconscious patient in semiprone position

effective. This procedure requires considerable practice before skill is attained and should not be delegated to a nurse inexperienced in the technique unless under supervision. It is less distressing for the patient if this procedure is carried out at frequent intervals of short duration; prolonged exposure to aspiration technique at lengthy intervals should be avoided. An oral airway may be introduced to assist in maintaining effective respiratory function. If so, it is important that the nurse realizes that the airway can become plugged with mucus; it must be removed when oral hygiene is being carried out and a fresh airway inserted.

Despite maintenance of correct position of the patient and adequate aspiration there are situations where respiratory embarrassment is such that other techniques must be employed. An endotracheal tube can be introduced or a tracheostomy performed (Ch. 6).

Care of the skin

The conscious patient confined to bed can do one of two things if he becomes aware of discomfort. He can change his position in bed or, if unable to do so, he can inform the nursing staff of his problem. The unconscious patient can do neither. Here, an awareness of the patient's needs by the nurse is of the utmost importance.

Changing the patient's position in bed has already been mentioned in maintaining adequate respiratory function. It also serves the double purpose of ensuring that one area of the body will not be subjected to the harmful effects of pressure over a prolonged period. Routine care of skin and pressure areas (Ch. 14) is particularly important as the patient's skin is in constant danger of contamination from vomit, urine and faeces; these contaminants should be removed at once and the area washed. Any soiled linen must be removed and clean linen supplied. A bed-bath should be given each day. Any evidence of reddening or an actual break in the continuity of the skin must be reported at once. The special care necessary if pressure sores occur is described in Chapter 14.

Under no circumstances should hot water bottles be placed in the bed of an unconscious patient, because of the danger of burns from direct contact or from water escaping unnoticed from the bottle. The nurse should also ensure that the patient's finger- and toe-nails are cut and filed. Unless contraindicated, the hair should be brushed and combed and arranged in an attractive style.

Care of the mouth

In many instances the unconscious patient tends to breathe through his mouth, which will become excessively dry. It may also become heavily coated with mucus. If an oral airway is in situ it is removed, the oral cavity gently but thoroughly cleaned every 2 hours and a fresh airway inserted.

Feeding

The following principles can be applied in considering the safest method of feeding the patient:

1. If the patient is conscious with both cough and swallow reflexes present he may be fed by the normal oral route.

2. If the patient is unconscious but cough reflex is present then feeding by nasogastric route is used.

3. If the patient is unconscious and both cough and swallow reflexes are absent intravenous feeding is essential.

Feeding by intravenous route

Various regimes may be advocated. Table 3.2 shows preparations totalling 5828 kJ which, if infused over a 24-hour period, will meet the patient's basic kilojoule requirements.

The specific responsibilities of the nurse in the care of the patient are as follows. Prior to the start of the infusion the site chosen must be shaved of hair and thor-

Table 3.2
An intravenous feeding regime

Preparation	Volume (litres)	Constituents	Kilojoules supplied	Advantages	Disadvantages
Intralipid 20%	½	Soya beans 10% Glycerol 2.5%	4200	Contains essential fatty acids and phosphorus; neutral pH	Expensive
Aminoplex 14	1	Synthetic amino acids	1428		
Glucose 50%★	½		4200	Normal physiological substrate essential for cerebral metabolism	Viscid and an irritant to veins. Must be given via large central vein. Hyperglycaemia with excessive loss of water in urine. Insulin must be given to ensure effective metabolism.
Normal saline 0.9%	½				Isotonic solution

Potassium 1.5 g added to each flask.
Parentrovite (vitamin B complex) given every second day.

★ Fructose 20% can be substituted for glucose 50%. It is less irritating and can be infused via a peripheral vein. Less water is lost in the urine. It does, however, carry risk of causing lactic acidosis and must be used with caution.

oughly cleaned. Strict observance of an aseptic technique must be given by both the doctor commencing the infusion and the nurse assisting. The infusion site must be inspected regularly for signs of inflammation. If for any reason blood or plasma are transfused (Ch. 8) the infusion apparatus must be changed before feeding recommences. The addition of any supplements (such as vitamins) to the infusion flask must be kept to a minimum as this will increase the risk of introducing a contaminant to the sterile solution.

Observations should be made to ensure that the rate of infusion is as prescribed and care taken that the flask is not allowed to empty completely before being changed. Should a flask empty, under no circumstances must it be replaced with a full flask until the doctor has examined the infusion tubing to see if air has entered. Fluid running through tubing which contains air will force the air into the venous circulation and expose the patient to the risk of formation of an air embolus.

Fungal infections are not uncommon and the application of an antifungal agent to the infusion site is advised.

The amount of fluid given from any flask should be recorded on the patient's fluid balance chart after the fluid has been infused.

Feeding by nasogastric route (Fig. 3.35)

The most important point to remember is that the unconscious patient must be nursed in either the lateral or semiprone position. Then, if vomiting of food occurs, the patient can maintain a clear airway. Ideally a disposable polythene catheter should be used. This is firmer than rubber and therefore easier to pass into the stomach. It also has the advantage of being less irritating to tissues than rubber and diminishes the volume of secretions.

The nostrils should be cleaned of any dirt or secretions. The upper third of the catheter should be lubricated avoiding the orifice of the catheter. It should then be

Figure 3.35
Nasogastric feed

inserted into a nostril and gently guided into the stomach. If the nurse experiences any resistance to the passage of the catheter force should not be used as this may result in damage to the delicate turbinate bone. The other nostril can be used or the catheter passed by the oral route. The nurse can satisfy herself that the catheter has not entered the respiratory tract by carrying out the following observations:

1. Looking for any evidence of cyanosis which would indicate respiratory embarrassment.
2. Listening for the sound of expirations whistling through the tube.
3. Making sure any aspirate obtained from the tube shows an acid reaction on litmus paper, indicating gastric contents.

The practices of placing the open end of the catheter in a bowl of water to see if bubbles appear, and of injecting water down the tube, which, if in the respiratory tract, will result in the patient coughing, are not recommended.

A spigot should be placed in the open end of the catheter. The catheter should then be brought across the cheek and behind the ear where it is secured by a piece of tape.

Before administering a feed the total contents of the stomach should be aspirated, measured, and the amount of aspirate recorded on the fluid balance chart. This will indicate how effectively the feed is passing from the stomach to the small intestine. If feeds are continued without assessing emptying ability of the stomach, the patient may regurgitate food which may then be inhaled. As the aspirate contains important electrolytes most of it should be returned to the stomach. If the amount of aspirate indicates that previous feeds are not being passed effectively, then medical advice should be sought.

The following regime is an example of one commonly used:

Water 15 ml hourly for 4 hours.
Water 30 ml hourly for 4 hours.
Water 60 ml hourly for 4 hours.
Milk 30 ml and water 30 ml hourly for 4 hours.
Milk 60 ml and water 30 ml 2 hourly for 4 hours.
Milk 90 ml and water 60 ml 2 hourly for 4 hours.
Milk 120 ml and water 90 ml 2 hourly for 4 hours.

If at the end of this 28-hour period the patient has tolerated the gradual increase in amount, an instant breakfast product 120 ml and water 90 ml should be given 2 hourly for the following 24 hours.

Special feeds consisting of milk, eggs, Casilan and a vitamin syrup are prepared by the dietitian. Usually the total feed for 24 hours is sent to the ward and this must be kept in the refrigerator to prevent the growth of bacteria. This special feed 120 ml and water 90 ml can be given 2 hourly for an indefinite period.

Drugs should, if possible, be given in liquid form. Powders or crushed tablets should be dissolved in a quantity of water from the diet allowance and given following the feed.

The part of the catheter entering the nose should be kept free from crust formation by the application of a lubricant. The catheter should be removed and a fresh one introduced into alternate nostrils every fourth day. Changing of the catheter should always take place immediately before a feed and following aspiration of stomach contents.

Observations of vital signs

The frequency with which these observations are made depends on the patient's condition and can range from 15-minute to 4-hourly intervals. Irrespective of the time interval the nurse should remember the following points.

As all patients who have sustained a head injury will suffer a degree of shock, the skin will tend to be cold and clammy.

The **hypothalamus,** a group of cells within the cerebrum forming part of the autonomic nervous system, may be damaged. As one of the functions of the hypothalamus is the control of body temperature, damage to it can result in marked variations in temperature during 24 hours. The patient may develop a chest infection with a resulting elevation of temperature. Infection entering the subarachnoid space will result in meningitis with an accompanying elevation of temperature. These changes will not always be apparent if the axillae or groins are used as the site for placing the thermometer. The nurse should therefore always use the rectum to register changes in temperature. It should be noted that, while in most patients evidence of a chest infection would indicate the use of semirecumbent or upright position, in the unconscious patient following head injury no change can be made from recommended positions.

The rate, rhythm and volume of the pulse and respirations should be observed and any change no matter how slight, must be reported.

The absence of a pulse beat can prove frightening to a young nurse who may immediately assume that arterial circulation has ceased. While this may be the case, it is not necessarily true. The fluctuation between systolic and diastolic pressure gives rise to the pulse beat. If no difference existed between systolic and diastolic pressures there would be no evidence of a pulse beat but circulation of blood would still be adequate.

Accuracy in recording blood pressure is essential (Ch. 7). The sphygmomanometer should be placed at a level corresponding to the level of the patient's heart and not on a table top well above the level of the recumbent patient.

The importance of observing pupillary reaction to light has already been discussed (p. 91). The patient should be informed of the procedure. Both eyes should be opened and the pupils observed for size and equality. The beam from the torch should then be directed on the pillow near the patient's head and gradually brought over the patient's face and finally to the eyes. Under no circumstances should the beam be directly focused on the eyes because, if there is existing damage to the eyes or surrounding tissue, a sudden involuntary closure of the eyelids can result in a haemorrhage. Light directed on one pupil should result in both pupils becoming smaller. The reaction should be tested with the light being directed into one eye, then, after allowing a short interval of time for the pupils to return to their original size, the procedure should be repeated with the light being gradually directed into the other eye. The observations should then be recorded and any change reported at once.

Care of the eyes

If unconsciousness results from an organic cause the corneal reflex is absent. As the secretion of tears is diminished and the patient cannot close the eyelids completely, the eye is exposed to irritation by dust particles and to excessive dryness. Regular observations should be made for evidence of inflammation; neglect can result in ulceration of the cornea (Ch. 12).

Crusts on the eyelids or eyelashes should be gently removed with sterile cotton wool balls soaked in normal saline. Each eye is treated separately using a fresh cotton wool ball for every application to the eye. The eyelids are gently closed and can be maintained in position by applying a small strip of tape or micropore over the eyelid and cheek. Great care must be taken when removing this strip as the delicate skin below the eye can be easily damaged. Eye shields made of X-ray film can be used to cover the eyes and afford protection from dust or other harmful substances.

Care of the urinary bladder

The unconscious patient usually suffers from incontinence of urine with the resulting increased risk of contamination of the skin. The nurse can help reduce this risk by offering the patient a bedpan or a urinal at regular intervals. It is important to remember that although the patient is unable to communicate his needs, he may be aware of his immediate environment, and it is possible to establish a bladder training regime. By observing the times at which the patient voids urine the nurse can plan the times at which to offer the bedpan or urinal.

Obviously contamination of the skin and bed linen will occur and the regime itself can be time-consuming, but the advantages to the patient cannot be overemphasized.

If bladder training is not possible, male patients may be kept dry by the use of Paul's tubing. A suitable length of the tubing is cut and one end is placed over the penis and secured if necessary with a strip of Micropore. The other open end is introduced into a urinary drainage bag which is secured by a holder to the bed below the level of the patient. To avoid irritation to the skin from the tubing a protective layer of petroleum jelly should be applied to the penis prior to application of the tubing.

The practice of placing a urinal in situ is to be discouraged. The patient is exposed to the dangers of damage to the surrounding skin from pressure by the urinal and contamination of the skin by spillage of urine.

Catheterization of the urinary bladder should not be contemplated unless absolutely necessary. It carries the grave danger of introducing infection into the urinary tract and adding a further embarrassment to the patient's chances of recovery. The following situations would, however, necessitate catheterization:

Development of retention of urine.
Administration of a diuretic such as mannitol (by intravenous infusion) in the treatment of cerebral oedema will result in a vast diuresis and an accurate record of the urinary output is essential.
If catheterization is carried out, a form of tidal drainage is desirable:
To prevent contamination of the skin with urine.
To produce regular emptying of the bladder and obviate the necessity of repeated catheterizations.
To assist in maintaining normal tone of bladder muscle.
To reduce the risk of infection.
To treat infection by the introduction of an irrigating antiseptic solution.
To reduce the exposure of the patient to physical and mental distress.

Care of bowel function

The principle of offering the patient a bedpan is equally applicable here. Constipation or impaction of faeces can be avoided by the administration of an enema every third day.

Care of the joints

Prolonged immobilization will result in a stiffening of the joints, often in an abnormal position. This complication can be avoided by ensuring that all joints are put through their full range of movements several times each day. The nurse can complement the work of the physiotherapist by performing these passive exercises at appropriate times during the day, for example following the patient's daily bed-bath. It is important, however, that the nurse is shown the correct method of carrying out these exercises by the physiotherapist before attempting to put them into practice. An overvigorous movement of the limbs of an unconscious patient can result in a tearing of associated muscles.

Reduction and control of temperature

A slight elevation of temperature is common in most patients following head injury and is not of any particular import. However, if the elevation is above 38°C it would suggest either infection or damage to the heat-regulating centre in the hypothalamus. The main danger is that this temperature elevation will increase the amount of oxygen required by the brain but, as there is not a corresponding increase in volume of air reaching the lungs, the volume of oxygen will not meet its needs. The result is a deterioration in the patient's level of consciousness. The nurse can employ the following techniques to reduce and control the patient's temperature.

The patient should be naked, a cradle placed in the bed and a sheet loosely draped over him. As far as possible a calm, noise-free atmosphere should be ensured. An electric fan can be placed next to the patient and cool air directed over his body.

Unless contra-indicated the fluid intake should be increased. This decision, of course, would rest with the doctor.

If the mechanism of sweating is absent, tepid sponging can be carried out thus allowing the loss of heat from the body by evaporation. If, however, the patient is sweating, the sweat must be removed from the skin by frequent sponging. Sweat allowed to remain on the skin will quickly cool and if the patient starts to shiver there will be a further elevation in temperature. Observations and recordings of temperature should be made every half hour.

Postoperative nursing care

The care necessary following surgery to evacuate an intracranial haematoma is basically the same as for the unconscious patient (p. 93). If a drain has been left in situ the amount and colour of drainage is observed and recorded. The dressing is inspected for staining and repacked with sterile material as required. The initial dressing should not be disturbed until removal of the drain, usually 48 hours following surgery. The surgeon may wish to carry out this procedure himself. The fresh dressing is not disturbed until the removal of sutures within 5 to 7 days.

The patient may experience a period of disorientation about the third postoperative day. The nurse must ensure that he does not disturb or remove the dressing. In certain instances a form of restraint may be used, such as application of splints to the arms, but this can result in the degree of disorientation becoming more marked and should never be employed without the written permission of the surgeon in charge.

The formation of crusts on the scalp can be dealt with following removal of sutures. A liberal application of petroleum jelly should be gently massaged into the scalp and the head covered with a towel arranged as a turban. The following morning the scalp should be shampooed and crusts can easily be removed. The female patient may well be self-conscious about her shaved head, and encouraging her to wear a wig or an attractively designed head scarf will do much to lessen her anxiety.

Treatment of fracture

If the patient has sustained a simple fracture no specific treatment is required. If it is a compound fracture, the scalp laceration is sutured and a course of antibiotic therapy is begun. A comminuted or depressed fracture can be dealt with following admission; however it is more common for the surgeon to wait until the patient has made a complete recovery from the effects of his head injury. Therefore treatment for this type of fracture usually takes place about 6 months following the injury.

The patient is readmitted to the neurosurgical unit. X-rays of the skull are taken to determine the site and the extent of the fracture. The patient is taken to the theatre where the scalp is shaved and then infiltrated with a local anaesthetic. The scalp is incised and bone fragments removed. Any blood clots or dead tissue are removed by suction. The bone defect can be closed in several ways: by utilizing fragments of bone that were removed or by inserting bone grafts or specially moulded plastic or metal caps. The scalp is then closed by sutures, and further X-rays are taken.

The postoperative care of the patient follows a pattern identical to that already described.

The course of head injuries

Fortunately most patients make a spontaneous recovery and can return to their homes and occupations with little if any change in their previous pattern of living. However, there are others who will suffer from some disturbance which may or may not be due to an organic condition. Only a brief summary will be given, as the number of disturbances which can arise are too varied to be dealt with here.

Post-traumatic epilepsy

This is divided into two stages:

1. **Early epilepsy.** Occurs 1–7 days following initial injury and usually takes the form of focal seizure (see p. 108). Commonly follows a depressed fracture or an intracranial haematoma. Approximately 25% of patients will develop status epilepticus (see p. 111). Anticonvulsant drugs are prescribed for 12 months to 18 months.
2. **Late epilepsy.** This usually occurs about 12 months following initial injury, but, in a small number of cases, the first seizure may be delayed for 4 years. Anticonvulsant drugs are prescribed for 18 months to 2 years.

Brain stem injury

The effect varies according to the degree of trauma. The patient may remain in a state of unconsciousness for months or years. If the injury is less severe the ability to balance and walk may be impaired.

Headaches

These may arise from the patient's anxiety on return to the outside world, particularly if he has difficulty in concentrating or remembering. Headaches can also result from scars on the scalp, but this is not common.

Severe brain damage

This can result in a deterioration in both patterns of behaviour and intellect.

The postconcussion syndrome

Although organic damage may have occurred this can be classifed as a neurotic condition. The disturbances the person complains of are far in excess of any which might arise following minimal organic damage. The symptoms are constant headaches, impairment of memory, intolerance of noise, fear of traffic and crowds, inability to sleep and vertigo. The patient may complain of a sensation of fear if placed in a situation similar to that experienced prior to his injury. The exact cause of this condition is still being debated, but it is most commonly seen in patients of previously low intelligence.

Post-traumatic vertigo

In this condition the patient feels either that he is spinning round or that his immediate external environment is spinning around him. He usually falls to the ground but there is no impairment of his conscious level. These attacks can persist for months following the initial injury but recovery will eventually take place.

Rehabilitation

It is generally accepted that the most important aspect in ensuring an adequate regime of rehabilitation is the nurse's approach to her patient. She must at all times display a cheerful, optimistic outlook on the patient's eventual ability to cope after leaving hospital. She must not, however, fall into the trap of being oversympathetic to any impairment of function experienced by the patient. A patient suffering from the postconcussion syndrome (p. 100) would play unmercifully on this well-meant but misguided approach.

It is most important that the patient should be allowed to develop both his physical and his mental capabilities to their fullest extent before leaving hospital. This aspect of care is not normally carried out in the acute neurosurgical unit. Following gradual ambulation the patient is transferred to a rehabilitation unit. The following members of the health team then have specific responsibilities for ensuring an adequate rehabilitation regime.

The **physiotherapist** begins active exercises which the patient must continue until recovery of impaired voluntary muscles has been achieved or no further improvement is anticipated.

The **speech therapist** deals with any speech defect which has arisen following injury.

The **social worker** collects information regarding the patient's home circumstances and any financial problems likely to arise during the period prior to the patient returning to work.

The **rehabilitation officer**, by co-ordinating with the social worker, physiotherapist, speech therapist, doctor and educational psychologist, determines whether the patient can return either to his former job or to a modified form of it. If not, suitable training is given which will prepare the patient for work geared to his needs.

The patient's own **doctor** is informed of the extent of injury sustained and the treatment given. He can then decide what further medical care is necessary from him. This may require the services of a district nurse who co-ordinates with the family doctor.

Education of the patient's family is vital. They must have a clear understanding of any deficits from which the patient is suffering or may suffer. Guidance should be given as to how they can best offer support during any difficult times. This will go far in preventing misunderstanding and a possible breakdown of relationships within the family circle.

Finally, the period of rehabilitation should not be hurried. If the patient is allowed to develop a sense of physical well-being there is less likelihood of a neurotic breakdown.

If the patient is a child the problems of rehabilitation are minimal. The main concern is that the child will overtire himself by too much activity. The parents should be advised to ensure that the child has regular rest periods. The family doctor will decide when attendance at school is permissible and this is better done in gradual stages — a few hours for the first week, then half a day for the following week and finally full attendance.

In all cases arrangements should be made for the patient to visit the out-patient department to see the surgeon 3 months following discharge from hospital.

Tumours

Tumours arise in the following areas:

1. The brain tissue.
2. The meninges.
3. The skull.
4. Peripheral and cranial nerves.

Figure 3.36
Common brain tumours

The brain tissue

a. Astrocytomas

These arise in the astrocytes and while occasionally they may be of a benign nature they are mostly malignant. They may occur in any age group and are the commoner type of brain tumour.

b. Ependymomas

Most occur in children from 8 to 15 years of age. The tumour usually arises in the floor of the 4th ventricle but may arise in the posterior end of the 3rd ventricle or at the cerebellopontine angle.

c. Oligodendrogliomas

These arise in the cerebral hemisphere and may infiltrate and become adherent to the dura mater. They occur mainly in adults.

d. Medulloblastomas

These arise in the vermis of the cerebellum and are highly malignant. They invade the 4th ventricle thus obstructing the flow of cerebrospinal fluid. The tumour may spread to the 3rd ventricle and seeding may occur in the subarachnoid space. Occasionally metastases occur in bones and lymph nodes. The tumour is more common in boys between the ages of 6 and 10 years. The anticipated life-span is 1 to 2 years. It can occur in adults when seeding is not a feature and therefore the prognosis is more favourable.

The meninges

Meningiomas

These tumours usually arise from a small area of the dura mater, and are essentially benign tumours. They are most common in adults especially middle-aged women.

The skull

Primary tumours of the skull are very rare and may be benign (osteomas) or malignant (sarcomas)

Secondary tumours of the skull are more common and arise as metastases from a primary growth in thyroid gland or bronchi.

Peripheral and cranial nerve tumours

Benign tumours may arise from peripheral and cranial nerve sheaths. A common example is an acoustic neuroma, a benign tumour of the eighth cranial nerve.

Features of intracranial tumours

The combination of headaches, vomiting and papilloedema known as 'the Classical Triad', is the most characteristic presentation of a tumour, although tumours may be present when the classical triad is absent.

Headaches

There is controversy over the cause of headaches. The two theories put forward are that they result either from a stretching of the dura mater or from abnormal tension in the walls of blood vessels.

Vomiting

This is due to interference to the reflex centre of vomiting in the medulla.

Papilloedema

The raised pressure of cerebrospinal fluid within the subarachnoid space is communicated to fluid within the optic nerve. As a result there is interference to the venous return and the optic disc swells and retinal veins distend.

Investigations

Plain skull X-rays

These may be helpful because a tumour may cause bone erosion. In a few instances a meningioma may invade the bone causing *hyperostosis*.

Spine and chest X-rays

These may demonstrate erosion of bone and may show a primary lesion such as a bronchogenic carcinoma (Ch. 6, p. 237).

Computerized axial tomography (CAT) or Electro medical industry (EMI) Scan

This is a non-invasive X-ray procedure which allows the densities of a transverse slice of the brain to be seen by producing an image at any given level. Any abnormality such as a tumour can therefore be detected. The scanner (Fig. 3.37) employs conventional X-rays but instead of using a film a computer reproduces a picture. While no specific preparation is necessary for this procedure, it is important that the patient remains still during the scan which takes about four minutes. It therefore may be necessary for a sedative or a general anaesthetic to be given. Occasionally the radiologist may inject intravenously an iodine contrast medium to enable some tumours to be more readily demonstrated.

Angiography

This may occasionally be undertaken to demonstrate the abnormal blood supply in tumours. Space occupying lesions may show displacement of the blood vessels (pp. 86–87).

Radio-isotope scanning

This procedure may be used in centres where computerized axial tomography is not available. A radioactive isotope is given intravenously, usually technetium (Tc^{99m}) pertechnetate. Any disturbance within the blood brain barrier allows this radio-

Figure 3.37
EMI scanner

Figure 3.38
Two different scans showing
(A) an infarct
(B) a tumour.

nuclide to pass through and accumulate in the oedema around the space occupying lesion. The patient preparation is minimal. An oral dose of 200 mg of sodium or potassium perchlorate is given 1–2 hours prior to intravenous injection. This drug stops the uptake of the isotope in the thyroid gland and empties the choroid plexus which would also accumulate the isotope. The examination is performed about 60–90 minutes after the injection of the isotope. The head is scanned using a rectilinear scan which detects the gamma rays emitted by the isotope. This can record the concentration of the isotope as dots on paper or a polaroid film. A gamma camera may also be used.

Cranial nerve examination

Examination of the cranial nerves may demonstrate abnormalities. Tumours involving the optic nerve pathway may produce a visual field defect. Hearing tests may be given to test the cochlear component of the acoustic nerve. The vestibular component is tested by irrigating the auditory canal with ice cold water. If there is no nystagmus or nausea, the vestibular function is impaired

Treatment and nursing care

Surgical excision of the tumour is the main aim although this is not always possible without causing disastrous neurological deficits; there is no justification for complete removal at the expense of disabling the patient totally. Biopsy of the lesion may be undertaken for histological report only. If the lesion is contained within a lobe of the brain, it may be possible to perform a lobectomy without further damage to functional areas. A subtotal removal of the tumour will reduce the size of the lesion and thus relieve the intracranial pressure for a time. Cystic tumours if accessible can be drained and completely removed. If *craniotomy* has been performed, routine postoperative care is given (p. 99). The patient will be nursed as any unconscious patient until fully recovered from the anaesthetic (p. 93). The nurse should in addition pay particular attention to neurological assessments (p. 90) and record her observations half hourly for 24 hours at least. Many tumours are highly vascular and therefore some bleeding may occur postoperatively causing an extradural or subdural haematoma (p. 89). Serial observations lead to the detection of this complication and allow measures to be taken to obviate their dangerous effects. As far as his condition allows the patient may be mobilized around the second postoperative day and encouraged to carry out everyday tasks for himself.

Posterior fossa operations may be performed to excise cerebellar tumours, or acoustic neuromata. In general the postoperative care is the same as that following craniotomy. In addition because of the possibility of swelling around the brain stem the respirations should be recorded quarter hourly and any fall below ten breaths per minute should be reported to the medical officer.

Management of cranial nerve palsies

Cranial nerve palsies may be present preoperatively or may occur as a result of posterior fossa exploration in an attempt to remove the tumour. The fifth, seventh, eighth, ninth and tenth cranial nerves are the ones usually involved (Table 3.1, p. 83).

One or more nerves may be affected.

Trigeminal nerve (fifth) dysfunction will cause sensory loss to one side of the face and eye. This anaesthetic eye is now much more liable to injury and it is necessary therefore for the nurse to protect it. Initially postoperatively a protective celluloid eye shield may be placed over it. Condensation occurring inside the shield will keep the eye moist and should only be removed to renew the dressing around the shield. If eye care is required, great care is taken to keep the eye tightly closed so that the cotton wool does not separate the eyelids and come in contact with the insensitive cornea. If the patient cannot feel dust he will not blink and therefore tears will not be produced to wash away any foreign substances. Protection must also be given to the patient prior to discharge. This may take the form of wing pieces fitted to plain glass spectacles or to the patient's own spectacles. These must be worn on all occasions when out-of-doors and in all circumstances where dust may go into the eye. The patient should be taught how to inspect and clean his eye, and to report to the doctor, should inflammation occur.

The *facial nerve* (*seventh*) may also be damaged. The motor component supplies the muscles of the face. Incomplete eyelid closure if combined with fifth nerve paralysis may further complicate the care of the anaesthetic eye. A tarsorrhaphy (p. 470) may be performed as a temporary or permanent measure. Here the outer margins of the upper and lower eyelids are sutured together. The tarsorrhaphy suture line is kept clean of discharge and crusts using sterile cotton wool balls soaked in normal saline, swabbing from the inner canthus out. Sutures are removed around the 14th day.

Damage to the ninth and tenth nerves, the *glossopharyngeal* and the *vagus* may cause swallowing difficulties. Instructions may be given that no oral fluids be given until the nerves are tested and proved to be functioning normally. Nurses may observe that the patient has difficulty in swallowing his own saliva and therefore requires gentle suction to alleviate his distress. A facial nerve palsy resulting in drooping of the angle of the mouth, combined with ninth and tenth damage will add to the patient's troubles. If swallowing is a problem, feeds will have to be given by other routes, for instance via a nasogastric tube (pp. 95–97) or by jejunostomy (Ch. 5). These cranial nerve palsies may not be present at the time of operation and indeed may only occur as the lesion enlarges. The nursing care of patients with space occupying lesion will depend very much on the symptoms occurring at that time.

Treatment of hydrocephalus

Hydrocephalus may occur at any time due to blockage of the cerebrospinal pathways by tumour invasion or by pressure and can be relieved by the insertion of a ventriculoperitoneal or atrial shunt (p. 135). Routine postoperative care should be instituted. Transient adynamic ileus may occasionally be a complication of peritoneal placement of tubing and the nurse should be aware of the clinical features of this. (Ch. 5, p. 215).

Radiotherapy is often combined with surgical treatment. This regimen will be started after the sutures are removed and the wound is well healed, and may continue over a period of 4 to 6 weeks. Life expectancy following radiotherapy may be increased from months to years depending on the grade of the tumour. Since a medulloblastoma metastasizes into the cerebrospinal fluid the spinal cord may also be irradiated as well as the cerebellum and fourth ventricle.

Patients undergoing radiotherapy are often extremely tired and may feel worse during the weeks of treatment. Bone marrow is irradiated therefore the patient's white blood cell and platelet counts fall, sometimes dramatically, requiring temporary cessation of treatment. This low count makes the patient very susceptible to minor infections and clotting defects. Nausea and vomiting may accompany radiotherapy. Patients should be encouraged to eat and drink small appetizing meals and plenty of high calorie drinks should be provided; anti-emetics may be administered prior to food. If the salivary gland is in the field of radiation production of saliva may be diminished and loss of taste may occur. Citrus sweets can be given to stimulate production and help maintain a moist mouth. When the spine is also irradiated, constipation may result and routine mild laxatives may overcome this. Patients should be made aware of the possibility of epilation and to avoid some of the embarrassment the patient and relatives are encouraged to choose a wig prior to surgery.

Skin reactions and care

Some redness and flaking of the skin, similar to sunburn, may develop but application of creams is not encouraged except on medical instructions. Washing of the area is permissible but the patient should be careful not to rub off the radiotherapy markings. If patients are treated with fast neutron therapy, (Cyclotron) they will develop marked skin reactions which heal 4 to 6 weeks following treatment if careful skin care is given. The skin reaction progresses from erythema to dry desquamation and occasionally to moist desquamation. Crusting and pigmentation may occur on healing. Epilation may be permanent.

Dry desquamation. Keep dry and exposed to the air if possible. Do not attempt to pick off the crusts.

Moist desquamation. Use normal saline or sterile water to clean the area and apply Graneodin ointment sparingly. If possible expose to the air. If a dressing is necessary choose a non-adherent dressing with micropore strapping which should be applied outside the treatment area.

Graneodin ointment may be used where crusting is heavy or the skin itchy. The following preparations are contra-indicated:

Eusol (Edinburgh University Solution of Lime).
Zinc and castor oil ointment.
Silver nitrate.
Acriflavine.
Oily and occlusive dressings.

Patients are reviewed weekly while the reaction is minimal.

Drug therapy

Some drugs may be given at different times during the progress of the tumour. Dexamethasone for instance helps to control the oedema that surrounds the tumour thus reducing the intracranial pressure. Cytotoxic therapy may be given in an attempt to destroy the cancer cells but because of difficulty in crossing the blood brain barrier, these drugs have not proved really effective.

Continuing care

Continuous support must be given to the patient's family from the time of diagnosis and especially in the terminal stages of the patient's illness. The patient should be encouraged to go home for short periods of time and good liaison with the community services is essential for this to work well. Relatives should be made aware that they can communicate with the hospital staff for advice or a 'chat' when the patient is at home and that readmission can be easily arranged. As the patient's condition deteriorates he should be kept comfortable and free of pain. Relatives should be encouraged to visit whenever they wish and help nurse their relative if they desire to do so. This may help relieve some feelings of guilt which may be present at not looking after the patient at home. The hospital chaplain may be involved with the relatives throughout the care of the patient. Terminal care of a child is also discussed (Ch. 15, p. 619).

Epilepsy

Definition

An epileptic fit is an intermittent disorder of cerebral function often associated with disturbance of consciousness, resulting from abnormal electrical discharge of cerebral neurones. Epilepsy may be classified according to whether the electrical discharge is generalized and involves both cerebral hemispheres, or is restricted to one part of the brain only. In the former case the epilepsy is described as being of the generalized type; in the latter, of the focal or partial type.

Clinical features

1. *Generalized epilepsy*

Grand mal (tonic/clonic epilepsy). The attack may be preceded by an **aura**. This may be a vague sensation of the patient's surroundings becoming more distant, or a feeling of being generally unwell. The aura may last from a few seconds to a minute or two. The next stage is a complete and sudden loss of consciousness. If the patient is standing, he falls to the ground. At this point the **tonic stage** commences and is characterized by a sustained contraction of all muscles of the body. This may result in air being forcibly exhaled through a partially closed glottis, causing the epileptic cry. During this phase there is no effective flow of air into and out of the lungs, and the patient may become cyanosed.

Tonic contraction of the muscle of the bladder wall during this stage gives rise to the characteristic urinary incontinence observed in this type of epilepsy. Contraction of the muscles closing the jaw may cause injuries to the tongue or the inside of the mouth. After about 30 seconds, the **clonic phase** ensues. Powerful symmetrical jerking movements are observed in all limbs. Rhythmic facial movements may cause an accumulation of frothy saliva at the mouth. After a minute or so, these movements subside and the patient lies in a relaxed and sleepy state which may last anything from a few minutes to several hours.

Petit mal. The term is often applied erroneously; many adults claiming to suffer from this condition actually suffer from temporal lobe epilepsy (see below). Petit mal is almost always a condition of childhood. It is best described as an absence attack in which the child suddenly stops what he is doing, and stares blankly ahead for a few seconds. He then continues what he was doing as if nothing had happened. These attacks may pass unnoticed and patients may often be considered by their schoolteachers to be daydreaming. The condition may only come to light when scholastic performance begins to fall. Very rarely petit mal may continue into adult life, but more commonly it subsides during adolescence. Patients who have had petit mal during childhood may develop grand mal in later life. It should be noted that true petit mal is associated with a characteristic EEG abnormality.

2. *Focal or partial epilepsy*

Jacksonian epilepsy. This form of epilepsy is associated with rhythmic, jerking movements involving the limbs of one side of the body, in some cases one limb only. Movements can last up to 2 or 3 minutes, and may not be associated with any alteration of consciousness. At the onset the jerking may be very localised, but spread to become more widespread. When the movements subside the affected limbs may be weak. This phenomenon is called *Todd's paresis*. The occurrence of this type of epilepsy implies an abnormal electrical discharge in the part of the brain controlling the limbs which show abnormal movements.

Temporal lobe epilepsy. This is the commonest type of focal epilepsy. The temporal lobe is concerned with psychological functions, and epileptic discharges in this part of the brain give rise to characteristic disturbances of thought or memory. Many patients describe a feeling of 'butterflies in the stomach' at the onset of an attack. The patient may then feel nauseated and complain of an abnormal, unpleasant taste in the mouth. Consciousness may be impaired such that the patient feels detached from his surroundings but remains aware of his situation. The phenomenon of déjà vu may be mentioned. This is the sensation of reliving a previous experience in an exceptionally vivid way.

Investigations

In assessing a patient with 'funny turns' which are considered to be of a possibly epileptic origin, an eye witness account is vital. This may come from a relative or friend of the patient, but equally from a nurse who may have observed an attack in the patient who has been admitted to hospital (p. 110). This is important as it is only from a good description of an attack by a third party that a doctor may be able to arrive at a precise diagnosis. Other causes of loss of consciousness must be differentiated from epilepsy as the treatment of these conditions may be quite different. These include hyperventilation, paroxysmal cardiac dysrhythmia, syncope and hypoglycaemia. This latter may cause an attack which is clinically indistinguishable from an epileptic fit, and the opportunity should be taken of checking the blood sugar in an undiagnosed patient having an attack of loss of consciousness in the ward or casualty department. It is also possible that the nurse's observations may lead the doctor to suspect that the attack may not have had an organic basis (that is hysterical).

In general the diagnosis will have been made on the basis of the patient's history in addition to an eye witness account of an episode. Further investigation is aimed at determining whether there is an identifiable cause for the epilepsy. This may, or may not, require specific treatment. The doctor will make a thorough physical examination. The desirability of estimating the blood sugar level during an attack has been mentioned.

A skull X-ray may show an area of calcification within the brain raising the possibility of the presence of an underlying structural lesion which may be the cause of epilepsy.

The electroencephalogram (EEG) is widely used in the management of epilepsy. This is a record of the electrical activity of the brain obtained from an array of recording electrodes placed on the scalp. It is important to realise that the EEG does not show abnormalities which are diagnostic of epilepsy except in the special case of petit mal already mentioned. A clinical diagnosis of epilepsy may be made despite a normal EEG. Sometimes abnormalities are seen in the EEG between attacks. If these are focal in origin a structural lesion is more likely and further investigation may be required.

In recent years the investigation of patients with epilepsy has been revolutionized by the development of the CAT scan (p. 86). This is becoming widely used in the investigation of epileptic patients; it may demonstrate a focal structural lesion in the cerebral hemisphere which could cause epilepsy. The likelihood of there being such a lesion is increased if the attacks have focal features. In children it may be the result of a birth injury. In young adults and in middle age, an underlying tumour may be found. This may be a primary tumour of the brain but more commonly it is a metastasis, for example, of bronchial carcinoma. Meningiomas may present with focal or generalised epilepsy. These are benign lesions which can be successfully removed surgically. Such patients should be identified as early as possible. As the patient becomes older, there is a higher incidence of cerebrovascular disease and the lesions may result in epilepsy. No such cause may be found for most patients suffering from epilepsy even after extensive investigation.

Management during a grand mal attack

The immediate nursing care necessary will be determined by the actual number of phases of the seizure through which the patient passes.

1. **The aura.** The patient should be laid on the floor. Dentures should be removed and a rolled handkerchief placed between the gums. As the aura may not occur or may be of short duration, it may not be possible to carry out all the treatment recommended. Under no circumstances should any attempt be made to force the mouth open to insert a gag once the tonic phase has commenced. Due to contraction of muscles any such attempt can result in damage to the jaw muscles, fracture of the lower mandible or damage to teeth.

2. **The tonic phase.** The patient should be moved from any immediate danger such as an open fire or articles of furniture. Tight clothing at neck, chest or waist should be loosened and shoes removed.

3. **The clonic phase.** The convulsive movements of the limbs should not be restrained. Ideally the nurse should guide the movements of limbs thus reducing the risk of injury by sudden contact with a hard object.

4. **The postepileptic coma.** The patient can now be transferred to his bed. Maintenance of a clear airway is the prime duty of the nurse, and correct positioning of the patient is essential. Removal of excessive secretions from the mouth and pharynx should be carried out. If contamination of the skin by urine or faeces has occurred, soiled clothing must be removed and the skin cleansed.

5. Reassurance should be given during the transient period of disorientation.

Nursing observations during an epileptic fit

Apart from providing the immediate necessary treatment, the nurse can be of inestimable value to the doctor in reaching a diagnosis if she has made certain observations during a seizure.

Most units dealing with patients suffering from epilepsy have a printed sheet of appropriate questions which the nurse should answer. It is essential that the nurse completes this form at the earliest opportunity as she may find it difficult to remember specific details later. She should not, however, attempt to fill in any part of the questionnaire during the seizure as her full attention must be given to the nursing care of her patient.

The following is a typical list of questions:

What was the time of the attack?
What was the frequency in relation to previous attacks
What activity was the patient engaged in prior to the attack?
Did he appear calm or upset?
Did he experience an aura? If so, what form did the hallucination take?
Did he emit a cry?
Did he fall?
Did he appear to lose consciousness? If so, how long did it last?
Was there a phase of muscle rigidity?
Was there a phase of muscle convulsions?
If convulsions occurred where did they start?
Did they spread to any other areas of the body?
Was he incontinent?
Was there any change in skin colour?
Was there evidence of bloodstained saliva?
In the case of the female patient is there a relationship between the onset of a seizure and the onset of menstruation?
What was the patient's pattern of behaviour following recovery?

Long-term management of epilepsy

1. General aspects

It is important that epileptic patients lead as normal a life as possible. There are inevitably some constraints, and it is unwise for patients with epilepsy to indulge in any form of climbing as severe injury may result should the patient have a fit while engaged in this pursuit. Epileptics should not swim unless they are under the observation of someone who is able to rescue them should they have an attack while in the water.

It should be remembered that patients with epilepsy are debarred by law from holding a driving licence unless they can show that they have been free of fits by day over a 2-year period. A heavy goods vehicle licence cannot be held by anyone who has had an epileptic fit after the age of 3 years. The regulations for drivers of public service vehicles are even more stringent. If at first sight these restrictions seem harsh, it is only necessary to consider the dangers to other road users of a person having an epileptic fit while driving a car or heavy goods vehicle. Patients with epilepsy should be discouraged from excessive consumption of alcohol. This makes the patient more likely to have a fit and may make drug treatment less effective.

2. Drug treatment

In general patients who have had more than one fit are started on treatment aimed at preventing further attacks. Anticonvulsant treatment has become less likely to cause troublesome side effects in recent years. The treatment recommended depends on the type of epilepsy, but it is important that the patient takes the recommended dose regularly in order to obtain the maximum benefit from treatment. The first drug which is usually used in patients with grand mal epilepsy is phenytoin (Epanutin). This can be given as a single daily dose, and is often most satisfactorily taken before retiring to bed at night. Phenobarbitone, primidone (Mysoline) and sodium valproate (Epilim) may also be used in this type of epilepsy. Petit mal is most successfully treated with ethosuximide (Zarontin). In recent years sodium valproate has also been found to be effective in this type of epilepsy. Focal or partial epilepsy is often most successfully treated with carbamazepine (Tegretol), but phenytoin is also effective in this type of epilepsy, and may be more effective than carbamazepine in post-traumatic epilepsy.

Status epilepticus

Status epilepticus is defined as the occurrence of two or more epileptic fits without the patient regaining consciousness between the attacks. This is a medical emergency, and is potentially life-threatening. The patient is likely to become hypoxic, and this may cause cerebral oedema. This makes it even more difficult to bring the epilepsy under control. It is therefore important that the condition is treated as soon as possible. Intravenous treatment is required, and is usually commenced with a bolus injection of a drug such as clonazepam (Rivotril) or diazepam (Valium). It is usually necessary to continue treatment with an intravenous infusion of one of these drugs. Sometimes an infusion of chlormethiazole (Heminevrin) or thiopentone sodium (Pentothal) is used as an alternative. It is sometimes necessary to give these drugs in such a dose as to cause respiratory depression and patients may, on occasion, require to be artificially ventilated.

Cerebrovascular accident

The main blood flow to the brain is from two internal carotid arteries and two vertebral arteries (Fig. 3.39). The vertebral arteries converge around the pons varolii to form the basilar artery, which in turn gives off the two posterior cerebral arteries. The internal carotids also give off branches, the two anterior cerebral arteries, joined together by the anterior communicating artery. The middle cerebral artery also leaves from the internal carotid. The posterior cerebral arteries communicate with the internal carotids through the posterior communicating arteries. This arrangement is in the form of a circle called the circle of Willis (Fig. 3.40). Normally, blood within the circle does not mix, that is basilar blood does not mix with blood from the internal carotids, but in disease a good cross circulation may develop and be all important for brain function.

Aetiology. Three main lesions, excluding trauma, may alter the blood supply within the brain. All are vascular in origin damaging nervous tissue by oxygen depletion. Cerebrovascular accident (stroke) is the term given to this damage.

1. Common carotid artery
2. Internal carotid artery
3. Anterior cerebral artery
4. Middle cerebral artery
5. Posterior communicating artery
6. Vertebral artery
7. Basilar artery
8. Posterior cerebral artery

Figure 3.39
Arterial blood supply to brain: lateral view

Internal carotid artery

Anterior cerebral artery

Anterior communicating artery

Posterior communicating artery

Middle cerebral artery

Posterior cerebral artery

Basilar artery

Anterior spinal artery

Vertebral artery

Figure 3.40
Circle of Willis: basal view

1. Cerebral thrombosis

Here atheromatous changes associated with arteriosclerosis occur within the cerebral circulation (Ch. 7) eventually causing complete blockage of the vessel lumen. This depletes the oxygen supply to the part of the brain supplied by the diseased vessel. Death of tissue, or infarction, may occur. The clinical features vary depending on:

1. The site of infarction.
2. The extent of vessel blockage.

Cerebrovascular accident from thrombosis is most commonly a disease of the elderly. Gradual occlusion causes a progressive deterioration in the patient's condition. Signs and symptoms occur and diminish with no lasting effect, but recur at intervals. Eventually, when the blockage becomes complete, deficits become permanent. Occlusion may affect any of the vessels of the circle of Willis, but most commonly the internal carotid and middle cerebral arteries. These supply the motor and sensory areas and internal capsule within the temporal and frontal lobes. The presenting feature is usually a hemiplegia. If the dominant hemisphere is affected (containing the speech centre), the patient may also have speech problems, such as expressive dysphasia.

2. Embolism

An embolus may also block cerebral blood vessels. In this case blocking occurs suddenly, the embolus having broken off, say, from vegetations around diseased heart valves such as those which occur in subacute bacterial endocarditis. Occasionally a thrombus may give off multiple emboli.

3. Haemorrhage

Primary intracerebral haemorrhage associated with arteriosclerosis and hypertension is almost always fatal. Patients are usually deeply comatose on admission. Subarachnoid haemorrhage may be due to an aneurysm or an arteriovenous malformation. There is spontaneous rupture of the aneurysm (weakness in the wall of an artery) into the subarachnoid space. Aneurysms tend to occur at the bifurcation of vessels within the circle of Willis. All age groups are affected. Rupture occurs suddenly and often at rest. There is intense headache, vomiting, photophobia and neck stiffness. There may be loss of consciousness and paralysis depending on the affected area. Untreated aneurysms may rebleed within 14 days causing further damage.

Recently it has been found that the use of an antifibrinolytic agent can decrease the risk of rebleeding. This is given initially intravenously and then orally preventing fibrinolysis of the thrombus in and around the aneurysm. This drug therapy is maintained until the time of surgery. The use of this drug allows a longer period of time to be spent on investigations and assessment prior to surgery.

In all three types if loss of consciousness extends over 48 hours the prognosis is poor. Care of the unconscious patient has already been given (pp. 93–99).

Investigations

Echoencephalography, lumbar puncture and angiography are performed. Scan, using radioactive isotopes, is injected into the venous circulation. As the isotopes break down they give off radiation which can be detected and measured. Brain tumours have a higher uptake of radioactive material. Occasionally tumours bleed giving features similar to cerebral thrombosis. Scanning is one means of investigating this problem.

Treatment and nursing care

If possible aneurysms are treated surgically by application of a clip to the aneurysm neck and/or wrapping the aneurysm with muslin.

The usual postoperative care is given. However, the patient requires constant care for at least 24 hours with temperature, pulse, respiration and blood pressure assessments being performed every 30 minutes, as well as assessment of conscious level. Any deterioration in conscious level, limb movements or pupillary reaction should be reported and, if necessary, specific treatment given. Deterioration may indicate:

1. **Cerebral vessel spasm.** A mild hemiparesis may become severe. Intravenous dextran 40, 500 ml daily, may improve this situation. Dextran is of low molecular weight which helps reduce erythrocyte 'sludging' when cerebral blood flow is slow.

2. **Oedema of cerebral tissue.** The aim of treatment is to reduce the water content of the brain. A solution with a high osmotic pressure given intravenously

will attract fluid to itself from the tissues, including brain tissue. As the blood volume increases a diuresis is inevitable. Such a solution is mannitol which, when given quickly, is very effective.

Steroids such as dexamethazone may also be given for their anti-inflammatory properties, thus restricting the development of oedema. Dexamethazone acts slowly and may therefore be combined with mannitol.

3. **Haematoma formation**. Pressure from the clot may alter conscious level. Surgical intervention may be required to evacuate it.

The rehabilitative treatment for hemiplegia is identical irrespective of the cause.

Nursing a patient with hemiplegia

The aim of rehabilitating a patient with hemiplegia is to restore a state of optimum effectiveness for that individual. Treatment is a team effort which requires contributions from physiotherapists, occupational and speech therapists, medical and nursing staff and the patient's family, who should be helped to understand the patient's problems and capabilities.

In the acute phase, care on admission may be directed to altered consciousness when the neurological and physical assessments of the patient's needs should be evaluated and appropriate care given. Rehabilitative care however can be aided even at this early stage if nursing support is directed at problems that exist or may develop. These are the onset of spasticity and loss of muscle tone as well as the possibility of sensory/perceptual problems.

Development of spasticity/loss of tone

Interruption of cortical influence at the time of injury, results in diminution of the activity to the anterior horn cell and therefore hypotonus develops in the affected side causing a flaccid paralysis. After a period of time reflex activity does recover to the extent of hypertonicity. Normal muscle tone is greater in the antigravity muscles and following a cerebrovascular accident the stronger muscles oppose the weaker muscles thus causing spasticity to develop and therefore possible contractures. The two main muscle groups affected are the shoulder and hip muscles. Spasticity developing in these causes adduction of the shoulder with forward flexion and extension of the leg, with backward rotation of the pelvis. From the acute stage the hemiplegic limbs should be carefully positioned in positions to oppose the developing spasticity (Fig. 3.41). An alternative to the lateral and supine positions is the upright position which may be used as the patient progresses (Fig. 3.42).

Figure 3.41A & B
Lying on affected side (shaded area)
1. The head is slightly forward, supported on a flat pillow with the trunk straight and in line with the neck.
2. The affected shoulder is brought forward with the palm of the hand upwards.
3. The underneath leg is straight from the hip and flexed slightly at the knee.
4. The uppermost leg is placed on one pillow.
5. A pillow is placed at the back for support.
6. Nothing should be placed in the hand or against the sole of the foot.

Figure 3.41C & D
Lying in the supine position
This position should be avoided
if possible as it encourages
increased abnormal tone.
1. The head is turned towards
   the affected side.
2. The shoulder is brought
   forward on a pillow with the
   arm raised above the head or
   supported at the side.
3. To prevent external rotation
   of the leg a pillow is placed
   lengthways under the pelvis
   and outer aspect of the thigh.
4. Nothing should be placed in
   the hand or against the sole
   of the foot.

Figure 3.42A & B
Sitting up in bed
1. When the patient is nursed in
   the upright position, the head
   and neck must be well
   supported by pillows.
2. The shoulder is brought
   forward using pillows and the
   arm slightly abducted and
   resting on pillows.
3. The pelvis may be raised
   slightly by placing a pillow
   lengthways under the hip and
   outer aspect of the thigh.
   Legs are straight.

Passive limb exercises should also be performed by nursing staff at frequent intervals (p. 47). Any excessive stimulation such as a pillow at the foot or a foam roll in the hand will increase spasm and should therefore be discouraged.

Without normal muscle tone, postural control is also lost so that the patient is unable to maintain equilibrium. Re-education of postural reflex mechanism, which normally develops from birth can begin whilst the patient is confined to bed. This involves encouraging the patient to roll from side to side, to 'bridge' the trunk, that is to lift the trunk from the bed, and gradually to support himself on his affected side and to maintain his balance sitting on the edge of the bed. Once this trunk control has been achieved in bed, the natural progression is to teach the patient to transfer from bed to chair and to sit correctly (Fig. 3.43).

Before walking can commence the patient must be taught to gain equilibrium in the standing position. This can be achieved by the patient observing himself in a mirror, standing in a standing frame and progressing to parallel bars. At this stage the physiotherapist can determine if any leg brace or walking aid will be required, and only when the patient is ready will walking practice start. Although training is individualized most patients require assistance and support on the affected side. Repeated practice is necessary in many patients and may take some time to perfect.

Loss of sensory/perceptual ability

This may become more of a barrier to rehabilitation than loss of motor power. There are various categories:

a. Distortion of body image may occur so that the patient may neglect the paralysed side or completely deny that the paralysed side belongs to him.

Figure 3.43A–E
Transfer from bed to chair
The nurse should:
1. Place chair parallel to head of bed on the patient's affected side (A).
2. Roll patient on to affected side (A).
3. Place one arm under affected shoulder resting her hand over the shoulder blade, the other arm is placed around the patient's legs. The patient is then brought into a sitting position by swinging legs over the side of the bed (B, C).

4. Encourage the patient to rock or wriggle to edge of bed.
5. Check patient's feet are flat on floor.
6. Stand in front of the patient and place her arms under patient's shoulders, resting her hands over scapulae. The patient should not grip hands behind nurse's neck to avoid injury (D).
7. Bend knees and keeping back straight, wedge patient's feet and knees with her own (D).
8. Lean slightly backwards, keeping patient's shoulders forwards, thus counter-balancing patient's weight, to bring the patient into the standing position (D).
9. Pivot patient around and lower into chair (E).

Figure 3.43F, G
Sitting in a chair
1. The chair should give adequate support to thighs and shoulders. It should allow the patient to sit well back to maintain the hips, knees and ankles at right angles. This position allows the body weight to be evenly distributed over both buttocks.
2. The head and neck are in line with the trunk and the affected shoulder is brought forward slightly and supported on a pillow on a table.

b. Spatial problems. Normally one relates or is aware of oneself in the surrounding environment. The patient with a spatial disorder as well as disregarding his affected side, neglects one half of his environment. When asked to draw a clock or house, he will draw the side with his unaffected field of vision. When eating, he will leave food on his affected side.

These two problems are common in right hemiplegic damage.

c. Occasionally the patient may fail to appreciate size, weight, shape and texture of articles, so that he does not recognize objects placed in his hand. He may also be unable to recognize known sounds or familiar sights.

d. Another form of sensory impairment is apraxia, where there is inability to execute a learned movement when no muscle weakness exists and the command is understood. For example, when a comb is placed in the patient's hand and direction given to 'comb your hair' this well known movement cannot be performed.

Closely related sensory perceptual problems are visual field defects due to interruption to the fibres of the optic nerve travelling to the occipital lobe in and around the tempero-parietal area (Ch. 12). This damage produces a visual loss in the fields opposite the lesion and is called a homonymous hemianopia (Fig. 3.44). Patients with right hemisphere damage have loss of vision in the left half of both eyes. This in combination with neglect and spatial disorientation can add to the rehabilitation problems. Patients should be encouraged therefore to look, or have their head turned, towards the affected side.

When sensory perceptual impairment exists the patient must constantly be made aware of the affected side and be positioned so that maximum sensory input occurs from the affected side. The patient should know where his limbs are positioned and they should be within his field of vision. Tactile sensation can be increased on the affected side by touching or stroking. References to right and left should be avoided, rather stimulate the affected side and give directions such as 'place your weak arm into the sleeve'. The nurse should approach the patient from the affected side and the bedtable should be placed on that side.

Language function may also be damaged or impaired; the speech centres and their connections are situated in the dominant hemisphere of the brain, normally the left side but occasionally the right in some left-handed people. The patient's inability to communicate but not necessarily to think rationally is affected. His speech may be unintelligible and it may be difficult for an inexperienced person to realise that intelligence is not affected. The speech disorder may be a difficulty in understanding the spoken word, called receptive dysphasia or being able to understand the spoken word but being unable to express oneself in answering, called expressive dysphasia.

Figure 3.44
Homonymous hemianopia

THE NERVOUS SYSTEM   117

Occasionally the speech disorder may involve a combination of both. A code for certain expressions, like 'yes' and 'no' should be established as early as possible to reduce the very great frustration the patient will feel because of his inability to communicate normally. It would be additionally demoralising for a person so affected to be treated as other than an intelligent adult. Sympathetic staff, relatives and the speech therapist all have a part to play in encouraging recovery of speech function (p. 655).

General aspects of care

Occupational therapy should also start early to avoid the patient becoming overdependent on nursing staff. While still confined to bed the patient should be encouraged to wash and feed himself and be provided with aids designed for the task, such as special cutlery and non-slip mats for crockery and basins.

Depression is common after cerebrovascular accident and positive reinforcement will improve the patient's morale when aids are used successfully, although much encouragement and practice is required.

As the patient progresses, ordinary daily activities like dressing will be taught and practised. Success here and the gradual return of independence help the patient to look to the future with optimism. When he is able, the patient will go to the occupational therapy department and be taught common necessary activities such as simple cooking, washing, ironing, getting in and out of the bath and so on. Tasks such as woodwork or knitting may be given to strengthen weak muscles. The speech therapist also works closely with the occupational therapist in the relearning of motor skills and relearning to write.

Prior to discharge, the occupational therapist, physiotherapist and medical social worker pay a home visit to assess if help is needed and what alterations are required, such as putting up handrails, removing loose carpets, and arranging for 'meals on wheels'. Even after discharge, treatment continues. The patient may attend a medical rehabilitation centre. Previous skills and interests may be utilized here if the patient must change his occupation.

Disorders of cranial nerves

While the cranial nerves may be involved in diseases associated with other structures, there are disorders specific to certain cranial nerves, and only those will be described (see Table 3.1 for cranial nerves and their functions).

Trigeminal neuralgia (5th cranial nerve)

The cause of this condition is not known. It usually occurs in middle and late life and is more common in women. The main symptom is an acute episode of severe pain which commences at a specific point of the face and then radiates through the affected area. The distribution of pain will depend on the division of the trigeminal nerve affected. Most frequently pain is localized initially to the second (maxillary) division but will in time spread to the first (ophthalmic) and third (mandibular) divisions. The pain is almost always confined to one side of the face. Although each acute episode may only last for seconds, the pain will persist for days or weeks and will increase in intensity. Attacks may be precipitated by food or fluids at extremes of temperature, exposure of face to cold wind, or touching a particular point of face, gums or teeth (trigger points).

Treatment and nursing care

During acute phases the aim of treatment is relief of pain by administration of drugs. A drug which is proving particularly beneficial is carbamazepine (Tegretol).

Sedatives may be ordered to ensure adequate sleep.

Relief from pain can also be achieved by the injection of alcohol into the affected division of the trigeminal nerve. The relief from pain may last for several months and treatment can be repeated.

However the only permanent cure lies in cutting the sensory root of the trigeminal nerve. Unless the three divisions are involved, a partial section is performed thus sparing divisions unaffected. As the after effects of this surgery are permanent, i.e. sensation of stiffness and numbness of affected area, it is recommended that surgery should always be preceded by an injection of alcohol. In this way the patient can be acclimatized to the permanent sequelae.

Prior to surgery, the patient should be mobile unless this is contra-indicated. Exposure to draughts or inclement weather should be avoided. As chewing may trigger off an attack of pain, food should consist of semisolids and fluids given at room temperature. If pain still occurs a nasogastric infusion of nutrients may be commenced. The tube should be passed via the nostril on the unaffected side of the face. As any form of pressure can trigger off an acute episode of pain, the patient may neglect to wash his face, shave or brush his teeth. The nurse must encourage the patient to perform these daily activities in spite of possible resulting discomfort. The face cloth should be of a soft material and water for washing or mouth rinsing should be lukewarm.

If the patient is a woman, it is of particular importance that the minimal amount of hair is shaved from her head. Remaining hair should be secured in an attractive style away from the site of operation. This attention may help to maintain morale.

The immediate preoperative care is as for any operation requiring a general anaesthetic. The operation for trigeminal root section is performed using an extra-dural approach and is a relatively safe procedure. Immediate postoperative care is as for any operation under a general anaesthetic. Specific observations should be made for any sign of facial weakness when the patient closes his eye or smiles, for evidence of facial oedema or the appearance of sordes. The patient is confined to bed for 24 hours following recovery from anaesthetic. When the patient realizes that eating is no longer accompanied by pain ensuring an adequate intake of nutrients ceases to be a problem. However, as there is now absence of sensation on the affected side of the mouth, the patient should be reminded to chew food on the opposite side to prevent biting the inside of the cheek. Hot food or fluid must be avoided to prevent burning of desensitized tissue. The patient must be told that he will no longer be aware of particles of food left in the mouth and a mouth rinse is essential after every meal.

If the ophthalmic division of the trigeminal nerve has been sectioned, anaesthesia of the cornea on the affected side will result following surgery. A Bullar shield will be fitted over the affected eye to protect it against entry of foreign bodies. If the patient wears spectacles, he will be visited by an optician who will fit a shield over the spectacle frame. It is vitally important that the patient is educated in the care of his eyes prior to discharge. He will be told that he will not feel particles entering the eye nor will debris be washed away by tears. He must therefore protect the eye, by wearing the special shield supplied on all occasions when out of doors and in any circumstances where debris may enter eye such as attending to a coal fire, sweeping or polishing. He must never rub the eye with fingers or handkerchief. If any discharge does develop he should use a small piece of moist cottonwool and wipe from outer surface of the lids while eye is closed. The eye should not be irrigated nor should drops or ointment be instilled. If inflammation of the eye does develop he must report at once to his doctor. His doctor will receive details of surgery performed from the surgeon and will be aware of possible complications to his patient.

Another form of treatment which may be considered is stitching the eyelids together by means of a nylon suture — tarsorrhaphy. No anaesthetic is required as the area is already insensitive. The suture is removed in approximately 14 days after which closure of the eye is usually secure.

The patient will be discharged about 7 days following surgery.

Facial paralysis — Bell's palsy (7th cranial nerve)

The cause is thought to be a viral infection. Another theory is that it is caused by a local ischaemia and oedema. The initial symptom is a feeling of discomfort behind an ear, which within hours is accompanied by a complete flaccid paralysis of the

Figure 3.45
Bell's palsy

affected side of the face. The patient is unable to close the eyelid, raise the eyebrow, smile or show his teeth and the mouth is displaced towards the unaffected side. As a result of these features the patient presents a grotesque appearance (Fig. 3.45). He experiences difficulty in swallowing food or fluid and loses sense of taste on affected side of tongue.

In the majority of cases the muscles regain their tone within 3–4 weeks and complete recovery can be anticipated in 3–4 months. However, in a minority of cases recovery may take 6–12 months and may not be complete.

Treatment and nursing care

The aim of treatment is the prevention of complications. Massage and electrical stimulation (faradism) may be used to stimulate and maintain muscle tone. Vasodilating drugs may improve circulation of blood supply to the affected area. Steroids have been prescribed to reduce oedema of the nerve. The use of a facial sling aids in preventing stretching of the weakened muscles, and by improving lip alignment, it facilitates eating (Fig. 3.46).

A malleable wire splint may be used to support the patient's mouth on the affected side. One end of the splint is hooked into the angle of the mouth and the other end is secured behind the ear. The wire is flesh coloured which reduces any embarrassment to the patient. The aim of nursing management is also towards alleviation of patient's disabilities and prevention of complications. The patient should be instructed to chew food on the unaffected side to prevent biting of cheek. Hot food or fluid must be avoided to prevent burning of insensitive area of mouth. As patient will be unaware of particles of food left in an insensitive area, a mouth rinse is essential after every meal. As difficulty on swallowing and partial loss of taste are particular features of this condition, anorexia can be prevented by ensuring that meals are small, attractively presented and of a semisolid and fluid consistency. Eye care is the same as that described in trigeminal neuralgia.

As the patient will react emotionally to his appearance, the nurse must adopt a positive attitude to a possible recovery. The patient's relatives and friends should be advised to adopt a matter of fact acceptance of his disabilities. Such steps should help to minimize adverse emotional reactions.

If recovery is not complete, the patient will be told of the possibility of anastomosis of the facial nerve with the eleventh and twelfth cranial nerves or alternatively of plastic surgery.

Ménières syndrome (8th cranial nerve). As this condition affects the acoustic nerve which is involved in both hearing and balance, it has been described in another chapter (see p. 506).

Figure 3.46
Facial sling

Multiple sclerosis

This condition is a common neurological disease disabling young adults and is a disorder of which there is considerable public awareness. There is, as yet, no known cause but it is thought that the disease has an immunological basis and that the immunological abnormality may be triggered by a virus or some other transmissable agent. It is quite possible that exposure to the agent may occur many years before the disorder causes the patient to seek advice.

The disease results in multiple areas of demyelination in the central nervous system; nerve fibres passing through the diseased area lose their myelin sheath. The lesions of the disease are restricted to the brain, spinal cord and optic nerve.

In young adults the disease tends to follow a relapsing and remitting course; in middle age a more slowly progressive form of the disease may be encountered the lesion being in the spinal cord. The patient develops a slight weakness and stiffness of the legs which becomes slowly worse as the years go by. The relapsing and remitting form of the disease is usually associated with lesions at characteristic sites in the central nervous system.

Lesions in the optic nerve (optic neuritis) give rise to episodes of blurring of vision in one eye persisting for a week or two before improving spontaneously. If the lesion is in the mid-brain the patient may complain of double-vision; again this tends to subside spontaneously.

Areas of degeneration lower in the brain stem may affect the vestibular system, and cause vertigo. The patient experiences a feeling of his surroundings going round and round and this is accompanied by nausea and vomiting. Lesions may occur in the cerebellum and make the patient unsteady when walking. Unfortunately the unsteady gait may give rise to unwarranted suspicions of alcohol intoxication. Weakness, or tingling in the legs or arms, suggest that these are areas of demyelination in the spinal cord.

The severity of disability in multiple sclerosis is extremely variable. Although the popular lay conception of a patient with multiple sclerosis is someone who is paralysed and permanently in a wheelchair, this is by no means always the case. Many people are able to continue in employment despite the disease. Indeed in many cases exacerbations are separated by many years without significant disability.

Treatment

There is, as yet, no curative treatment, although it is quite possible that in the future effective treatment may emerge. Increasing numbers of strategies are being advocated, in particular various dietary regimes including gluten free and sunflower seed oil supplements. Although some patients find these diets of help there is no objective evidence that they influence the course of the disease.

Steroid treatment has also been used in this condition. In acute exacerbations it is thought that it may bring about a more rapid improvement, but there is no evidence that the long-term outlook is improved. Long-term steroid therapy is to be discouraged as it is of no benefit and side-effects may only compound the problems of nursing a disabled patient.

Despite these rather negative considerations it is possible to help patients with multiple sclerosis, particularly those with chronic paraparesis. Painful muscle spasm may be alleviated by physiotherapy and drug treatment with anti-spastic drugs such as baclofen (Lioresal), and dantrolene sodium (Dantrium). Patients often have problems with control of their bladders and bowels. They may complain of urgency and frequency of micturition; the small contracted bladder and frequent passage of small quantities of urine predispose to urinary tract infection. It is important that these infections are promptly treated and the urgency may be relieved by drugs such as paptrin. Some patients may be incontinent of urine.

Patients with less severe paraparesis may experience difficulty in walking due to a tendency to trip over uneven pavements. This is a manifestation of foot drop and such patients may be helped by the provision of a simple polythene support splint to support the ankle.

In recent years stimulation of the spinal cord by permanently implanted electrodes has been suggested in the management of pain, spasticity and urinary incontinence for patients with multiple sclerosis.

Although there is no cure for multiple sclerosis it will be seen that it is still possible to alleviate some symptoms of the disease. Most patients find it helpful to attend a hospital clinic from time to time at which difficulties may be discussed. This is also useful for patients in the early stages of the disease or while the diagnosis is not confirmed. It may not be possible to make a firm diagnosis until some years have elapsed following the first episode. A number of self-help groups are being formed and some patients may choose to join them.

Nursing care

The aims of treatment are to assist the patient in achieving his maximum physical capacity and optimum psychological adjustment to his condition. If the patient suffers double vision (diplopia), an eye patch can be worn and his head positioned to make the best use of remaining vision. If partially sighted his ability to read can be enhanced by use of large print books, talking book or magnifying glass; the patient's name can be entered in the register for the blind or partially sighted. The handicap accompanying tremor may be reduced by the use of lead shot wrist bands and by positioning the patient's elbows between the chair and his body. A wing chair and high backed wheel chair should be provided for maximum comfort. At meal times the patient should be given his own table. A feeding cup with lid should be provided, forks should be avoided and if possible food which can be picked up with the fingers should be served. Smoking should be permitted only when a member of staff or a relative is with the patient as a cigarette may be dropped with disastrous results. If the patient has speech problems, the nurse should phrase sentences so that patient need only reply 'yes' or 'no' and should resist the temptation to complete the sentence for the patient, or to anticipate his requests. If speech is non-existent, a communication chart and, if the patient can write, a scribble pad and pencil should be provided. Physiotherapy is necessary to strengthen non-affected muscles and to ensure maximum use of those weakened by the disease. Adequate support of paralysed limbs is essential especially if paralysis is flaccid. Flat heeled shoes should be worn and aids such as calipers, tripods, Zimmer and wheel chair provided as required. The occupational therapy department will supply bath aids. The application of ice to limbs gives sufficient relief from spasms to enable limbs to be put through a full range of movements. The stimuli provoking spasm can be reduced by using a cage to relieve the weight of bed clothes, ensuring bladder and lower colon are emptied of contents and observing measures necessary to prevent any breaks in the continuity of the skin. The use of drugs such as diazepam and nitrazepam aid in reducing spasms.

The patient should be encouraged to void urine every 2 hours. Tapping over the bladder area and applying pressure over the suprapubis may help in initiating micturition. If the problem is increased, frequency of micturition the use of Paul's tubing, incontinence pads, incontinence pants and uridoms must be considered. As a last resort catheterization of the urinary bladder will be necessary if the patient's skin is becoming damaged by incontinence of urine. The patient should be encouraged to defaecate at the same time each day, preferably after breakfast. Senokot should be given on two evenings a week followed by a sodium phosphate enema; manual evacuation of faeces may be necessary. Oral fluids should be in excess of 3000 ml per day. If the sensory pathways are involved certain precautions are necessary to prevent injuries, for example the temperature of the bath water must be determined, the patient should avoid direct heat from a fire, hot water bottles should not be used. Stockings should be intact and free fitting, and protective felt boots provided. If a plastic foot-drop splint is used the area under the splint should be observed for signs of pressure. Constant visual reassurance regarding the size, shape and position of limbs and body is the only support the nurse can offer the patient who suffers the distressing symptom of altered body image. Patients who have an altered body image and a paralysis require frequent change of position when in bed.

. Prior to the patient's discharge from hospital action should be taken to ensure that his home circumstances are as ideal as possible. Patient may attend a day centre and when at home receive visits from district nurse and health visitor. The local authority social work department may be able to give assistance such as the services of a house help, meals on wheels or Aids to Daily Living (Ch. 20). His house may require alterations, perhaps to allow a wheelchair to be used, or it may be possible to arrange for ground floor accommodation. Financial help in the form of a heating allowance, mobility allowance and attendance allowance are entitlements in the United Kingdom.

The patient's family may become exhausted as a result of caring for him at home and the patient can be admitted to hospital to allow the family to have a period of rest.

The life expectancy of a person with multiple sclerosis is 15 to 20 years. Death is usually due to renal failure, bronchopneumonia or involvement of vital centres within in the brain.

Parkinson's disease

This is a common disorder of the elderly. The most widely known feature of this condition is the tremor (Fig. 3.47) which is present at rest, tending to disappear on action. It is a fairly coarse tremor involving particularly the thumb and forefinger, hence the descriptive term of 'pill rolling' (Fig. 3.48) preferred first by Dr James Parkinson, a London general practitioner, in 1817. It is not, however, the most disabling feature of the disease, as patients who are troubled by the tremor alone can often cope surprisingly well.

The most disabling feature of the disorder is hypokinesis, a difficulty in initiating movement which can be seen when watching a patient with Parkinson's disease get up out of a chair. Initiation of movement is hesitant and everyday tasks such as dressing and eating meals, become extremely slow and laborious. Drooling of saliva is a distressing feature. Swinging arms when walking and similar automatic movements disappear and the patient walks with a distinctive stooped posture and shuffling foot steps (Fig. 3.49). The face becomes immobile and expressionless. Friends and relatives may form a false impression that the patient is demented. Hand writing is commonly affected; letters become small and spidery and consequently difficult to read.

In recent years it has become apparent that Parkinson's disease is caused by a degenerative process leading to a loss of pigmented cells in the substantia nigra. These cells connect the basal ganglia with higher centres and depend on the neurotransmitter substance, dopamine, to pass impulses on to other cells. This degenerative process results in a decrease in dopamine content in the pathways involved and is an important factor in the pathogenesis of the clinical features of this disease. The fall in dopaminergic activity leads to increased activity in pathways which depend on acetylcholine as a neurotransmitter. The effects of the disease on both these pathways is of importance when considering the drugs to be used in treatment.

Treatment

Dopa preparations

The most commonly used drugs in the treatment of Parkinson's disease are those which increase the level of dopamine in the basal ganglia. Dopamine cannot be given orally as it would be broken down in the digestive tract before it could be absorbed into the blood stream. Its precursor, dopa, can, however, be given and is absorbed into the circulation, and leads to increased levels of dopamine in the basal ganglia. When this treatment was first used pure levodopa was given, but this had unwanted systemic side-effects. In recent years it has been possible to overcome these side-effects by combining the levodopa with a substance which does not enter the brain and serves to prevent the unwanted side-effects of the dopa in the body. Such combined preparations are marketed under the names Sinemet and Madopar. These drugs are well tolerated and are widely used in the treatment of patients with Parkinson's disease. They seem particularly to help the hypokinesis, but do not help the tremor to the same extent. If a patient is taking too high a dose of either levodopa or one of the combined preparations, involuntary movements or abnormal posturing of the limbs may be observed. Sometimes patients who have been on this treatment for many years develop the so called on-off phenomenon, where there are frequent and sudden changes from a severely Parkinsonian state to well controlled state throughout the day. This appears to be a complication of long-term treatment, and is often difficult to treat. Its cause is controversial at the present time.

Figure 3.47
Tremor

Figure 3.48
Pill rolling

Figure 3.49
Parkinsonism

Anticholinergic drugs

Anticholinergic drugs such as benzhexol (Artane) have been less used since the advent of the dopa preparation. They are still helpful, however, particularly for patients in whom tremor is the predominant feature. They tend to help this manifestation more than the dopa preparations, but are by contrast not as helpful as dopa for hypokinesis. Anticholinergic drugs may cause side-effects such as dryness of the mouth and exacerbation of glaucoma. Occasionally they may cause confusion and frank psychosis as a side-effect.

Other drugs

Bromocriptine is a newer drug which has effects similar to dopamine which is, of course, the missing substance in Parkinson's disease.

Although it is theoretically a very attractive drug to use in the treatment of this disorder, its use has not been as successful as might have been hoped, and its place in treatment remains controversial.

Amentadine hydrochloride (Symmetrel) was first used as an anti-viral drug. It was noted that it had no significant effect in this regard, but that it tended to help patients with Parkinson's disease. This drug has since been used in the treatment of Parkinson's disease and can be quite useful in some circumstances. Unfortunately its effect seems to last for a few months only, and it is not maintained in the long term.

Nursing care

The patient is normally admitted to hospital for 2 to 3 weeks until stabilization of drug therapy is achieved. He must be kept as active as possible and encouraged to maintain his independence. Sitting upright in bed is discouraged as the patient tends to slide down so he should be seated in a chair and supported by pillows. The nurse should ensure that he has a plentiful supply of tissues to cope with excessive salivation. The diet should be light and semisolid, and additional fluids should be given to compensate for that lost in saliva. Drugs are given in five small doses daily immediately following meals; this has been found to reduce the incidence of nausea. Regular observations must be carried out for signs indicating side effects to drug therapy. The blood pressure must be recorded four hourly with the patient in recumbent and upright positions. As delusions of persecution are a possible side effect the nurse must realize that a display of aggression towards her by the patient is outwith his control. Her reaction must be one of firm but sympathetic understanding of her patient's needs. The patient's tremor can be made less obvious if he or she is allowed to carry something for example a newspaper or a handbag. A programme of physical therapy is essential and will involve the physiotherapist, the nurse and the patient's relatives. Specific exercises have been designed to improve efficiency of muscles and prevent deformities and they will be demonstrated to the nurse and the relatives by the physiotherapist so that all parties will play a role in the rehabilitation programme. In particular, the patient must be encouraged to perform again and again any motor activity that he finds especially difficult. The use of zips rather than buttons will make dressing or undressing that much easier. Walking aids are of little value, but the trolley type of Zimmer is helpful in some cases. The patient and his family must be informed of the nature of illness in order that they are best prepared to participate in the programme of treatments.

Surgical treatment. Before dopa preparations became available, surgical treatment of Parkinson's disease was widely used. This involved stereotacxic surgery in which a lesion was made in the ventrolateral nucleus of the thalamus by means of a probe passed into that structure. Such treatment is only very rarely necessary now, and is only used in special centres with experience of the technique.

Drug-induced Parkinson's disease

It should be noted that treatment with certain psychotrophic drugs can produce a syndrome very similar to Parkinson's disease as a side-effect. These tend to be drugs of the phenothiazine group such as chlorpromazine (Largactil) and thioridazine (Melleril) and butyrophenones such as haloperidol (Serenace). These drugs tend to be used to treat patients suffering from psychosis such as hypomania and schizophrenia. It may be necessary to continue treatment of the psychiatric disorder with these drugs despite the appearance of drug induced Parkinsonism. In the circumstances the Parkinsonian features are best treated with one of the anticholinergic drugs.

Peripheral neuropathy

Motor and sensory fibres may be involved in this diffuse disorder of the peripheral nerves. The first symptoms usually appear at the extremities of the limbs. Involvement of the sensory fibres causes a sensation of tingling in the toes and feet followed by similar sensory disturbances in the fingers and hands. Involvement of motor fibres in the leg leads to foot drop with consequential difficulty in walking because of a tendency to trip over uneven objects. Involvement of the motor fibres in the arm gives rise to difficulty in the use of the hand for fine tasks such as sewing and knitting. Many cases of peripheral neuropathy are chronic, but not disabling. On occasion, however, chronic peripheral neuropathy can cause severe disability and patients may be admitted to investigate the possibility of underlying causes such as diabetes, autoimmune disorders, and latent carcinoma. A proportion of cases of peripheral neuropathy have an hereditary basis and a number of commonly used drugs may cause this disorder as a side-effect.

In some cases neuropathy is an acute illness often following a virus infection. In this instance a patient may experience a rapidly progressive weakness of all limbs starting in the feet and ascending, sometimes over a period of only a few hours, to the extent that paralysis of the intercostal muscles may occur; this obviously results in respiratory failure and artificial ventilation of such patients is necessary. This condition is known as the Guillain-Barré syndrome, and there is no known medical treatment. All the resources of modern intensive care are required to care for the patient while he is tetraplegic and dependent on the ventilator.

This is an example of a condition in which standards of nursing care are a particularly important determinant of a successful outcome. Few disorders offer such a challenge to the nurse in the management of a severely disabled patient, unable to do anything for himself, dependent on the ventilator, but at the same time retaining full awareness of his surroundings and able to hear and understand what is going on around him.

The physiotherapist has a particularly important role during this period both with regard to the respiratory management and execution of passive movements of the arms and legs to prevent the development of contractures. The nurse must know the exercises carried out by the physiotherapist to ensure continuity of care is maintained. The use of corticosteroids has previously been advocated in this condition to speed up the recovery process. It is now thought that these drugs do not have any beneficial effect, and may be harmful.

Motor neurone disease

This condition may, on occasions, mimic a peripheral neuropathy involving the motor system. It is, however, a degenerative disorder in which there is selective loss of the nerve cells of the motor system resulting in progressive weakness and wasting of all limbs. It is virtually always fatal. The average duration of the illness from the first symptoms is about 3 years. The terminal stages are usually characterized by bulbar palsy in which there is involvement of the muscles controlling swallowing. This leads to more difficulty in swallowing (dysphagia) and the patient becomes even more thin and wasted from the resulting poor nutritional state. He is eventually unable to swallow his own saliva which tends to drool from the sides of the mouth. The speech becomes slurred and indistinct and attempts to swallow food and drink often result in aspiration. Aspiration pneumonia, the most common immediate cause of death in such patients is the consequence of dysphagia.

Despite extensive research, there is little clue as to the cause of this unfortunate disease, and regrettably there is no effective treatment. The only help which can be offered to unfortunate sufferers is support and any symptomatic treatment which it may be possible to offer.

Myasthenia gravis

This is an uncommon disorder, but it is important because it often affects young people and effective treatment is available. It most commonly involves women in the third decade of life, but can occur in either sex at any age. It is a disorder of the neuromuscular junction and the symptoms and signs vary from time to time within a day. The various manifestations characteristically become worse as the day progresses. The ocular muscles are commonly involved giving rise to a drooping of the eye lid (ptosis) and/or double vision (diplopia) (p. 477). Involvement of the muscles controlling the tongue and swallowing mechanisms cause slurring of speech (dysarthria) and difficulty in swallowing (dysphagia). These features may become more apparent as the patient continues to talk, or as a meal progresses. Loss of muscle power accompanying the onset of fatigue may occur in muscles of the shoulder girdle or hip joint. Involvement of the respiratory muscle is sometimes seen and this is potentially fatal; artificial ventilation may be required.

Treatment

Although anticholinesterase drugs such as neostigmine (Prostigmin) and pyridostigmine bromide (Mestinon) may give some symptomatic relief they have no effect on the underlying disease process, which is an autoimmune response against the neuromuscular junction. This disturbance of immunity can be suppressed by corticosteroids. The necessity for high dose corticosteroid treatment in the long term may be reduced by concurrent administration of azathioprine. Abnormalities of the thymus gland may be detected in patients with myasthenia gravis and they are often improved after surgical removal of the thymus gland (thymectomy). Plasmaphoresis has been used in recent years but its place in the treatment of this disorder remains controversial.

'Crises' may occur in patients with myasthenia gravis, resulting both from undertreatment and over-treatment with anticholinesterase drugs. These events constitute acute medical emergencies and should be managed by physicians with experience in treating myasthenia gravis. Patients with myasthenia gravis should be able to refer themselves to their parent neurological unit should any complications arise because the supervision of personnel experienced in dealing with myasthenia makes possible the identification of problems at an early stage before they become life-threatening.

Nursing care

The main aim of the nurse is to help the patient to adjust to the constraints imposed upon him by the disease process.

She should emphasize the need to avoid any prolonged exposure to physical or emotional stress, and the importance, for the patient, to plan his periods of rest carefully.

As he will suffer a degree of dysphagia, his food should be of a semisolid or fluid consistency. Naso-gastric feeding may be inevitable when dysphagia is severe. Some patients however, tolerate solid food following the commencement of drug therapy. The patient's degree of mobility will be determined partly by the number of voluntary muscles affected by the disease, and partly by his response to drug therapy. The nurse's role is to offer him support in meeting those activities of daily living with which he is experiencing difficulty. It is essential that the patient and his relatives are made aware of the drug regime; that is they should all know the medicine, the dose the time it is to be taken and the importance of maintaining accuracy and punctuality. They should also be aware of any adverse reactions associated with the drug or drugs prescribed.

The nurse must ensure that both the patient and his relatives know the action they must take should a 'crisis' occur following the patient's transfer home.

Spinal lesions

Spinal lesions can result from pathology within the cord (intrinsic — for example demyelinating) or outside the cord (extrinsic). Extrinsic pathology may lie within or without the meninges.

Causes of spinal lesions

These are given in Table 3.3.

Table 3.3
Causes of spinal lesions

Cause		Example
Congenital		Spina bifida
Acquired	1. Traumatic	Fractures
		Dislocations
		Gunshot and stab wounds.
	2. Infective	
	a. Acute	Abscess
	b. Chronic	Poliomyelitis
		Syphilis
	3. Neoplastic	
	a. Benign	Neurofibroma
	b. Malignant	
	i. Primary	Ependymoma
	ii. Secondary	Deposits from breast cancer.
	4. Degenerative	Cervical spondylosis.
		Prolapsed disc.

Note: This table does not include demyelination since the aetiology is unknown.

General features of spinal lesions

The features depend on the level and severity of the lesion but usually all functions of the cord — motor, sensory, and autonomic — are affected to a greater or lesser degree. The motor signs depend on whether the upper or lower motor neurone, or both, are involved (Fig. 3.11, p. 75). Damage to the upper motor neurone will result in spastic weakness and increased reflexes below the level of the lesion. Lower motor neurone damage presents as profound muscle wasting, flaccid weakness and depressed or absent tendon reflexes at the level of the lesion.

Different sensory tracts convey different types (modalities) of sensation, pain, temperature, touch and proprioception. The type of sensation lost will depend on the tract or tracts affected. If sensory roots are affected all form of sensation will be impaired.

Since the spinal cord ends at the level of the first lumbar vertebra, any lesion below this level, such as protrusion of a lumbar intervertebral disc, can only produce root lesions resulting in lower motor neurone weakness and impairment of all forms of sensation.

Investigations

Plain X-ray

This is the simplest form of investigation and may demonstrate fractures, dislocations and carcinomatous deposits in the vertebrae. Secondary deposits invading the vertebral column tend to arise from a primary carcinoma of the breast, kidney or prostate. Osteophytes (bony outgrowths) and narrowing of the intervertebral disc spaces are often demonstrated on X-ray in cases of cervical spondylosis.

Lumbar puncture

Since the spinal cord is encased within the meninges it is possible to obtain a sample of cerebrospinal fluid by lumbar puncture.

Lumbar puncture may be necessary for one of the following reasons:

1. To estimate CSF pressure (occasionally to remove some CSF to reduce the pressure) and to demonstrate any blockage of the subarachnoid pathways.

2. To obtain CSF for diagnostic purposes, say, for confirmation of a subarachnoid haemorrhage or meningitis. Immediately after subarachnoid haemorrhage the CSF is bloodstained. After a time it becomes xanthochromic (yellow in colour) due to the breakdown of red blood cells. In meningitis the CSF may be turbid. If meningitis is suspected a specimen of CSF will be sent to the laboratory for estimation of cell, protein, chloride and glucose content, culture of organisms and antibiotic sensitivity tests. CSF stagnating below a spinal block may be yellow in colour and will have an increased protein content.

3. To instil drugs in cases of infection.

4. For contrast radiography. A contrast medium, such as air for outlining the ventricular system or a dye for spinal myelography, may be injected.

The nurse can do much to alleviate the anxiety of the patient by explaining the lumbar puncture procedure to him. Usually the lumbar puncture is performed with the patient in the left lateral position. The legs are drawn up and flexed on the abdomen, the head and neck are flexed towards the chest wall. This flexes the vertebral column separating the vertebral spines so as to facilitate entry of the lumbar puncture needle. The nurse should hold the patient in this position during the procedure (Fig. 3.50). The level chosen is usually the space between the second and third or third and fourth vertebrae. As the spinal cord ends above this level there is no risk of damage to the cord.

As one of the indications for lumbar puncture is to estimate CSF pressure a calibrated manometer can be fitted to the spinal needle. Normally CSF pressure varies from 60 to 180 mm of water and is affected by pulse and respiration. The flexed position also increases the pressure; therefore, the pressure should be measured with the patient in a relaxed position after entry of the lumbar puncture needle. Increased pressure may be due to a space-occupying intracranial lesion such as an abscess, neoplasm or blood clot, brain swelling or hydrocephalus.

If blockage of CSF pathways is suspected, Queckenstedt's manoeuvre may be performed (Fig. 3.51). This shows whether or not there is an unobstructed CSF pathway between the lumbar and intracranial subarachnoid space. The nurse will be asked to compress both jugular veins; if done correctly this causes no discomfort. Pressure on the jugular veins causes an increase in the intracranial venous sinus pressure. This pressure rise is transmitted to the CSF in the subarachnoid space. If there is no subarachnoid blockage, there is free rise and fall of the CSF in the

Figure 3.50
Positioning patient for lumbar puncture

Figure 3.51
Queckenstedt's manoeuvre

manometer. If there is a partial blockage there may be sluggish rise and fall, and in complete blockage pressure on the jugular veins will cause no rise in the CSF pressure.

Following lumbar puncture the patient is nursed flat or head down for 24 hours. This should lessen the likelihood of headache which may result from removal of CSF from the subarachnoid space, or later leakage of CSF following withdrawal of the lumbar puncture needle. If headache is severe, analgesics may be prescribed. Some patients may have difficulty in micturition because of their unaccustomed position. If so it may be permissible to allow the patient up to use a commode. The decision is the doctor's and will depend on the patient's condition. If there is any indication of increased intracranial pressure a close watch must be kept on conscious level, pupils, pulse, respiration rate and blood pressure (vital signs). In extreme cases where there is great pressure increase the sudden reduction of pressure may cause part of the temporal lobe to slip through the tentorial hiatus and impact against the brain stem or may cause the cerebellum to be pushed into the foramen magnum. This causes deterioration in conscious level and alteration in vital signs and may cause respiratory arrest.

Myelography

This consists of injecting a radio-opaque iodine substance which is heavier than CSF. The patient is placed on a tilting X-ray table. A lumbar puncture is performed , a quantity of CSF is withdrawn and a smaller quantity of contrast medium is injected into the subarachnoid space. Since this is heavier than CSF, by tilting the X-ray table it can be made to run along the whole spinal subarachnoid space, outlining any abnormalities.

Irregularities of the theca or spinal block will be observed using the X-ray image intensifier and X-ray films can be taken of the level. The dye is removed following the procedure and the patient is nursed flat for the following 24 hours. The care is the same as for lumbar puncture.

A water soluble dye may demonstrate more clearly the outline of the nerve roots and could be used in preference to the iodine dye. The patient sits upright for six hours following this and then may be allowed up. The upright position is used following radiculogram as occasionally the water soluble dye may act as an irritant to the cord and brain.

Traumatic spinal lesions

Fracture or dislocation of the vertebral column may damage the spinal cord in several ways:

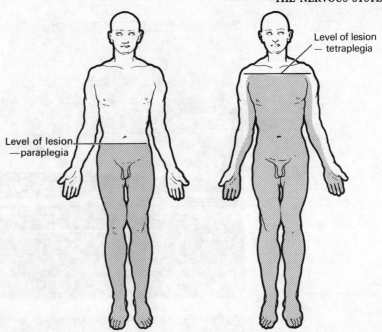

Level of lesion
— tetraplegia

Level of lesion
—paraplegia

Figure 3.52
Left: Paraplegia
Right: Tetraplegia

1. Concussion.
2. Contusion.
3. Laceration.
4. Compression.
5. Damage to blood supply.

Clinical features depend on the level and severity of the lesion. If the whole of the cord is damaged there will be complete paralysis and loss of sensation below the level of the lesion. A thoracic or lumbar lesion will result in paralysis of the lower limbs (**paraplegia**). A cervical lesion results in paralysis of all four limbs (**tetraplegia**) (Fig. 3.52). In both paraplegia and tetraplegia the autonomic system is also involved so that bladder, bowel, vasomotor and sexual functions may be lost. Lesions of the conus and nerve roots result in paralysis of the lower motor neurone type.

Paraplegia and tetraplegia

At the time of injury the patient presents with a flaccid paralysis. Autonomic control is lost resulting in retention of urine and faeces. Sympathetic paralysis results in postural hypotension, troublesome at the stage of mobilization. A patient with a high cervical lesion has respiratory problems, since the diaphragm is paralysed. Diaphragmatic breathing is preserved in lower cervical lesions because the diaphragm is controlled by the phrenic nerve derived from cervical segments three, four and five.

Nursing a patient with paraplegia

The treatment of spinal injury in the acute phase aims at stabilization of fractures, reduction of dislocations and prevention of further complications such as pressure sores, limb contractures and urinary tract infections.

Initially the aim is to correct spinal deformity by positioning, which is most conveniently achieved by nursing the patient on a Stryker frame (Figs 3.53 and 3.54). This treatment will not undo cord damage but it will lessen the risk of further damage. The patient is nursed on the frame on a layer of pillows suitably placed to maintain his spine in the best position (usually hyperextension) for correction of the deformity. He should be turned every 2 hours. Only two nurses are required for this procedure. The patient may be nursed on the frame for 8 to 12 weeks.

Alternatively, the patient may be nursed on a Stoke Egerton or an ordinary hospital bed on pillow packs. The Stoke Egerton bed operates electrically and turns the patient from one side to the other. Pillow packs are disposed so that the bony

Figure 3.53
Patient on a Stryker frame

Figure 3.54
Turning a patient on a Stryker
frame

prominences (sacrum, trochanters, heels and shoulders) are supported. Pillows
should be placed under and between the legs to avoid pressure on the condyles of
the knee and the malleoli of the ankles. The disadvantage of nursing a patient on
a bed as opposed to a frame is that, four or five nurses are required to lift and turn
the patient in 'one piece', maintaining proper alignment of the vertebral column.

Care of the skin

Due to his lack of sensation the paraplegic is not aware of discomfort. The nursing
staff must turn the patient every 2 hours to relieve areas of prolonged pressure, thus
minimizing the risk of pressure sores. The skin should be inspected at every turn
and any area which is red or broken should be relieved of pressure until healed. The
skin is kept clean by daily baths and by washing the pressure areas more often if
necessary. Even when artificial methods are used to relieve pressure, for example
a ripple mattress (a device which constantly redistributes the patient's weight),
turning should not be omitted — such devices are no substitute for regular turning.
Sheets must be kept dry, crumb- and wrinkle-free. Hot water bottles or electric
blankets should never be placed in the bed since the patient can be burned without
experiencing any discomfort. (There is great temptation to use them as paralysed
extremities are very cold.) For the same reason, once mobilized the patient must

be warned against sitting too close to fires, radiators or unlagged hot water pipes; handling hot water taps; using too hot water; and so on. The slightest break in the skin may take a long time to heal. A high protein diet and correction of anaemia, if present, are necessary if sores are to heal.

Care of limbs

In upper motor neurone lesions, return of reflex activity and tone is usually noticeable about 6 weeks after injury causing the flaccid paralysis to become spastic. In a conus or cauda equina lesion the legs and bladder remain flaccid since it is the lower motor neurones which are damaged. With return of reflex activity the patient may develop flexor or extensor spasms. Untreated spasms may give rise to permanent deformities of the limbs due to contractures of the muscles. Contractures can be prevented by careful positioning in bed and by putting the joints through their full range of movements twice daily. The patient may be nursed face down if he has severe flexor spasms. Pressure sores tend to increase spasm. Antispasmodics such as baclofen (Lioresal) and diazepam (Valium) may be of considerable value in the control of spasm.

Care of the urinary bladder

Renal failure is a common cause of death in paraplegics. Initially the bladder is flaccid. Overdistension must be avoided either by continuous bladder drainage or intermittent catheterization. Strict aseptic technique must be practised.

In upper motor neurone lesions, if the continuous method is being used, when reflex activity returns (or in any case in 6 weeks), the catheter is clipped and released at 2-hourly intervals. The patient may have a bizarre sensation of bladder fullness or he may experience headache, flushing or sweating. The catheter is withdrawn and attempts made to initiate reflex bladder evacuation by stimulating 'trigger spots' — tapping over the lower abdomen or rubbing the vulval area. If reflex evacuation is achieved, an injection of a drug such as carbachol is given resulting in further voiding. The residual urine is measured by reintroducing the catheter. Subject to obtaining satisfactory residuals (less than 60 ml) the catheter is left out for progressively longer periods and may eventually be dispensed with altogether, as indeed may the carbachol injections.

The patient should endeavour to empty his bladder regularly, say, every 2 to 4 hours, before the onset of sensations of fullness, headache or sweating. Great patience and perseverance are necessary to achieve such automatic bladder function. It may take many months, but it is a worthwhile achievement since bladder emptying is likely to be fairly complete. It is also more socially acceptable.

In conus and root lesions the bladder remains flaccid and autonomous bladder emptying may be achieved by straining and suprapubic compression. These patients tend to have greater residuals and are therefore more prone to infection. Surgery may be necessary to achieve relaxation of the internal and external sphincters. If neither automatic or autonomous bladder function is achieved an in-dwelling catheter will be necessary, carrying with it a higher risk of infection and calculus formation.

Once the initial oliguria of the first fortnight has passed a high fluid intake (3–4 litres) must be encouraged. Catheters are changed daily at first, then at longer intervals. Permanent in-dwelling catheters are changed monthly, and urine is sent for culture regularly. A concentration of organisms of 10^6/ml or greater is usually treated irrespective of whether or not there is constitutional upset. Organisms of lesser concentration require no treatment, unless there is systemic upset.

It is important to assess renal and bladder function at regular intervals after discharge from hospital. The procedures undertaken include intravenous pyelography, measurement of residual urine volumes, estimations of blood urea, creatinine and serum electrolytes.

Care of bowel function

Digital evacuation is performed initially by the nursing staff. Once the patient is mobilized he is taught to transfer to the toilet seat from his wheel-chair and to evacuate his own bowels by straining or by digital evacuation. Digital check should always be carried out to ensure that the rectum is emptied. Laxatives and/or suppositories may be necessary as may periodic enemas.

Sexual function

Although this aspect of paraplegia is very rarely raised by the patient it is nevertheless a cause of anxiety to many.

Females. Paraplegic women can conceive and bear children normally. They do not, however, have the normal sensations of sexual intercourse.

Males. Some men with upper motor neurone lesions may get reflex erections but of those only a few ejaculate, so that the chances of fathering a child are remote. During intercourse the female must be the active partner. In conus or root lesions erection and ejaculation are impossible.

A group entitled SPOD (Sexual Problems of the Disabled) has recently been set up by the National Fund for Research into Crippling Diseases, to study and to give advice on this difficulty. Information is available from the Committee on Sexual Problems of the Disabled, 49 Victoria Street, London SW1.

Mobilization

Transfer from a Stryker frame or pillow packs is usually possible 8 to 12 weeks after injury. Gradually the number of pillows under the head and shoulders are increased. Due to sympathetic paralysis patients with high lesions frequently suffer from dizziness and fainting attacks and it may be some time before they can tolerate the upright position. When the patient can sit upright he is supported with his legs over the edge of the bed and taught sitting balance in front of a long mirror. He is then transferred to a wheelchair. Dependent feet may develop oedema and to alleviate this condition elastic stockings may be necessary. In the physiotherapy and occupational therapy departments, the patient is taught feeding; toilet and dressing procedures; transfer from bed to chair, chair to toilet seat; and so on. In transfer the weight is taken by the arms, and upper limb musculature must be developed to enable the patient to do these manoeuvres. In the wheel-chair the patient sits on a 5–10 cm foam cushion and is advised to raise his buttocks off the cushion every 15 minutes to lessen the risk of ischial pressure sores.

Excessive reflex sweating is common. Sheepskin seat covers are useful to absorb sweat.

Rehabilitation

Rehabilitation starts from the moment the patient is diagnosed as paraplegic. The patient may find it very difficult to accept that he may never walk again. He may be very depressed, frustrated and aggressive. The aggression is a defence mechanism and may be directed towards members of staff or close relatives. It is a way of getting rid of pent-up emotions. Psychological support from the whole team is necessary. Relatives also require help and advice. The medical social worker can help with financial problems as well as by assessing the home situation with the occupational therapist. Change of accommodation may be necessary. The living room, bedroom and bathroom should be on ground-floor level. Doors may need to be widened, ramps provided at outside doors, furniture rearranged and even kitchen fittings lowered.

The disablement resettlement officer can arrange for assessment, retraining and placement in suitable employment. He can also arrange for the provision of a special car and an allowance.

Ideally the district nurse is invited by the ward team to visit the patient in hospital in order to become familiar with the patient and any special care necessary.

The patient should not be without his hobbies, relaxations and pastimes. In hospital the patient should be encouraged to engage in swimming, archery, table tennis, and so on, all of which strengthen arm muscles, as well as providing the stimulus of competitive sport.

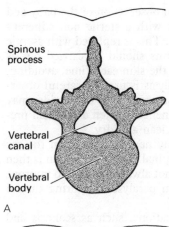

Spinous process

Vertebral canal

Vertebral body

A

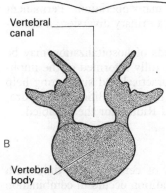

Vertebral canal

B

Vertebral body

Figure 3.55
Spina bifida
(A) Normal vertebra
(B) Failure of neural arch to close

At the end of the patient's stay in hospital — amounting to a year or more — it is hoped the patient will have gained some measure of independence and that he will again be integrated in home and society.

Spina bifida

Neural tube defects comprise a large percentage of congenital abnormalities, the most common in Great Britain being spina bifida. This defect is subdivided into:

1. Spina bifida occulta
2. Spina bifida cystica: a. meningocele
b. myelomeningocele

There is failure of the vertebral arch to close in the midline (Fig. 3.55) thus allowing meninges or meninges and cord to prolapse through the gap. These defects can occur anywhere within the vertebral column, the most common site being in the lumbosacral area. The vertebral arch normally closes by the twelfth week of gestation.

Spina bifida occulta. This as the term implies is a hidden lesion. Detailed examination of the new born infant (p. 588) may enable the midwife or doctor to detect this. There may be a slight dimpling of the skin and a tuft of hair may be present. A slight gap may be felt on palpation of the vertebral spines. Spina bifida occulta is usually of no significance and may not produce neurological symptoms. Occasionally, however there may be an underlying sinus leading to a lipoma or demoid cyst. This may become infected or the nerve roots may be compressed by the lesion. Surgical exploration and excision usually gives good results.

Spina bifida cystica. a. *Meningocele.* In this abnormality the meninges herniate through the gap and lie on the surface of the back. The skin may not cover the defect completely. The middle is usually translucent and cerebrospinal fluid can be seen. There is danger therefore of the meningocele rupturing and greater risk of meningitis occurring prior to surgery (Fig. 3.56).

b. *Myelomeningocele.* This is by far the commonest and most serious type of spina bifida. As well as meninges herniating, the spinal cord and nerve roots are also contained in the sac, and are adherent to it. Again skin covering is imperfect often consisting of a thin arachnoidal membrane with an even greater risk of rupture and infection. A myelomeningocele involving the lumbosacral region causes a flaccid paralysis of legs, bladder and bowel (Fig. 3.57) (Fig. 17.11, p. 589).

Vertebral body   Spinal cord   Meninges

Meningocele

Figure 3.56
Meningocele

Figure 3.57
Myelomeningocele

Spinal cord   Meninges

Myelomeningocele

Vertebral body

Treatment and nursing care

Aspects of nursing care include prevention of infection, maintenance of body temperature and careful observation of bladder and bowel function. Closure of the defect will be carried out as early as the child's general condition permits, should operation be the course decided upon. The infant is nursed without clothing in an incubator, in the prone position. This allows maximum observation of the baby and prevents pressure on the lesion. The area is covered with a sterile non adherent dressing or sterile gauze soaked in sterile normal saline. This is replaced with aseptic technique as often as is necessary. Changing of napkins should be carried out as often as required with careful cleansing and drying of the skin each time, avoiding, as far as possible, contamination of the lesion. If paralysis is present careful observation on bladder and bowel emptying is necessary. Compression of the bladder may be required to avoid overdistension. Dribbling incontinence is often a problem pre- and postoperatively and the skin requires to be kept clean and dry.

Surgical closure of the lesion aims at separating any neural tissue from the sac and after exploration of the canal replacing it into the spinal canal. The lesion is then closed by direct closure or by a rotation skin flap. It is not always possible to improve motor or sensory function and the infant may remain paralysed requiring careful skin, bladder and bowel care.

A child with spina bifida may have other complications, such as scoliosis and talipes; closure of the spina bifida cystica may be first of many operations. Permanent dribbling incontinence causing excoriation may require a urinary diversion, a ureterostomy, to avoid skin breakdown.

The parents should be made aware that long periods of hospitalization may be required. Through counselling sessions they should be fully informed of the implications of this handicap. Advice can be given of the practical and supporting help provided by listed charitable organizations principally the Spina Bifida and Hydrocephalus Society, The Disabled Living Foundation and Riding for the Disabled.

Hydrocephalus

This condition is caused by a gradual accumulation of cerebrospinal fluid with associated dilatation of the ventricular system. The condition occurs in combination with spina bifida cystica which may be present at birth or develop following closure of the lesion. Other causes include aqueduct stenosis, closure of the aqueduct between the third and fourth ventricle and complications from an accidental or non accidental injury. Measurement of the occipital — frontal circumference is carried out and an increase above the normal limits may indicate the presence of hydrocephalus.

Other signs of developing hydrocephalus are:

1. A tense and bulging fontanelle. Increase in CSF pressure displays the suture lines thus allowing the head circumference to increase and a normal slack fontanelle to become tense.
2. The scalp veins become engorged due to interference with intracranial venous drainage.
3. The infant may also develop 'sunsetting' of the eyes. This occurs with midbrain compression impairing upward and outward gaze (Fig. 3.58).
4. As the intracranial pressure increases the infant shows signs of irritability and malnutrition due to reluctance to feed and projectile vomiting.

These clinical features occur before drowsiness and other neurological deficits as the intracranial pressure is temporarily relieved by the increasing head circumference. Should hydrocephalus develop later in life after closure of the anterior fontenelle, e.g. following subarachnoid haemorrhage or be secondary to a space occupying lesion then the clinical features are of raised intracranial pressure. (p. 92).

Figure 3.58
Sunsetting

Investigation

Computerized axial tomography will be performed which may demonstrate enlargement of the ventricular system (p. 103).

Treatment and nursing care

Preoperatively the infant is given good nursing care to prevent skin breakdown, by changing position frequently. Areas at risk are in the parietal regions of the skull,

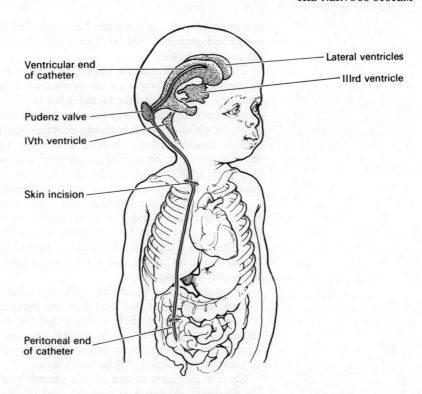

Ventricular end of catheter

Lateral ventricles

IIIrd ventricle

Pudenz valve

IVth ventricle

Skin incision

Peritoneal end of catheter

Figure 3.59
Ventriculoperitoneal shunt

Lateral ventricles

Ventricular end of catheter

Pudenz valve

Atrial end of catheter in R. atrium

Figure 3.60
Ventriculo-atrial shunt

Ventricular catheter (proximal end)

Pudenz valve

Distal end

Shunt system

Figure 3.61
Pudenz valve

upper and lower limbs which may require to be wrapped in cotton wool if the baby is very irritable, to prevent excoriation due to hyperactivity. Nasogastric tube feeding may be necessary to prevent further malnutrition and to ensure adequate fluid intake.

A shunt procedure is the operation of choice. This consists of diverting the CSF from the lateral ventricles to another area where it can be absorbed. Commonest is the ventriculoperitoneal shunt (Fig. 3.59), the distal end is placed in the subphrenic space, or the ventriculo-atrial shunt (Fig. 3.60), the distal end of which is threaded into the internal jugular to the right atrium. The valve used in the shunt system is either the Pudenz (Fig. 3.61) or Spitz-Holter.

Postoperatively the child is observed carefully for signs of shock or haemorrhage, the incision being checked for leakage of spinal fluid. Records of TPR are maintained and deep breathing encouraged. The child is positioned on the side opposite to operation to prevent pressure being applied to the valve. Accurate recordings of intake and output should be maintained, the child occasionally requiring intravenous fluids and nutrition.

The anterior fontanelle should be observed for bulging or excessive depression indicating an ineffective or an overactive shunt. The shunt valve is not pumped routinely. Continuing care includes the teaching of the parents to recognize complications that may arise at any time e.g. the shunt system may become blocked, kinked or as the child grows the tubing requires lengthening. Very quickly the child will develop raised pressure, becoming irritable and drowsy. The effectiveness of the shunt system can be judged by medical and nursing staff. A valve that is difficult to depress indicates the distal end is blocked, whereas a valve that remains concave indicates ineffectiveness of the ventricular end.

Gradually the nurse can teach the parents to feed, hold and bathe their baby, to express his bladder, aid him in his bowel evacuations, exercise his limbs, pump his shunt (if necessary) and to recognize the early signs of raised intracranial pressure. By encouraging them to take an active part in looking after their baby they will learn to feel confident in their own abilities to provide him with adequate care in spite of his physical handicap.

When the infant is feeding well, the shunt is working satisfactorily, and when medical and nursing staff feel that the parents are able to meet his needs, he will be discharged home. Before doing so, the community nursing services must be contacted and also the family general practitioner. They should arrange to visit as soon as the baby arrives home, so that they can give assurance to the parents, that they can be contacted if difficulties arise.

Close supervision of the child's growth and developmental progress is made by the paediatrician and psychologist, and guidance and support given to the parents to help them understand the severity of the problem, the consequences of surgical treatment and the future of their child.

Figure 3.62
Section of vertebral column showing ligaments

Anterior longitudinal ligament

Intervertebral disc

Body of vertebra

Posterior longitudinal ligament

Intervertebral foramen

Supraspinous ligament

Interspinous ligament

Ligamenta flava

Figure 3.63
Normal lumbar vertebrae and intervertebral discs

Prolapsed lumbar intervertebral disc

The spinal cord is enclosed within the neural arch of the vertebral column. The vertebrae are movable bones held in their respective positions by ligaments placed around the vertebral column, which limit to a certain extent the possible movements of individual vertebrae (Fig. 3.62). Between each vertebral body is a cartilaginous intervertebral disc held in place by a fibrous band, the annulus fibrosis, which also holds the vertebrae together. The vertebral column as a whole has a variety of movements — flexion, extension, rotation and lateral flexion. The majority of these movements, however, occur in the lumbar region because the rib cage reduces thoracic movement; therefore the lumbar area carries the total weight of the body and any object the person may carry. Figure 3.63 shows normal lumbar vertebrae and intervertebral discs.

Aetiology

In more than half the cases of disc protrusion there is a history of trauma, either direct or indirect, which places a strain on the spinal ligaments and annulus causing laxity so that the disc extrudes. The lumbar levels affected are usually lumbar 4(L4) and lumbar 5(L5) or lumbar 5(L5) and sacral 1(S1). When a disc prolapses it compresses the spinal nerve leaving from the intervertebral foramen below (Fig. 3.64). Therefore a disc protrusion between L5 and S1 compresses the first sacral nerve.

General features

The patient may have had backache or sciatic pain on and off for years due to increasing pressure on the lumbar or sacral nerves. Acute lumbar disc protrusion occurs suddenly: the patient lifts an object awkwardly and feels something 'give' in his back. Initially he may be unable to straighten up and feels a shooting pain down his leg. This pain is termed sciatica. Scoliosis may develop in an attempt to ease the pain, the spine flexing towards the affected side. Coughing and sneezing increase the pain.

The distribution of pain depends on the affected nerve. In fifth lumbar nerve compression, the pain radiates along the back of the thigh and leg crossing into the foot towards the great toe, whereas pressure on the first sacral nerve causes pain in the lateral aspect of leg and foot and into the small toe. Since it is a lower motor neurone lesion there may be minimal wasting and motor power loss of the muscles affected.

Investigations

1. General examination may reveal a scoliosis.
2. Straight leg raising increases pain due to stretching of the sciatic nerve.
3. Pain can also be induced by pressing the appropriate intervertebral space.
4. Plain X-rays may show narrowing of the disc spaces, and myelography (p. 128) should demonstrate disc prolapse.

Treatment

If treated conservatively with bed rest, traction and analgesics most lesions resolve. Some, however, require surgical excision if the pain persists or a neurological deficit develops for example due to compression of the nerves to the bladder and bowel. A laminectomy is performed in which the lamina of the neural arch is removed and the prolapsed disc excised.

Pre- and postoperative general care is the same as for any operation. In turning the patient from side to side it is usually easier and less traumatic for the patient if he is rolled face down instead of on to his back. The problem of difficulty in micturition may arise, and a careful note should be made of the amount of urine passed. If the disc prolapsed centrally on to the cauda equina, compressing nerves to the bladder, the problem may have existed preoperatively and will not resolve immediately postoperatively. In this case the care is as for paraplegia until tone has been recovered (p. 129).

Depending on the surgeon, the patient is mobilized in 1 to 3 days and physiotherapy is begun. The patient is taught to re-use weakened muscles to maintain correct posture and to lift objects correctly. Sutures are removed 7 to 10 days postoperatively.

SUGGESTED ASSIGNMENTS

1. Patients who have suffered severe brain damage due to head injury may have both behavioural and intellectual deterioration. In a young child this will present an educational problem.

Figure 3.64
Prolapsed lumbar intervertebral disc

a. List the difficulties which you think the child's teacher might encounter.

b. When a suitable opportunity arises, ask a teacher involved in the education of such children what problems he or she encounters.

c. Now compare these with your previously prepared list and note the validity of your comments.

2. Paralysis of the dominant hemisphere of the brain may affect the individual's ability to understand the spoken word and/or to express himself orally. This defect is one of the commonest sequelae to a cerebrovascular accident.

a. Keep a written account of how you have attempted to communicate with a group of patients suffering from dysphasia.

b. When given the opportunity, discuss your methods with patients who have recovered from this disability.

c. From the comments given, evaluate how effective your methods have been.

FURTHER READING

Bickerstaff E R 1978 Neurology, 3rd edn. Hodder and Stoughton, London

Hickey J V 1981 The clinical practice of neurological and neurosurgical nursing. Lippincott, Philadelphia

Jennet B, Galbraith S 1983 An introduction to neurosurgery, 4th edn. Heinemann Medical, London

Jennet B, Teasdale G 1981 Management of head injuries. Davis, Philadelphia

Reid C 1983 A primer of neuroanatomy, 2nd edn. Lloyd Luke, London

Chapter Four
Nutrition

This chapter provides information to explain the importance of nutrition to the nurse herself and therefore to patients. Nutrition cannot be seen in isolation from other subjects studied in the nursing curriculum. It is essential to relate a basic study of nutrition to subjects such as physiology, sociology and psychology in order to obtain an overview of their interrelationships and consequently an understanding of the problems occurring when it becomes necessary to change the established patterns of nutrition either in order to promote health and prevent illness, or to assist in the recovery from illness.

It is a professional responsibility of the nurse to promote constructive nutritional practices through health education, to apply the principles of the social sciences to nutritional decisions and to involve the patient in the health care programme from conception to completion where the patient's ability permits. Attitudes, values and beliefs and consequently behaviours can be resistant to change. The nurse has the task, from her knowledge of the patient, of identifying the nutritional choices available to that patient within the constraints of his condition. The dietitian and the patient will select priorities within these choices so that optimum health through nutrition becomes available and attainable.

NUTRITION IN HEALTH

Nutrition is defined by the American Medical Association as 'the science of food, the nutrients and other substances therein, their action, interaction and balance in relation to health and disease, and the process by which the organism ingests, digests, absorbs, transports, utilizes and excretes food substances. In addition, nutrition must be concerned with social, economic, cultural and psychological implications of food and eating.'

Dietetics is defined as 'the interpretation and application of the scientific principles of nutrition to the human subject in health and disease' (British Medical Journal 1945 2: 617).

Nutrition is concerned with what is eaten and how the body uses food for growth, development and maintenance.

Nutrients are substances that nourish the body. Food is made up of different nutrients that are needed for growth and health. The amounts of nutrients needed by the body may vary according to age, sex, build, activity and state of health. An excess, deficit or an imbalanced intake of nutrients may be detrimental to health.

A knowledge of nutrition is, therefore, essential because the maintenance of a person's health depends on the ingestion and absorption of foods containing the appropriate amounts of energy and all the nutrients. The complex bodily activities — ingestion, digestion, absorption, assimilation and excretion — must be physiologically normal because any alteration in function may require dietary modifications to be made. A careful nutritional assessment is necessary before dietary decisions are made either in consultation with the patient or for him when he is unable to make decisions for himself.

Diet is the term used to describe the total solid and liquid intake of any individual. This term is often incorrectly used to mean *diet therapy* which is treatment through prescription of a specific diet. A balanced diet is one which prevents deficiency diseases by providing all the essential nutrients in the optimum proportions for a given individual. In Britain a diet is considered to be balanced when it contains the 'recommended' intake of each nutrient. These nutrient intakes have been recommended by national and international bodies and appear, for example in the Department of Health and Social Security Report, 1969. The constituents of a balanced diet are:

Proteins.
Carbohydrates.
Fats.
Mineral salts.
Vitamins.
Fibre (roughage).
Water.

Energy is produced as the result of the metabolism of proteins, carbohydrates and fats, and in dietetics it is measured in kilojoules (kJ). In 1960, the International System of units was introduced (S.I. units). The *joule* replaced the calorie as the unit of energy (in whatever form). It is a convenient unit of measurement because units of energy can be expressed in whole numbers by adding a prefix:

Kilo (kilojoule) = × 1000
mega (megajoule) = × 1 000 000
1 g carbohydrate provides 17 kJ
1 g fat provides 37 kJ
1 g protein provides 17 kJ

and with this information and the weight of nutrients in a portion of food, the total kilojoule content can be estimated.

The larger amount of food required daily is expressed in megajoules — 10 mJ (10 000 kJ).

The energy requirements are conditioned by:

1. Age — more energy is needed during periods of growth.
2. Optimum weight — depends on height and bone structure of an individual.
3. Sex — women need fewer kilojoules than men.
4. Well-being — disorders of physical or mental health can alter energy requirements.
5. Climate — energy requirements increase in cold climates when the body loses heat to the environment and decrease in hot climates.
6. Activity — the main factor in determining energy requirements. If the body does not receive enough food to provide energy for work, it will utilize its own tissues (usually fat). On the contrary if food is eaten in excess of energy needs it will be stored in the body as fat. Energy intake should balance output.

Table 4.1 gives some commonly accepted levels for various individuals.

Table 4.1
Daily energy requirements

Activity level	Men (kJ)	Women (kJ)
Sedentary	10 500	8800
Moderately active	12 500	10 500
Active	14 750	12 500
Very active	17 850	15 750
Pregnant (last 3 months)		11 500
Lactating		12 500

Sociological aspects

The availability, preparation and eating of food does more than simply provide the required nutrients for maintaining health. Eating is a social activity and food holds both social and psychological significance for most people. However, seen in the social context food can be a contribution to nutritional disorders such as obesity. Alternatively, enforced dietary therapy may alter established eating patterns producing responses leading to non-compliance or discontinuation of therapeutic dietary recommendations. It is the role of the dietitian in conjunction with doctors and nurses to educate the public to develop healthy eating patterns or when necessary to provide nutritional therapy in the least disruptive way.

The student of sociology will understand the term *socialization*. It is the acquisition and adoption of knowledge, values, attitudes and beliefs that are considered the norms of a particular culture or sub-culture within society. Throughout the life-span of an individual behaviours are adopted because of the influence of the groups most closely in contact with the individual at a given time. In nutritional matters the influence of the family is predominant. Decision-making regarding food matters is the province of the mother. She will have an influence on what foods are 'good' for the child. She will set the pattern of buying and the presentation and timing of meals. The child may be punished if he does not eat certain foods and rewarded with food, perhaps sweets, for good behaviour.

When the child reaches school age other influences may change his nutritional preferences. At present the trend in many schools is to provide a cafeteria-type of service and this may encourage the schoolchild to rely on snacks to satisfy hunger and appetite. He will also begin to be influenced by the practices of his friends who may have very different nutritional backgrounds. He may begin to question the meals produced in his own home because he prefers those which he has had at a friend's home.

In adolescence, further influences occur. Male and female styles tend to become established. Some foods are preferred by women, for example muesli, fruits and salads, probably because of the desire to be slim and healthy and to conform to fashion trends and media pressure. Men, on the other hand, develop a preference for foods such as steak, meat pies, chips and beer as these are seen as manly foods. Both are forms of behaviour which are adopted without conscious decision. Health education regarding nutrition should be directed towards acquiring a knowledge of nutritional needs and taking a conscious decision to eat appropriately to maintain optimum health.

Later in middle-life and into old age nutritional habits may alter because of changing circumstances, for example when members of the family leave home, the mother and father may eat out more often and experiment with foods from other cultures. Conversely, in old age economies rather than preferences may be the determining factors in the choice of food and nutritional advice is now being directed at how to budget on a small income and still provide nutritious foods in variety.

Factors influencing food choice

Figure 4.1 illustrates five of the main factors which determine food choice.

Availability and acceptability

The types of food available will vary from country to country, and from region to region. This is not now primarily because of geographic location but a result of tradition because foods can now be imported from many different countries.

The type of food grown is governed by the climate which will sustain it: therefore, the types of crops that can be grown will determine the availability of food and help to set the patterns of eating. Political influence such as Britain's membership of the European Economic Community (E.E.C.) can also determine the importance attached to different foodstuffs, and their availability. Cultural factors are also important. Certain foods are not acceptable to some religious or ethnic groups who prefer to retain their traditional selection patterns and eating practices.

Figure 4.1
Factors influencing food choice

Economics

The pattern of food consumption is dictated by the level of family income. It is very difficult to be adventurous with food on a restricted budget. This occurs, for example, in times of high unemployment where the total family income is derived from State benefits. Income may also be lower in households where the wife is the sole breadwinner. In more fortunate families, wives are also working and contributing to the household income and consequently patterns of expenditure are very different. Convenience foods are being used more often, fast-food restaurants are useful although not now cheaper, and because travel is relatively cheap, these families are often holidaying abroad and developing a more positive attitude to unusual foods.

The price of food to the consumer may be directly dictated by government policy. This has been the case since Britain joined the E.E.C. where certain agreements were made to sustain the price of foods. Some foods such as lamb and butter are still imported from Commonwealth countries, and consequently their price has increased greatly. Seasonal variations in the price of fruit and vegetables especially influence their consumption and play a part in creating the eating pattern.

Individual preferences

Some foods are associated with pleasant events, such as birthdays, Christmas, personal anniversaries and make people feel better and happy. Certain events provoke the need for a celebration. Food is psychologically important and the focal point on such occasions. Other foods may be associated with unpleasant childhood memories and be avoided thereafter.

Individuals through genetic and cultural influences develop their own preferences for certain foods. These may be preferences associated with the choice, taste, texture, colour or presentation of the food. Some people become extreme in their eating patterns and develop food fads. This is particularly prevalent in North America where the proliferation of diets of all kinds has almost become a cult.

Some people are unable to exercise full choice over what they eat because it is necessary to learn to live within a therapeutic dietary regime. Diabetics and children with inborn errors of metabolism, for example, must live their lives with their dietary choices limited.

Social factors

Many mothers are now working either part-time or full-time and this has a direct influence on the pattern of meals within the family. Meal-times tend to be less regular, convenience foods are utilized more often and generally less fresh meat, fish and vegetables are prepared.

Both men and women may be in employment which involves shift work which again alters eating patterns and may reduce the desire for food. Working conditions may encourage the use of packed lunches and canteen meals; both of which may or may not be adequate nutritionally.

In times of high unemployment role reversal often occurs. The wife may remain gainfully employed while the husband is made redundant. The wife becomes the breadwinner and the husband prepares the meals. The income level will often be reduced and the family will adopt new nutritional routines.

Food has significance also to social status. Among social groups certain foods are not acceptable because they imply low social status, for example fish and chips, while other food such as game and salmon are considered high status foods. Foods from other cultures may or may not be acceptable depending on the individual's view of the status of that culture.

The body resembles a biological clock. If its rhythms are upset persistently by factors such as transcontinental air travel, changes from day to night duties in employment and alterations in shift working, it is recognized that performance will be affected.

British dietary patterns have been slow to change but the effects of government policies, importation of new and different foods, the increase in travel and the development of a multi-ethnic society are having an impact on traditional nutritional patterns.

Health education and nutrition

Health is defined by the World Health Organization (W.H.O.) as 'the state of complete physical, mental and social well-being and not merely the absence of disease or infirmity.'

Food, activity, recreation and sleep are all necessary to maintain health. A well-nourished person should be the correct weight and height for his age and build, his skin and hair should be healthy, posture erect, disposition pleasant, appetite good and he should give a general impression of alertness. When health is good, the individual is able to resist most infections.

When the body is supplied with insufficient nutrients it suffers from nutritional deficiency. When this is the cause of ill-health it is described as *primary deficiency*, but when nutritional deficiency occurs as the result of another disorder it is termed *secondary nutritional deficiency*.

Malnutrition is incorrect nutrition caused by a dietary deficiency or excess of one or more nutrients.

In order to prevent nutritional deficiency and malnutrition, the maintenance of good nutrition can be encouraged through Health Education. This is not a simple task because the health educationalist is competing for public attention against the flood of information (often incorrect) that is produced by advertising companies and the media and by the claims of food faddists.

Education about nutrition must be taught by people with a proper understanding of nutrition. The best place to start would be by promoting good practices within

Figure 4.2
Promotion of nutrition through health education

Figure 4.3
The food groups

Figure 4.4
An adequate diet

Group 1	Cereals	4 servings, particularly whole grain, fortified or enriched grain products
Group 2	Meat & meat products	2 servings
Group 3	Milk & dairy foods	2 servings—adult 4 servings—teenager 3 servings—children
Group 4	Fruit & vegetables	4 servings
Group 5	Non-dairy fats & foods	Energy needs of individual will determine amount needed

the family. This advice could be supplemented or reinforced in a number of areas where a carefully selected nutrition educational input could be included.

The inclusion of nutrition in the school curriculum as a subject in its own right or as an adjunct to biology would provide a better understanding of the advantages of good nutrition. Teachers would require some guidance on this topic if they were not experts in the subject.

Nurses, medical practitioners, health visitors and nutritionists all have a contribution to make to community health education. The health visitor is in a particularly important position because of her role with families and very young children. In health clinics it should be possible to organize group teaching sessions to promote a positive approach to nutrition.

The media (newspapers, radio and television) have an extensive audience and exert considerable influence. Most people regularly buy a particular newspaper and listen to selected radio or television programmes. Each is a powerful agency and may be used to promote educationally sound nutritional comment, but too often the content is restricted to giving recipes or discussing controversial dietary issues.

A planned programme of nutrition information, discussions about nutritional issues and the availability of services could be promoted by any of the media. This may not create an attitude change but would provide accurate information to the individual so that he can, when necessary, discuss dietary matters in an informed way with dietitian, doctor or nurse. Subsequently he may be persuaded more readily to adopt good nutritional habits and be more amenable if therapeutic dietary modifications become necessary.

The Health Educational Council was established in 1968. It has the responsibility for health education through national branches and carries out educational campaigns in all aspects of health education including nutrition. Many publications are available including leaflets on nutrition.

It is recognized in the new programme of nurse training in Scotland that health education should be seen as a continuing theme. The nurse should, in whatever field she eventually chooses to work, see herself as a teacher promoting positive attitudes whether in the community or in hospital. The nurse in hospital often has the role of educating the patient to accept and adopt a dietary pattern for life, for example because of diabetes or coeliac disease. Emphasis should be placed on leading as normal a life as possible within the limits of the dietary restriction. The nurse can also suggest that the patient makes use of the developing expertise of self-help groups such as the British Diabetic Association or the Coeliac Society where up-to-date information and advice can be obtained following discharge from hospital.

The whole emphasis of nutritional education must be placed on teaching not preaching. The public become confused when so much emphasis is placed on the nutritional food values and recommended daily intake of all the nutrients. People go to the supermarket or local shops to buy food not nutrients. An easy-to-use guide for food selection has been made through the use of the Food Groups. Figure 4.3 shows the five main food groups which can supply an adequate intake of nutrients when taken in the appropriate amounts. The average daily amounts that are recommended in Figure 4.4 will provide a nutritionally adequate diet. This allows for personal choice within a carefully devised teaching framework. Selection from Groups 6–8 will provide enjoyment if taken in moderation.

Nutritional assessment

The basic processes of nutrition take place within the cell. Each cell receives nutrients from the bloodstream via the tissue fluid and returns the end products of metabolism to these fluids for subsequent excretion. In nutrition, therefore, the evaluation of the food eaten and consequently nutrient intake is crucial. The purpose of nutritional assessment is to measure the relationship between the dietary intake of nutrients and the physiological responses of the body both in health and disease.

There are four main methods of conducting a nutritional assessment:

1. Dietary assessment
   a. A 24-hour recall of food eaten by the person is required. This means that an ability to remember will be necessary.

b. A dietary history may be taken by the dietitian or a dietary diary may be kept. Both these methods involve a longer period of time, usually 7 days, to account for variations in intake patterns such as weekend meals. The dietary history or diary is useful in validating the 24-hour recall response.

2. Biochemical assessment

This is an analysis of nutrients and their metabolites or enzymes. It includes haemoglobin estimation, assessment of levels of glucose in the blood or urine, full urinalysis and faecal analysis.

3. Clinical assessment

This involves a complete physical examination to determine any clinical signs of nutritional deficiency as well as to assess nutritional status, for example emaciation or obesity.

4. Anthropometry

Various body measurements are made such as height, weight and skinfold thickness.

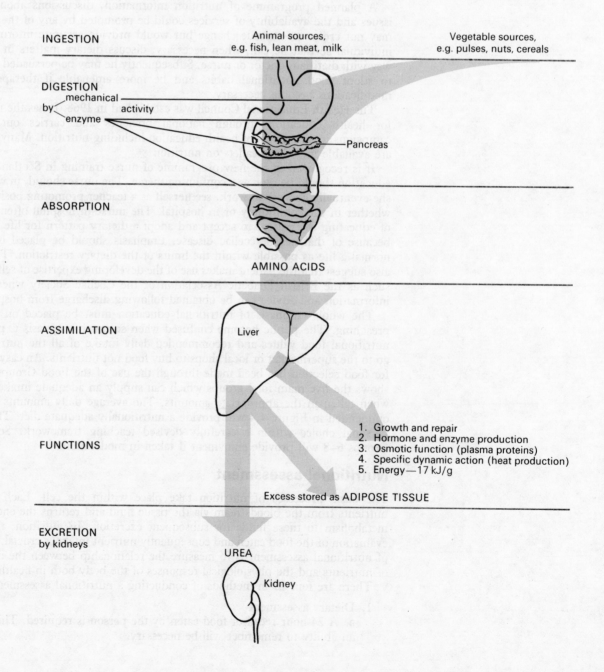

Figure 4.5
Proteins

FOOD COMPONENTS

Proteins (Fig. 4.5)

These complex substances are composed of **carbon, hydrogen, oxygen, nitrogen, sulphur** and **phosphorus**; rich sources are lean meat, fish, egg whites, cheese, milk, pulses, nuts and cereals. Digestion occurs as a result of their combination with gastric, pancreatic and intestinal enzymes, which break down the complex protein into a number of different amino acids; in this form they can be absorbed across the wall of the small intestine.

In the liver, various amino acids are combined to form complex molecules required by the body, or are synthesized into other amino acids not available in the diet. Any excess over need is taken up by the liver; the nitrogenous substances are formed into urea and excreted by the kidneys, the remainder of the molecule being oxidized to form carbon dioxide (excreted by the lungs) and water (excreted by the kidneys). If oxidization does not occur, conversion into carbohydrate can take place. As a result energy can be produced or, alternatively, the carbohydrate can be converted into fats which are stored as adipose tissue.

Classification

Proteins are classified according to their biological value:

1. Those of animal origin, which contain all of the essential amino acids are called first class proteins. The body requires approximately 22 amino acids in a specialized combination in order to manufacture human protein and is able to produce all but eight of them. These are known as essential amino acids and must, therefore, be ingested in the diet.

2. Those of vegetable origin lack or are very low in any one of the essential amino acids and are termed second class proteins.

Animal proteins promote growth and maintenance to a greater extent than proteins of vegetable origin and, therefore, the human diet should contain a proportion of animal protein. About half the total protein ingested each day should consist of first-class protein. Excess amino acids cannot be stored in the body and they will be used most effectively if a range of amino acids is supplied at each meal together with the correct amount of energy-providing foods. Animal and vegetable protein can be given together in meals such as breakfast cereal and milk, or as a roll and cheese.

Methionine and lysine have been made commercially. In America special loaves have been produced containing lysine, and in the developing areas of the world some protein mixtures have methionine added. These are not necessary in Western countries where the protein intake is adequate.

Functions of proteins

1. Proteins provide basic materials for growth, maintenance and repair of body tissues. As all cells have a protein component, the dietary needs are increased during periods of growth, or following injury (including surgical wounds) when repair with new cell formation is required. The healthy adult requires approximately **55 to 85 g per day**, or 10 % of total energy intake. The amount of protein in dairy products is variable, but the following approximations may be helpful: one large egg 7 g (mainly in the white); two slices of lean meat 35 g; one average helping of macaroni cheese 20 g; 500 ml of milk 20 g. More detail of this and other components discussed below may be obtained from specialist dietetic texts. The growing child needs about five times this amount in proportion to his body weight.

2. Proteins are constituents of all hormones and enzymes.

3. Proteins are the source of the blood proteins and cells that have a vital function in immune response mechanisms and in maintaining the osmotic pressure within the circulation.

4. Proteins have a specific dynamic action by which the metabolic process produces more heat from the same quantity of food (without alteration in thyroid

function). This is of importance in cold climates, where a diet high in protein plays a significant role in maintaining an adequate body temperature.

5. In the absence of an adequate total intake of kilojoules or any excessive protein intake over need, energy and heat will be produced by *gluconeogenesis* in the liver. Energy yield: 17 kJ per g.

Proteins are the only dietary sources of nitrogen. The body is said to be in nitrogenous equilibrium, or **nitrogen balance**, when the nitrogen intake equals the nitrogen lost in the excreta over a measured period of time.

When the intake of nitrogen is greater than the amount excreted, the individual is described as being in a state of **positive nitrogen balance**. Positive nitrogen balance is necessary for normal growth; growth will be stunted if a child's nitrogen intake does not exceed his nitrogen loss — hence the statement made earlier that the proportion of dietary protein to body weight for a growing child should be five times greater than the proportion for an adult.

If the intake of nitrogen is less than the output, the person is said to be in a state of **negative nitrogen balance**. An inadequate intake of protein, and therefore of nitrogen, may have many causes including economic: most protein foods are more expensive than carbohydrates. Excessive loss of protein from the body may result from pathological conditions, such as burns (Ch. 14) or some renal diseases (Ch. 9). Protein deficiency results in poor healing of wounds, muscle wasting with subsequent loss of power, oedema due to changes in osmotic pressure resultant upon loss of plasma proteins, and an increased vulnerability to a cold environment and possibly also to infection. The low-protein diet of many elderly people in Great Britain is partially responsible for the increasing number who become victims of *hypothermia* each winter.

From this discussion, it can be seen that the nurse has a responsibility to ensure an adequate protein intake to maintain her own health and resistance to infection. Also she must endeavour to assist her patients, who are often anorexic, to ingest a suitably presented form of protein to meet the demands of their individual circumstances.

Carbohydrates (Fig. 4.6)

These are composed of **carbon, hydrogen** and **oxygen** in variable proportions; the more carbon molecules present, the more complex the substance and consequently the longer it takes to break down and become available for absorption. Sources are all cereals and their manufactured products, pulses, root vegetables including beetroot, cane sugar and anything to which it has been added, honey, fruits and milk.

Digestion begins in the mouth for cooked starches only; the breakdown of uncooked starch commences in the small intestine due to the activity of pancreatic and intestinal enzymes which also act on the cooked starches until a simple molecular form is reached, which can be absorbed through the mucosa of the small intestine. If required immediately, glucose is metabolized in the cells (the presence of insulin being necessary to enable it to enter the cell) and heat and energy are produced, water and carbon dioxide being the waste products. If not required for immediate energy needs, glucose can be converted into glycogen and stored as such in the liver and muscles or converted into fat stores. As glycogen can be converted rapidly back into glucose, eating can be discontinuous and even fairly prolonged fasting can be undertaken without impairment of mental function. The brain, although only one-fiftieth of total adult weight, utilizes one-fifth of all absorbed glucose and appears to acquire all its energy from this source and not from fat sources. Any ingested carbohydrate which is not broken down into glucose will be excreted as waste (see Roughage, p. 156).

Classification

Classification of carbohydrates is by molecular complexity.

Monosaccharides are simple sugars and are the form in which carbohydrates are absorbed into the bloodstream through the gut wall. Glucose (from honey), fructose

INGESTION Cereals, root vegetables, cane sugar, honey, fruits and their manufactured products

DIGESTION

by mechanical activity

by enzyme

Pancreas

ABSORPTION MONOSACCHARIDES

INSULIN

ASSIMILATION CARBOHYDRATE

Cell

Liver

GLYCOGEN

Muscle

1. Produce heat and energy—17 kJ/g
2. Necessary for intracellular metabolism of fats
FUNCTIONS 3. Stored as adipose tissue
4. Protein sparer
5. Bulk—cellulose, in diet

EXCRETION by gut INDIGESTIBLE CELLULOSE

Figure 4.6
Carbohydrates

(from fruits) and galactose (from milk) are monosaccharides; carbohydrates which arrive in the stomach in this form will be absorbed through the stomach wall, the only energy sources except alcohol which are, and thus provide a useful source of 'instant energy'.

Disaccharides are more complex, being two molecules combined together, therefore requiring a one-stage breakdown process before absorption can occur. Lactose (from milk) and sucrose (from cane sugar) are common dietary sources.

Polysaccharides. Main forms of polysaccharides are starch, glycogen and cellulose; readily available sources are cereals, pulses, liver, root and leafy vegetables.

Polysaccharides comprise the tough and fibrous structure of cereals, grains, vegetables and fruits. Some polysaccharides are instantly broken down to monosaccharides but this depends on their structure. Polysaccharides are complex substances made up of many thousands of linked glucose units.

Starches are found enclosed in the cellulose walls of grains and vegetables. To make starches digestible they are broken down by grinding or cooking.

Glycogen is the form in which carbohydrates are stored in the liver or muscles and used as a source of energy in an emergency.

Cellulose is synonymous with the terms fibre, roughage and bulk. Cellulose is indigestible and passes through the alimentary tract unchanged. It is insoluble in water but because of its resistance to digestion and its water-binding capacity it furnishes bulk in the digestive tract and stimulates peristaltic action.

Functions of carbohydrates

1. To produce heat and energy when combined with oxygen in the cell. Energy yield: **17 kJ per g**.
2. To participate in the intracellular metabolism of fats.
3. To form adipose tissue which protects organs and insulates the body from cold. The greater proportion of subcutaneous fat in women compared with men offers them protection from exposure to adverse weather conditions.
4. To act as a protein sparer: insufficient intake of carbohydrate will result in utilization of protein for energy with a subsequent impairment of specific protein function. This role is of special significance in untreated diabetes mellitus (Ch. 11), when cells (though not the body as a whole) are starved of carbohydrate, resulting in the muscle wasting and weakness of which the patient complains. It is also the reason why patients suffering from acute glomerulonephritis (Ch. 9) are normally given 100 g of carbohydrate daily. It is common practice for these people to be advised to restrict their fluid intake to 500–600 ml of water each day and to reduce protein drastically. Some carbohydrate must be taken to meet energy needs. In its absence body protein would be converted to supply energy and consequently nitrogenous wastes would be produced, so defeating the aim of the regime. Subsistence on a diet containing no protein, restricted water and a small quantity of carbohydrate should result in a fall in blood urea and at the same time decrease the load on renal function. This regimen is only suitable for short periods.

5. To provide roughage (see p. 156).

The average daily requirement of carbohydrate is about 55% of total energy intake, usually **400 to 500 g per day**. Of particular importance to those with a tendency to be overweight, it is worth noting that one rounded teaspoonful of white sugar contains 8 g of carbohydrate; one average slice of fruit cake 20 g; a slice of bread 10 g. Because the sources of carbohydrates are usually the cheaper foods, hungry people and adolescents who seem never to be satisfied generally 'fill up' on them. This may develop into undesirable eating habits which are hard to change when activity decreases. The excess is then stored as fat and the process leading to obesity starts (p. 168).

Inadequate intake of carbohydrate may produce ketosis (p. 152) from incomplete fat metabolism. This produces symptoms of nausea, impairment of mental function and confusion as a result of neuronal deprivation; muscle wasting and weight loss as a result of utilization of proteins and fats for energy; and general lassitude due to inadequate catabolism and energy production. The mechanism of hunger usually prevents these symptoms from becoming severe, as a meal or a snack would normally be taken to raise the blood sugar and replace the glycogen stores which are being utilized to maintain an adequate blood glucose level. It should be remembered, however, that many patients are required to fast for prolonged periods for diagnostic or therapeutic purposes. Postoperative nausea may be due as much to an overprolonged preoperative fast (plus operation time itself) as to any anaesthetic drug or operative manipulation that has been involved. A low blood sugar level also prolongs the period, and increases the severity, of postoperative hypotension and increases the risk of infection. Unless specifically requested, the preoperative fasting period should not exceed 6 hours.

Many patients are also maintained for some days on intravenous therapy, which may incorporate only low concentrations of dextrose solutions as sources of energy. As a guide 2 litres of 5% dextrose will yield rather less than a quarter of the normal carbohydrate intake; this takes no account of other energy sources which would normally be ingested nor of the patient's energy requirements.

The nurse herself may have noticed that, when hungry, she is less efficient, less able to respond rapidly to changing situations, more easily tired and less tolerant with her patients. If both nurse and patient are irritable, interpersonal relationships may suffer.

Fats or lipids (Fig. 4.7)

These are composed of **carbon, hydrogen** and **oxygen** in complex molecules.

Fats are the most concentrated energy source in the diet. After oxidation, they provide twice the number of kilojoules per gram provided by carbohydrates or proteins, e.g. 1 g of fat yields 37 kJ and therefore permits large increases in energy intake without creating too much bulk or the need for frequent ingestion.

Fat slows the secretion of hydrochloric acid, reduces muscular contractions and the rate of digestion and, therefore, prevents the fast return of hunger. Sources are cream, butter, cheese, fat meat, oily fish, some fruits for instance nuts and olives, and some vegetable sources such as sunflowers and corn. These last are common sources of cooking oils.

Digestion of fats begins in the small intestine where bile and lipase, a pancreatic and intestinal enzyme, emulsify the dietary fat into fatty acids and glycerol. These are converted into triglycerides in the cells of the wall of the small intestine and are then absorbed into the lacteals, thence to the lymphatic system and general circulation.

The liver then combines each triglyceride molecule with a protein molecule to form a lipoprotein, which is more readily transported round the body. In adipose tissue, fats are stored as triglycerides, the conversion process requiring the presence of carbohydrate in the cell. The protein molecule is now available for other purposes.

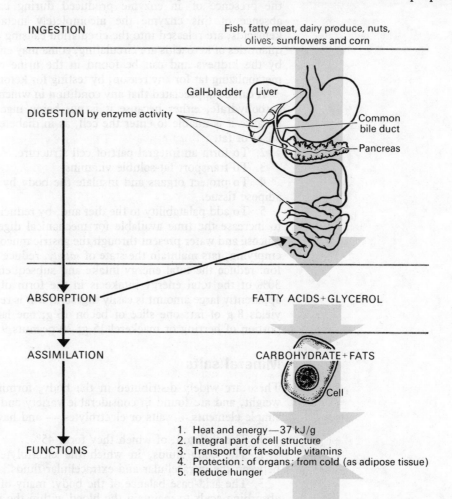

INGESTION — Fish, fatty meat, dairy produce, nuts, olives, sunflowers and corn

DIGESTION by enzyme activity

Gall-bladder — Liver — Common bile duct — Pancreas

ABSORPTION — FATTY ACIDS + GLYCEROL

ASSIMILATION — CARBOHYDRATE + FATS — Cell

FUNCTIONS
1. Heat and energy—37 kJ/g
2. Integral part of cell structure
3. Transport for fat-soluble vitamins
4. Protection: of organs; from cold (as adipose tissue)
5. Reduce hunger

FAT STORE

Figure 4.7
Fats

The energy needs of the body are met by utilization of fatty acids, the form in which triglycerides are mobilized from adipose tissue. Deposits of adipose tissue are in a continuous state of change. Energy needs are met from these stores and not from circulating fat. If energy needs become greater and the dietary intake of carbohydrate is not increased, no further deposition of fat occurs and the rate of mobilization of the stored fat accelerates. This is the rationale behind the management of obesity.

Classification

Lipids, when metabolized, fall into three groups:

1. The **triglycerides**, including fatty acids, may be stored in the body; they are sources of energy and fulfil a protective function.

2. The **phospholipids** are an integral part of cell structure and circulate in the blood; in the latter situation they are a means of transport for fatty acids.

3. The **sterols**. Cholesterol, the more important, is concerned with the transport of fatty acids; ergosterol has a role in vitamin D synthesis. The androgenic hormones and adrenocortical hormones are closely related to this group (hence the name steroids).

Functions of fats

1. To produce heat and energy. Fats yield **37 kJ per g** and therefore permit large increases in total energy intake without creating too much bulk or the need for frequent ingestion. The complete metabolism of fats in the cell is dependent upon the presence of an enzyme produced during carbohydrate metabolism. In the absence of this enzyme the incompletely metabolized products of fat, called ketoacids, are released into the circulation causing acidosis and nausea. If very large quantities of ketoacids are circulating, coma may ensue. These ketoacids are excreted by the kidneys and can be found in the urine of persons who are incompletely metabolizing fat for any reason, by testing for ketones using the appropriate reagent.

It can be appreciated that any condition in which the body is unable to metabolize carbohydrate, either because it is not being ingested, as in anorexia nervosa, or because it is unable to enter the cell, as in diabetes mellitus, will affect the metabolism of fat.

2. To form an integral part of cell structure.

3. To transport fat-soluble vitamins.

4. To protect organs and insulate the body by contributing to the formation of adipose tissue.

5. To add palatability to the diet and, by reducing the speed of gastric emptying, to increase the time available for mechanical digestion and the absorption of any glucose and water present through the gastric mucosa. By reducing the rate of gastric emptying, fats maintain the state of *satiety*, reduce the desire to eat again and therefore reduce the total energy intake and subsequent risk of obesity. Approximately 30% of the total energy intake is in the form of fat: **80 to 100 g per day**. This apparently large amount is easily ingested, if it is realized that one small pat of butter yields 8 g of fat; one slice of bacon 16 g; one large egg (mainly the yolk) 6 g; a portion of herring or mackerel 15 g; 20 peanuts 9 g.

Mineral salts

These are widely distributed in the body, forming approximately 4% total body weight, and are found in considerable variety and proportion. They are present as simple elements — salts or electrolytes — and have general functions related to:

1. The skeleton, of which they form 45%.

2. The body fluids, in which the electrolytes maintain the osmotic balance between the intracellular and extracellular fluids.

3. The acid-base balance of the body: many of the complex salts are capable of absorbing acids to maintain the blood within the range of pH 7.2 to 7.4.

Some minerals are found in quantity and must therefore be ingested in quantity;

these are sodium, potassium, calcium, iron, chlorides, magnesium, phosphorus and sulphur. Traces of iodine, copper, zinc, fluoride, cobalt and manganese are also found, but assessment of intake is rarely necessary as a normal diet would include adequate quantities.

Sodium

Functions of sodium

1. To give, with calcium, rigidity to bone.
2. To exert an osmotic effect by its presence, as an electrolyte, in the extracellular fluids.
3. To assist in maintaining the acid-base balance in the body. The salts of sodium which influence this balance are sodium bicarbonate, sodium carbonate and sodium phosphate.
4. To make the diet more palatable.

This last 'asset' results in the daily ingestion of about 20 g per day, but health could be maintained adequately if intake was **2 to 5 g per day**. Sodium is readily available in fish, meats and nearly all manufactured foods, is used as a preservative and is freely added to food as a condiment at table or in cooking.

In health, sodium imbalance rarely occurs because the excess intake is excreted by the kidneys and the necessary quantities are retained as a result of the action of aldosterone on the renal tubules. In occupations where severe sweating occurs, such as mining or smelting, fluid replacement without additional sodium will produce sodium depletion.

Conditions in which aldosterone activity is impaired, for instance Addison's disease (Ch. 11), or in which excessive sodium is lost, as in diarrhoea and vomiting, result in loss of sodium from the circulation with subsequent hypotension, muscle cramps, weakness and collapse. (It should be remembered that the heart is a muscular organ whose efficiency is dependent upon the concentrations of sodium and potassium on either side of the cell membranes.) Sodium retention causes oedema due to the increased osmotic pressure in the extracellular fluid. If sodium intake is reduced, the amount of water retention possible must also be reduced. As oedema is a feature of congestive cardiac failure and as it can be seen that the average daily intake of this mineral far exceeds need, the simple measure of restricting added salt in cooking and at table, combined with the avoidance of foods preserved in salt, may greatly influence the patient's progress.

Potassium

Aldosterone influences the excretion of potassium by the kidneys and a daily intake of **2 to 5 g** of potassium is adequate. Fish, meat, vegetables and some fruits, especially citrus fruits and grapes, are rich sources of this mineral. Pathological conditions attributable to inadequate potassium intake are unknown.

Functions of potassium

1. To maintain osmotic balance between intracellular fluid (in which it is present in relatively high concentrations) and extracellular fluid.
2. To exercise an important role in muscle contraction (notably the heart) and nerve conductability.

Retention of potassium may occur as a result of renal disease, or Addison's disease; a raised serum potassium level is a characteristic feature of these conditions. The nurse should appreciate the need to discourage the intake of fruit juices by such patients and seek alternatives to meet their fluid needs. Depletion of body potassium, from diuretic therapy, severe diarrhoea with desquamation of intestinal mucosa, diabetic (hyperglycaemic) coma, or inability to absorb potassium due to prolonged use of liquid paraffin as a laxative will cause potassium to leave the cells and enter the circulation, thus giving rise to high serum potassium levels. Muscle cramps and cardiac irregularities will ensue. It is important to note that rapid changes in serum potassium levels, which can occur, for example, when infusing potassium in intravenous solutions, can cause severe cardiac arrhythmia or sudden death due to ventricular fibrillation. As the nurse is responsible for the regulation of the rate of intravenous infusions within the time span ordered by the medical staff, she should be aware of the special dangers of irregular flow when potassium is added to the fluid and avoid them.

Calcium

Calcium is absorbed in the gut, stored in the bones and excreted by the kidneys under the control of parathormone. This is activated by a negative feed-back mechanism; when the serum calcium level drops, the hormone is released and raises the serum calcium by (a) increasing absorption, (b) increasing solubility of the stored calcium in bone so that it enters the circulation and (c) reducing excretion.

Functions of calcium

1. Calcium forms a major part of bones and teeth (Fig. 4.8). Its presence is especially important during their formation in fetal life and childhood, and for their subsequent maintenance and repair.
2. It maintains neuromuscular stability.
3. It is essential for the clotting mechanism of blood (see Ch. 8).

Daily requirements are **1 g per day**, but this should be exceeded during pregnancy and childhood. Sources are milk, cheese, eggs, cereals, soft-boned fish (for instance, pilchards, of which the bones are eaten) and green vegetables.

Deficiency may result from a poor diet or failure to absorb calcium adequately from the gut. Absorption of calcium is increased in the presence of proteins and vitamin D, whilst unabsorbed fatty acids and phytic acid (a compound of carbo-

DIETARY INTAKE   Proteins (+vitamin C)   Calcium (+vitamin D)   Sodium

Absorption

Balance dependent upon:

Small intestine

Excretion of waste

Kidney

Parathyroid gland secretion (parathormone)

Adrenal cortex (mineralocorticoids and glucocorticoids)

Formation of matrix therefore more required if growth or repair occurring

Mineral deposition

Strength

Figure 4.8
Bone development

hydrate metabolism) hinder calcium absorption. The deficiency produces rickets, osteomalacia, tetany and bruising. Tetany may be the first evidence of the accidental removal of one or more of the parathyroid glands during surgery of the thyroid gland, with consequent reduction in parathormone secretion (see Ch. 11).

Retention of calcium results from a parathyroid tumour, which continues to secrete parathormone despite a high serum calcium level causing renal calculi, dental caries and osteomalacia. The clotting mechanism is not affected (except possibly in the newborn producing haemolysis), as the amount of calcium required is not quantitative for this function and clotting will occur provided the serum calcium level is not **below** normal levels.

Iron

This is necessary for the formation of haemoglobin (Fig. 4.9). Normal daily requirements of **12 mg** should be increased during pregnancy; women during their menstrual years should ensure that this level is maintained. Red meat, liver, egg yolks, oatmeal, pulses, green vegetables and chocolate are rich sources; two slices

Figure 4.9
Erythrocyte and haemoglobin formation

of calves' liver yields 9 mg of iron; 100 g of dark chocolate 4 mg. The absorption of iron is increased in the presence of proteins and vitamin C, whereas oxalic acid (found in rhubarb) and phytic acid interfere with its absorption.

Deficiency due to failure of absorption, lack of adequate intake or excessive loss results in *hypochromic microcytic* anaemia. Female nurses should recognize the need to maintain an adequate iron intake so that deficiency is avoided with its consequent fatigue, loss of efficiency and accident proneness. The frequency with which iron-deficiency anaemia is found in the elderly, who form an increasingly large proportion of the patient population, should be borne in mind when planning nursing care, with particular reference to the problems of wound healing and the prevention of trauma.

Chlorides, magnesium, phosphorus and sulphur

These are present in quantity in all living matter and therefore do not present a dietary problem.

Of the trace elements mentioned previously, the role of two is of special significance to certain social groups.

Iodine

This mineral is found in seafood and in vegetables grown near the sea. It is a constituent of the thyroid hormones and is therefore concerned with general metabolism. Before the development of rapid and refrigerated transportation methods, land-locked areas such as Derbyshire and Switzerland had a restricted supply of this mineral, and iodine deficiency with simple goitre formation resulted. To overcome the problem, iodine was added to all table salt by the processors, but this practice is no longer necessary.

Fluorine

This mineral may play a valuable part in the prevention of dental caries (and the resultant digestive problems of poor mastication) because of its role in the formation of bone and dental enamel. It is found naturally in many areas of the world in drinking water, and can be added artificially to promote dental health. Such mass medication is not acceptable in some societies, and in some areas weekly mouth-washes with fluoride solutions for schoolchildren are substituted.

Vitamins

These are classified according to source, that is fat-soluble and water-soluble vitamins. The fat-soluble vitamins are A, D, E and K; the water-soluble vitamins are the B complex group and vitamin C. Utilization of vitamins is affected by various factors: the availability of the substance (it may be present but in an unabsorbable form) or the inability to digest the fats in which the fat-soluble vitamins are found. Some substances in food, termed **antivitamins**, may be taken up by the body and may block the activity of the true vitamin at its site of action in enzyme systems. Another factor is the availability of **provitamins**: these are substances which can be converted by the body into specific vitamins. Finally, the gut normally contains bacterial flora capable of synthesizing significant amounts of some vitamins.

Roughage

Cellulose is one of the three most important polysaccharides in man's diet, the other two being glycogen and starch. Like the others, it is formed from several glucose molecules linked together, but man is unable to break this down and so it remains undigested within the lumen of the gut. It forms the bulk of faeces and plays an important role in stimulating peristalsis. The highly refined diet of the Western world, low in roughage, is thought to be a significant factor in the high incidence of diverticulitis. A chemical product of cellulose, *methyl cellulose*, which is inert,

Table 4.1
Fat-soluble vitamins — A, D, E, K

Vitamin	Daily requirement	Functions	Dietary or other sources	Deficiency symptoms
A (retinol) Precursor-carotene is converted to Vitamin A in walls of small intestine	750 μg	1. Assists in the synthesis of mucous secretions which prevent epithelial tissues from hardening. 2. Maintains normal vision in dim light. Visual purple (rhodopsin), present in the rods of the retina is decomposed in bright light and restored by Vitamin A. 3. Promotes good tooth structure by producing ameloblasts (enamel-producing epithelial cells). 4. Promotes normal growth in children.	Animal sources — liver, chicken, kidneys, eggs, whole milk, butter, fish liver oils, fortified margarine. Plant sources — (precursor) carrots, leafy green and yellow vegetables, fruit.	Follicular hyperkeratosis. Xerophthalmia. Nyctalopia (night blindness, poor adaptation to dim light). Prone to infection of mucous membranes. Poor tooth formation.
D (calciferol)	2.5 μg — 10 μg	1. Aids normal skeletal development. 2. Facilitates absorption of calcium and phosphorus.	Action of ultra-violet rays of sunlight on skin. Dietary sources — eggs, butter, oily fish, cod-liver oil. Artificial sources — produced by irradiation of plant sterols — medications, fortified margarine.	Rickets in children. Osteomalacia in adults. Poor teeth. Lowered blood calcium and phosphorus levels. Poor posture.
E (tocopherols)	20 mg	1. Helps in formation and function of red blood cells. 2. May protect red blood cells from haemolysis. 3. Protection of essential fatty acids. 4. Anti-oxidant.	Vegetable oils, green leafy vegetables, wholegrain cereals, wheatgerm, egg yolk, nuts.	Not recognized.
K (phytomenandione)	Very small amount met by dietary intake and bacterial synthesis.	Assists in the formation of prothrombin in the liver. Necessary for the coagulation of blood.	Green leafy vegetables, wheatgerm.	Prolonged clotting time of blood. Haemorrhagic disease of the newborn.

tasteless and bulky because of its hygroscopic action, is used therapeutically to increase the bulk of ileostomy excretions; it can also be given to persons prescribed weight-control diets to reduce hunger pangs.

Water

All plant and animal life is composed of a high proportion of water. The maintenance of water balance depends on intake, the various means by which fluid is lost from the body and the controls. Intake is regulated by the thirst mechanism, which is activated by a series of neurosecretory mechanisms that monitor the osmolality of the blood. When thirsty, fluids are taken into the body and the antidiuretic hormone from the posterior pituitary is released to increase the reabsorption of water from the distal convoluted tubules of the nephrons.

Fluid is lost from the body in measurable quantities via the kidneys and in the faeces. Insensible loss through the skin can become an important mechanism in maintaining fluid balance if the environmental or body temperature is raised; water vapour is also lost in expiration.

Control of fluid loss is exerted mainly in the kidney, but the formation of urine, which is a means of excreting many waste products, requires a sufficient intake of fluid to dilute the waste products adequately.

Table 4.2
Water — soluble vitamins — B complex, C

Vitamin	Daily requirement	Functions	Dietary sources	Deficiency symptoms
B₁ (thiamine)	0.4 mg for every 4200 kJ of intake	Necessary for complete metabolism of carbohydrate.	Meat (especially pork). Liver. Nuts. Wholegrain and enriched cereals and bread. Brown rice and wheatgerm. Milk, dairy foods, eggs. Brewer's yeast.	*Beriberi* with symptoms: polyneuritis anorexia, fatigue depression irritability pain, weakness and inco-ordination of leg movements abnormal carbohydrate metabolism.
B₂ (riboflavin)	1–2 mg	Necessary for cell oxidation and reduction processes and efficient use of carbohydrates, proteins and fats.	Wholegrain and enriched cereals. Milk, dairy foods. Liver. Eggs. Leafy vegetables. Liver concentrates.	Greasy, scaly skin. Stomatitis. Cheilosis. Bloodshot eyes, blurred vision. Glossitis.
B₃ (niacin, nicotinic acid nicotinamide)	10 mg	Essential for tissue oxidation and needed by central nervous system to maintain mental health.	Meat, especially liver and kidneys. Fish and poultry. Wholegrain and enriched cereals. Pulse vegetables. Nuts. Milk and eggs.	*Pellagra* with symptoms: depression or dementia dermatitis diarrhoea.
B₆ (pyridoxine)	Trace.	Important in metabolism of amino acids. Regulation of nervous system.	Lean meats. Wholegrain cereals, dried yeast. Walnuts, leafy green vegetables.	In infants, convulsions.
B (folic acid)	Trace. Increased need in pregnancy.	Essential for development of red blood cells.	Green leafy vegetables, yellow fruits and vegetables, yeasts, meats nuts, milk.	Megaloblastic anaemia.
B₁₂ (cyanocobalamin)	Trace.	1. Necessary for formation and maturation of red blood cells (see Fig. 4.9). (It is the extrinsic factor and requires the intrinsic factor produced by the oxyntic cells of the stomach for its absorption.) 2. Needed for functioning of all cells particularly of bone marrow, nervous system and gastrointestinal system.	Animal sources — liver, kidneys, fish, beef, milk and dairy products.	*Macrocytic anaemia* due to: 1. inadequate intake of Vitamin B₁₂ (e.g. vegetarians) 2. deficiency of intrinsic factor (e.g. Addisonian pernicious anaemia, total gastrectomy) 3. bacterial or parasitic interruption of normal absorption in alimentary canal 4. malabsorption syndrome.
C (ascorbic acid)	30–70 mg	1. Production of collagen. 2. Necessary for growth and tissue repair. 3. Aids absorption of iron by reducing ferric iron to ferrous iron in gastrointestinal tract. 4. Formation of red blood cells in bone marrow.	Citrus fruits, tomatoes, leafy green vegetables, potatoes, small berry fruits.	1. Weakness, proneness to infection, pains in limbs and joints. 2. *Scurvy* — prolonged deficiency.

Summary of the functions of nutrients

A nutrient must be capable of one of the following:

1. Providing heat and energy — the 'go' foods: carbohydrates, fats, B vitamins.
2. Building and repairing tissue — the 'grow' foods: protein, calcium, vitamins A and D.
3. Regulating body processes and vitality — the 'glow' foods: iron and vitamin C.

In terms of food groups (Fig. 4.3) the functions are:

Group 1
For energy, production of heat and to reduce hunger.
Groups 2 and 3
For growth and repair.
Group 4
For general health and vitality.
Group 5
For concentrated energy and warmth.
Groups 6, 7 and 8
To add variety and give pleasure.

Presentation of meals

Food is important to every patient and it is the nurse's responsibility to ensure that meals are served under hygienic conditions, that the patient receives the correct diet and that the food is attractively presented to the patient.

Many hospitals now have a menu selection system which allows the patient to select foods from a wide choice of items daily for each meal to suit his individual preferences, or it may be used as a guide for the patient who requires to follow a specific dietary regime. Foods suitable for these diets are indicated by a code letter — D = diabetic, P = low protein, F = low fat, R = reducing (Fig. 4.10). This

Figure 4.10
Sample menu

GENERAL HOSPITAL

WARD
NAME

MONDAY 1   BREAKFAST

☐ PORRIDGE   D.R.P.F.
or
☐ RICE CRISPIES   D.R.P.F.
or
☐ CORN FLAKES   D.R.P.F.
or
☐ ALPEN   P,F.

☐ MORNING ROLL   D.R.P.F.
or
☐ WHITE BREAD   D.R.P.F.
or
☐ BROWN BREAD   D.R.P.F.

☐ MARGARINE   D.R.P.F.
or
☐ BUTTER   D.R.P.F.

☐ MARMALADE   P.F.

CODE –
D=DIABETIC   F=LOW FAT
P=LOW PROTEIN   R=REDUCING

SOME MODIFICATION MAY BE NECESSARY
FOR SPECIAL DIETS

GENERAL HOSPITAL

WARD
NAME

MONDAY 1   LUNCH

☐ TOMATO SOUP   D.P.F.
or
☐ FRUIT JUICE   D.R.P.F.

☐ STEWED STEAK & VEGETABLES   D.R.P.F.
or
☐ HAGGIS   D.P.
or
☐ CHEESE, EGG & POTATO NEST   D.P.R.
or
☐ VEAL & HAM PIE   D.P.

☐ CREAMED POTATO   D.R.P.F.
and/or
☐ CHIPPED POTATO   D.P.
☐ CABBAGE   D.R.P.F.
and/or
☐ TURNIP   D.R.P.F.
☐ PUREED VEGETABLE   D.R.P.F.
☐ SALAD   D.R.P.F.

☐ STEAMED JAM ROLL   P.
☐ CUSTARD   D.P.F.
or
☐ BAKED RICE PUDDING   D.P.F.
or
☐ FRESH FRUIT   D.R.P.F.
or
☐ CHEESE & BISCUITS   D.

SCRAMBLED EGG, and JELLY or ICE CREAM
can be provided as alternatives at Lunch and
Supper.

GENERAL HOSPITAL

WARD
NAME

MONDAY 1   SUPPER

☐ ASPARAGUS SOUP   D.P.F.

☐ HOT GAMMON & PINEAPPLE   D.R.P.F.
or
☐ POACHED EGG & SPAGHETTI   D.R.P.F.
or
☐ CHICKEN SANDWICH   D.R.P.F.

☐ BOILED POTATOES   D.R.P.F.
☐ BROCCOLI   D.R.P.F.

☐ TRIFLE   D.P.F.
or
☐ CHEESE & BISCUITS   D.R.

☐ WHITE BREAD   D.R.P.F.
or
☐ BROWN BREAD   D.R.P.F.
☐ BUTTER   D.R.P.F.
or
☐ MARGARINE   D.R.P.F.
☐ JAM   P.F.

enables the patient to make an informed choice and not feel different from the other patients in the ward. Special therapeutic diets require consultation with the dietitian, but he will try to provide the amended diet in the most palatable way for the patient.

Nurses are not now responsible for the preparation of food and in many hospitals a 'plated' service is in operation (e.g. the Gannymede system). The nurse must still check every meal for accuracy against the pre-selected menu and ensure that appropriate utensils are provided to suit the needs of individual patients. Modified cutlery or aids may be required or the patient may need to have his food cut up for him.

Ill patients require oral hygiene and careful positioning prior to meals. The patient should have the opportunity to empty his bladder and wash his hands, and the environment should be made as conducive to eating as possible by removing any unpleasant objects from sight before the meal is served.

Skill, patience and care are necessary in order to feed a patient successfully. The nurse must take account of the rate at which the patient is able to eat and when he prefers to take fluids. She should sit down beside the patient if assisting in the feeding and make eating a pleasant, social occasion for him.

After the meal, the nurse must record the amount of fluid taken and report to the nurse in charge if food has been left or refused.

Preparation and care of food

Cooking

Cooking of food by any method may change the nutritional value by rendering some components less absorbable or by splitting coarse fibrous coatings, such as are found on pulses and cereals, enabling the digestive enzymes to act upon the starch and protein they contain. Meat fibres are converted into gelatin — tougher (that is, more fibrous) meat takes longer to reach this stage. Meat tenderized in this way is more readily digested.

The method of cooking used may destroy some of the nutritional value of food; minerals and water-soluble vitamins may be lost in large quantities when the cooking water is discarded — hence the value of steaming or using minimum quantities of water when cooking vegetables. The loss that results from washing rice in societies where it forms a major part of the diet is sufficient to cause beriberi.

The most easily destroyed nutrient is ascorbic acid. Its decomposition occurs as a result of oxidation. The process is more rapid in the presence of heat, enzyme action, alkalis, traces of copper and free access to atmospheric oxygen. As storage in the body is not possible, care must be taken to protect sources of this vitamin from copper cooking pots, prolonged cooking, 'keeping warm' (even standing in strong sunlight) or standing uncovered.

Obviously cooking may increase the nutritional value of a diet. Salt may be added to enhance flavour and other additives may increase palatability so that intake is encouraged. Using oils for frying increases the vitamin and energy intake. For oedematous patients it may be necessary to use salt substitutes in cooking and at table, and alternative methods of food preparation must be practised if the obese individual is to lose weight.

By producing and maintaining a temperature high enough to kill micro-organisms, cooking serves a preservative and protective function. But this asset can be negated by careless food handlers with unclean personal habits or by using dirty equipment or inappropriate storage methods.

Storage

Storage methods are geared to the prevention of contamination by vectors and to the provision of an environment in which micro-organisms will not multiply (Ch. 1).

Preservation

Refrigeration (short term) and freezing (longer term) are suitable for many foods and do not adversely affect nutritional value. It is important to note the advice of manufacturers regarding the maintenance of equipment and the length of time for which specific foods may be stored. Once defrosted, frozen foods are subject to the same deterioration and contamination risks; usually they may not be refrozen.

Canning of goods, whole or evaporated to reduce bulk, involves an airtight container which is then sterilized by heat. Provided the tin is undamaged and the canning process is carried out correctly, goods preserved in this way retain their food value almost indefinitely. If the tin is damaged, micro-organisms can enter; if the sterilization process fails, any micro-organisms in the tin will multiply producing gases and the 'blown' tin.

Smoking, pickling and salting all produce environments not conducive to growth and multiplication of micro-organisms. Drying is an effective means of preservation since all living organisms require water to sustain life; however, storage in a safe place is necessary to avoid contamination from mice and rats.

Food legislation

Two principles govern the legislation of food in the member states of the European Economic Community:

1. Protection of health.
2. Prevention of fraud (to protect the purchaser and the manufacturer).

Nationally, each member country has its own food legislation. The Food and Drugs Act 1955 was the main piece of legislation in England and Wales, and there is similar legislation in Scotland and Northern Ireland. This legislation makes it an offence to sell food which is not of the quality demanded, to label food falsely, to add to or remove from food substances that would render it harmful to health, or to sell unsound food. Many regulations supporting these main provisions and recommendations are made by the Food Standards Committee and the Food Additives and Contaminants Committee.

PHYSIOLOGICAL CHANGES INFLUENCING NUTRITIONAL NEEDS

Under certain circumstances it may be necessary to adjust the intake of one or all the components of the balanced diet to meet changes in body needs. The presentation of the diet may be modified in infancy, childhood and old age. Modifications may be necessary to meet changing physiological needs in healthy individuals or the changes arising from pathological processes.

The rate of growth of all tissues demands a large supply of proteins for cell structure, calcium for bones and iron for the formation of large numbers of red blood cells to provide oxygen for the anabolic process. Vitamin supplements, notably of vitamins A and D, may be of value, especially in deprived areas.

Infancy

The nutritional needs of infants are met by feeding with milk (p. 592). Human milk meets the needs of the normal baby. If this is not available other milks may be used but only after being modified. This is to ensure that they will be easily digested by the infant and will have the correct proportions of protein, fat, carbohydrate and minerals. Babies fed on unmodified milks may suffer brain damage as a result of *hypernatraemia*. There is also a grave risk of infection if fresh milk is used.

Cow's milk is the obvious alternative to breast milk in this country and can be obtained easily in fully modified form with vitamins and sugar already added. There are both liquid and powder preparations available.

Goat's milk may be used if there is a history of allergy to cow's milk. It is fairly easy to obtain but should be used only under medical supervision. It is essential to ensure that the milk is free from infection especially as regards brucellosis.

Childhood and adolescence

During adolescence the increased energy needs must be met as well as the protein and mineral needs for the final growth spurt. The temptation is to increase the carbohydrate content of the diet on the grounds of economy. Although understandable, this solution increases the problem of teenage acne and may initiate obesity or promote the liking for sweet things, which will persist when physical activity decreases.

Adulthood

Women, because of their physiology, are prone to iron deficiency anaemia throughout their menstruating years. The use of the contraceptive pill, with the resulting reduction in menstrual flow, and the smaller average family size, with less strain being placed on a woman's iron stores, have reduced the severity of the problem but not its frequency in society as a whole.

During pregnancy, the needs of the developing fetus will be met at the expense of maternal needs, especially of the minerals iron and calcium. A diet rich in these should be advised and iron and folic-acid supplements supplied to meet the high demands for these by the fetus.

During lactation, large quantities of nutrients are lost from the maternal stores. However, in the later stages of pregnancy a woman increases her deposits of adipose tissue and does not need to 'eat for two' in terms of carbohydrates and fats. Proteins must be ingested in large quantities, however, since they cannot be stored. Equally, calcium and vitamins must be taken in, either from the diet or from supplements. An adequate fluid intake is also necessary if the needs of the thirsty baby are to be met satisfactorily.

SOME PATHOLOGICAL STATES INFLUENCING NUTRITIONAL NEEDS

Modifications to diet will be necessary if pathological processes interfere with the ability to digest, absorb, assimilate or excrete all or any components of the normal balanced diet. An understanding of the physiology of digestion and absorption and of the assimilation and excretion processes and their controls, together with a comprehension of the nature of the various pathological processes (such as inflammation or tumours), will ensure that the nurse sees the specific modification of the intake as a logical part of a patient's therapy.

Table 4.3
Special milk preparations

Type of preparation	Name	For treatment of:
Low protein	Prosparol	Renal disease
Low sodium	Edosol	Cardiac failure
Low calcium	Locasol	Hyperparathyroidism
	Low Calcium Milk Food	
Low lactose	Galactomin	Galactosaemia
	Nutramigen	
	Low Lactose Milk Food	
Low phenylalanine	Minafen	Phenylketonuria
	Lofenalac	
	Albumaid	
Soya bean	Velactin	These are free of milk proteins
	Formula S Soya Food	and suitable for treating children
	Wysoy	who seem allergic to caseinogen
		and lactalbumen
Low fat	Cow and Gate Separated	Obesity
	Milk Food	
	Medium Chain	
	Triglyceride (MCT) Oil	

Diseases requiring dietary modification as part of therapy are discussed in the relevant chapters for example, see diabetes mellitus in Chapter 11.

Pathological conditions in the young child in which dietary modifications are therapeutic require **special milk preparations** to meet specific needs. Many firms produce various suitable products, available by prescription only. Some examples are given in Table 4.3.

DISEASES OF MALNUTRITION

Malnutrition — or bad nourishment — is a term which describes a range of pathological conditions whose causal factors are related to an intake of food (or its availability in the body) which is unsuited to the body's needs. The treatment, therefore, is concerned with establishing the cause and applying dietary modifications as appropriate. Some of these disorders may result from genetic defects, by which the normal metabolic processes are blocked, while others result from a developing hypersensitivity to specific nutrients.

The deficiency diseases are conditions in which one particular dietary component is available in insufficient quantity; the disorders in this group commonly found in Great Britain are discussed below, but others of significance elsewhere are kwashiorkor and scurvy. Subnutrition is another aspect of malnutrition, in which one or more of the major energy providing foods is inadequate; examples are anorexia nervosa (see p. 574 and Ch. 16), those suffering from malabsorption syndrome (see p. 191), or starvation. A major nutritional disorder in which excessive amounts of food (principally carbohydrates) are ingested is obesity (see p. 169).

It should not be thought that these three groups are mutually exclusive. Persons suffering from subnutrition may well be more profoundly affected by one specific deficiency which general re-feeding will not rectify. It is also not uncommon for obese people, whose dietary intake is often grossly distorted, to suffer from a deficiency disease, usually iron deficiency anaemia.

Rickets

This disease of calcium and phosphorus metabolism results from an insufficient intake or synthesis of vitamin D and, additionally, inadequate calcium in the diet. Increasing costs of the foods which would supply these nutrients and overcrowding in industrial cities, combined with diets high in cereals and low in milk and milk products, have produced an increased incidence particularly among immigrant populations.

Clinical features

The growth rate of the child is greater than the speed at which he can form bone, and hard bone produced by adequate quantities of mineral deposits is not achieved.

Lack of calcium also affects muscle tone and the child is restless, pale and flabby. He has a distended abdomen (due to weak abdominal muscles and intestinal fermentation from the high carbohydrate content of the diet) and tends to sweat excessively, especially over the scalp. The normal milestones of sitting up, crawling, standing, walking and eruption of teeth are delayed; the 'soft' teeth are vulnerable to caries and the 'soft' bones to deformity once weight-bearing occurs. Deformity of the chest is accompanied by both a prominent sternum and spinal deviations; in the female, pelvic deformities may cause serious difficulties later at childbirth.

Delayed milestones, a fretful, sweaty baby and poor dietary history, combined with radiological evidence and a raised serum alkaline phosphatase level, will establish the diagnosis. Early recognition and treatment will prevent irreversible bony deformities.

Treatment

Treatment depends on establishing an adequate intake of calcium in the diet and a therapeutic dose of vitamin D. This ranges from 1000 to 8000 iu daily and should be continued until the serum alkaline phosphatase level returns to normal, after which the vitamin D dose should be gradually reduced to the prophylactic level of 400 *iu* daily. It can be given as cod-liver oil, halibut-liver oil or calciferol, depending on the quantity which would be required to give the prescribed dose. It is important to improve the environment of the child; often he is overdressed and his mother may need tactful education to allow him to be outside in the sunshine as much as possible and to continue the improved diet once he appears well. It is in this area that the nurse in the community can play a vital role, as well as by noting any early symptoms.

Osteomalacia (Fig. 4.11)

This is the adult counterpart of rickets. Calcium and vitamin D are deficient with a resulting failure to lay down calcium in the organic matrix of bone; therefore the ratio of calcium phosphate to matrix is reduced. In Eastern countries it occurs in women who live on a high cereal diet with little milk, who rarely go out into the sunshine and who by repeated pregnancies (and lactation) are depleted of calcium. In Western societies it is more common as a secondary feature of chronic renal disease or some form of malabsorption.

Clinical features

Bone pain and tenderness may be prominent and the gait is uneven due to pain in tarsal and metatarsal joints. Spontaneous fractures may occur, and iron deficiency anaemia is usually present. Diagnosis is made on clinical evidence — the radiological appearance of generalized rarefaction and the presence of pseudofractures, which are pathognomonic of osteomalacia.

Treatment

Treatment is based upon dietary correction or the addition of calcium lactate to the diet in countries where dairy produce is not readily available. Vitamin D in doses up to 50 000 *iu* daily must be given. Bony deformities do not respond to medical treatment and will require surgical correction.

NORMAL Collagen fibres
Calcium deposits } equal proportions

OSTEOPOROSIS Normal ratio collagen:calcium
but BOTH reduced

OSTEOMALACIA Collagen normal but
reduced calcium

Figure 4.11
Osteoporosis and osteomalacia

Osteoporosis (Fig. 4.11)

In this condition, which is the most common nutritional bone disease found in clinical practice, there is atrophy of bone leading to a reduction of the total quantity of bone. Thus the ratio of calcium phosphate to matrix is normal. It may be localized as a result of inflammation or neoplasm or, more commonly, immobilization. Hence the bedridden, the elderly, the patient whose movement is reduced by pain (as in rheumatoid arthritis) or splinting will be prone to this condition. The importance of early mobilization, active (and where necessary passive) physiotherapy and adequate pain relief should be noted as a part of nursing care, especially of the elderly.

Generalized osteoporosis is associated with the reduction of androgen formation and occurs more commonly in women and at an earlier age due to the abrupt nature of the menopause. Malnutrition, with associated abnormal protein metabolism, and endocrine disorders such as Cushing's syndrome, thyrotoxicosis and acromegaly exacerbate the condition. Corticosteroid therapy over prolonged periods is also associated with this condition. Osteoporosis in the young is generally found in conjunction with hypofunction of the gonads.

Diagnosis and treatment

Diagnosis is made on the history and radiological appearances. Blood chemistry is all normal. Treatment is aimed at:

1. Relieving pain, which may be severe and incapacitating.
2. Preventing deformity, especially of the spine, which may damage the cervical, thoracic or lumbar nerves.
3. Reducing the demineralization of bone by increasing mobility.
4. Enhancing the opportunities for adequate bone formation by a good mixed diet, rich in calcium and protein.

Supplements of calcium and vitamin D may help. The administration of hormones (oestrogens, androgens and other anabolic agents) leads to the relief of pain and an increased sense of well-being. There is no evidence that any of the above measures increases the amount of bone laid down, but it appears that the progress of the disease is arrested.

Prevention

Prevention is the important factor, as this is a slowly progressive disease. An active life and a well-balanced diet which includes a pint of milk daily would be the appropriate approach. As advancing years are associated with the onset of many chronic conditions which affect appetite and mobility, their adequate management and the appreciation of these factors in the patient's future well-being will reduce the degree of osteoporosis from which the elderly may suffer.

Nutritional anaemia

Anaemia occurs where there is prolonged loss of blood or a dietary deficiency of the nutrients necessary for the formation of red blood cells — iron, protein, copper, folic acid and vitamins B_6 and B_{12} and C. A deficiency of any one nutrient may cause anaemia but an iron-deficiency anaemia is common in all age groups (Ch. 8).

Nutritional anaemia is more common in infancy due to growth requirements and in old age due to a poor dietary intake of iron. The clinical presentation in the latter age group may be fatigue and pallor, an increased susceptibility to infection, mental confusion and anorexia which will exacerbate the problem. Anaemia may present where there is an adequate dietary iron intake but an increased loss due to persistent bleeding such as menstrual loss, or an increased demand for iron as in pregnancy.

Careful dietary review is necessary and an adequate intake of foods containing rich sources of iron should be recommended. Good sources of iron are cocoa, liver, kidneys and shellfish. The diet may require to be supplemented by elemental iron in order to speed up the recovery process.

Phenylketonuria

This is a condition in which, due to a genetic defect, the enzyme necessary to convert phenylalanine, a protein substance, to tyrosin is missing. The blood levels of phenylalanine rise above the normal 1 to 2 mg/ml and these high levels damage the developing brain, resulting in severe mental retardation. Though a rare condition (1 in 10 000 births) and incurable, it is possible by dietetic means to prevent the brain damage, which only occurs once milk feeding is established and consequently high levels of phenylalanine enter the blood.

Diagnosis

Early diagnosis is essential. This is made by estimating the level of phenylalanine in the infant's blood, usually between the seventh and tenth day of life. (A minimum of 48 hours must have passed since the commencement of milk feeding.) This blood test is called the Guthrie test.

Treatment

Treatment is aimed at keeping the blood level of phenylalanine below 5 mg/100 ml and is achieved by feeding the baby with a low phenylalanine preparation (Minafen). Change to mixed feeding of non-phenylalanine foods usually occurs early, since the milk preparations have an unpleasant taste and smell. Regular Guthrie tests are the most reliable monitor of the child's condition, but a quick estimation can be made by testing the urine with Phenistix for the presence of phenylpyruvic acid, which will occur if the blood level of phenylalanine rises above 15 mg/100 ml. Ingenuity on the part of the mother and encouragement and support from medical and nursing staff are necessary to ensure that the child takes his diet. The management of the diet requires expert advice, as the number of proprietary foods, such as soups, to which protein substances have been added is enormous and limits choice. It is very expensive.

It is possible that only the developing brain of the young child is vulnerable to the effects of high phenylalanine levels, and therefore a gradual return to a more normal food intake may be possible once the child is about 10 years of age. The major practical difficulty in testing this theory lies in the inability to measure reliably intellectual ability. Mental deterioration, should it occur after the introduction of normal diet, is likely to be slow. It may, therefore, be impossible to diagnose before irreversible damage has occurred.

Cystic fibrosis

Clinical features

The baby with this condition may present before 3 months of age suffering from 'failure to thrive', or 'malabsorption syndrome'. He is likely to be irritable, pale in appearance, with a ravenous appetite and yet static weight or actual weight loss, abdominal distension and offensive, fatty stools. The condition is caused by a **genetic defect** which results in the absence of the pancreatic enzymes, amylase, lipase and trypsin. Digestion is impaired, absorption cannot take place and the child is hungry. He will also exhibit signs of calcium and vitamin deficiency.

Diagnosis

It is important that other causes of malabsorption are excluded, and the nurse plays a vital role in assisting in various diagnostic tests. A **sweat test**, in which a piece of filter paper is placed on a carefully cleaned part of the child's arm or thigh and enclosed by a polythene square, may be carried out. It must be kept in place for half an hour, and is then sent for estimation of sodium content. Sweat from a child with this condition will contain an abnormally high level of sodium (above 60 mEq/litre). **Stool collections** will be required, and great skill is necessary to achieve this from such a young baby; they are sent for estimation of fat content and tryptic activity. Estimation of tryptic activity is performed on juices removed from the duodenum. This entails passing a radio-opaque tube via the nose or mouth into the duodenum. After checking that it is appropriately sited, the tube is aspirated and juices sent for analysis. As the tube may take some time to pass through the pylorus, great patience must be exercised by the nursing staff. The child must be fasted prior to the test, and prevented from removing the tube before the test is completed.

Management

Once diagnosed, the management of this condition is to replace the missing enzymes by using Pancrex, which can be sprinkled on to food, and by dietary modification. This involves a low fat diet, as the digestion and absorption of proteins and carbohydrates are reduced in the presence of much fat in the intestines. Alfonal and the Cow and Gate Separated Milk preparations both provide a fat content of 0.1%. It is necessary to increase protein and carbohydrate intake to meet energy needs, and the fat-soluble vitamins A, D and possibly K must be given as water-soluble supplements. Unfortunately, the other aspect of this disease, the viscosity of mucus, especially in the respiratory tract, is less easily managed. These patients suffer from recurring, severe respiratory infection and most die in their early teenage years.

Coeliac disease (gluten-induced enteropathy)

The main pathological finding in coeliac disease is an abnormal mucosa in the small intestine due to a sensitivity to gluten resulting in malabsorption of nutrients. It is not known precisely why gluten induces this damage and flattening of the villi of the small intestine but the agent responsible for the damage has been identified as gliadin, a polypeptide fraction of gluten. Gluten is found in the temperate grains, wheat, rye, oats and barley.

Clinical features

Coeliac disease may be diagnosed in any age-group but commonly becomes apparent in the early years of life following the introduction of cereals to the diet. The child who has previously been healthy ceases to put on weight, becomes irritable, growth is retarded and the disorder is characterized by the passage of pale, bulky, offensive stools. The abdomen becomes distended and gradually iron deficiency anaemia develops. Diarrhoea may also be a symptom.

In adults, the presentation of the disease may be different. The disease presents with symptoms of anaemia — tiredness and lethargy, loss of weight and possibly diarrhoea. Diagnosis may be more difficult to establish initially because of the vague symptoms, but any patient with unexplained weight loss and symptoms of anaemia should undergo investigations for malabsorption.

Confirmation of coeliac disease may be made by examining a specimen of small intestine histologically. This is obtained by the use of a Crosby capsule (p. 183) which is a fine tube with a metal capsule attached which is capable of obtaining a small specimen of jejunal mucosa for examination or, if the patient has difficulty in swallowing the capsule, a specimen of the jejunal tissue may be obtained during endoscopy using biopsy forceps.

Treatment

Treatment is aimed at elimination of gluten from the diet. All products containing wheat, rye, oats or barley or their derivatives are excluded. This means that foods commonly used such as bread, cakes, biscuits and some cereals cannot be taken. Care must be exercised in the buying of manufactured products as many of these have additives containing gluten. Specially-prepared gluten-free flour, biscuits and pastas are obtainable on prescription. Initially the dietitian will advise which foods may or may not be eaten and also which fluids may be drunk because lemon barley water and certain beers contain gluten. Patients with coeliac disease can be encouraged to make their own bread, cakes and puddings using gluten-free flour. The Coeliac Society provides a useful booklet of information and recipes, and also regularly updates a leaflet on manufactured products which are gluten-free which is a useful guide for shopping.

Most patients respond after a month or more on a gluten-free diet but may require iron and vitamin supplements initially. Patients who do not respond should have a very careful dietary assessment carried out as they may inadvertently be eating foods which contain gluten. This dietary modification is palatable and does not present as great a problem in some ways as the management of phenylketonuria. It is, however, expensive, and may need to be continued for life, as it is doubtful if complete recovery ever occurs.

Anorexia nervosa (Fig. 4.12A)

This condition presents as a desire by the person, usually an adolescent girl or young woman to achieve and maintain an abnormally low body weight. There may be a history of obesity in the family or the girl may have been through a phase of obesity when she was teased and taunted. The girl is often intelligent and obliging and the emergence of the desire for slimness may be related to stressful situations such as school examinations. Food in the home is usually plentiful and both parents and the girl will often deny anything is wrong until the condition is very serious. Special regimes of treatment in a psychiatric hospital with regular observation and support will help the person towards achieving a target weight. The difficulty is to maintain the desired weight once the patient has been discharged from hospital. Bunch (1974) has commented on the distortion of body image and 'the vigour and stubbornness with which the often gruesome emaciation is defended as normal and right and the only possible protection against the dreaded fate of being too fat.'

Anorexia bulimia

Sometimes the eating patterns will consist of eating binges when large quantities of totally inappropriate or bizarre foods are bought and consumed. This is followed by

Figure 4.12
(A) Anorexia nervosa
(B) Obesity

Obesity (Fig. 4.7B)

induced vomiting or excessive purging and these practices are hidden from the family or friends. Specialist treatment is required and it is recognised that those patients who have a previous history of anorexia nervosa have a poorer prognosis in the treatment programme.

Obesity (Fig. 4.12B)

Obesity is the most common disease of malnutrition in the Western world. It results from ingesting more energy foods than are required for the energy expenditure; the excess is stored as fat. The term obesity is generally applied if the individual's weight is 10% in excess of the standard weight shown in Table 4.4. (The weights shown in this table include an allowance of 7 to 9 lb for men and 4 to 6 lb for women, to take account of clothing worn when weighed.)

Associated factors

There are many factors which may affect the regulating mechanism of appetite and produce obesity:

1. **Age and sex**. In childhood the sex ratio of obese subjects is equal. After puberty, obesity is much more common in women, especially after pregnancy and the menopause.

2. **Pregnancy**. Part of the weight gain during pregnancy is due to an increase in adipose tissue which serves as a store against the demands of lactation. This may not be lost after the baby is born or weaned, and with each subsequent pregnancy, the woman's weight at the time of conception will be greater than on the previous occasion.

3. **Economics**. Most cheap meals are formed largely of carbohydrates. These satisfy the appetite less readily than protein and fatty foods, so an increased quantity is eaten — hence the greater number of obese people in the lower economic groups.

4. **Eating habits**. Many obese people are nibblers, and people concerned with food preparation are particularly vulnerable. Obese people appear to be stimulated to eat more by habit than in response to stomach contractions due to hunger.

5. **Physical activity**. Scientific advances, which have provided mechanized household equipment and transport, enable work to be done without as much energy expenditure as in the past. The advent of sedentary leisure occupations like the cinema, television and radio, and our growing cities which discourage walking as an occupation, all increase the likelihood of obesity.

6. **Psychological factors**. Unhappy people may find solace in overeating and consequently become obese. On the other hand, there are many obese men and women who appear to lead happy, full lives.

7. **Genetics**. Although genetic factors may play a part, it is probable that environmental factors are more important, such as family custom and eating habits.

8. **Endocrine factors**. Many endocrine diseases are associated with weight gain, but it is unlikely that they are a cause of obesity.

9. **Overfeeding in childhood**. Fat babies tend to become fat adults. Fat cells which are formed in early childhood tend to refill rapidly, even after dieting has reduced their size. These unfortunates fight a constant battle against becoming overweight.

Consequences of obesity

Why treat obesity? The reduction of body weight will not remove any of the causative factors, but the obese person will feel better, look better and survive longer if his weight is reduced to the standard for his height and build.

Aesthetic considerations, which mean that the obese person finds it difficult to dress well and look attractive, may add to the burden of mechanical disabilities from which obese people suffer.

Mechanical problems result from the excessive weight the skeleton is being asked to support and transport. Flat feet and osteoarthrosis of the knees and hips are common. Muscular tissue is infiltrated with fat, giving rise to uterine prolapse,

Table 4.4

Desirable weights of adults according to height and frame (*from* Macleod J 1981 Davidson's Principles and Practice of Medicine, 13th edn. Churchill Livingstone, Edinburgh)

Height			Desirable weight in kilograms and pounds (in indoor clothing), ages 25 and over					
without shoes			Small frame		Medium frame		Large frame	
metres	ft	in	kg	lb	kg	lb	kg	lb
Men								
1.550	5	1	50.8–54.4	112–120	53.5–58.5	118–129	57.2–64	126–141
1.575	5	2	52.2–55.8	115–123	54.9–60.3	121–133	58.5–65.3	129–144
1.600	5	3	53.5–57.2	118–126	56.2–61.7	124–136	59.9–67.1	132–148
1.625	5	4	54.9–58.5	121–129	57.6–63	127–139	61.2–68.9	135–152
1.650	5	5	56.2–60.3	124–133	59–64.9	130–143	62.6–70.8	138–156
1.675	5	6	58.1–62.1	128–137	60.8–66.7	134–147	64.4–73	142–161
1.700	5	7	59.9–64	132–141	62.6–68.9	138–152	66.7–75.3	147–166
1.725	5	8	61.7–65.8	136–145	64.4–70.8	142–156	68.5–77.1	151–170
1.750	5	9	63.5–68	140–150	66.2–72.6	146–160	70.3–78.9	155–174
1.775	5	10	65.3–69.9	144–154	68–74.8	150–165	72.1–81.2	159–179
1.800	5	11	67.1–71.7	148–158	69.9–77.1	154–170	74.4–83.5	164–184
1.825	6	0	68.9–73.5	152–162	71.7–79.4	158–175	76.2–85.7	168–189
1.850	6	1	70.8–75.7	156–167	73.5–81.6	162–180	78.5–88	173–194
1.875	6	2	72.6–77.6	160–171	75.7–83.5	167–185	80.7–90.3	178–199
1.900	6	3	74.4–79.4	164–175	78.1–86.2	172–190	82.7–92.5	182–204
Women								
1.425	4	8	41.7–44.5	92–98	43.5–48.5	96–107	47.2–54	104–119
1.450	4	9	42.6–45.8	94–101	44.5–49.9	98–110	48.1–55.3	106–122
1.475	4	10	43.5–47.2	96–104	45.8–51.3	101–113	49.4–56.7	109–125
1.500	4	11	44.9–48.5	99–107	47.2–52.6	104–116	50.8–58.1	112–128
1.525	5	0	46.3–49.9	102–110	48.5–54	107–119	52.2–59.4	115–131
1.550	5	1	47.6–51.3	105–113	49.9–55.3	110–122	53.5–60.8	118–134
1.575	5	2	49–52.6	108–116	51.3–57.2	113–126	54.9–62.6	121–138
1.600	5	3	50.3–54	111–119	52.6–59	116–130	56.7–64.4	125–142
1.625	5	4	51.7–55.8	114–123	54.4–61.2	120–135	58.5–66.2	129–146
1.650	5	5	53.5–57.6	118–127	56.2–63	124–139	60.3–68	133–150
1.675	5	6	55.3–59.4	122–131	58.1–64.9	128–143	62.1–69.9	137–154
1.700	5	7	57.2–61.2	126–135	59.9–66.7	132–147	64–71.7	141–158
1.725	5	8	59–63.5	130–140	61.7–68.5	136–151	65.8–73.9	145–163
1.750	5	9	60.8–65.3	134–144	63.5–70.3	140–155	67.6–76.2	149–168
1.775	5	10	62.6–67.1	138–148	65.3–72.1	144–159	69.4–79	153–174

Based on weights of insured persons in the United States associated with lowest mortality (*Statist bull Metrop Life Insur Co* 40. Nov.–Dec. 1959)

abdominal herniae and varicose veins. The deposition of excessive amounts of fat in the subcutaneous tissues around the rib cage interferes with its free movement, giving rise to recurrent chest infections.

Many **metabolic disorders** are associated with obesity: diabetes mellitus, gout, atherosclerosis and cholelithiasis are all more common in overweight people. Patients with these disorders are also prone to their complications — peripheral neuropathy, hypertension, and cerebrovascular accidents.

Cardiovascular problems, especially angina, are more common among the obese because of the increased amount of effort required to move an overweight body. The coronary arteries may develop atheromatous plaques, predisposing to cardiac failure.

Generally speaking, obese people are **more accident prone** than persons of normal weight. The excess tissue prevents a good grip and the obese person readily drops things, spills kettles of boiling water or trips over things. Because of his increased bulk and tendency to mechanical disorders the obese person cannot rapidly avoid danger as can other people. Finally, the complications of obesity, combined with slow wound healing, make the obese patient a **poor anaesthetic and surgical risk.**

All these factors mean that the expectation of life for the obese individual is reduced. A man of 45 years who is 11 kg above standard weight has a reduced life expectancy of 25%.

Management

The nurse can play a vital role in the management of obesity both in hospital and in the community. Primarily, the patient must be motivated to lose weight and to maintain a standard weight once it is achieved. This motivation may be based on very individual factors, but every effort must be made to reinforce it and to support the patient with advice and encouragement during the times when the goal appears more remote.

It is important that the members of the patient's intimate circle do not sabotage these efforts, either psychologically (the husband who says he likes his wife plump) or physically by encouraging the ingestion of prohibited foods. Another vital factor in successful weight reduction is that the supervisors have a realistic goal in time and make sure the patient is aware of it. Other factors, such as the need to recognize that the initial dramatic weight loss will not be repeated each week and that premenstrual tension and fluid retention may temporarily increase weight despite adherence to the dietary regime, should be explained so that the patient is not unnecessarily depressed by temporary set-backs and abandons treatment.

As the cause of obesity is an increase of food intake over energy expenditure, the aim of treatment is to change eating habits, so that weight is lost, and to increase the amount of exercise. This will permit a reasonable energy intake while still achieving the primary objective.

Although small amounts of excess adipose tissue can be lost by 'crash' dieting, this method is unsuitable for the obese person. The diet must be sufficiently satisfying to ensure that the ill-effects of *ketosis* or excessive tiredness do not occur, which would interfere with daily activities, impair interpersonal relationships and reduce motivation to the point where the attempt at weight reduction is discontinued. The diet must be flexible to allow variety and economic food buying, and also to reduce the temptation to cheat. Each failure makes further attempts less likely to succeed.

To avoid these complications and to allow a sufficiently prolonged period under close supervision for habit changes to take place, it is wise to allow the patient a diet which provides between **4000 and 4500 kJ per day.** The average middle-aged housewife requires about 9250 kJ per day, and would then be short of approximately 5000 kJ per day, which she will obtain from her adipose tissue. A weekly weight loss of approximately 1 kg is possible on this regime (based on the physiological fact that the energy value of adipose tissue is approximately 31.5 kJ per g) and should be the aim.

To attempt to change habits outside the normal environment is short-sighted — the patient is best treated in an out-patient setting. Education and support in practical and psychological terms form the basis of success. It is often helpful to make a graph on which the patient's progress can be charted; if the gradations on the ordinate are fixed so that even a small weight loss looks significant, it has a good psychological effect, even for those patients who know and understand exactly the ruse that has been practised!

The balance of the diet is altered to meet the physiological needs. The carbohydrate intake is reduced to 100 g per day. This reduction appears very drastic to the patient, since overindulgence in these foods is the most common cause of obesity. Protein intake of 60 g per day is adequate for the patient's needs and negates the argument often raised in defence of obesity, that reducing diets are expensive. If these two components are taken in these quantities, only 40 g of fat may be ingested if the total energy intake is not to exceed that stipulated.

As this is a new pattern of behaviour for the patient, it is desirable that energy-producing constituents in the diet be weighed in the early stages. The amount of time spent on explanation and discussion of a suitable dietary regime is never wasted. Frequent discussion of difficulties and repetition of advice and encouragement are all worthwhile. It may be helpful to reduce salt intake, especially during the premenstrual period; vitamin supplements should not be necessary, as most vegetables supply few kilojoules and can therefore be taken freely. Iron supplements may be worthwhile: most obese patients are middle-aged women who also tend to be slightly anaemic.

Although the control of diet is the corner-stone of treatment, other factors can influence its success. An increase in daily exercise is desirable, and walking (often the most strenuous activity possible for obese people) requires a steady energy output. A minimum of 3 miles a day should be encouraged. **Regular daily exercise** is more valuable and less dangerous than spurts of intense activity at intervals.

Exercise in combination with a low carbohydrate intake is effective in increasing weight loss for two reasons. Firstly, an increase in energy demands requires the mobilization of triglycerides from the fat stores; secondly, because of the reduced carbohydrate intake, the ability to convert lipoproteins into triglycerides and store them is reduced. The use of skin calipers to measure this reduction in skin fold thickness is only valid if practised by an expert, using the same area of tissue on each occasion.

Drug therapy as an adjunct to diet has some place, especially in the treatment of the relapsed obese person. How much of the effect is psychological and how much physiological is difficult to say. In some cases the side-effects of drugs make them unsuitable for the patient. The addictive properties of amphetamines have led to their withdrawal, but there are other anorectic agents available. Metformin, for example, is particularly suited to the needs of the obese diabetic patient, since it is thought that this drug (one of the biguanide group) increases the uptake of glucose in muscle. Another drug which has undergone successful controlled trials is fenflur-amine: it is thought that this drug increases the breakdown of fat and decreases the synthesis of triglycerides, thus reducing the fat depots. All drugs should be used with caution and their use does not obviate the need for strict adherence to the dietary regimen.

The role of surgery in the treatment of obesity is doubtful. It is possible that operations on the small intestine which involve bypassing segments of the gut and so reducing the absorptive surface available may be of value. Such procedures, however, neither treat the cause of obesity nor bring about the necessary long-term changes in eating habits. Only in severe, intractable cases, and with due consideration of the special risks of surgery to which obese persons are vulnerable, should such measures be considered.

Overeating destroys more than hunger — efforts to sustain and encourage those who endeavour to apply the remedies and avoid destruction are more than gratifying.

SUGGESTED ASSIGNMENTS

1. An elderly lady is convalescing at home following a cerebrovascular accident. She has limited mobility and refuses to accept the meals-on-wheels service. Her only source of income is her old age pension. What advice could this lady be given to ensure that her nutritional needs are met on this limited budget?

2. A group of young women are embarking on a 25-mile sponsored walk to raise funds for a particular charity.
   a. What are the approximate energy requirements for each person for the day?
   b. Plan two packed meals that will meet the nutritional requirements for that day.

3. What dietary advice would you give to a recently widowed, elderly man?

4. A child of 6 months is diagnosed as suffering from coeliac disease. What advice and practical support would you offer his family in the immediate and long-term future?

5. A 45-year-old woman is 155 cm tall and weighs 100 kg.
How would you establish her standard weight? How would you assist her to achieve and maintain this?

FURTHER READING

Beck M E 1980 Nutrition and dietetics for nurses, 6th edn. Churchill Livingstone, Edinburgh
Craddock D 1978 Obesity and its management, 3rd edn. Churchill Livingstone, Edinburgh
Macleod J (ed) 1981 Davidson's principles and practice of medicine, 13th edn. Churchill Livingstone, Edinburgh
McLaren D S 1981 Nutrition and its disorders, 3rd edn. Churchill Livingstone, Edinburgh
Ministry of Agriculture Fisheries and Food 1975 Manual of nutrition. HMSO, London

FOR REFERENCE

Bunch H 1974 Eating disorders, obesity, anorexia nervosa and the person within. Routledge and Kegan Paul, London·
Davidson Sir Stanley, Pasmore R, Brock J F, Truswell A S 1979 Human nutrition and dietetics, 7th edn. Churchill Livingstone, Edinburgh
Department of Health and Social Security 1969a Recommended intakes of nutrients for the United Kingdom. Reports on Public Health and Medical Subjects no. 120. HMSO, London
Department of Health and Social Security 1969b The fluoridation studies in the United Kingdom and the results achieved after eleven years. Reports on Public Health and Medical Subjects no. 122. HMSO, London
Ministry of Agriculture, Fisheries and Food 1970 Report on claims and misleading descriptions. HMSO, London
Pasmore R, Robson J S 1976 A companion to medical studies, 2nd edn. Blackwell Scientific, Oxford, vol 1

Chapter Five
The gastrointestinal tract and the abdomen

Many gastrointestinal disorders when diagnosed can be cured or controlled by dietary or drug therapy without the patient having to be hospitalized. Therefore it is likely that the nurse in training may only care for these patients when they have been admitted to hospital during an acute exacerbation of a gastrointestinal disorder or when complications require surgical correction.

ANATOMY AND PHYSIOLOGY

The gastrointestinal tract

The gastrointestinal tract is a muscular tube about 9 metres in length (Fig. 5.1). It includes the mouth, pharynx and oesophagus, which lead to the stomach. From the

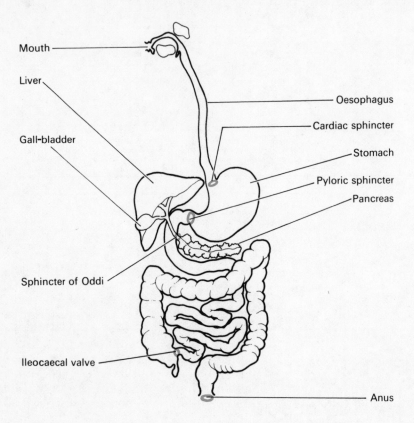

Figure 5.1
The gastrointestinal tract

Outer fibrous elastic
(or serous) coat

Muscle coat

Loose submucous coat

Mucous
membrane lining

Figure 5.2
Cross-section of gastrointestinal tract

stomach it continues as the duodenum, jejunum and ileum, known collectively as the **small intestine**. It proceeds as the caecum. ascending, transverse, descending and sigmoid colon known collectively as the **large intestine**. The tube continues and becomes the rectum, then ends as the anal canal. The tract is under autonomic nervous control, is lined throughout with mucous membrane (Fig. 5.2) and is constructed in such a way that the different parts can play their separate roles. The various glands associated with the tract are the salivary glands, the pancreas and the liver. These glands empty their secretions into the tract and are necessary for its proper functioning. The functions of the gastrointestinal tract are **ingestion, digestion** and **absorption** of food, and the **elimination** of semisolid waste. The various sphincters of the tract enable the timely passage of intestinal content.

When food is ingested the action of the teeth, tongue and muscles in the sides of the mouth reduce it to small particles. This chewing action stimulates increased flow of saliva containing the enzyme amylase and digestion begins. The food is formed into a soft bolus which can be swallowed. It passes through the cricopharyngeal sphincter down the oesophagus into the stomach by peristaltic movement. The oesophago-gastric sphincter prevents regurgitation of food and gastric acid into the oesophagus.

The stomach is the expanded part of the tract and the oesophagus enters its upper end just below the diaphragm. The stomach has three zones: the fundus, the body and the antrum. The parietal cells producing acid and the chief cells producing pepsin are concentrated in the fundus and body of the stomach. The antrum secretes alkaline mucus and the hormone gastrin. There are two phases. Initially, the vagus nerve stimulates the flow of gastric secretion in response to the sight, taste and smell of food. This is the **cephalic phase**. When food passes into the antrum the hormone gastrin is released into the blood and further stimulates gastric secretion. This is the **gastric phase**.

The action of the gastric muscles and secretions reduces the food to a semisolid, partially digested state called **chyme**. This is stored in the stomach before passing through the pyloric sphincter into the small intestine at a rate which will allow further digestion and absorption. Intestinal secretion and hormones are produced when chyme enters the duodenum. The hormones stimulate the secretion of pancreatic enzymes, cause contraction of the gall-bladder and relaxation of the sphincter of Oddi. Bile from the liver which has been stored in the gall-bladder flows into the duodenum along with the pancreatic enzymes, and the further breakdown of fat, carbohydrate and protein occurs. The food is now in a fluid alkaline state. Once this stage is reached the absorption of chemicals and nutrients can take place across the specially constructed walls of the small intestine into the blood. Residue passes on through the ileocaecal valve into the large intestine. Large quantities of water are absorbed mainly through the walls of the caecum and ascending colon. By peristalsis the residue then moves through the transverse to the sigmoid colon where further water absorption takes place. This gives the residue, faeces, its normal semi-solid consistency. The entry of faeces into the rectum causes the desire for defaecation and there is relaxation of the internal anal sphincter. After the first few years of life the external anal sphincter comes under voluntary control, and defaecation occurs at will.

Accessory organs

The salivary glands

Saliva is a thin watery solution containing salts and an enzyme called amylase which splits cooked starch. It is produced by three pairs of salivary glands: the parotid, the submandibular and the sublingual, whose ducts open into the mouth. There is a continuous flow of small amounts of saliva which cleanses and lubricates the mouth and tongue. In response to the sight, smell, taste or thought of food an increased amount of saliva is produced. The mechanical breakdown of food which is then mixed with saliva in the mouth is the start of the process of digestion.

The pancreas

The pancreas is a large gland which has an exocrine and endocrine function. The exocrine or external secretion of the pancreas contains the enzymes **trypsinogen, amylase** and **lipase** and alkaline salts. When acid chyme enters the duodenum the hormone secretin is released to stimulate and maintain the secretion of pancreatic juice into the duodenum. Its function is to neutralize the acid from the stomach and to continue the digestion of protein, carbohydrate and fat. The endocrine or internal function of the pancreas is the production of the hormones glucagon and insulin which circulate in the blood and regulate carbohydrate metabolism (Ch. 11).

The liver, biliary tract and gall-bladder

The liver is the largest gland in the body and is indispensable to life. One of its many functions is the production of **bile** (Fig. 5.3). The liver is composed of a large number of lobules from which pass small bile ducts. These unite with similar ducts to form the largest hepatic ducts. The bile secreted by liver cells passes from the hepatic ducts to the cystic duct and is then stored and concentrated in the gall-bladder. When fatty foods are present in the duodenum the hormone **cholecystokinin** causes contraction of the gall-bladder and relaxation of the sphincter of Oddi. The bile then passes down the bile duct and enters the duodenum along with the pancreatic secretion. One of the functions of bile is emulsification of fats by the bile salts. It also provides a means of excreting the pigment bilirubin, an end-product of the breakdown of red blood cells.

After the absorption of nutrients and chemicals from the intestinal tract into the blood, it is transported via the portal vein to the liver. There some substances are altered, some stored and others passed into general circulation to reach the tissues of the body.

The peritoneum

The stomach, small and large intestine, liver, pancreas and gall-bladder are contained in the **abdominal cavity**. The peritoneum, the serous membrane which

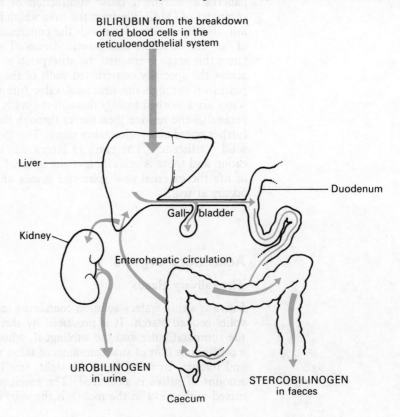

BILIRUBIN from the breakdown
of red blood cells in the
reticuloendothelial system

Liver

Duodenum

Gall-bladder

Kidney

Enterohepatic circulation

UROBILINOGEN
in urine

STERCOBILINOGEN
in faeces

Caecum

Figure 5.3
The formation and excretion of
bile

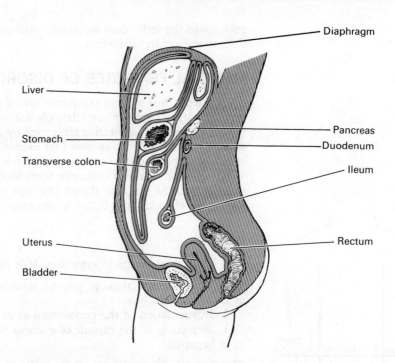

Figure 5.4
The peritoneum

lines the cavity, covers and supports the abdominal viscera (Fig. 5.4). The **peritoneal cavity** is the potential space between the two layers of peritoneum.

The blood vessels and nerves to the small and large intestine are supported by thickened folds of peritoneum called the mesentery, the transverse mesocolon and pelvic mesocolon. The large fold in front of the abdominal viscera is the omentum. This supports blood and lymph vessels and is capable of isolating infection within the peritoneal cavity.

Further support for the abdominal viscera is provided by the muscles of the anterior abdominal wall, the pelvic muscles and the diaphragm.

AETIOLOGY

Aetiology of disease varies from one level of the tract to another and it is not proposed, therefore, to provide a comprehensive list of influencing factors. The following points are of particular relevance:

Diet

As discussed in Chapter 4, dietary imbalance may occur in a variety of ways and may cause disturbance of gastrointestinal function.

Poor food hygiene

This, and deficient sanitation, are associated with poor social conditions, over-crowding and lack of health education. Inflammatory gastrointestinal infections are, however, still relatively common in affluent communities where there is little excuse for laxity in standards of cleanliness. Fashionable restaurants and, even more regrettably, hospital kitchens are among the offenders.

Psychosocial factors

The influence of **emotional** factors on gastrointestinal tract disorder is universally accepted. Anxiety and continuous tension can predispose to mechanical upsets such as acute vomiting and diarrhoea. The incidence of structural breakdown as in peptic ulceration is high in people subject to stressful conditions.

Cigarette smoking and the **ingestion of alcohol** tend to aggravate, complicate and predispose the individual to certain gastrointestinal disorders, especially malignant disease and peptic ulceration.

GENERAL FEATURES OF DISORDER

The patient's history and symptoms are of particular importance since the signs of gastrointestinal disorder are relatively few.

'**Indigestion**' is a collective term used by patients to describe many of their symptoms. True indigestion, as found for example in pancreatic insufficiency when there is failure to produce the necessary digestive enzymes, is very rare.

'**Dyspepsia**' is also a collective term used, it must be admitted, by medical and nursing staff, to describe almost any type of abdominal discomfort associated with the taking of food. It is better to use more specific terms.

Pain

Pain is the most common symptom. It is caused by either:

1. Strong contractions of smooth muscle, giving rise to colic such as intestinal or biliary colic.
2. Inflammation of the peritoneum as in appendicitis.
3. Stretching of the capsule of a viscus when the organ within becomes swollen, as in hepatitis.

The character of the pain may vary and patients may differ in the description of their pain; these varying accounts can be misleading. Nonetheless, the site of the pain is of significance and the nurse should be able to report whether it is, for example, epigastric, umbilical or hypogastric (Fig. 5.5). Symptoms of local or generalized rigidity or tenderness are commonly associated with abdominal pain.

Another related phenomenon is that of referral; of pain from the diseased area to some distant region. The mechanism of this is not quite clear.

The nurse should note the degree and the duration of pain, its relationship, if any, to meals and whether or not the taking of food aggravates or relieves pain.

Figure 5.5
Regions of the abdomen

Flatulence

Under normal circumstances ingested air is rapidly eructated from the oesophagus and stomach. In some conditions, such as pyloric stenosis, the patient may complain of excessive amounts of 'wind' which may also be foul smelling. Gas accumulating in the colon whether ingested or resulting from imperfect digestion is passed via the rectum.

In the postoperative patient gas cannot be eructated normally and some passes into the intestines. It becomes trapped, causing distension of the upper colon, and discomfort results. It will only be relieved when the patient becomes mobile. Therefore, it is important to ensure some movement even when the patient continues to rest in bed.

Heartburn

This is a sensation of burning behind the lower end of the sternum and is often accompanied by regurgitation of fluid into the pharynx. The causes are many but the burning sensation suggests gastric acid reflux at the lower end of the oesophagus.

Alteration in eating habits

The desire to eat (appetite) is often diminished. This loss of appetite is known as **anorexia** and will result in weight loss. Persistent refusal to eat for psychological reasons is termed **anorexia nervosa** (Ch. 4). Some patients may omit certain items of diet in the belief that they disagree with them. This is characteristic of people suffering from peptic ulceration who may, as a result, develop signs of nutritional deficiency. Such deficiencies may also arise from persistent vomiting.

Nausea

The feeling of sickness is experienced mostly in the epigastrium. The accompaniment of salivation, sweating and pallor usually indicates that vomiting is to follow.

Vomiting

This is a reflex act caused by a wide variety of stimuli, too many to list comprehensively. They include unsuitable food, many systemic diseases and psychological disorder. The reflex can to some extent be suppressed by taking deep breaths through the mouth or by holding the breath.

Alterations in bowel habit

These are manifest by diarrhoea or constipation due to altered peristaltic activity. However, they may or may not have an underlying organic cause. Dietary indiscretion or deficient food hygiene play an important part in the disorganization of gastrointestinal tract function, hence the importance of health education in the community.

Diarrhoea

Acute diarrhoea may be due to infection or overindulgence in fatty foods.

Chronic diarrhoea is a common symptom of a large number of diseases, particularly those affecting the colon, such as ulcerative colitis.

Constipation

Acute constipation is likely to be organic in origin; it is present, for example, in intestinal obstruction.

Chronic constipation is often due to faulty eating or toilet habits. In hospital the usual practice is to record the number of bowel movements a patient has each day. Abnormalities of stools must be noted and reported with care.

Intestinal haemorrhage

Melaena, blood in stools, and haematemesis, blood in vomitus, are extremely serious symptoms indicative of some structural erosion within the gastrointestinal tract. Such symptoms always merit immediate investigation.

Dysphagia

This is the term used to describe difficulty in swallowing. It is a symptom of many disorders, including painful conditions of the mouth and throat, compression of the oesophagus — for example by an enlarged thyroid gland — and a growth or disease of the oesophagus itself, in particular from carcinoma and inflammatory conditions.

As can be seen, many symptoms of gastrointestinal disorder cause both acute physical distress and social embarrassment; therefore, mental depression is a common sequel.

INVESTIGATIONS

Gastrointestinal studies tend to be exhausting and very lengthy. Patients already fatigued by disease processes require the utmost consideration and care when undergoing investigation.

Analysis of gastric content

Gastric aspirate

This is obtained by using a radio-opaque Levin tube passed through the nasal cavity into the antrum of the stomach. The position of the tube should be checked by the accepted method in the ward, for example, by using litmus paper. Some doctors like to check the position fluoroscopically.

Intubation is usually performed in the early morning following an 8- to 10-hour fast. In the normal fasting subject the amount of gastric-secretion rarely exceeds 100 ml. Volumes in excess of this amount occur in gastric hypersecretion, pyloric obstruction and duodenal regurgitation.

Gastric acid secretion

Definite variations in hydrochloric acid content are present in some diseases; therefore the quantitative assessment of gastric acid secretion is of diagnostic importance.

The patient is fasted overnight and left to rest in bed in the morning. A Levin tube is passed, its position checked and the fasting juice aspirated. With the patient lying comfortably in the left lateral position gentle suction is applied to the tube to provide continuous aspiration. After 1 hour this resting juice is collected and a gastric stimulant is given. The most suitable gastric stimulant is pentogastrin (Peptavalon), a synthetic polypeptide structurally related to gastrin. It is given subcutaneously in a dose of 6 μg per 1 kg body weight. The gastric juice is then collected for 1 hour. The volumes are measured, the juice titrated and the output of acid calculated. The results are of value in deciding the type of surgery needed.

The total absence of hydrochloric acid is termed achlorhydria and is uncommon except in patients with pernicious anaemia or in those who have undergone extensive gastric surgery.

Collection of stools

Stool collections for 3 or 5 days may be ordered in the event of suspected malabsorption syndromes, especially in cases of steatorrhoea, which indicates abnormal fat digestion. Faecal fat estimations are made while the patient's daily fat intake is being controlled by the dietitian.

Radiology

Plain films

Supine and erect films of the abdomen are indicated in cases of suspected intestinal obstruction or ileus in order to demonstrate distended loops of bowel and fluid levels. Free gas may be seen under the diaphragm following perforation of a duodenal ulcer, or indeed any part of the alimentary tract. Gallstones and renal stones may sometimes be demonstrated on plain films.

Barium meal

The main indications for this examination are suspected gastric or duodenal ulcer, gastric carcinoma and hiatus hernia. The examination is normally carried out in the morning and it is essential that the patient should have had nothing to eat or drink since the previous evening. The mucosa of the oesophagus, stomach and duodenum are coated with barium and the lumen distended with air. The patient is then positioned by the radiologist and X-ray films taken under television control to demonstrate any lesions that may be present. Many radiologist give 20 mg i.v. Buscopan (hyoscine-N-butylbromide) in order to make the stomach and duodenum hypotonic during the examination. This may cause some blurring of vision and the patient should be told not to drive a car until this effect, which usually lasts for less than an hour, has worn off.

Small bowel barium studies

This technique may be used to investigate suspected malabsorption, Crohn's disease or tumours of the small bowel. The preparation of the patient is the same as for a barium meal. Some radiologists give the barium by mouth taking frequent X-ray films until the whole small bowel has been examined whilst others prefer to intubate the duodenum with a special nasogastric tube and instil the barium into the small bowel. Most examinations should be completed within an hour using modern rapid transit barium.

Barium enema

The purpose of this examination is to demonstrate polyps and tumours of the colon, diverticular disease and ulcerative and Crohn's colitis. These lesions are shown by coating the mucosa with barium and distending the lumen of the colon with air. X-ray films of the colon are taken in various positions as determined by the radiologist. In order to carry out a satisfactory barium enema the colon must be completely free of faeces. The bowel may be prepared either with water washouts or with an enema containing a colonic activator such as veripaque (dihydroxyphenylisatin). 3 g of veripaque are mixed with 1½ litres of warm water and this is run into the colon at least one hour before the barium examination. The patient spends the interval between the preliminary cleansing enema and the barium enema in the toilet in order to ensure complete evacuation of the colon. There is no need to fast the patient for this examination.

Sinography

A sinogram may be helpful in demonstrating the site and extent of a sinus track or fistula between the bowel and abdominal wall. For this procedure a fine Portex or Foley catheter is introduced down the sinus track and a water soluble contrast medium injected. X-ray films are taken when the full extent of the sinus or fistula has been demonstrated.

Cholecystography and cholangiography

Oral cholecystography is indicated if gall-stones are suspected. The patient is given a light meal the night before the examination. The contrast medium is taken by mouth in tablet form and thereafter the patient is given nothing to eat or drink until after the X-ray examination the following morning.

If the gall-bladder fails to concentrate the contrast then an **infusion cholangiogram** may be performed in an attempt to show the gall-bladder and bile ducts. While the intravenous infusion of the contrast medium is in progress the nurse should observe the patient for any sign of an allergic reaction.

During cholecystectomy most surgeons routinely perform **operative cholangiography** in theatre to make sure that there are no residual stones in the bile ducts.

If the patient is jaundiced the oral and intravenous contrast media will not be excreted by the liver. In such cases the biliary tract may be outlined by **percutaneous transhepatic cholangiography** which involves passing a thin needle through the skin and into the liver under local anaesthesia. Contrast medium is injected into the bile ducts to show the cause and site of the obstruction. After such an examination the patient is usually given a broad spectrum antibiotic; regular checks on the pulse and blood pressure are made by the nurse as the examination carries a small but definite risk of biliary peritonitis, intraperitoneal bleeding and ascending cholangitis.

An alternative method of examining the biliary tract is by **endoscopic retrograde cholangiopancreatography**. At this examination a fine catheter is passed into the bile ducts through a fibreoptic endoscope under X-ray control and contrast medium injected to outline the bile ducts. This examination has the added advantage that the pancreatic duct can also be X-rayed following cannulization and the injection of contrast medium.

Arteriography

This is occasionally of value in demonstrating vascular abnormalities of the alimentary tract and tumours of the liver and pancreas. The examination is performed by passing a catheter from the femoral artery into the aorta and taking rapid serial films following the injection of contrast medium. Following the examination regular checks should be made to ensure that there is no bleeding from the puncture site in the femoral artery and the pulse and blood pressure should also be checked regularly by the nurse.

Ultrasonography

Detail of the anatomy of the liver, gall-bladder, bile ducts and pancreas can now be demonstrated by means of ultrasound examination. This examination, which is described more fully on page 378, has the advantage that is is non-invasive and is therefore without risk to the patient. No special preparation or after care is required except that patients for gall-bladder examination should fast.

Nursing care

The nurse can be of great assistance when an ill patient is being X-rayed, particularly if an intravenous infusion is being administered. The patient will also require help and support when turning into the various positions required by the radiologist and radiographer.

Endoscopy

Endoscopy is the examination of the inner lining of an organ, such as the colon or stomach, by direct vision using a special illuminated tube or fibreoptic instrument.
The procedure may be:

1. Diagnostic, to observe, photograph and obtain a biopsy of tissue.
2. Therapeutic, for example, to dilate strictures or remove foreign bodies.

Preparation of the patient

This varies according to the organ which is to be examined and the type of anaesthesia required. Upper endoscopy involves the use of a local anaesthetic throat spray but general anaesthesia may be necessary for patients who are very apprehensive or unable to co-operate.

In some instances, for example during oesophagoscopy, the patient is unable to speak. Although the procedure may not be painful it is uncomfortable and can be alarming. Therefore the patient should be given an explanation of the preparation and procedure necessary for his examination.

Patients who are to have upper endoscopy carried out, fast for at least 6 hours prior to examination. Five minutes before the procedure begins the throat is sprayed with local anaesthetic, Diazepam 20 mg is given intravenously, and if the patient is under 60 years of age Buscopan is also given.

Oesophagoscopy

Figure 5.6
Left: Oesophagoscope
Right: Oesophageal biopsy forceps

Oesophagoscopy is the examination of the oesophagus using a metal oesophagoscope (Fig. 5.6) or a fibreoptic instrument which is passed through the mouth and down the oesophagus to the cardiac sphincter. The nurse should stay with the patient and hold his hand as this is his only way of communicating when the instrument is being passed. Any sudden movement at this stage could damage the oesophagus.

Bouginage. Dilatation of oesophageal stricture can be carried out via an oesophagoscope. The patient is prepared as for upper endoscopy. Graduated dilators (ranging in size from 21 mm to 45 mm) are used.

Due to the risk of trauma, aftercare of the patient is extremely important. Frequent observation of pulse and blood pressure is carried out for the first 12 hours. Initially the patient is given nil orally, but mouthwashes during this time will be greatly appreciated. After approximately 6 hours the patient may be given sips of water, iced, but previously boiled. If tolerated, free fluids are introduced. Following examination by the physician a soft diet may be recommended.

Gastroscopy/duodenoscopy

Gastroscopy is the examination of gastric mucosa using a flexible fibreoptic instrument (Fig. 5.7). It can be controlled so that it is possible to examine the pylorus, duodenum or postoperative reconstruction. Biopsy can be obtained under direct vision.

After care of patients having upper endoscopic examination

When the procedure has been completed the patient must not eat or drink until his swallow reflex has recovered from the local anaesthetic, usually in about 4 hours. In the few days following he may be hoarse or complain of a sore throat; this can be relieved with warm gargles. Patients who are investigated as out-patients should be allowed time to recover before being escorted home by a friend or relative.

Proctoscopy

This is the examination of the anus and rectum using a metal or plastic proctoscope which is about 8 cm long and 2 cm in diameter. The patient is allowed a light breakfast on the morning of the test. Preparation of the rectum varies; patients who are not suspected of having inflammatory disease may be ordered a small enema to clear faecal matter which would obscure the examiner's view of the rectal mucosa. For this examination the patient is helped into the left lateral position with his knees drawn up. He should be adequately covered. The nurse should help him maintain this position and encourage him to relax by taking deep breaths.

After examination the patient is allowed to rest.

Sigmoidoscopy

The examination of rectal and sigmoid mucosa using a sigmoidoscope, which is a metal tube 25 cm long and 1.5 cm in diameter; is called sigmoidoscopy. Preparation for this examination is as for proctoscopy. The patient is examined in the knee-chest or left lateral position; though uncomfortable, the procedure should not be painful. During sigmoidoscopy air may be pumped into the colon to distend the lumen and allow a better view of the mucosa. This may cause pain; therefore the nurse should observe the patient carefully since he may feel faint.

After this tiring examination the patient is allowed to rest and have a light meal, especially if he is an out-patient.

Colonoscopy

This examination (Fig. 5.8) is gradually replacing sigmoidoscopy mainly due to the versatility of the fibroscope which allows an extended view to the level of the caecum. Preparation of the patient may, in some circumstances, need to be more extensive and include colonic washout. It may be performed under general anaesthesia.

Biopsy

Removal of a small portion of tissue for microscopic examination is termed biopsy.

A biopsy of the small intestine can be taken using the Crosby capsule. This apparatus consists of a small hollow capsule with a side hole; inside there is a circular, spring-loaded blade. The capsule is attached to a long thin polythene tube. When suction is applied to the tube, mucosa is pulled into the side hole of the capsule and the spring-loaded blade severs the trapped tissue.

Preparation of the patient involves fasting overnight and receiving an explanation of the procedure. On the day of the examination the patient is asked to swallow the capsule. This can be made easier if he sits in the upright position. The doctor may prescribe a drug such as Maxolon to stimulate peristalsis and prevent nausea. The time taken for the capsule to reach the small intestine depends on motility and the state of the pyloric sphincter. When the capsule reaches the antrum (estimated by markings on the tube) the patient is asked to lie in the right lateral position for 2 hours. The presence of bile-stained duodenal juice in the tube indicates entry of the

Figure 5.7
Oesophago-gastroduodenoscope in use

Figure 5.8
Colonoscopy

capsule into the duodenum. The position is checked fluoroscopically before the biopsy is taken. The capsule is withdrawn, opened and the tissue carefully removed. The apparatus is checked to ensure that it is complete.

Biopsy of the small intestine may be necessary during the investigation of malabsorption syndrome.

DISORDERS OF THE ORAL CAVITY

Glossitis, inflammation of the tongue, in acute and chronic forms is frequently caused by deficiency of substances essential for the metabolism of healthy cells such as iron and vitamins of the B group (Ch. 4). The shiny, smooth and often painful tongue is due to the surface being denuded of papillae. Chronic inflammation leads to leukoplakia characterized by snowy-white patches on the tongue and sometimes on cheeks and gums. Painful, tender fissures develop later and become sites of chronic infection or malignant changes.

Halitosis (offensive breath) may result from dental disorders or the excretion of odour from the gastrointestinal tract or lungs. In addition to its clinical significance it is socially embarrassing.

Stomatitis or inflammation of the mouth appears in many forms. The commonest type is thrush.

Thrush (moniliasis)

This condition occurs readily in infants (Ch. 17) and the fungus is easily transmitted by inadequately sterilized feeding bottles or poor hygiene of nursing or medical staff. In adults it occurs either during debilitating illnesses when resistance to infection is low, or in those receiving corticosteroid or antibiotic therapy when normal bacterial flora are diminished.

Clinical features

The yeast-like fungus, *Candida albicans*, forms ivory-white patches on the mucous membrane of the mouth, tongue, palate or pharynx. These patches coalesce to form an easily detached membrane which, when wiped off, leaves a bleeding excoriated surface. The membrane is easily recognized when examined under a microscope.

Treatment

The condition is uncomfortable rather than painful. Two-hourly mouth care is carried out very gently using weak solutions of sodium bicarbonate. An oral suspension of nystatin may be prescribed; this is applied locally by being held in the mouth for several minutes. Fruit juices are most useful in stimulating the flow of saliva to cleanse and bathe the mouth.

As the condition is easily transmitted the patient's feeding utensils are reserved for his use only and are sterilized afterwards.

DISORDERS OF THE OESOPHAGUS

Oesophagitis

Any substance causing injury and irritation to the oesophageal mucosa produces oesophagitis.

Corrosive poisons

The consequences of wittingly or unwittingly ingesting corrosive substances are dramatic. Severe burning sufficient to cause collapse is felt throughout the length of the oesophagus. The mucosa becomes ulcerated.

Treatment

This involves identifying the poison and giving oral preparations immediately to neutralize the effect. The healing process produces scar tissue which may result in oesophageal narrowing and stricture formation.

Foreign bodies

Almost any small object may be swallowed by a young child, irritate the mucous membrane and produce pain. Obstruction by a radio-opaque foreign body such as a fish bone is readily seen on X-ray examination, but other materials may not show up at all. Oesophagoscopy is carried out to locate and remove the foreign body.

Oedema

Swelling resulting from mucosal trauma may cause temporary oesophageal stricture and accompanying dysphagia. A soft diet and a plentiful fluid intake must be encouraged until the swelling subsides and normal diet can be resumed.

Reflux oesophagitis

This may occur in an acute form after repeated vomiting. However, inflammation caused by regurgitated gastric acid secretion quickly decreases as the vomiting subsides and the associated pain disappears. In some conditions, such as hiatus hernia, reflux of gastric juice occurs repeatedly causing chronic irritation, ulceration, eventual stricture formation and dysphagia in several cases.

Stricture formation

This may follow ingestion of corrosive poisons or foreign bodies or a severe case of reflux oesophagitis. After inflammation and oedema have settled, the resulting stricture is amenable to dilatation (see bouginage, p. 182).

Hiatus hernia

The diaphragm has several openings through which herniation of abdominal viscera into the thorax can occur. The commonest and most important is the oesophageal hiatus.

Aetiology

Age is important, for hiatus hernia is commoner in middle and later life, probably because muscle tone diminishes with age and the hiatus becomes more lax. The condition occurs more frequently in women. Increased intra-abdominal pressure in pregnancy and obesity predisposes to it, as do some chest deformities, for instance those associated with *kyphosis*. In children the condition is due to congenital short oesophagus.

Clinical features

In adults hiatus hernia may be symptomless if the cardiac sphincter remains in a normal position (Fig. 5.9 *top*).

After taking food, a feeling of substernal discomfort may be experienced owing to distension of the hernial sac. Heartburn is the cardinal symptom and is typically associated with any change of posture which increases intra-abdominal pressure, for example stooping, lifting or straining. Patients tend to be awakened from sleep and pain is only relieved by sitting upright. A feeling of food sticking in the oesophagus is a common complaint. Regurgitation of food into the mouth occurs unexpectedly, especially during exercise immediately after a meal.

Careful enquiry into the patient's history and a clear description of the site and character of the pain and its relationship to posture make diagnosis almost certain. A barium meal examination will demonstrate the hernia (Fig. 5.9 *bottom*) and on oesophagoscopy the inflammatory changes characteristic of reflux oesophagitis can be seen.

Oesophagus

Cardia

Oesophago-gastric angle

Cardia

Loss of oesophago-gastric angle causing reflux into the oesophagus

Figure 5.9
Top: Normal
Bottom: Hiatus hernia

Complications which may arise are peptic ulceration within the hernial sac or, more rarely, bleeding.

Treatment

The majority of middle-aged patients respond well to medical treatment. In obese patients reduction of weight with consequent reduction in intra-abdominal pressure relieves symptoms. Similarly the hernias of pregnancy disappear after parturition.

Prevention of reflux at night is assured if patients are encouraged to sleep in a semi-upright position with the head of the bed raised on blocks. Tight clothing should not be worn. A bland diet is advised, and during acute stages antacid medications are given frequently for the immediate relief of heartburn and to protect the inflamed oesophageal mucosa from further damage by gastric acid.

Persistent oesophagitis and the intractable pain associated with ulcer and stricture formation are only relieved by surgery. The purpose of surgery is to reduce the hernia, strengthen the hiatus and restore the oesophago-gastric angle.

Achalasia (cardiospasm)

This is the condition of deranged oesophageal motility. As a result of this nervous disturbance, the cardiac sphincter fails to relax and allow entry of food into the stomach. Progressive dysphagia with persistent vomiting are the outstanding symptoms. Treatment involves selective division of the sphincter muscle (Heller's operation).

Carcinoma of the oesophagus

This malignant growth; occurring usually in middle-aged or elderly patients, produces a progressive dysphagia.

Clinical features

At first, difficulty is experienced when swallowing solids. Finally even fluids cannot be tolerated, with resultant dehydration, wasting and anaemia from lack of nourishment. The constant regurgitation is distressing and carries the risk of aspiration pneumonia. The stricture is demonstrated on barium swallow X-ray and diagnosis of malignancy is confirmed by oesophagoscopy and biopsy examination. Pain is a late symptom.

Treatment

Radiotherapy is effective in causing regression of the tumour.

Oesophagectomy a severe mutilating operation, involves removing a large section of the oesophagus and anastomosing the remainder to the stomach below.

Palliative therapy. The aim of palliative treatment is to provide the patient with adequate nourishment. Because of the stricture, it is often impossible to pass a nasogastric tube into the stomach. It is sometimes possible to pass a tube such as an *MB tube* through the growth to allow partial freedom from dysphagia. Failing this a gastrostomy is performed: a small opening is made into the stomach and a catheter is inserted for feeding purposes.

DISORDERS OF THE STOMACH AND DUODENUM

Incapacitating conditions of the stomach and duodenum are common in the Western hemisphere and, since they often affect people in their middle years, they have important social and economic implications.

Gastritis

Inflammation of the mucous membrane lining of the stomach is termed gastritis.

Acute gastritis generally results from some gross dietary indiscretion or ingestion of contaminated food. In most cases the intestine is also inflamed (gastroenteritis).

Chronic gastritis presents a more serious clinical problem and is likely to be encountered in patients who habitually enjoy highly seasoned foods, overindulge in alcohol or have a raised acid secretion. Symptoms are similar to those of peptic ulceration and the patient is treated medically as for this condition.

Peptic ulceration

The term peptic ulceration refers to an ulcer formed on any mucosal surface exposed to the irritating effects of gastric hydrochloric acid and the enzyme pepsin.

Aetiology

The areas affected are the lower end of the oesophagus, when it is subjected to acid reflux, the stomach and the duodenum. Peptic ulcers may occur in areas brought into contact with gastric juices following gastric surgery. The incidence of ulcer disease is lower in women than in men and this apparent immunity is increased during pregnancy. It is possible, therefore, that hormonal substances increase normal mucosal resistance. Heredity is a well-recognized factor as is the association of peptic ulcer with patients in blood group O. It is also recognized that emotional factors play an important part in the development of an ulcer.

The ingestion of alcohol and certain types of food as well as cigarette smoking tend to aggravate ulcers.

Clinical features

Pain and discomfort, often described as burning in character, are usually felt in the epigastric region and at specific times in relation to meals. Localized tenderness and rigidity are felt directly over the ulcer site. Food eases the pain caused by most peptic ulcers but relief is more lasting in the case of duodenal ulcer. Vomiting is likely when pain is severe and always affords some measure of relief. If appetite remains good, weight loss is uncommon. Heartburn is experienced in most cases.

Ulcers may be acute or may follow a chronic course with the patient complaining of long-standing but intermittent dyspepsia. These recurring attacks, often preceded by emotional stress, tend to become more frequent and severe before the patient seeks medical advice.

Investigations

Diagnosis is usually made on barium meal examination which shows an ulcer crater.

Gastroduodenoscopy may be performed to confirm the presence of an ulcer and, more important, to determine whether the lesion is malignant or benign. A biopsy is therefore taken during endoscopy.

Gastric secretion tests are carried out: normal acid levels are usually found in patients with gastric ulcer, while excessive amounts may be found in those with duodenal ulcer. A finding of achlorhydria excludes the possibility of simple peptic ulcer. Examination of faeces may reveal the presence of occult blood.

Course and complications

The uncontrolled symptoms of peptic ulceration affect the patient's life at home and at work. From time to time he will have acute exacerbations of the disease and complications may arise. Common complications are:

1. **Pyloric stenosis**. The formation of scar tissue and of inflammation around the pyloric sphincter may cause delayed emptying of the stomach resulting in stasis of gastric content.

2. **Perforation** of an acute or chronic ulcer (p. 189) will allow the irritating gastric or duodenal content to drain into the peritoneal cavity resulting in peritonitis (p. 211).

3. **Haemorrhage**. Severe haemorrhage occurs if the ulcer erodes a large blood vessel producing the alarming symptom haematemesis.

4. **Malignancy**. There is the risk of malignant changes occurring in chronic gastric ulceration (p. 211).

Treatment and nursing care

Medical treatment

The aims of medical treatment are the relief of symptoms, the healing of the ulcer and the prevention of complications.

1. **Bed rest**, whether at home or in hospital, is the single most effective part of patient care. Ambulation is allowed for toilet or bathing purposes only; otherwise, the patient must be afforded all the physical and mental rest possible in order to relieve pain and hasten the healing process. Since stress is a contributory factor in the hypersecretion of acid the patient is advised to avoid anxiety; sedatives may be prescribed for the very anxious person.

2. Bland, small, frequent meals may be prescribed — some authorities consider them a means of neutralizing gastric acid. Although a particular **dietary regime** may ease the patient's pain there is no evidence that any specific diet assists healing. The continuing presence of occult blood in faeces proves this point.

3. **Drug therapy** plays an invaluable role in treatment by neutralizing and inhibiting acid output and reducing spasm and inflammation.

Antacids such as aluminium hydroxide or magnesium trisilicate can be taken between meals to neutralize gastric acid and relieve pain. These preparations must be fast-acting, harmless, palatable and — above all — cause no interference with bowel function or the acid-base balance of the body.

Anticholinergic drugs depress gastric motility and acid secretion by inhibiting the vagus nerve stimulus. Prescribed in addition to diet and antacid therapy, drugs such as propantheline (Probanthin) help to prevent pain, particularly during the night. Carbenoxoline (Biogastrone), an oral preparation derived from extract of liquorice, is found to have some effect on ulcer healing in the ambulant patient. It is thought to reduce inflammation around the ulcer.

4. Since there is evidence to suggest that cigarette smoking inhibits healing **smoking is discouraged**.

Healing takes 4 to 6 weeks according to the initial severity of the condition. However, at the end of a week following medical treatment symptoms should subside; gradual return to normal activity is then permitted. Thereafter, management involves the prevention of recurrence. Regular, non-irritating meals with interjacent milk drinks are recommended and the avoidance of alcohol, cigarette smoking and stress situations are advised.

Unfortunately, there is no sure means of maintaining healing or preventing relapses, therefore surgery is recommended when medical treatment fails, when complications occur or when there is any suspicion of malignant change.

Surgical treatment

The aim of surgical treatment, for those who do not respond to medical treatment, is the reduction of acid secretion. This may be achieved by diminishing vagal stimulation to the parietal cells of the stomach by severing some branches of the vagus nerve, (highly selective vagotomy) (Fig. 5.10 *left*). Another means of reducing acid production is by removing the antrum, the gastrin-secreting area of the stomach, by performing antrectomy (Fig. 5.10 *right*).

Postoperative complications. Following gastric surgery, the majority of patients can again enjoy normal digestive function and good health. Regular out-patient examination is advised, however, to detect and treat any late postoperative complications. These include:

Nutritional disorders. The alimentary canal has considerable adaptive powers following surgery, but sometimes, because of gastric resection, food is not prepared properly for its onward passage through the tract. Also, when a drainage procedure has been carried out, unprepared food may leave the stomach at a rapid rate.

Figure 5.10
Left: Highly selective
vagotomy
Right: Antrectomy

Undigested food cannot be absorbed and deficiency diseases with weight loss will result.

Anaemia. This is a late complication associated in particular with partial gastrectomy. The anaemia may be due to malabsorption of iron or failure to produce the intrinsic factor.

Dumping syndrome. The usual complaint is of epigastric fullness, giddiness and extreme fatigue occurring during a meal or immediately afterwards and when the patient is in an upright position. It is probably due to the sudden distension of the jejunum. The symptoms are eased if the patient eats dry meals, avoids hot fluids and rests immediately after eating. Explanation of symptoms does much to allay the patient's anxiety. If symptoms do not subside corrective surgery may be necessary.

Perforated peptic ulcer

This is an abdominal emergency of sudden onset and with early signs of acute peritonitis. Perforation of the ulcer allows gastric contents to drain into the peritoneal space. It may also erode a blood vessel and cause severe haemorrhage.

Clinical features

The patient is pale, tense and afraid to move because of the intense pain. Respirations are shallow and rapid. The abdomen is held rigid and does not move on breathing. The pulse is rapid and of poor volume.

The patient complains of severe, generalized, abdominal pain which may be referred to his shoulders because of the presence of gas and irritant fluid under the diaphragm. Haematemesis will indicate erosion of a major blood vessel.

Investigations

The patient's history is important: he may already be known to have a peptic ulcer. X-ray of the abdomen in the supine and erect positions will show air under the diaphragm in most cases.

Nursing observation and records

Pulse and blood pressure.
Degree of pain and signs of circulatory collapse.

Treatment and nursing care

Pain is relieved and the patient prepared for surgery to repair the perforation and control bleeding.

A nasogastric tube is passed to aspirate gastric contents before and after the operation. Intravenous infusion is started to replace fluid, electrolyte and blood loss. The operation is usually a simple closure of the perforation and ligation of the eroded blood vessels.

In the postoperative period gastric suction and intravenous infusion are continued until the patient is free of pain, has no abdominal distension and no signs of toxaemia. Antibiotics may be prescribed if chest infection or peritonitis complicate the postoperative period.

There is usually a dramatic improvement in the patient's general condition. If this is maintained oral fluids and then light diet can be introduced about the fourth day after surgery. Stitches are removed and the patient is allowed home about the tenth day.

Because of the possible recurrence of complications most patients are reviewed at a later date for elective surgery. This may be vagotomy and gastroenterostomy for duodenal ulcer or partial gastrectomy for gastric ulcer.

Gastric carcinoma

Carcinoma of the stomach is the commonest malignant tumour of the gastrointestinal tract.

The condition is commoner in men than in women and mostly occurs in middle age. The cause is unknown but the incidence of malignant change is greater in those patients who have a previous history of chronic gastritis and peptic ulceration.

Clinical features

Early symptoms of dyspepsia, usually vague, are readily dismissed and the patient may seek medical advice only when the tumour is advanced and there are signs of extensive spread. Epigastric pain resembling that of peptic ulcer but lacking the characteristic relationship to meals may occur alone or accompanied by nausea, vomiting, anorexia, weight loss and constipation. An abdominal mass easily palpable suggests an advanced unresectable tumour. Gastrointestinal bleeding is a feature found in one-third of patients. Coffee-grounds vomiting and melaena indicate a slow but constant ooze of blood from the lesion. Anaemia is always present.

Investigations

Diagnosis is confirmed by a combination of radiology, gastroscopy and biopsy. Barium meal examination shows a filling defect caused by the tumour (Fig. 5.11).

Figure 5.11
Defect in the stomach outline
indicative of malignant tumour

Treatment

Management of gastric carcinoma is by immediate surgery where possible and involves either partial or total gastrectomy. When the growth is widespread no resection may be attempted, but accessible areas of tumour may be removed thereby affording considerable symptomatic relief from obstruction and haemorrhage. Radiotherapy is of little value in these circumstances.

DISORDERS OF THE SMALL INTESTINE

Regional enteritis (Crohn's disease)

This is a non-specific inflammatory process affecting the whole thickness of the intestinal wall. It may occur in single or multiple segments and most commonly affects the ileum. There is thickening of the submucosa, ulceration and hypertrophy of the muscle wall causing narrowing of the lumen of the intestine. As the ulceration heals, scar tissue formation prevents absorption of nutrients and also causes strictures. The inflammatory process may affect the mesentery and lymphatic system in the area.

The disease usually occurs between the ages of 20 and 30 years. It affects men and women equally and may take the form of an acute or chronic illness.

Clinical features

The patient with chronic regional enteritis has a history of general ill health, weight loss and anaemia. Intermittent colicky pain associated with diarrhoea may occur three or four times daily. The stools often contain mucus, pus and undigested food; there can be fistula formation and intestinal obstruction. In acute regional enteritis, the patient has severe abdominal pain low on the right side. He may have a moderate fever and mild diarrhoea.

Investigations

A barium meal and follow-through X-ray will show the areas of the small intestine that are affected. A barium enema is also performed to assess any involvement of the colon.

Nursing observations

Temperature, pulse, respiration and blood pressure.
Fluid intake and output.
Character and frequency of diarrhoea.
Early signs of intestinal obstruction, such as abdominal distension, pain, vomiting and dehydration.

Course and complications

The inflammatory and fibrotic changes in the mucosa of the small intestine prevent the normal absorption of fat and protein. This causes deterioration in the patient's general health. Oedema and congestion can result in adhesions between loops of bowel or other abdominal organs and lead to the formation of fistulae or abscesses. Intestinal obstruction may occur due to strictures caused by adhesions or narrowing of the small intestine lumen.

Treatment and nursing care

The patient has a chronic debilitating disease and will require sympathetic nursing care to help him accept this and adjust his way of living. General health can be improved by attention to diet, which should be bland, high calorie and high protein with iron and vitamin supplements. During an acute phase the patient is nursed in bed. He may require intravenous replacement of fluids and electrolytes if diarrhoea becomes a problem. Steroid drugs may be prescribed to reduce acute inflammation during relapses. Antibiotic therapy will be prescribed if there are signs of infection and abscess formation. Antispasmodic drugs will help to relieve pain associated with diarrhoea.

Although treatment is essentially conservative, complications such as intestinal obstruction, abscess or fistula formation will require surgery. Grossly affected segments can be excised leaving as much normal intestine as possible for the absorption of nutrients.

Rehabilitation and community care

Because the patient has a chronic illness a great deal of support is required. Patient and family should be educated in maintaining nutrition. Ideally the help of a dietitian to explain the preparation of special diets and supplements should be made available. Although the patient should be encouraged to become employed, within the limitations imposed by the illness, financial support may be needed — particularly to help finance the diet required to maintain his general health.

Malabsorption syndrome

The term can be applied to any disorder of the gastrointestinal tract which impairs the digestion and absorption of one or a number of nutritional substances. However the term usually refers to conditions where there is multiple malabsorption. The conditions may be grouped in the following way:

Incomplete digestion — from either a lack of pancreatic enzymes, as in pancreatitis, or absence of bile salts due to biliary tract obstruction (p. 205). It may also be the result of gastric surgery such as gastrojejunostomy when chyme leaves the stomach and enters the jejunum without being mixed with the enzymes and bile salts in the duodenum.

Impaired absorption — caused by either inflammatory conditions of the small intestine, such as regional ileitis (p. 190), or bacterial invasion of this part of the tract, which is usually sterile. It may occur as a result of gastric surgery, for example in the blind end of the duodenum following some types of gastrectomy.

Congenital malformation of the mucosal lining of the small intestine as in coeliac disease, will reduce the area and ability of the small intestine to absorb.

Clinical features

Signs of malnutrition — glossitis, anaemia, weight loss and bone disease — are evident. There may be abdominal distension and the patient often complains of diarrhoea with pale, bulky, offensive stools.

Investigations

The patient's history of any previous gastrointestinal surgery.
Barium meal and follow-through X-ray.
Biopsy of small intestine (p. 183).
Faecal fat estimations.
Glucose tolerance test.
Blood levels of various substances, such as urea.
Urine collection.

Treatment

This depends on the cause of malabsorption. Surgery may be necessary to relieve biliary tract obstruction and to correct the blind loop following gastric surgery. Specific treatment will be required for conditions such as regional ileitis, pancreatitis and coeliac disease.

Intestinal obstruction

Intestinal obstruction develops when the contents of the gastrointestinal tract cannot pass through the lumen of the small or large intestine. This may be caused by mechanical, adynamic or vascular disorders of the tract.

There are three categories of mechanical obstruction:

1. Extramural obstruction caused by pressure outwith the wall of the intestine.
2. Mural obstruction caused by an abnormality of the intestinal wall causing narrowing of the lumen.
3. Intraluminal obstruction due to tumour or foreign body within the lumen of the intestine.

Extramural obstruction is most commonly caused by the formation of adhesions following surgery or inflammatory disease. These strands of tissue may constrict the intestine or provide a focus for rotation or kinking of the gut; this condition is called volvulus. Another cause of obstruction may be that part of the intestine becomes trapped within a hernial sac. Pressure exerted on the wall of the intestine by tumour in an adjacent organ could occlude the lumen so causing obstruction.

Mural obstruction may result form the healing and scarring process of some inflammatory disease or from malignant growth within the wall of the intestine causing narrowing of the lumen.

Intraluminal obstruction may be caused by a bolus of meat or fruit, a large gallstone or by tumour within the lumen of the intestine.

Adynamic **obstruction** results from any condition which impairs peristalsis; severe pain or handling the intestine during surgery can result in paralysis of the intestine.

Vascular disease of the mesentery such as mesenteric embolus will prevent adequate blood supply to a segment of the intestine causing loss of function.

Obstruction causes distension of the immediately proximal part of the intestine. This is due to the accumulation of gas derived from swallowed air (which is normally passed through the tract) and produced by bacterial decomposition of stagnant intestinal content. The pressure exerted by the accumulated gases stops the absorption of fluids and electrolytes from the lumen of the gut.

Clinical features

Symptoms vary according to the level at which the obstruction has occurred. High obstruction in the small intestine will produce symptoms more rapidly than obstruction lower down the intestinal tract. The four classical features are pain, vomiting, abdominal distension and constipation.

Pain. The first reaction of the intestine to obstruction is to produce more and more powerful contractions, hyperperistalsis, which causes waves of abdominal colic. In obstruction of the small intestine the waves of pain occur every 2 to 3 minutes: in the large intestine every 10 to 20 minutes.

Vomiting. As time passes the affected intestine becomes weak and distended by the collection of fluid. When the fluid level reaches the stomach the patient begins to vomit: at first stomach contents, bile-stained fluid and later, faeculent fluid.

Distension. The exhausted distended intestine becomes adynamic and distension increases.

Constipation. As a result of hyperperistalsis the patient may have diarrhoea, but as the adynamic state is reached there will be absolute constipation and absence of flatus.

The patient appears pale, tense and afraid. Signs of dehydration such as thirst, dry furred tongue are apparent.

Investigations

Physical examination, auscultation of the abdomen may elicit hyperactive bowel sounds.

X-ray of the abdomen with the patient in the erect and supine position will show gas patterns and fluid levels.

Observations and records

Temperature, pulse, respiration and blood pressure.
Fluid balance.
Amount of pain.
Character of vomitus.

Course and complications

The patient's general condition deteriorates rapidly. Gross dehydration may lead to peripheral circulatory failure. The accumulation of gas produced by bacterial decomposition of stagnant intestinal content causes increased distension. This prevents the absorption of fluids and electrolytes. The affected part of the intestine may become necrotic if its blood supply becomes strangulated. Due to the increasing pressure there is the possibility of perforation of the intestine.

Treatment and nursing care

A combination of conservative and surgical treatment is employed to relieve obstruction, correct dehydration and electrolyte imbalance and remove the cause.

A nasogastric tube is passed to enable the gastric content to be removed. This will relieve vomiting and prevent aspiration pneumonia (Ch. 6). The amount and nature of the aspirate must be recorded. Intravenous infusion of fluid electrolytes and plasma are necessary to correct dehydration which may have reduced the blood volume. Pain relief will allow rest and lessen apprehension. Emergency surgical treatment may be required to remove the cause of obstruction when there is risk of strangulation.

Obstruction of the small intestine can be relieved by the release of strangulation or adhesions and, if necessary, resection and anastomosis of the necrotic segment or excision of the tumour. This will restore continuity and allow normal flow of intestinal content. Postoperative management is explained on pages 214–215.

Obstruction of the large intestine is usually treated in three stages:

1. Decompression of the intestine by temporary colostomy (p. 197). In some cases resection of the cause of obstruction, for example carcinoma of the colon, may be done at the same time.

2. Resection of the cause of obstruction a few weeks after the decompression operation. The patient's general condition can be improved in the time before resection (p. 201).

3. Closure of colostomy at a later date when healing of the resection is satisfactory.

DISORDERS OF THE LARGE INTESTINE
Appendicitis

This is an inflammatory condition of the appendix. The cause has not yet been defined but it may result in obstruction of the appendix lumen by hardened faeces or a foreign body. The obstruction impairs circulation and results in lowered resistance to organisms normally present in the bowel such as E. coli. The condition is more frequent in males and usually occurs in older children and young adults.

Clinical features

There is sudden onset of pain in the umbilical area, anorexia, nausea and vomiting. The pain then becomes sharp in the area halfway between the umbilicus and the right ileum. These symptoms, occurring suddenly in an otherwise healthy person, are typical of acute appendicitis. There may also be a moderate rise in temperature and a change in bowel habit.

Investigations

Abdominal palpation may elicit other symptoms such as guarding and tenderness in the right lower abdomen. Rectal examination is carried out. It may produce pain in response to pressure high on the right of the rectum.

Nursing observations and records

Records of temperature, pulse and respiration are kept by the nurse. The general condition of the patient and the degree of pain he has should be observed and recorded. Any changes in his condition must be reported promptly.

Course and complications

As the disease progresses, abscess formation may occur around the appendix and in the pelvis. Total obstruction of the appendix will result in its becoming gangrenous and then rupturing. This will cause generalized peritonitis.

Treatment and nursing care

When appendicitis is suspected, the patient is admitted to hospital immediately. He will be confined to bed until investigations and observations have been made. An operation may be required shortly after admission, and for this reason the patient is given nothing to eat or drink. A nasogastric tube may be passed and intravenous infusion started. The patient is given frequent mouth care and helped into a comfortable position in bed. If the patient is a child the doctor will inform the parents and request their permission to operate, once the diagnosis has been confirmed.

The appendix is usually removed through a small incision in the right side of the lower abdomen. Drains are inserted only when there is evidence of abscess formation or if the appendix has ruptured.

Following surgery, the symptoms disappear and normal bowel function soon returns. Fluids and food can then be given as desired. The patient is allowed out of bed the day after operation. Moving out of bed and standing can cause anxiety and wound pain. The nurse who is helping the patient at this time should therefore assess his condition before encouraging him to take short walks. Early discharge from hospital may be arranged if home circumstances are suitable and community care is available. Provision is made for the removal of sutures in the patient's own home or in the out-patient department. Normal activity should be resumed within 2 to 4 weeks.

When it has been necessary to insert a wound drain, the patient should be nursed in an upright position to encourage free drainage. The character and amount of drainage should be observed and dressings changed when necessary. The patient should have plenty of fluids and may be given antibiotics. Attention to skin and mouth will help to make the patient comfortable. He will be discharged from hospital when he has recovered from the acute phase of his illness and is able to be up and about. If necessary dressings can be changed by the community nurse or the patient's own doctor.

Ulcerative colitis

Ulcerative colitis is an inflammatory disease of unknown origin involving the mucosa and submucosa of the large intestine. The incidence is highest among young adults, especially young women. Although the cause is unknown, it is thought that psychological factors play a part in the disease process.

Initially, the mucosa of the rectum and the sigmoid colon becomes swollen and congested. The mucosa bleeds easily and patchy ulceration occurs where the mucous membrane has been eroded. The condition may spread to other regions of the colon and may involve the caecum. The disease is progressive with periods of remission and of acute exacerbation.

Clinical features

The onset is insidious with abdominal discomfort, mild diarrhoea, blood in the stools and possibly anal excoriation. The symptoms then become more defined with loose stools and frequent urgent discharge of blood and mucus. In the acute stage, the patient has pain, weight loss, fever and general debility. The profuse diarrhoea causes severe fluid and blood loss. The patient, understandably, may display signs of emotional disturbance and depression.

Investigations

Examination by direct vision of the rectum (proctoscopy) and the sigmoid colon (sigmoidoscopy), during which a biopsy of mucous membrane can be obtained.

Barium enema to assess the extent of ulceration.

Haematological examination to assess haemoglobin, electrolyte and protein loss.

Nursing observations and records

Degree of anxiety and mental stress.

Accurate records of fluid intake and output.

Stools — amount, frequency, consistency and presence of blood or mucus.

Course and complications

At first only inflammatory changes occur; ulceration follows later. In the chronic condition the thickened oedematous mucosa may undergo changes which produce pseudopolyps. The continuous healing process and formation of scar tissue cause loss of both elasticity and absorptive capability of the colon; secondary infection may supervene. The loss of fluid, electrolytes, blood and protein from the colon into the faeces causes dehydration, anaemia and weight loss.

The spread of infection from the colon to the systemic and portal circulation causes bacteraemia and toxaemia. The muscle coat of the colon is affected only when secondary infection occurs. This causes loss of muscle tone and leads to fissure formation, dilatation of the colon and risk of perforation. Malignant changes and tumour formation may occur when the disease is long standing and severe.

Treatment and nursing care

The aims of nursing care during an active phase of the disease are to understand and support the patient during this exhausting illness and to ensure the provision of adequate rest, warmth and nutrition. The patient will require meticulous attention to his personal hygiene and should be nursed in a well-ventilated environment.

Medical treatment

Distressing diarrhoea can be controlled by drugs which will slow down the hyperactive colon. The addition of bulk such as bran or cellulose to the diet will reduce the amount of fluid loss. Anaemia and loss of protein can be corrected by giving the patient a high protein diet with iron supplements. Losses during an acute exacerbation may require blood replacement and intravenous infusion to correct the electrolyte balance.

Anti-inflammatory drugs such as Salazopyrin can be given in tablet form during periods of remission to prevent relapse. In severe cases cortisone may be prescribed and can be given in several forms — orally, by intramuscular injection, or by local application using suppositories and retention enemata.

A sympathetic, hopeful attitude towards the anxious and depressed patient will improve morale considerably. He can then be helped to recognize and cope with any emotional stress which may have caused the exacerbation of the disease.

It is important that the patient and his relatives are made aware that the condition will not be cured but only alleviated when the patient returns home. They should be guided in how to maintain good nutrition and helped to understand the disease and accept the patient's behaviour. The anxious patient will require encouragement to continue a fairly normal life between active phases of the disease. Socioeconomic problems may be solved with the help of a medical social worker thus relieving these causes of anxiety. Careful follow-up of the individual as an out-patient is essential because of the possibility of malignant changes in the colon. Early detection of other complications may prevent them from reaching serious dimensions.

Surgical treatment

Surgery will be indicated if medical treatment fails to control the symptoms. Recurrent acute exacerbations may make life intolerable for the patient. The operations which may be performed are subtotal colectomy or total colectomy with establishment of an ileostomy (p. 201). The patient is admitted to hospital and specific preparation is given to help him accept that he will have a permanent stoma. Many of the patients are from a fairly young age group. Their age and the relief obtained from the distressing symptoms of ulcerative colitis allow them to adapt to the situation and resume their normal place in society.

Diverticular disease

A diverticulum is a herniation of the mucosa through the muscle wall. Multiple diverticula (Fig. 5.12) may occur anywhere in the gastrointestinal tract. It is an acquired condition mainly affecting the colon. **Diverticulosis** only implies that diverticula exist. When diverticula become inflamed because of faecal impaction and

Figure 5.12
Cross-section of the colon showing diverticula

Figure 5.13
Narrowed lumen of the colon caused by diverticulitis

infection, the condition is known as **diverticulitis** (Fig. 5.13). It is considered a deficiency disease of Western civilization where the diet has become refined and of low residue. The lack of bulk in the diet requires increased pressures in the colon to transport faeces. This increase in pressure is thought to be the cause of herniation through the muscle coat.

Clinical features

Diverticulosis may be asymptomatic or there may be some history of dyspepsia and change in bowel habit.

Diverticulitis causes lower abdominal distension and pain. There may be recurrent attacks of acute pain and fever with a history of increasing constipation.

Investigations

Barium enema.
Sigmoidoscopy.

Nursing observations and records

Stools frequency, consistency and appearance.
Temperature, pulse and respiration.

Course and complications

Diverticulitis may resolve spontaneously, leaving only mild symptoms, or it may progress to an acute stage. In the acute phase the swollen and thickened colon becomes adherent to nearby structures with the possibility of formation of fistulae between colon and bladder or vagina. Peritonitis can occur following the formation of pericolic abscess or by perforation of the diverticulum. The lumen of the colon may become narrowed resulting in intestinal obstruction.

Treatment and nursing care

A mild form of the disease can be treated at home. The patient is given advice on the prevention of constipation and the constituents of diet that can help this condition. The ingestion of unrefined foods and plenty of fluids and the addition to foods of bran or a cellulose product are advised since they add bulk to the diet. Antispasmodic drugs may be prescribed to relieve pain.

During an acute attack, the patient may be nursed in hospital because of the need for early recognition of the dangerous complications. While the patient has pain and pyrexia, he requires bed rest. During this time a fluid diet is given. Parenteral antibiotic drugs may be prescribed to control infection and inflammation. When the patient has recovered from the acute attack, he can resume the treatment advised for the mild condition.

Recurrent exacerbations of this disorder can distress and debilitate the patient and for this reason elective surgery may be advised. If an operation is decided on, the patient is prepared for surgery (p. 201). The diseased part of the colon is excised and continuity re-established by joining the two ends of healthy colon. This operation is known as a colectomy.

Patients with complications such as intestinal obstruction and perforation require immediate surgery. A temporary colostomy will be made to relieve obstruction (Fig. 5.14 — *Stage 1*). This will divert the faecal stream away from the grossly affected section of the colon. A second operation will be performed later when the patient's general condition has improved and there has been time for the preparation of the colon for surgery. At this point, a colectomy will be performed (Fig. 5.14 — *Stage 2*). When this has healed satisfactorily, a third operation will allow the colostomy to be closed (Fig. 5.14 — *Stage 3*).

Stage 1

Stage 2

Stage 3

Figure 5.14
Stage 1: Temporary colostomy
Stage 2: Resection of the affected area of the colon
Stage 3: Closure of colostomy

Hirschsprung's disease

This is a congenital condition caused by abnormal nerve fibres and the absence of ganglion cells in the mesenteric and submucosal plexus of the colon. This abnormality always involves the distal end of the rectum and extends proximally for varying lengths. Two types are described: short segment Hirschsprung's disease when the area of aganglion cells extends from the internal anal sphincter to the mid-sigmoid region of colon; long segment Hirchsprung's disease when the area of aganglionosis may involve the entire colon and may extend into the small intestine. The result is failure of the affected segment to maintain peristalsis. Contents of the colon do not pass through the affected segment and this causes distension of the normal colon.

Clinical features

The condition is first noticed by the absence or delay in the normal passage of meconium shortly after birth and loose stools during the early weeks of life. During the first year of life there is abdominal distension and severe constipation with passage of small, ribbon-like stools. The condition may be severe enough to cause anorexia, vomiting and intestinal obstruction.

Investigations

X-ray of abdomen and small barium enema.
Rectal examination. Rectal manometry.
Biopsies of rectum and colon to establish the level at which normal nerve cells are present.

Nursing observations and records

The passage of meconium (or its absence) at birth and the character of subsequent stools should be noted and recorded. Weight should be recorded regularly. Signs of dehydration and abdominal distension should be looked for specifically.

Course and complications

The condition causes chronic, severe constipation and abdominal distension. The child fails to thrive and may develop acute intestinal obstruction.

Treatment and nursing care

Some infants require surgery for the relief of intestinal obstruction within days of birth. A temporary colostomy is made; fluid and electrolyte balance is maintained during the 24 hours following surgery by intravenous infusion via a scalp vein. Nutrition is then re-established by slow introduction of oral feeding. Careful observation and recording of fluid intake, fluid output and faecal output are important. The skin around the colostomy must be kept clean and dry to prevent excoriation. At this stage the mother can be involved in the care of her child. Practical experience, and education in the care of her child's colostomy and nutritional needs, should enable her to manage confidently when the child is discharged from hospital. Major surgery to resect the affected segment of colon will be delayed until the child is about 18 months of age. Children with less severe symptoms can be managed by observation and regulation of bowel habit by diet, aperients and enemata if necessary.

Follow-up

Regular health and developmental assessment should be carried out by a paediatrician. Support and education in nutrition and stoma care should be provided as the needs arise.

Carcinoma of the colon and rectum

A carcinoma of the large bowel is a malignant tumour arising from the mucous membrane. There is no known cause of malignant tumours, but benign polyps and ulcerative colitis are predisposing factors in some instances. Carcinoma may occur anywhere in the large colon although it is most commonly found in the caecum, sigmoid colon or rectum. The tumours are usually slow growing. They may be either (1) the polypoid type which projects into the lumen of the colon or (2) the annular type which grows around the lumen, causing a stenosing ring-like stricture (Fig. 5.15).

The spread of carcinoma is usually by direct invasion or by the lymphatic and venous drainage of the colon. Tumour cells are carried to the liver via the mesenteric and portal veins then into the circulation to produce secondary metastases elsewhere. There is increasing incidence of tumour with age: it is most common over the age of 50.

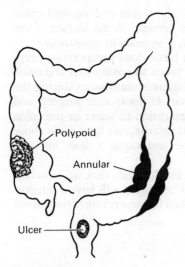

Figure 5.15
Types of carcinoma of the colon and rectum

Clinical features

Carcinoma causes symptoms which differ according to the site of the tumour.

A tumour in the caecum or ascending colon is usually polypoid. There the colon is wider and the faeces more fluid so that obstruction rarely occurs. The symptoms of the patient are usually anaemia, melaena as a result of gradual bleeding from the tumour surface.

In the sigmoid colon there is a high incidence of the annular type of tumour. The resulting stricture leads to partial obstruction which causes alternating constipation and diarrhoea with abdominal pain. Accompanying the change in bowel habit may be rectal discharge with blood and mucus. Complete obstruction can occur due to total occlusion of the lumen by tumour or by the impaction of faeces above the tumour.

A tumour in the rectum also gives rise to changes in bowel habit and the passage of blood and mucus per rectum. In addition the patient has a constant feeling of fullness in the rectum. A patient in the advanced stages of the condition may show signs of intestinal obstruction, perforation or complications arising from secondary metastases.

Investigations

Barium enema.
Rectal examination.
Colonoscopy

Nursing observations and records

Bowel habit.
The presence of blood and mucus or occult blood in stools.
Fluid intake and output.
Signs of dehydration, abdominal distension and haemorrhage.

Course and complications

Obstruction of the flow of fluids and nutrients will prevent absorption and cause abdominal distension because of accumulation above the level of the obstruction. Eventually there will be copious vomiting of the intestinal content producing dehydration and loss of nutrients. The patient will appear very debilitated and in great pain.

Treatment and nursing care

Surgical removal of the tumour following early diagnosis gives good results. The operation, called a colectomy, consists of resection of the tumour and the adjacent lymph nodes and restoration of the continuity of the colon. In low rectal or advanced tumour of the sigmoid colon, removal of the anal canal, rectum and sigmoid colon is necessary. The open end of the remaining colon is brought to the surface of the abdomen and an artificial anus established — that is, a permanent colostomy.

The success of the surgery depends very much on meticulous preoperative preparation of the patient (p. 201). Special care must be taken to ensure that the colon is cleansed by colonic lavages; it is customary to administer antibiotics during the 5 days prior to surgery. Peristalsis is inhibited for about 48 hours after surgery, and if faecal matter has not been removed the normal absorption of water in the colon will cause the faeces to become hard. When peristalsis returns, this hard mass above the site of the operation may tear the suture line and cause a leak into the peritoneum.

If there is intestinal obstruction the colon cannot be cleansed, making a preliminary operation necessary to relieve the obstruction. The patient will have a temporary colostomy which may be closed at the later date when his general condition allows the appropriate surgical procedure to be performed.

Haemorrhoids

The term haemorrhoids refers to dilatations of the terminal parts of the haemorrhoidal veins lying in the submucosa of the upper anal canal. They are classified as first, second and third degree. First degree haemorrhoids project into the lumen of the anal canal and become congested during defaecation. Second degree haemorrhoids are larger and tend to prolapse. Third degree haemorrhoids are completely prolapsed (Fig. 5.16). Both men and women can be affected by this painful condition. The predisposing factors are thought to be conditions which obstruct the haemorrhoidal venous drainage, such as chronic constipation and pregnancy; haemorrhoids may be secondary to tumours in the pelvis or rectum.

3rd degree haemorrhoid

Site of ligation and excision of haemorrhoid

Figure 5.16
Haemorrhoids

Clinical features

The first symptoms of haemorrhoids are local discomfort, prolapse and rectal bleeding during defaecation. With second and third degree haemorrhoids, the patient experiences pain, bleeding and anal discharge which causes pruritus. He may suffer from anaemia due to slow loss of blood over a period.

Investigations

History of bowel habit and physical examination.
Digital examination of anal canal and rectum.
Proctoscopy and sigmoidoscopy.

Course and complications

Congested, prolapsed haemorrhoids can become thrombosed and cause the patient great distress. Third degree haemorrhoids, which have prolapsed through the external anal sphincter, become oedematous and strangulated. This very painful situation completely incapacitates the patient as he is unable to walk or sit down.

Treatment and nursing care

The kind of treatment given depends on the severity and cause of the symptoms. In less severe conditions advice should be given to the patient about diet and regulation of bowel habit — to avoid straining at defaecation. Careful and frequent anal cleansing will help prevent pruritus. Rest in bed, local heat or hot baths can alleviate the pain caused by difficult defaecation.

Second degree haemorrhoids can be treated by injection therapy. A sclerosing agent such as 5% phenol in oil is injected into the submucosa around the haemorrhoid; the resulting inflammatory reaction causes fibrous changes which obliterate the veins.

Third degree haemorrhoids are treated by surgical excision with ligation; this operation is called haemorrhoidectomy. The patient is prepared for anaesthesia and operation in the usual way.

During the first 24 hours after surgery, careful observation of pulse and blood pressure is necessary. Haemorrhage may result from a slipped ligature and the blood loss will be concealed if it gathers in the anal canal.

Patients often have severe pain following haemorrhoidectomy. This can be relieved by careful positioning and support in the most comfortable position possible and by giving prescribed analgesic drugs. On the day after surgery, the patient is usually allowed out of bed; he may have supervised warm baths and may use a bidet to ensure cleanliness and to relieve pain.

If spontaneous bowel action does not occur an aperient may be given on the third evening after surgery. Following each bowel action the area is cleansed as noted above and, if necessary, a dressing is applied and held in place with a T bandage.

The patient may be anxious about the first bowel action and needs careful nursing as he may suffer considerable pain and feel faint. The passage of a stool of normal consistency following haemorrhoidectomy prevents stricture of the anal canal.

Follow-up

When discharged from hospital, the patient is advised to avoid constipation by taking a diet with adequate roughage and fluids. He may be given a mild aperient to be taken until regular bowel habit has been established.

Figure 5.17
Colostomy

Nursing care of the patient undergoing surgery of colon or rectum

Preoperative management

In addition to the routine physical and psychological care necessary before any operation, those who are to have surgery of the colon or rectum need special care to provide the best possible conditions for the process of healing. This objective may be achieved by ensuring that no faecal matter remains in the colon and by reducing the number of bacteria present.

During the 4 days before operation, the patient is given a high protein, low residue diet with plenty of fluids. The surgeon may want colonic lavages and a broad spectrum antibiotic to be given preoperatively. The patient and his relatives will require explanations of the operations and its attendant procedures. They should be allowed to express their anxieties and should be helped to come to terms with them.

On the day of operation, a nasogastric tube is passed allowing aspiration of the intestinal fluids and gases, which will accumulate due to the inhibition of peristalsis. This inhibition is the result of anaesthesia and of the handling of the intestine during surgery and usually persists for 24 hours after operation. To prevent damage to the bladder, a self-retaining catheter is inserted to allow free drainage of urine.

Special psychological preparation is of great importance for those patients who are having surgery which results in the formation of an opening from the intestinal tract on to the abdominal wall (colostomy [Fig. 5.17] or ileostomy [Fig. 5.18]).

The surgeon will explain the operation and its consequences to the patient. It is then the nursing staff's responsibility to give the patient concerned the opportunity to ask questions. Issues such as diet, sport, the reaction of a partner, holidays may cause the individual concern. At this stage it may be possible to introduce the patient to the stoma care nurse, a clinical specialist, or to a representative of the Colostomy/Ileostomy Association. Many areas prefer to invite the patient to discuss forthcoming self management with a former patient who is coping with a stoma successfully; if possible, patient and visitor should be matched for age, social group and sex. A selection from the various appliances available may be demonstrated, the patient being allowed to examine and handle these.

Careful preparation at this stage goes a long way to helping the patient come to terms with his stoma postoperatively. Emphasis is placed on the improved quality of life.

Figure 5.18
Ileostomy

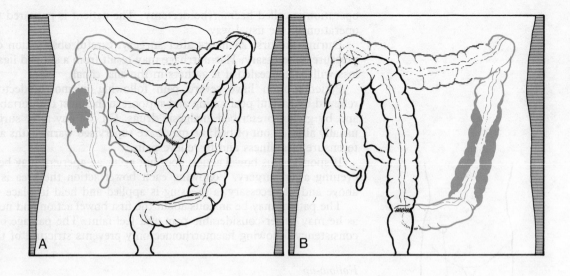

Figure 5.19
(A) Right hemicolectomy and ileotransverse anastomosis
(B) Left hemicolectomy
(C) Excision of rectum and formation of colostomy
(D) Proctocolectomy and formation of ileostomy

Operations on the colon and the rectum

Right hemicolectomy (Fig. 5.19A)

Restoration of continuity by anastomosing ileum to transverse colon.

Left hemicolectomy (Fig. 5.19B)

Restoration of continuity by end-to-end anastomosis between transverse colon and rectum.

Abdominoperineal excision of rectum (Fig. 5.19C)

Establishment of permanent colostomy in left iliac fossa.

Total proctocolectomy (Fig. 5.19D)

Excision of anus, rectum and colon. Establishment of ileostomy.

A stoma made in the terminal part of the ileum which is brought to the surface of the abdominal wall is known as an ileostomy. This can be a temporary or permanent means of draining the small intestine when there is disease of the colon.

Postoperative management

In the postoperative period, routine care is given with, in addition, observation of the stoma. It is important to notice if the circulation appears adequate and if there are signs of prolapse of the stoma into the abdominal cavity. At this time, there is very little intestinal activity with very small amounts of altered blood and mucus being discharged. When peristalsis does return the discharge is fluid and profuse. A well-fitting appliance is necessary to prevent excoriation of surrounding skin. Careful cleansing of the skin around the stoma and the application of a specially formulated adhesive to prevent leakage from the appliance are of great importance. Excoriation of the skin will cause the patient pain and distress. Whenever the patient's general condition allows, he should be gently encouraged to become involved in the care of his stoma.

Ileostomy

The particular problems associated with an ileostomy are caused by the normally semifluid contents of the small intestine. An ileostomy bag must be worn continuously and must be close-fitting to prevent the effluence coming in contact with surrounding skin as this would cause gross excoriation. Regulation of an ileostomy is difficult but the consistency can be varied by diet and the use of hydrophilic colloids. Before being discharged from hospital the chosen long-term management should be established. Careful follow-up is necessary to provide support and advice on diet, skin care and appliances.

Bacillary dysentery

Dysentry is an inflammatory disease of the colon and rectum which may be caused by bacterial or protozoan infection. Bacillary dysentery results from infection by *Shigella* organisms. The mucosa of the colon becomes inflamed and oedematous with superficial ulceration. The spread of infection is by personal contact or by food contaminated from unwashed hands. It is therefore possible to have an epidemic of the disease in large communities where sanitation is inadequate. The incubation period is between 1 to 7 days. The health authorities must be notified of any incidence of the disease.

Clinical features

The symptoms vary in severity from mild diarrhoea lasting about 3 days to a grossly debilitating illness. In the acute form the patient is febrile, dehydrated and has generalized abdominal pain with incontinence of blood-stained stools.

Investigations

Bacteriological examination of stools and rectal swabs.
Blood culture.

Nursing observations and records

Stool content and frequency.
Signs of dehydration.
Fluid intake and output records.

Course and complications

It is possible for some people to become carriers of the disease after complete recovery from an attack. A carrier, although symptomless, can spread the disease to others.

Treatment and nursing care

During a mild attack the patient can be nursed at home. He is advised to take plenty of fluids, drugs may be prescribed to control diarrhoea and antibiotic therapy instituted to suppress infection. He must be made aware of the need to prevent spread of the infection. Careful cleansing of the lavatory and handwashing after defaecation are essential.

A severe attack requires efficient barrier nursing. The patient is admitted to hospital for bed rest during the acute stage. Loss of fluids and electrolytes resulting from profuse diarrhoea can be replaced by intravenous infusions. Specimens of stool should be sent promptly for examination and should be collected with due precaution against spread of infection. The appropriate antibiotic therapy can then begin. Although symptoms subside and the patient recovers he cannot be declared free from infection until three consecutive stool cultures are negative.

DISORDERS OF THE LIVER

Viral hepatitis

Inflammation of the liver is known as hepatitis and the most common cause is viral infection. Normal liver cells take in bilirubin from the plasma; the cells then conjugate and excrete it into the biliary ducts (Fig. 5.3, p. 176). Inflamed liver cells are unable to carry out this function properly so that an excess of unconjugated bilirubin is left circulating in the blood, producing prehepatic jaundice. Failure to excrete bilirubin into the biliary ducts causes stasis within the liver and an excess of conjugated bilirubin in the circulation. This results in jaundice with symptoms similar to obstruction of the biliary tract.

There are two types of viral hepatitis — infective and serum.

Infective hepatitis

This is the most common liver disorder in Great Britain and other Western countries. The source of the virus is the human blood and faeces of an already infected person or healthy carrier of the disease. The incubation period is 10 to 40 days. The disease can be transmitted by ingestion of contaminated food or water; when the virus reaches the intestine it is absorbed into the blood. There is a higher incidence of the disease among children and people living in crowded communities where epidemics are more likely to occur.

Clinical features

There is a period of up to a week during which the patient complains of general malaise and experiences anorexia and low-grade fever. After this period jaundice appears from the increased levels of bilirubin in the blood and may become very marked within a few days. Urine becomes darker and stools paler in colour. The liver is tender and may become slightly enlarged. At this stage there may be a slight prolongation of prothrombin time. The course of the disease is 3 to 6 weeks. Some patients find that pruritus causes considerable discomfort.

Acute inflammatory changes may occur in the liver and result in liver cell necrosis, but usually the patient recovers completely.

Investigations

Examination of serum, for example, levels of bilirubin.

Treatment and nursing care

Treatment is aimed at resting the liver and supporting its function during the period of natural recovery. The patient can be managed at home and should be kept at rest until the serum bilirubin levels fall. No special dietary regime is thought necessary but the daily intake should include adequate protein and glucose. Alcohol, which, in health, is detoxicated by the liver, must be avoided for 6 months. Jaundice is usually present for 2 to 6 weeks; the patient can resume normal activities about 3 weeks after jaundice has faded. In patients who have jaundice due to intrahepatic cholestasis the jaundice persists for 7 to 20 weeks. A diet high in protein and low in fat is usual with vitamin K supplement. A common sequel to the disease is posthepatitis syndrome. The patient complains of malaise, is easily tired, has mild anorexia with fat intolerance and some depression. This may be related to other postviral infection syndromes such as that following influenza. No special treatment is required but the patient should be reassured that the liver is normal.

Community care

Prevention of the spread of infective hepatitis includes attention to general and personal hygiene. Special precautions must be taken for the safe disposal of urine and faeces from an infected patient. The virus is usually present in all the members of the patient's household and it is recommended that each person has a prophylactic intramuscular injection of gamma globulin. Such precautions may prevent or lessen the severity of an attack of infective hepatitis but are of little value in serum hepatitis.

Serum hepatitis

This is a less common but more severe form of viral hepatitis. The incubation period is about 3 months and the virus is transmitted by infected serum. Various body fluids such as saliva, vaginal discharge, seminal fluid and serous exudate have also been implicated. The condition can occur as the result of accidental innoculation during medical, surgical or dental procedures, blood transfusion, contaminated injection equipment, tattooing or laboratory accidents. It has been found that patients with serum hepatitis display specific antigens in their plasma. These antigens are highly infective protein particles. Initial infection may be followed by a persistent carrier state, so special care must be taken when nursing those who have positive serum. Patients who present with acute symptoms of serum hepatitis must be nursed in an isolation unit. The outcome of acute serum hepatitis may be either complete resolution, massive liver necrosis, chronic hepatitis, or resolution with scarring.

DISORDERS OF THE BILIARY TRACT
Gall-stones

Gall-stone formation is known as **cholelithiasis** and is thought to be a condition related to the Western pattern of living. It has become a common disease, with increasing incidence over the past 25 years. The stones may consist of pure bilirubin, cholesterol or a combination of both with some calcium deposits. While they are in the gall-bladder they may be entirely asymptomatic; problems arise when the stones move out into the cystic duct, where they tend to become impacted and cause inflammation of the gall-bladder or **cholecystitis**. A stone which has reached the bile duct and become impacted will obstruct biliary drainage (Fig. 5.20). This results in biliary colic and jaundice. Trauma from stones in the biliary tract causes stricture formation. Impaction of a stone or stricture at the sphincter of Oddi will prevent bile and pancreatic secretion from entering the duodenum.

The formation of gall-stones is thought to occur more frequently in women of child-bearing age.

Clinical features

The patient may have a history of dyspepsia and a special aversion to fatty foods. Pain occurs in the right epigastrium and radiates to the subscapular area. Typically, it is of sudden onset, colicky and very severe. Obstruction of the bile duct or the sphincter of Oddi results in high levels of bilirubin circulating in the blood. This produces a yellow tinge of the skin called jaundice, very dark coloured urine and pale, fatty stools.

The patient who is suffering from an acute attack of biliary tract disorder appears

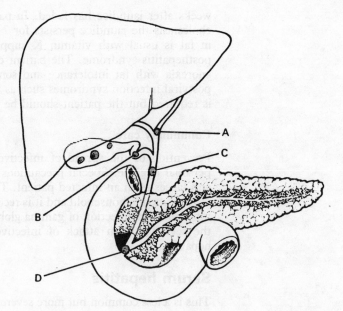

Figure 5.20
Sites of biliary tract obstruction
due to gall-stones
(A) Hepatic duct
(B) Cystic duct
(C) Bile duct
(D) Sphincter of Oddi

restless, in pain, nauseated and dehydrated. The jaundiced patient may have coagulation defects caused by inability to absorb fat and fat-soluble vitamins, including vitamin K.

Investigations

History and clinical examination.
X-ray of abdomen.
Examination of blood, urine and stools.
Cholecystogram to demonstrate gall-bladder appearance and function.
Cholangiogram to estimate biliary duct function and to show the presence of stones or stricture.
Ultrasound.

Nursing observations and records

Temperature, pulse, respiration and fluid balance.
Colour of stools, urine and skin.

Course and complications

Most patients with acute cholecystitis recover within a few days with conservative treatment. Recurrent episodes may occur and some have serious complications. Ascending infection in the hepatic ducts will cause cholangitis which will obstruct the flow of bile from the liver. Impaction of a stone in the gall-bladder neck or cystic duct will result in stasis of bile, infection and the possibility of pus formation in the gall-bladder which will distend and may eventually rupture resulting in peritonitis. Obstruction of the bile duct or the sphincter of Oddi prevents the flow of bile and pancreatic secretions into the duodenum. This will cause pancreatitis and inability to absorb protein, carbohydrate and fat.

Treatment and nursing care

During the acute inflammatory stage the patient is confined to bed and is more comfortable when nursed in a well-supported, upright position (Fig. 6.13, p. 225).

Medical treatment

Specific care of these patients includes the relief of pain using drugs to relieve spasm;

this may allow the obstructing stone to be passed into the duodenum. The patient has nothing orally, thus avoiding the normal stimulus to the gall-bladder to contract. Hydration is maintained by intravenous infusion.

Surgical treatment

When the patient has recovered and the signs and symptoms of inflammation have disappeared, surgery may be advocated to prevent the serious complication of biliary tract obstruction. The diagnostic procedures cholangiogram and cholecystogram are performed and the gall-bladder, which is the source of gall-stones, is removed. The operation is fairly common and is known as **cholecystectomy**.

The patient has routine preparation for theatre. Special preparation includes estimation of the prothrombin index, particularly if the patient has had biliary obstruction which has prevented the absorption of vitamin K. A nasogastric tube is passed before surgery as the procedure is less distressing to the patient at this stage. During the operation a cholangiogram is performed following the removal of the gall-bladder. This is to ensure that the bile duct is patent. Any exploration of the bile duct, which may be necessary as a result of the cholangiogram, will cause oedema and it therefore becomes necessary to insert a T tube drain to allow free flow of bile from the liver. At the end of the operation the patient will have a drain at the site of the gall-bladder to prevent the formation of haematoma and also a T tube drain in the bile duct if it has been explored (Fig. 5.21). General postoperative care is described on page 215.

Management of T-tube drainage following exploration of bile duct. Initially there will be free drainage of bile into the collecting bag attached to the drain. After a period of 48 hours the drain is clamped off for short periods and the patient is observed for signs of increasing pain, which indicates obstruction. If this occurs free drainage must be resumed immediately. When there is no adverse reaction to the drain being clamped off then this should be continued for longer periods each day until there is very little or no bile draining into the collecting bag.

Observation of stools and urine will also indicate whether or not proper flow of bile has been re-established. Usually after 10 days a postoperative cholangiogram is performed to confirm patency of the duct and then the T tube may be removed.

Follow-up. The patient who has a straightforward cholecystectomy will probably leave hospital after 10 days. At this stage he should be having a normal diet. One month after the operation he is reviewed at a follow-up clinic and should be ready to resume normal activity.

Figure 5.21
(A) Drainage tube in gall-bladder bed following cholecystectomy
(B) Site of T tube drain following exploration of the bile duct

DISORDERS OF THE PANCREAS

Diabetes, a disease of the pancreas related to its endocrine function, is described in Chapter 11.

When malignant tumours arise in the pancreas they are usually rapidly fatal; involvement of the head of the organ causes obstructive jaundice. Other important and serious conditions of the pancreas are the result of inflammatory processes.

Pancreatitis

Alcohol and gall-stones are thought to be the main causes of this inflammatory disease which may affect either sex and usually occurs between the ages of 40 and 70 years; it may be acute or chronic.

Acute pancreatitis

The predisposing causes are obstruction to the flow of pancreatic secretions in the pancreatic duct or at the sphincter of Oddi. The obstruction may be due to the presence of impacted gall-stones, tumour or inflammatory changes caused by regurgitation from a chronically infected biliary tract. Alcohol in excess is thought to produce spasm of the sphincter of Oddi and to stimulate the pancreas to produce excessive amounts of secretions. The damming back of pancreatic enyzmes within the gland results in vascular damage, necrosis and autodigestion of the pancreas. However normal function can be restored when the precipitating factors have been removed.

Clinical features

Typically there is a sudden onset of acute abdominal pain usually in the epigastrium and penetrating through to the back. The pain is persistent and may last for days; the patient has tachycardia, pyrexia and is hypotensive. Nausea and vomiting are common and there may be abdominal distention due to ileus. The patient looks very ill and develops signs of obstructive jaundice.

Investigations

Pancreatic function tests

1. The degree of duct obstruction and the excretory ability of the gland can be estimated by the levels of serum amylase and lipase. In acute pancreatitis the levels will be high in blood and urine.

2. Pancreatic function can be measured by taking specimens of duodenal aspirate and blood samples before and after giving intravenous injections of secretin and pancreozymin.

Radiology

Plain X-ray of the abdomen may demonstrate the presence of gall-stones, any other condition that may cause acute abdominal pain such as perforated peptic ulcer or acute cholecystitis may then be excluded.

Ultrasonography

Endoscopic retrograde cholangiopancreatography (ERCP) may aid diagnosis of those patients who do not have a history of alcohol abuse.

Surgery

Laparotomy may be necessary to confirm the diagnosis because the clinical features are very similar to those of a perforated ulcer.

Nursing observations and records

Effects of pain upon the patient.

Pulse and blood pressure.

Accurate records of fluid intake and output.

Observations of signs of adynamic ileus, a possible result of constant acute abdominal pain.

Observation of stools — steatorrhoea will occur because absence of lipase causes malabsorption of fat.

Observation of urine — glycosuria may be present due to a temporary diabetic state.

Course and complications

When the acute phase subsides and the cause of inflammation has been diagnosed, the patient may require surgery to remove the obstruction or may need treatment for alcoholism if this was a predisposing factor. Recurrent acute inflammatory changes may result in the formation of fibrosis and the destruction of acinar and islet tissue. This state of chronic pancreatitis will eventually produce symptoms of malabsorption and diabetes due to the reduction of exocrine and endocrine function of the pancreas.

Treatment and nursing care

Medical treatment

Conservative treatment in the acute stage is aimed at:

1. **Treatment of shock.** Bed rest and total nursing care. In severe shock plasma transfusion may be necessary to correct dehydration and electrolyte imbalance.

2. **Relief of pain.** Adequate control of pain may be difficult; morphine is seldom used as it causes spasm of the sphincter of Oddi and there is the risk of the patient becoming addicted since only opiates give relief.

3. **Inhibition of pancreatic secretion.** This can be achieved by continuous gastric suction to prevent gastric acid entering the duodenum, so stopping the production of secretin. Pancreatic and gastric acid secretion can also be reduced by drugs which prevent stimulus through the vagus nerve, for instance probantheline bromide.

4. **Prevention of infection.** Antibiotics may be given intramuscularly to prevent secondary infection of damaged tissue.

5. **Parenteral nutrition** may be necessary if this disease lasts longer than a week.

Surgical treatment

This is aimed at the relief of obstruction and at increasing drainage. Obstruction due to impacted gall-stones or from inflammation due to regurgitated bile from a chronically infected biliary tract can be relieved by removal of stones and the gall-bladder. Increased drainage can be effected by first demonstrating the stricture of the pancreatic duct by an operative pancreatogram, then subsequently by reconstructing drainage. The pancreatic duct can be anastomosed to the duodenum, by-passing the sphincter of Oddi. If the duct has become narrowed, a polythene tube can be inserted to increase drainage.

Total pancreatectomy may be necessary for the relief of intractable pain of acute recurrent pancreatitis. This radical operation requires immediate insulin replacement and oral pancreatic supplements at meal-times.

Chronic pancreatitis

Alcohol abuse is the main cause of chronic and relapsing pancreatitis. Those affected are usually middle aged and have a history of years of excessive drinking before the onset of symptoms. Obstruction and dilatation of the ducts and fibrotic changes in the pancreas are usually established before symptoms appear. The gland may become diffusely fibrosed with calculi and cyst formation within the ducts. The eventual calcification and necrosis of endocrine cells and islets of Langerhans results in permanently impaired function.

Clinical features

The patient has a history of recurrent attacks of mild to moderately severe pain in the epigastrium radiating through to the back. The onset of the attack is usually sudden and is precipitated by overindulgence of alcohol during the preceeding 24 hours. There is nausea, vomiting and jaundice.

Investigations

As for acute pancreatitis.

Nursing observations

Assessment of the degree of pain.
Record of fluid intake and output.
Observation of stools for steatorrhoea.
Observation of urine for glycosuria.

Course and complications

The eventual calcification and necrosis of exocrine cells and the islets of Langerhans. Permanently impaired pancreatic function results in diabetes and malabsorption. The formation of pancreatic cysts results in persistent pain.

Treatment and nursing care

Mild attacks of the disease can be treated with analgesics and light diet. The need for complete abstinence from alcohol should be emphasised to the patient. More severe attacks require hospitalization to assess and treat complications such as diabetes. Malabsorption of fat and protein requires pancreatic enzyme replacement therapy to reduce steatorrhoea and prevent weight loss.

DISORDERS OF THE PERITONEUM

Ascites

The fluid of the peritoneal cavity acts as a lubricant and allows the abdominal organs to glide smoothly over one another. Excess fluid in the cavity is termed ascites. Most commonly, ascites complicates conditions which increase venous pressure in the abdomen, such as congestive cardiac failure (Ch. 7), liver cirrhosis or portal vein thrombosis. Because of the high venous pressure, fluids leave the capillaries and enter the peritoneal cavity. Although rare, tuberculosis and malignancy of the peritoneum may also cause ascites.

Clinical features

Symptoms of the underlying condition are accompanied by a progressive and regular distension of the abdomen. Pressure symptoms such as dyspnoea are troublesome.

Treatment and nursing care

The underlying cause must be treated first. To relieve the distressing pressure symptoms abdominal paracentesis is carried out. Following local anaesthesia with ligno-caine 2%, a small trochar and cannula are inserted through the abdominal wall into the peritoneal cavity. Maintaining strict asepsis fluid is withdrawn and a specimen is sent for pathological examination. Since there is risk of the patient collapsing when a large quantity of fluid is withdrawn from the body, careful check is made of his pulse and general condition during the procedure.

Peritonitis

This is an inflammation of the peritoneum which is usually due to invasion by micro-organisms. Infection may be blood-borne as part of a generalized septicaemia. More commonly, however, rupture or perforation of some diseased abdominal organ causes a breach in the visceral peritoneum and allows infected material to spill into the cavity. The local infection may spread rapidly causing generalized peritonitis. A similar result may follow the use of corticosteroid drugs when the normal reaction to inflammation is inhibited. Any abdominal organ is then susceptible to inflammation, perforation and contamination of the peritoneal cavity by bacteria.

Clinical features

The onset of peritonitis may either supervene on the symptoms of an existing disease or occur dramatically, as in the case of perforated peptic ulcer. Less frequently it results postoperatively from breakdown of an anastomosis. Pain is acute, severe and continuous, rapidly spreading over the whole abdomen which becomes tender and rigid. Peristalsis is inhibited. The vomiting that occurs initially becomes more frequent and ultimately contains faecal material. As the state of collapse becomes more severe, the abdominal rigidity gives way to a less painful distension. The patient lies motionless, eyes sunken, face pale and anxious looking. The skin is cold and clammy, pulse rapid, blood pressure and temperature lower than normal. Urinary output is diminished.

Treatment and nursing care

Intravenous fluid replacement and antibiotic therapy are initiated immediately whilst continuous gastric suction, via a nasogastric tube, is established to relieve vomiting. The greater the amount recovered, the less the peritoneal contamination. No fluids are allowed orally.

A nurse in constant attendance can do much to allay anxiety and make such observations of the patient as will indicate any change in the course of the condition. Blood-borne peritonitis is treated medically and should respond well to intensive antibiotic therapy. Peritonitis due to perforation of some abdominal organ is more complicated and requires surgical treatment. A rising pulse, hypothermia, increasing pallor and collapse indicate that medical therapy is ineffective and surgical repair must be carried out immediately. If the peritonitis is localised, prognosis is much more favourable. However, in a generalized peritonitis, the condition is usually so severe and acute that the outcome is often fatal.

Such catastrophies can be avoided if threatening abdominal conditions are resolved before peritonitis is established.

DEFECTS OF THE ABDOMINAL WALL

Hernia

A hernia is the protrusion of an organ from its own cavity. A hernia of the anterior abdominal wall can be caused by congenital weakness of the supporting muscles. Alternatively it can be due to physical strain at work or strain produced by some disease such as chronic bronchitis, enlarged prostate gland or chronic constipation. Inadequate wound healing because of infection or poor physical condition may also result in the development of a hernia. If the organ can be returned to its cavity the hernia is termed **reducible**; if the size of the defect in the muscle does not allow the organ to be returned it is said to be **irreducible**.

Clinical features

The patient or the mother of a small child may notice a swelling at the site of the hernia (Fig. 5.22). This swelling or lump may enlarge when the patient coughs, strains or lifts heavy objects. There may also be some local discomfort which disappears when the patient lies down.

Figure 5.22
Common sites of hernia of the anterior abdominal wall

Incisional   Umbilical
Epigastric
Inguinal   Femoral

Strangulated inguinal hernia

Figure 5.23
Strangulated hernia

Course and complications

Initially, a sac of peritoneum protrudes through the weakened area and a loop of intestine may follow as the area enlarges. The hernia may become irreducible as a result of inflammatory adhesions or because of constriction of the protruding organ by the narrow opening into the hernial sac. If the blood supply to the organ becomes impaired the hernia is said to be strangulated (Fig. 5.23). This causes severe pain, nausea, vomiting and abdominal distension. The damaged part of the intestine becomes necrotic and intestinal obstruction ensues.

Treatment and nursing care

Surgical repair of the hernia, while the patient is in reasonably good physical condition, will prevent serious complications. The operation is called herniorrhaphy. During the preoperative period, any physical condition which will cause extra strain on the newly repaired tissue should be corrected. The herniating structure is returned to its cavity and the defect in the supporting muscle is sutured. A patch may be used to strengthen the muscle wall and prevent recurrence of the hernia. During the postoperative period, early recognition of symptoms which may cause greatly increased intra-abdominal pressure will prevent disruption of the repaired tissue. The nurse can help the patient to support his wound during sneezing, coughing or postoperative vomiting. Signs of bladder or abdominal distension should be reported immediately. The patient may be in hospital for 7 days, but if home and community care are adequate, he may be discharged within 2 to 3 days of the operation.

Community care

On discharge from hospital, the patient is advised to refrain from strenuous exercise for at least 3 weeks.

NURSING CARE OF THE PATIENT WITH A GASTRO-INTESTINAL DISORDER

When planning nursing care for the maintenance or restoration of health, it is important to consider the self-esteem of the patient. Disorders of the gastrointestinal tract often produce symptoms which intensify the physical and emotional distress caused by illness. For example, the apprehension and embarrassment experienced by the patient with diarrhoea and vomiting must be recognized. Observant, sympathetic nursing care can lessen the discomfort of the patient and those around him by ensuring privacy and proper ventilation and by preventing or dispelling offensive odour.

Psychological care

Anxiety may be allayed by giving the patient a simple explanation of nursing procedures and the part he has to play, so gaining his confidence and co-operation. Explanation and support during diagnostic and therapeutic procedures will help the patient to cope with a situation which he may find unpleasant and exhausting.

Since emotional disturbances also predispose to some gastrointestinal tract disorders, it is important that nurses in the course of their duties approach patients with a reassuring and optimistic attitude. They should be encouraged to express and share their stressful problems.

Physical care

The physical care of the patient includes the maintenance of respiratory and circulatory functions and the provision of an adequate fluid and nutritional intake.

Nutrition

The normal way to take nourishment is by oral ingestion. Some patients may be prevented from eating and drinking because of symptoms such as pain, nausea and vomiting. At this time intravenous infusion may be given to prevent dehydration and electrolyte imbalance. Satisfactory nutrition can be achieved by feeding via a nasogastric tube or by a tube opening into the jejunum, a jejunostomy. Others may have disorders which cause inflammatory changes, preventing digestion and absorption of nutrients. The only alternative for these patients is to be fed via the circulatory system, **parenteral nutrition**. In this situation the nutritional and biochemical requirements of the patient are estimated on a daily basis. The physician, with the aid of the biochemist, prescribes the nutrient solution for the individual's needs over 24 hours. Administration is achieved by cannulation of a large central vein. The doctor passes a catheter (most commonly via the subclavian vein) until the tip lies just above the right atrium of the heart. This procedure is carried out aseptically, preferably in the operating theatre. An X-ray is taken to check the position of the catheter.

Nursing care of the patient being fed parenterally requires skill and understanding. The patient's general condition and morale is likely to be low, therefore much encouragement will be necessary. There are several hazards associated with administration of nutrients parenterally, one of the most sinister being the risk of septicaemia. Great care must be taken by all involved to prevent the introduction of infection.

Many patients have been maintained solely on parenteral feeding for over a year, by which time the underlying condition has healed or corrective surgery has been possible. For the majority of patients parenteral nutrition is only required for a week or two. In either situation successful treatment may be life saving.

The mouth

Inspection of the mouth and pharynx reveals signs of systemic illness as well as local disease and must be carried out thoroughly as part of basic nursing observation. The appearance of the tongue in particular provides valuable information about the state of the gastrointestinal tract. The healthy tongue is pink and is kept moist by saliva which continually bathes the inside of the mouth.

A dry tongue is common in patients who mouth-breathe or who have lost excessive amounts of fluid and have become dehydrated. In dehydration, salivary secretion is diminished as body fluids are concentrated in vital areas and the patient experiences thirst. Often, for medical or surgical reasons, oral fluids are forbidden; therefore, thorough, regular mouth care must be provided in an effort to keep the mouth clean and comfortable.

A brown, furred tongue may indicate irregular oral toilet or inadequate elimination of waste — for example, renal insufficiency — but it usually accompanies underhydration. Frequent mouth care will help to cleanse and remove odour and unpleasant taste. Many patients during their treatment have a nasogastric tube inserted or are not permitted to eat or drink. If thirst is a problem, sucking small pieces of ice may afford relief, provided that too much fluid is not swallowed.

Observation of excreta

Vomitus

The volume and time in relation to food intake must be noted as well as the colour, presence of undigested food, frank or altered blood. In vomitus, blood changed by digestive juices has the appearance of coffee grounds.

Faeces

Stool consistency and regularity of bowel movement vary with the amount and type of food ingested. The faecal mass may be hard and dry when peristalsis is diminished, watery and offensive when the tract is inflamed and peristalsis is increased, or soft and ribbon-like in appearance when disease affects the lower bowel.

The faeces should not be unduly offensive and if they are bacteriological examination must be carried out to exclude the presence of pathogenic organisms. With this possibility in mind, specimens for observation and examination must be managed with care to prevent spread of infection (Ch. 1). Offensive stools are also likely in conditions of abnormal protein digestion when putrefaction occurs in the large intestine producing an unpleasant odour. Observation of the colour of stools is an extremely important aid to diagnosis. The normal brown stool becomes pale during a milk diet and dark when meat or iron containing preparations are ingested. When the biliary tract is obstructed the stool is clay-coloured due to the absence of bilirubin; excess of bilirubin produces dull green faeces. Bleeding within the tract may produce the typical black melaena stool. The presence of blood may be confirmed by using Occultest reagent tablets. Small quantities of blood may not be detected by the normal inspection, but this occult (hidden) blood will also react with Occultest reagents. In order to validate examination results three stool specimens are obtained on consecutive days. A melaena stool may, for example, be produced due to ingestion of blood following a tooth extraction thus giving a false sign of organic change.

The skin

The maintenance of an intact skin can prevent further discomfort and infection. This is of particular importance when the patient is confined to bed as the deprived tissues are at risk and easily damaged. By relieving pressure and keeping the skin clean and dry, damage may be avoided. When diarrhoea, faecal soiling or anal discharge exist, careful cleansing of the surrounding skin will prevent pruritus and excoriation. The use of a bidet or bath is the most efficient means of ensuring cleanliness and comfort.

Control of pain

Pain, in varying degrees of severity and character, is present at some time in most illnesses. Tolerance and reaction to pain vary from person to person and may be influenced by factors such as personality, cultural background or state of debility. The nurse's responsibility is to observe and make the patient as comfortable as possible. Reporting of observations can help the doctor prescribe appropriate treatment. Relief of pain permits diaphragmatic breathing, improves respiratory function and facilitates movement thus helping to prevent venous stasis and complications such as deep vein thrombosis.

Preoperative management

The nursing care of a patient having surgery should be directed towards meeting the varying physical, emotional and social needs of the individual. In this way each patient may be prepared to withstand the physiological and psychological stresses effected by anaesthesia and surgery.

The patient should be in the best possible physical condition before operation. For this reason examinations of the respiratory, circulatory and urinary systems are made to detect any coexisting disorder which may cause complications during or after surgery. The strange environment and procedures which are encountered when the patient comes into hospital may cause fear, depression or anxiety. Other stressful factors are pain, the uncertainty about survival, and doubts about retaining personal identity. In some patients this anxiety may reduce their understanding of the effects of surgery or of alternative treatment. The consequences of psychological stress result in physiological stress which may delay recovery. By giving the patient adequate information and allowing time to discuss socioeconomic problems, stress may be minimized. Indications are that patients who are carefully prepared in this way are more likely to make an uncomplicated recovery.

Postoperative management

In the immediate postoperative period when the patient has not yet fully recovered from the effects of anaesthesia an observant nurse can help to prevent the development of complications.

Frequent regular recording of blood pressure and pulse rate will indicate the state of the patient's circulatory system. Changes such as an increased pulse rate and a fall in blood pressure are signs of haemorrhage and must be reported immediately. The patient's colour and breathing pattern must be noted and attention drawn to deviations from normal. Shallow, inadequate ventilation may be due to the effects of drugs on the respiratory centre or the muscles of respiration and may result in respiratory failure. Noisy rapid breathing is usually caused by obstruction in the respiratory tract possibly by the tongue or a collection of secretions. Because of this possibility most patients are nursed on their side so that the tongue falls forward and secretions drain away.

Wounds and drains should be looked at as soon as possible so that the nurse can assess any further blood loss.

Any intravenous infusion should be inspected to ensure that the needle is in the vein and that the fluid is being administered at the correct rate.

As the patient regains consciousness he should be reassured and calmed. A restless patient can cause damage to his wound and may injure himself. Pain is another cause of apprehension and restlessness; therefore effective analgesia is necessary to give the patient much needed rest, relaxation and sleep.

The body's natural reaction to injury of any sort is to rest. This loss of function is apparent following surgery of the gastrointestinal tract and results not only from the surgical procedure itself but also from trauma associated with disturbance of the abdominal organs. Peristaltic action is lost because of post-traumatic paralysis or adynamic ileus.

Adynamic ileus

This loss of function may be:

1. Transient following for example, a simple appendicectomy.
2. Persistent following major surgery.
3. Present later if the repaired intestinal tract again becomes disordered.

Clinical features. There is absence of bowel sounds, faeces and flatus. Abdominal distension ensues due to the accumulation of intestinal gas and secretions. This causes discomfort and pain.

Vomiting will result when the stomach becomes dilated with an accumulation of gastric and intestinal secretions and gases.

Treatment includes intravenous replacement of fluids, nutrients and electrolytes; decompression of the intestinal tract by intermittent aspiration via a nasogastric tube. Decreasing amounts of aspirate suggest that normal function is returning.

Accurate records of fluid intake and output are necessary for the assessment of fluid replacement. Nothing is given by mouth until peristalsis is resumed. Restricted fluids are then allowed and the amount gradually increased as normal function returns.

Healing of abdominal wounds

This is normally straightforward provided that the wound is not contaminated or subjected to undue tension. Most uncomplicated wounds are exposed after 3 days and the patient is encouraged to bath or shower daily. Healing is fairly well established in 10 days and sutures can be removed.

Wound infection. A tense, painful and inflamed wound suggests that infection is present in the deeper tissues. In most cases, bacteriological examination of any discharge reveals the offending organism and a course of an appropriate antibiotic accompanied by aseptic wound care should effect speedy healing. Sometimes wound probing is required to open pockets of pus which should then be allowed to drain freely.

Regional abscesses may form in the pelvis or, less frequently, in spaces under the diaphragm (subphrenic abscess). Signs of infection persist long after surgery and necessitate drainage of the abscess.

Wound dehiscence (burst abdomen). This is a very alarming complication of abdominal wound healing which may occur about 10 days after surgery. The wound suddenly leaks serosanguinous fluid and subcutaneous and deeper layers of the wound edges separate allowing loops of intestine to appear on the surface of the abdomen. It is due to poor healing of the tissue which may be the result of:

1. Poor general health, anaemia, malnutrition and vitamin C deficiency.
2. Stress and strain during the postoperative period, for example from coughing or vomiting.
3. Wound infection and poor drainage procedures or the premature removal of sutures.

Treatment. As soon as possible the prolapsed intestines are wrapped in sterile towels soaked in warm saline. Meanwhile the operating theatre is alerted. A nurse in constant attendance can help to allay the anxiety produced by this dramatic event. The patient is prepared for theatre and the wound resutured under general anaesthesia. The degree of fluid loss and circulatory collapse is minimized if prompt treatment is provided.

Surgery is a traumatic experience for any patient but a confident, optimistic nurse can do much to avert anxieties, depression and apathy.

Early ambulation gives encouragement to most patients, but for those whose progress is hindered some light occupational or recreational therapy may be required.

SUGGESTED ASSIGNMENTS

Projects

1. Select a unit where there is a planned early discharge scheme for surgical patients. Find out how continuity of care is ensured and how the interests of the patient are safeguarded. If possible follow up one or two patients whom you know in consultation with the community nurse.

2. Where is the nearest stoma clinic for your area? What are its functions? If there is a stoma nurse what are her duties?

3. Choose two (or three) patients with a similar common disorder, for example peptic ulceration, on whom you could carry out a small comparative study. Headings under which you make your observations should be your own but could include previous history and circumstances which aggravated symptoms, reactions to admission to hospital, response to nursing care and treatment, length of stay, your own conclusions.

Discussion topic

Consider the hazards of living in an overcrowded environment with poor sanitation and its relevance to disorder of the gastrointestinal tract.

FURTHER READING

Bouchier I A D 1982 Gastroenterology, 3rd edn. Bailliere Tindall, London

Bonaparte B H 1981 Gastrointestinal care: a guide for patient education. Appleton Century Crofts, New York

Gillespie I E, Thomson T J 1983 Gastroenterology: an integrated course, 3rd edn. Churchill Livingstone, Edinburgh

Grant A K, Skyring A 1981 Clinical diagnosis of gastrointestinal disease. Blackwell Scientific, Oxford

Read E A, Harvey R F, Naish J M 1981 Basic gastroenterology including diseases of the liver, 3rd edn. Wright, Bristol

Chapter Six
The respiratory system

The many diseases that may affect the respiratory system can cause both acute and chronic illness. Often the early symptoms of illness are unobserved or ignored. The disease may then slowly progress to become a chronic condition. The high incidence of disability caused by chronic respiratory illnesses indicates that they are a major health problem. Health education can help by advocating means of prevention, early detection and treatment of disease.

ANATOMY AND PHYSIOLOGY

The respiratory system comprises passages and organs by means of which oxygen (O_2) is absorbed into the blood and carbon dioxide (CO_2) is excreted. The lungs are situated within the thoracic cavity (Fig. 6.1). Breathing is achieved by increasing and decreasing the size of the cavity. Enlargement of the thoracic cavity occurs as a result of nerve stimuli to the intercostal muscles and the diaphragm which cause them to contract, thus increasing the size of the cavity and drawing air into the lungs (inspiration) (Fig. 6.2). When the muscles relax the elastic recoil of the lungs expels the air (expiration). **Respiration** is the inspiration of air containing a relatively high proportion of O_2 and the expiration of air containing an increased amount of CO_2. The process of respiration is controlled by a group of nerve cells in the medulla oblongata known as the **respiratory centre**.

Figure 6.1
The lungs

Dead space air

Figure 6.2
Inspiration
The arrows indicate the direction
of chest expansion

Bronchiole

Alveolus

Air saccule

FROM
PULMONARY
ARTERY

Arteriole

Pulmonary
capillaries

Dilated alveoli

Venule carrying
oxygenated blood

TO PULMONARY VEINS

Figure 6.3
Structures enabling the diffusion
of O_2 and CO_2

The respiratory centre is influenced by the level of CO_2 and O_2 in the blood. High levels of CO_2 and low levels of O_2 stimulate the respiratory centre, causing an increase in the rate and depth of respiration in an attempt to 'wash out' or reduce the level of CO_2. Conversely, low levels of CO_2 diminish the stimulus to the respiratory centre, causing respiration to become slow and shallow. The maintenance of normal levels of oxygen and carbon dioxide in the blood depends on an adequate amount of oxygen in the inspired air and efficient respiratory and circulatory systems.

CO_2 passes from the blood in the capillaries to the alveoli in the lungs and O_2 is passed from the alveoli to the capillary blood. This gaseous exchange is known as **diffusion**. The structures which enable it to take place are shown in Figure 6.3. The carriage of oxygen through the lung tissue is dependent on an effective circulatory system. Lungs contain 3000 ml of air; this is the **vital capacity**. With each inspiration 400 ml of air enters the upper respiratory tract; of this amount, 150 ml (known as the **dead space air**) is held in the passages of the upper respiratory tract and the remaining 250 ml reaches the lungs for diffusion. This amount is known as the **tidal volume** and is necessary for normal metabolic function (Fig. 6.2). All tissues, including the medulla oblongata, require adequate oxygenation to maintain their normal function.

AETIOLOGY

The high incidence of respiratory disorder in temperate climates, especially in the United Kingdom, is associated with air pollution, cigarette smoking and cold, damp, foggy weather. These unfavourable conditions greatly aggravate any infective or allergic inflammatory changes present in the respiratory tract. The gravity of the situation in many countries has led to greater control of atmosphere pollution and of working conditions in occupations where dust and irritants are a problem.

Inflammation, increased secretion and infection prevent adequate alveolar ventilation and diffusion of gases. When these conditions become chronic there is a continuously lower percentage of O_2 in the blood (anoxaemia) and a higher percentage of CO_2 in the blood. Under these abnormal circumstances the respiratory centre is no longer influenced by the constant high percentage of CO_2 but by the low percentage of O_2 in the blood. In this situation great care must be taken to administer only the prescribed amount of O_2. Too high a percentage of O_2 in the blood will result in respiratory failure. If pulmonary oedema is present due to failure of the left side of the heart to transfer blood from the pulmonary veins, the diffusion of gases will also be inadequate (Ch. 7).

Trauma to the respiratory centre or to the muscles of respiration may prevent ventilation and necessitate the use of positive pressure ventilators. Failure of ventilation may also occur during the early postoperative period when obstruction of the airway or the effect of drugs on the respiratory centre may cause respiratory failure. Interruption of nerve pathways to the muscles of respiration in neurological diseases such as poliomyelitis and myasthenia gravis will also cause respiratory failure. Failure can also be of cardiac origin, for example following cardiac arrest when breathing usually stops within 30 seconds requiring immediate ventilation of the lungs by artificial means. Local spread of bronchial carcinoma embarrasses respiratory function by causing obstruction, collapse of a lobe or pleural effusion.

The accumulation of silica, asbestos fibre or coal dust results in **pneumoconiosis**. This is a collective term for a group of diseases caused by mineral dusts, which are progressive, and which produce fibrotic changes in the lungs; the pleura may also be involved. Recently there has been considerable concern regarding the role of blue asbestos in causing mesothelioma of the pleura; this is a malignant condition.

GENERAL FEATURES OF DISORDER

Cough

Cough is the most common symptom of respiratory disease and is a means of keeping the respiratory tract clear. The cough reflex is stimulated by any irritant touching the lining of the tract. The respiratory centre is the controlling factor in this reflex action, which causes forced expiration of mucus or foreign bodies. A cough may be dry or may produce sputum. Dry, unproductive coughing can be painful and exhausting to an ill patient and therefore a cough suppressant may be prescribed. A productive cough should not be suppressed but can be made less exhausting by giving an expectorant, a medication that loosens secretions.

Sputum

In health, sputum is not produced; it results from inflammation, infection or congestion, and may occur in varying amounts. Sputum produced by irritants is clear, white and mucoid; when infected sputum will be purulent (yellow or green) or mucopurulent; it may also contain blood.

Haemoptysis

The production of bright red, frothy blood from the lungs is usually associated with lung disease and vigorous coughing. The severity of the haemoptysis varies greatly from a few bloodstained streaks in the sputum to a very large haemorrhage that may be fatal.

Chest pain

Pain associated with respiratory disease may be:

1. Retrosternal pain made worse by coughing but not by deep breathing and most commonly caused by tracheitis.
2. Lateral or posterior chest pain usually occurring on inspiration; it is sharp and stabbing, increasing on deep breathing and coughing.

Dyspnoea

Difficulty in breathing that produces obvious changes in the normal respiratory pattern is called dyspnoea. It results from any obstruction to air intake, such as excessive secretions, spasm of air passages or the presence of a foreign body or tumour. Any condition affecting either the respiratory centre or the thorax, such as trauma to the chest wall, will also cause dyspnoea.

Hypoxia

Hypoxia is shortage of oxygen. It may be due to shortage of oxygen in the inspired air or to lung diseases which prevent oxygen reaching the blood.

Finger clubbing

This is a characteristic feature of lung abscess, bronchiectasis and bronchial carcinoma; the cause is not known (Fig. 6.4).

Cyanosis

This is blue discolouration of the skin or of the mucous membranes. It results from an abnormally high proportion of haemoglobin which has not combined with oxygen in the circulation. It is associated with the conditions causing hypoxia.

Pleurisy

Pleurisy is the term used to describe inflammatory changes occurring in the pleura. It is one of the symptoms of pneumonia, tuberculosis, malignant invasion of the pleura and pulmonary infarction. There are two forms of pleurisy. **Dry pleurisy** is characterized by a sharp, stabbing pain on deep breathing and coughing which restricts respiration. **Pleurisy with effusion** is caused by changes in the pleura which prevent the normal secretion and reabsorption of pleural fluid. This causes fluid to collect in the pleural space and inhibits lung expansion, necessitating pleural aspiration (thoracentesis).

Empyema

Is a condition in which there is infection causing pus formation in the pleural space.

Pneumothorax

Pneumothorax is the condition in which air is present in the pleural space, thus preventing normal lung expansion. This may result from chest trauma or be spontaneous. **Spontaneous pneumothorax** occurs when the rupture of a small air sac or bulla beneath the surface of the visceral pleura allows air to enter the pleural space. The collapse of the affected lung can cause displacement of the heart towards the opposite side. The resulting pressure on the opposite lung inhibits its expansion. If, as a result of chest trauma, blood is also present in the space the condition is known as **haemopneumothorax**.

The patient who has a spontaneous pneumothorax presents with a sudden onset of breathlessness and tightness in the affected side of the chest. Moderate or severe dyspnoea will occur according to the degree of displacement of the heart. On physical examination there will be absence of breath sounds on the affected side of

Increased curvature of nail

Swelling of fingertip

Figure 6.4
Finger clubbing

the chest. X-ray of the chest will demonstrate the edge of the collapsed area of lung and the degree of displacement.

Treatment is aimed at the re-expansion of the lung by introducing a thoracic catheter and connecting it to an underwater seal drainage bottle. Air can be removed by placing the catheter in the upper intercostal region, but if it is placed lower, air and serosanguinous fluid can be drained from the pleural space (Fig. 6.5). When there is only air present in the pleural space a **Heimlich valve** (Figs 6.6 and 6.7) may be inserted.

These are aseptic procedures carried out under local anaesthesia.

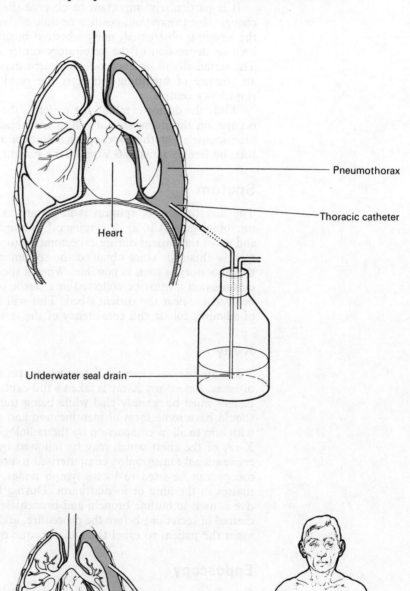

Figure 6.5
Underwater seal drainage

Pneumothorax

Thoracic catheter

Heart

Underwater seal drain

Figure 6.6
Heimlich valve

Figure 6.7
Heimlich valve in use

INVESTIGATIONS

Clinical examination

During the clinical examination the comfort and safety of the patient is the nurse's main concern. The patient requires an explanation of the procedure, reassurance, warmth and privacy. He will also need help and support while moving into suitable positions for the clinical examination. When the patient has been settled comfortably and well supported with pillows, his temperature, pulse and respirations should be taken and recorded accurately.

It is particularly important to observe the rate and depth of **respirations**. Any changes due to exertion, position or time of day should be noted and reported. When the airway is obstructed, noisy laboured breathing will result; this is called **stridor**. Pain or depression of the respiratory centre causes shallow inadequate breathing. The terminally ill or unconscious patient may develop periods of *apnoea* — that is an absence of breathing which is the result of a deficient blood supply to the respiratory centre.

While the doctor is taking the patient's medical and family history and details of occupation the nurse should collect instruments for examination including sphygmomanometer, stethoscope, ophthalmoscope and syringes for venepuncture: she will then be free to assist and support the patient during palpation and auscultation.

Sputum

The investigation of sputum is important as treatment is based on the results of microbiological (Ch. 2) or cytological examination. It may be necessary to support and assist the patient during expectoration to ensure that an adequate sputum specimen is obtained. Once obtained the specimen must be clearly labelled and sent to the laboratory as soon as possible. When a specimen is being sent for microbiological examination it must be collected in a sterile container. A wax carton should always be available near the patient's bed. This will allow general observations to be made of amount, colour and consistency of the sputum.

X-ray

There are various types of X-ray procedures included in the investigations of chest diseases. Before any X-ray is taken a full explanation to the patient is necessary. The patient must be warmly clad while being transported to the X-ray department; he should have some form of identification and all his previous X-rays should be sent with him to allow comparison by the radiologist. Initially all patients have a straight X-ray of the chest which may be followed by more specialized techniques such as conventional tomography, computerised tomography scan or bronchography. Fluoroscopy can be used to locate lymph nodes, movement of the diaphragm and of masses in the lung or mediastinum. During bronchography a special radio-opaque dye is used to outline bronchi and bronchioles. It is important that the bronchi are cleared of secretions before the procedure, and afterwards the physiotherapist should assist the patient to expel the radio-opaque dye from the bronchi.

Endoscopy

Examination under direct vision can be carried out during bronchoscopy, *thoracoscopy* or *mediastinoscopy* (Fig. 6.8). Preparation for these examinations includes explanation of the procedure and reassurance, as the patient may be very apprehensive. There are two types of bronchoscope, rigid and flexible fibreoptic (Fig. 6.9A, B). The examinations may be performed under either general or local anaesthesia, but the patient is usually required to fast to prevent regurgitation and inhalation of stomach content. The patient wears clothing which is warm and which can be easily removed. Identification bands are applied, premedication given, any prostheses and valuables are removed and stored in a safe place and he is allowed to rest. Notes and X-rays must accompany the patient to the diagnostic theatre. Following bronchoscopy under local anaesthesia the patient must not have anything

Figure 6.8
Position of the patient for
bronchoscopy

Figure 6.9
(A) Rigid bronchoscope
(B) Flexible fibroptic
bronchoscope

by mouth until cough and swallow reflexes have returned. Mouth care should be
carried out to make the patient more comfortable. Following thoracoscopy the
patient may return to the ward with an **underwater seal drain** to facilitate the re-
expansion of the lung (see p. 221 and Fig. 6.5).

Biopsy

Biopsy of lung tissue may be taken during thoracoscopy, transbronchial during bronchoscopy and larger specimens can be obtained during thoracotomy. Pleural biopsy
can be through the chest wall using an Abram's needle (Fig. 6.10). Lymph nodes
can be biopsied during mediastinoscopy. These biopsies are sent for pathological

Figure 6.10
Abram's biopsy needle

examination and great care should be taken when labelling; in particular, the **site** of the biopsy should always be noted.

Pleural aspiration

Specimens of pleural effusion can be obtained during therapeutic or diagnostic pleural aspiration. The specimen is sent for microbiological or *cytological* examination. In order to withdraw fluid from the pleural cavity the patient must sit in the upright position so that fluid in the pleural cavity will drain towards the base. The most recent X-rays, showing fluid levels in the chest, must be available to enable the doctor to decide where to introduce the aspiration needle (Fig. 6.11). The main concern of the nurse during pleural aspiration is to position, support and reassure the patient. Whenever possible the patient should be in the upright position, sitting either on the side of a bed or astride a chair with his feet supported and his arms and head resting on a bedtable or the back of the chair. In this position the shoulders and arms are raised, the rib-cage elevated, the intercostal spaces increased, thus facilitating the introduction of the aspirating needle into the pleural space. Observations of pulse, respirations, colour and pain are made during the procedure. To prevent the aspirating needle puncturing the visceral pleura the patient is asked to remain quite still and not to cough without warning, and if possible not to cough at all. At the end of the procedure an occlusion dressing is applied over the site of the aspiration and the amount of fluid is measured and recorded. Specimens of pleural fluid that have been collected in sterile containers must be labelled accurately before being sent to the microbiology laboratory.

Figure 6.11
Pleural aspiration

Respiratory function tests

Lung function tests involve the use of a **spirometer** (Fig. 6.12) to measure the volume changes within the lungs during inspiration and expiration. A spirometer consists of a drum inverted inside another drum which contains water. A tube is passed through the drums and ends above the water level. The drum is balanced with a weight. As the patient breathes in and out volume changes are recorded on the calibrated spirograph paper.

One of the most commonly performed tests is that used to measure, in individuals, the volume of air that can be expired forcefully at one, two or three seconds

Figure 6.12
Spirometer

after full inspiration. Forced expiratory volume after one second following full inspiration is expressed as FEV.

Blood tests

Examination of arterial blood will demonstrate the amount of circulating haemoglobin and therefore its oxygen-carrying capacity. Samples will also be analysed to estimate the percentage of oxygen and that of carbon dioxide in the blood.

NURSING CARE OF THE PATIENT WITH RESPIRATORY DISEASE

The nursing care of the patient with a respiratory disorder must be directed to meeting his physical, psychological and social needs. One must consider the clinical features of the disease and in this way choose the most effective means of relieving the patient's discomfort. It must also be remembered that the patient's needs and dependence will relate directly to the severity of his illness.

The objective, when planning a patient's physical care, should be the maintenance of cell functions. The assistance of a physiotherapist is always desirable and may be life-saving. The aims when meeting this objective are:

1. To maintain the best possible ventilation.
2. To maintain circulation.
3. To maintain a balance of body fluids.

1. **The maintenance of the best possible ventilation** can be achieved by nursing the patient in a warm, well-ventilated environment. This will provide an adequate supply of oxygen from the atmosphere and reduce the possibly of cross infection. Mechanical ventilation can be improved by nursing the patient in the upright position supported with a back-rest and pillows (Fig. 6.13). This position will ensure the best possible chest expansion unhampered by the pressure of abdominal organs under the diaphragm. The aid of a physiotherapist is essential to remove secretions which may be obstructing alveolar ventilation. The purpose of physiotherapy is to remove bronchial secretions, improve gaseous exchange and decrease sputum, so preventing further bronchopulmonary infection. The methods used by the physiotherapist to achieve this end will be breathing exercises, chest percussion, vibration and postural drainage. If this fails it may be necessary to remove secretions by suction through a rigid type bronchoscope. It is important that the patient himself is taught to breathe and expectorate effectively.

2. **The maintenance of an adequate circulation** will ensure an adequate flow of oxygenated blood to the tissues. This can be achieved by assisting venous return, which will prevent the formation of deep venous thrombosis and decubitus ulcers.

Figure 6.13
Upright position in bed

Venous return is promoted during physiotherapy to the chest and by leg exercises, which may be active or, if the patient cannot move without assistance, passive. The maintenance of circulation allowing adequate oxygenation to the body tissues will, in conjunction with turning the patient to relieve pressure on vulnerable areas, prevent the formation of decubitus ulcers.

3. **The maintenance of fluid balance** is necessary for the well-being of the body's internal environment. The balance will be disturbed if the intake of fluids does not replace that lost from the body by the kidneys, lungs and skin, especially if the loss of water by skin and lungs is increased because of pyrexia and increased respiration rate. Accurate records should be made of all fluids taken orally or parenterally and of those lost from urinary or alimentary tract, aspiration or drainage from wounds. An accurate record of fluid balance can be used to assess the amount of replacement fluids necessary to prevent dehydration. Normally fluid balance is maintained by diet and fluid intake. During illness the metabolic rate is increased and therefore the diet should contain increased kilojoules, protein and fluids (see Ch. 4).

Patients who have respiratory diseases may be admitted to hospital in a critical condition. They will require a great deal of reassurance and support initially while in this stressful situation and unusual environment. These diseases can be progressively incapacitating. The patient should be made aware of and helped to accept his limitations. As his condition may alter his life pattern and those of his dependents considerably, he should know that support will be available. While in hospital medical and social service personnel can be alerted and can continue to provide help and support if necessary after discharge from hospital.

Care of the patient having oxygen therapy

Patients with a low oxygen concentration in their blood, that is **anoxia**, will have impaired metabolic function. An oxygen supplement will therefore be necessary and can be administered by various types of equipment. When the anoxia is due to insufficient gaseous exchange oxygen can be administered by mask, nasal catheter or oxygen tent (Ch. 18). The oxygen can be obtained from an oxygen cylinder or from a system of pipes from a central supply. The administering apparatus is connected to the oxygen source by tubing which allows the oxygen to pass through a flow meter and a humidifier (Fig. 6.14). The nurse can then administer the prescribed amount of humidified oxygen. Most oxygen masks are disposable and can be adjusted to fit the patient comfortably. A high concentration of oxygen can be given by using a closed mask such as the Polymask. When an accurate percentage of oxygen supplement is required, as in some chronic respiratory conditions, a mask

Figure 6.14
Administration of oxygen by
Ventimask and oxygen cylinder

such as Ventimask will be required (Fig. 6.15). This mask is available in three models which deliver 24%, 28% and 35% O_2 respectively.

Nasal cannulae (Fig. 6.16) provide a rather unpredictable O_2 concentration but an O_2 flow rate of 2L/minute will usually provide an O_2 intake of about 30%. The advantage of this method of O_2 therapy is that the patient can communicate and take food uninhibited by a face mask. Even though the oxygen is humidified the patient may feel dry; therefore oral and nasal hygiene are very important for his comfort. Since oxygen supports combustion, relatives and neighbouring patients must be warned of the hazard of fire and therefore the danger of smoking in the vicinity of any patient who is receiving O_2 therapy.

Figure 6.15
Ventimask

Oxygen supply

Figure 6.16
Nasal cannulae in use

Care of the patient with underwater seal drainage

To allow re-expansion of the lung or lobe following chest surgery, trauma or spontaneous pneumothorax, a thoracic catheter is introduced into the pleural space and connected to an underwater seal drainage bottle.

Under local anaesthesia a trocar with a cannula attached to it is introduced through an intercostal space. The sterile catheter is then passed through the cannula into the chest and the cannula is withdrawn. The catheter is held in place by a stitch and attached to the drainage tube and bottle. This allows air to leave the pleural space, prevents its re-entry and permits the re-expansion of the lung or lobe (Fig. 6.5, p. 221).

The patient is nursed in the upright position and care is taken to prevent traction or compression of the drainage tubing. To prevent water entering the chest cavity the tubing **must** be clamped firmly before raising the bottle from floor level. The bottle stopper must be firmly in place to prevent ascending infection of the pleural cavity. During inspiration the pressure within the chest is reduced and the water level in the tube rises. On expiration the water level falls. This is often termed 'swinging' and demonstrates that the tube is patent. When no 'swinging' is observed this fact should be reported immediately. X-ray will demonstrate when lung re-expansion has been achieved and the catheter can be removed using aseptic technique; an occlusion dressing is then applied. When a more rapid removal of air from the pleural space is necessary a low pressure suction pump is used.

Care of the patient with a tracheostomy

A tracheostomy is an opening made into the trachea to facilitate breathing. The indications for tracheostomy are failure of respiratory function due to upper respiratory tract obstruction and conditions affecting the respiratory centre or muscles of respiration. Today it is more often an elective rather than an emergency procedure and is usually performed under general anaesthesia. The selection of the tracheostomy tube is very important as there are various types and sizes. Examples are:

Jackson tubes.
Cuffed siliconised PVC tubes.

Jackson tubes are silver and each has an inner tube which can be removed for cleaning. This type of tube provides an airway and a means of removing secretions when there is obstruction above the trachea and when assisted ventilation is not required. The PVC tube has a fitting which can be attached to the ventilating machine. The cuff, when inflated, seals the area between the trachea and the tube (Fig. 6.17) and thus allows **positive pressure ventilation** and prevents aspiration from either the upper respiratory or the gastrointestinal tract. For patients who need assisted ventilation for only a short time, an endotracheal tube may be passed, to avoid the hazards of a tracheostomy. In addition to the basic nursing care required for all patients, there are some specific nursing responsibilities for tracheostomy patients; these are: to maintain a clear airway, to prevent infection or trauma and to ensure adequate humidification of inspired air.

Maintaining a clear airway

This can be achieved by turning the patient from one side to the other (if this is

Upper respiratory tract

Tracheostomy tube
with inflated cuff

Reduced dead space will
allow more efficient ventilation

Figure 6.17
Tracheostomy tube in situ

Figure 6.18
Aspiration via tracheostomy tube

possible), by physiotherapy to the chest and by aspiration of bronchotracheal secretion (see below).

Preventing infection

The aspiration of bronchotracheal secretion is an aseptic procedure performed to prevent descending infection. If the patient is conscious, he should be given a reassuring explanation to allay apprehension. Prior to aspiration, oral hygiene is carried out and oropharyngeal suction is used to remove secretions from the area above the tracheostomy tube. The aseptic procedure of bronchotracheal suction is then begun, using a catheter which will not occlude the tracheostomy tube. The ventilator is disconnected during aspiration, therefore the procedure must be done deftly and quickly. Suction should only be applied when withdrawing the catheter (Fig. 6.18) and this can be controlled by a Y connection attached to the suction catheter to prevent trauma to the lining of the trachea and bronchi. Secretions from the other side can be removed by turning the patient and repeating the aseptic procedure. It is important to use an aseptic technique when changing tracheostomy tubes or dressings to prevent infection.

Humidification of inspired air

Air entering the tracheostomy bypasses the humidifying area of the respiratory system. It is therefore necessary to provide an alternative source of moisture to avoid the drying of the secretions and mucosa. There are various types of humidifier which can be attached to ventilating machines. A small disposable humidifying filter may be fitted to a tracheostomy tube when assisted ventilation is not required.

Special aspects of nursing care

Patients with assisted ventilation may not necessarily be unconscious but they are totally dependent on nursing staff. The conscious patient may be apprehensive and requires a great deal of psychological support. He will be unable to talk while the tracheostomy or endotracheal tube is in use and therefore should be given an alternative means of communication, such as a bell or a note book. He may also be anxious about eating and drinking and should be told how the nurse will care for his needs. If respiratory failure is due to chest trauma, for instance, the patient may be conscious but unable to tolerate or synchronize with the ventilator. In such circumstances heavy sedation may be necessary to allow effective ventilation.

While a patient is being cared for with a mechanical ventilator (Fig. 6.19) he must be under constant supervision. The patient's relatives will also need help and advice, particularly concerning his communication problems.

Figure 6.19
Patient on intermittent positive pressure (IPP) ventilator

COMMON DISORDERS OF THE RESPIRATORY SYSTEM
Coryza

Coryza, or the common cold, is a droplet infection caused by a virus; most people succumb to it at least once a year.

The symptoms of the common cold, which usually appear suddenly, are dry throat, nasal congestion causing thin, watery discharge and sneezing. There may be a moderate rise in temperature, the voice may become husky and the eyes watery, and the sense of taste or smell may be diminished. Often a cough develops, which may become productive.

The common cold usually lasts 7 to 10 days but may be complicated by sinusitis, otitis media, laryngitis, tracheitis or simple bronchitis.

Treatment is directed towards relief of symptoms and prevention of complications and of spread of infection to others. The patient requires a warm, well-ventilated environment, preferably not in close contact with others who may become infected. Nasal decongestants will reduce swelling and allow increased air flow. A dry mouth and throat will be soothed by hot drinks. To prevent excoriation of nasal skin, soothing cream can be applied with soft, easily disposed of tissues.

Influenza

This is an acute viral infection, affecting any age group, that occurs especially during the winter months. It is a febrile illness of sudden onset starting with general malaise, headache, backache and joint pain. There may be a painful, unproductive cough, conjunctivitis and enlarged lymph glands.

The course of the disease is about 4 to 5 days but may be prolonged by secondary bacterial infection of the lower respiratory tract.

The patient should be isolated in a warm, well-ventilated environment. While he is febrile and suffering from anorexia, fluids must be encouraged. A linctus may be given to control a dry, unproductive cough. Steam inhalations will provide moisture to the upper respiratory tract (Fig. 6.20).

Steam outlet via mouthpiece

Air inlet

Figure 6.20
Nelson steam inhaler
The steam which is inhaled through the mouth condenses on the bronchotracheal mucosa and stimulates the expectoration of secretions.

Bronchitis

Bronchitis is a general term describing an inflammatory condition of the bronchi. It may be acute or chronic.

Acute bronchitis

Inflammation of the bronchi may result as a complication of an upper respiratory infection such as coryza, influenza or measles.

Clinical features

There is mild elevation of temperature, a feeling of soreness behind the sternum, general malaise and an unproductive cough which may become productive due to secondary infection. The infection may spread downwards to the bronchioles.

Nursing observations

Four hourly recording of temperature, pulse and respirations.
Observation of amount and colour of sputum, which is usually abundant and purulent.

Investigations

A specimen of sputum — sent for culture and sensivity of organisms.
Chest X-ray.

Course and complications

Gradual improvement in 4 to 8 days occurs in the majority of cases. However, those patients who smoke or live in areas of high atmospheric pollution may have a prolonged illness. Infection descending to fine bronchi and bronchioles becomes a serious complication in young children, debilitated patients and those suffering from chronic bronchitis.

Treatment and nursing care

Bed rest is necessary while the patient is pyrexial and having antibiotics. Pain caused by the inflammation can be relieved by medicated steam inhalations and an unproductive cough can be eased by the administration of a cough suppressant drug.

Rehabilitation and community care

Most patients only need advice about rest and diet during the convalescent period.

Chronic bronchitis

This is a progressive denegerative disease affecting the mucous membrane and cilia of the bronchi; it is caused by irritants associated with industrial pollution or the personal pollution of cigarette smoking. An acute exacerbation of the condition can be precipitated by viral or bacterial infection.

The changes which occur during the course of the disease greatly reduce the number of cilia and destroy normal function. The mucous glands enlarge and the increased amount of secretions block bronchioles and impair alveolar ventilation. As a result of infection fibrosis and stenosis of bronchioles occur (Fig. 6.21).

Clinical features

The patient will have a chronic cough, wheeze and tightness of the chest, especially in the morning before bronchial secretions have been expectorated. The sputum is usually thick, tenacious and mucoid, often copious, and may become purulent due

Narrowing of bronchiole preventing adequate alveolar ventilation

Collection of mucus preventing adequate gaseous exchange

Figure 6.21
Chronic bronchitis

to secondary infection. The patient may be cyanosed and dyspnoeic even at rest, cyanosis and dyspnoea becoming more evident on exertion. Chest expansion is poor and expiration is slow and difficult, leading to a higher level of carbon dioxide in the blood.

Nursing observations

Temperature, pulse and respiration.
Sputum, amount and colour.

Investigations

Chest X-ray
Respiratory function tests.
Microbiological examination of sputum.

Course and complications

The symptoms slowly progress over the years and eventually lead to emphysema and right-sided cardiac failure (see Ch. 7). Loss of elasticity of lung tissue prevents adequate expiration and may be the cause of the typical 'barrel chest' of the chronic bronchitic. The respiratory centre is no longer stimulated by high levels of CO_2 but by the lower than normal level of oxygen. This is very important to remember when administering oxygen because to overoxygenate the patient would result in a higher than normal level of oxygen in the blood. There would then be no stimulus to the respiratory centre and the patient would go into complete respiratory failure, requiring assisted ventilation with a positive pressure ventilator.

Treatment and nursing care

Bed rest is essential. Nursing care is as described on page 225. There should be careful administration of oxygen using a Ventimask which allows a regulated percentage of oxygen to supplement the atmospheric air. The percentage of oxygen and the length of time the patient requires oxygen therapy will be prescribed by the doctor following analysis of arterial blood samples. Antibiotic therapy will depend on the culture and sensitivity report on the sputum specimen.

Drugs which dilate the bronchi, especially salbutamol, are more effective when given by inhalation. In acute exacerbations they may be administered by an intermittent positive pressure ventilator with oxygen-enriched air over a period of 3 minutes four times daily.

Chest physiotherapy and the use of drugs to reduce the viscosity of mucus help to prevent the accumulation of excess mucus which would obstruct the airway.

Rehabilitation and community care

The patient must be well supported in the community as it may be necessary for him to change his whole life-style, housing and means of livelihood. Attendance at follow-up clinics to assess his condition should be encouraged. He should also continue physiotherapy and he and his family should be instructed in the use and dangers of oxygen therapy.

Pneumonia

Pneumonia is a general term describing an inflammatory condition of the lungs. There are two types: specific pneumonia, caused by a particular organism, and aspiration pneumonia, a secondary descending infection affecting lungs with an existing abnormality.

Specific pneumonia

Specific pneumonia can be caused by bacteria, viruses or mycoplasma (see Ch. 1) affecting one or more lobes. Young adults are more commonly affected by this type. The incidence is higher in winter and the spread is by droplet infection. The affected lobe becomes consolidated with exudate in the alveoli. When liquefaction of the exudate occurs, the infected material is either absorbed or expectorated.

Clinical features

The onset of the condition is sudden with the temperature rising to 40°C within a few hours; the patient may have rigors. General malaise, anorexia and headache accompany the pyrexia. The patient is dyspnoeic, he may have pleuritic pain and a painful, unproductive cough. The patient is made particularly uncomfortable by hot, dry skin and mouth. Herpes simplex may be present on or near the lips. The painful cough, caused by the inflamed pleura and consolidation, disappears when resolution occurs, allowing copious amounts of rusty-coloured sputum to be expectorated.

Nursing observations

Sputum, amount and colour.
Temperature, pulse and respirations.

Investigations

Chest X-ray.
Sputum for microbiological examination and sensitivity of any cultured pathogens.
Blood for culture and sensitivity.

Course and complications

There is usually a quick response to antibiotic therapy and a corresponding fall in temperature, pulse and respiration. With resolution other symptoms gradually abate, usually within 7 days. Complications which may occur are pleural effusion, emphysema and lung abscess.

Treatment and nursing care

The patient needs bed rest; nursing care is as described on page 225, with particular attention to oral hygiene and the care of herpes simplex. Pain can be relieved by local heat and analgesics, while antibiotics will reduce temperature and toxic symptoms. Oxygen therapy may be prescribed during the early stages of the disease and given via a Polymask. Fluids must be encouraged especially when there is pyrexia and the possibility of the patient becoming dehydrated. Efficient expectoration and chest expansion can be achieved with the aid of physiotherapy.

Rehabilitation

This is a debilitating disease requiring a fairly long convalescence to return the patient to health.

Aspiration pneumonia

Any abnormality in the respiratory system predisposes the lungs to invasion, even by organisms of low virulence. Generally, infections reach the alveoli by aspiration of infected material from the upper respiratory tract. An acute reaction may be the result of a breakdown in the normal defence mechanism of the respiratory tract due to unconsciousness or ineffective coughing, particularly following an operation. Bronchial obstruction by a foreign body or carcinoma will also prevent efficient drainage of secretions.

This condition can affect the young, the elderly and the debilitated and has a high morbidity rate.

Clinical features

There are signs of acute bronchitis with a gradual rise in temperature, pulse and respirations, dyspnoea and cyanosis. Cough is severe with purulent sputum. The course of the disease is longer than in specific pneumonia and the patient is often drowsy, lethargic and confused as a result of cerebral anoxia.

Nursing observations

Temperature, pulse and respiration.

Investigations

Chest X-ray.
Sputum for culture and sensitivity.
Blood for culture and sensitivity.

Course and complications

The bronchi become inflamed and the alveoli collapse or become consolidated and therefore gaseous exchange is greatly reduced. A bronchus may become obstructed by a plug of mucus, causing *atelectasis* of the affected lobe. Bronchiactasis will occur if there is incomplete resolution of the consolidation.

Treatment and nursing care

The treatment and nursing care is as previously described (p. 225), with special care necessary during the period of confusion when the patient is unable to co-operate. It is particularly difficult to ensure an adequate diet and fluid intake for this patient, who may be both aggressive and resentful. As the patient may be very young or elderly and debilitated, particular attention must be given to skin care especially for those who are incontinent. Oxygen can be administered to a baby in an incubator, to a young child in an oxygen tent (Ch. 18) and to adults by an oxygen mask or nasal cannula. Physiotherapy is essential in the management of this patient.

Rehabilitation and community care

Rehabilitation and community care depend upon the age of the patient and the underlying cause of the aspiration pneumonia. If the cause is unknown, diagnostic investigations will have been carried out in hospital and treatment instituted. Generally the patient's return to health is prolonged and the elderly may require long-term nursing care either in hospital or in the community if their home conditions are suitable.

Bronchiectasis

In this disease the small bronchi become permanently dilated as a result of obstruction. This can be caused by acute pulmonary infection or a bronchial tumour causing collapse of a lobe. When the lobe collapses the alveoli and bronchi dilate to take up the space. If infection occurs this dilatation is permanent due to loss of elasticity caused by fibrotic changes. The condition may exist without symptoms until there is infection of the dilated bronchi; then the symptoms vary according to the degree of infection present.

Clinical features

Usually the patient presents with a history of recurrent cough and sputum which are more troublesome in the morning. The reason for this symptom is that lower lobes are more frequently affected and the change in position from arising stimulates the need to cough up the copious secretions that have collected during the hours of sleep. Haemoptysis can occur as a result of vigorous coughing which may rupture distorted blood vessels. Typically the patient who has suffered from this condition for some years has a decline in general health. A very common feature of this disease is finger clubbing.

Nursing observations

Sputum, amount and colour.
Temperature, pulse and respiration.

Investigations

Bronchography, sputum culture.

Course and complications

Complications of the disease have been greatly reduced by the emergence of antibiotic drugs. However, recurrent pulmonary infection such as pneumonia, emphysema and haemoptysis may occur.

Treatment and nursing care

When the bronchiectasis is confined to one lung, surgery may be advocated and the affected lobe removed. However, if bronchography demonstrates extensive damage, surgery may not be possible. Medical treatment will be aimed at the control of infection and the drainage of sputum. The choice of antibiotic drugs will depend on the sensitivity of the cultured organism. During winter months it may be possible to prevent acute infection by giving the patient long-term antibiotic therapy. The method used to remove sputum efficiently is called **postural drainage**. It involves placing the patient in a position most suitable for drainage by gravity from the affected area (Fig. 6.22A, B, and C).

Rehabilitation and community care

The patient should be helped to understand the importance of a balanced diet with a high fluid intake. He should be advised to avoid chest infections and to continue breathing exercises, including postural drainage when necessary. These measures will help to prevent exacerbations of the condition. A light, outdoor occupation and leisure time spent in fresh air and sunshine will be beneficial to him.

Asthma

Asthma is a disease characterized by recurrent attacks of dyspnoea and wheezing. This is due to a temporary narrowing of the small bronchi caused by muscular spasm and oedema of the mucosa.

There are two clinical types of asthma: extrinsic and intrinsic.

Extrinsic asthma occurs in children who have a family history of allergic disease. Attacks of asthma may be precipitated by a hypersensitivity to certain *allergens* or as a result of psychological stress.

Intrinsic asthma occurs in later life in a person who has neither a personal nor a family history of disease caused by allergens. No obvious allergic factor is isolated when the disease does occur.

Clinical features

There is a history of periodic attacks of dyspnoea and of wheezing, especially on expiration. Adults experience a feeling of tightness on waking and sometimes during the night. These episodes may be the result of inhaled or ingested allergens, or of emotional stress. The patient adopts the upright position and the accessory muscles of respiration are used in an attempt to increase expiration. The attacks may last several hours and leave the patient physically and emotionally exhausted.

Figure 6.22A
Position used to facilitate the
removal of secretions from right
upper lobe and upper segment
of left upper lobe

40 cm elevation

Figure 6.22B
Position used to facilitate
removal of secretions from right
middle lobe

50 cm elevation

Figure 6.22C
Position used to facilitate
removal of secretions from right
lower lobe

Nursing observations

Signs of alterations in respiratory pattern and anxiety.

Investigations

Sensitivity tests to identify the allergen.
Identification of psychological factors.
Investigation of personal and family history — important in reaching a diagnosis.

Treatment of the acute attack

A vigilant nurse will notice at once when an attack is imminent, and, by initiating prompt treatment, will often avert the development of a severe attack. The patient is nursed in the upright position supported by pillows. A pillow on a bed table placed in front of the patient will support him in the optimum position during the acute episode. Psychological reassurance may be given by the presence of a calm nurse. When the attack has subsided, hot sweet drinks can be given to replace fluids lost due to increased metabolic rate during the attack. In a more prolonged, severe attack drugs may be necessary to relax the bronchial spasm.

A bronchodilating drug such as salbutamol can be given by inhalation using a nebulizer (Fig. 6.23), and oxygen therapy may also be prescribed to raise the oxygen content of the blood. Oedema caused by inflammatory changes can be controlled by the anti-inflammatory effects of steroid therapy.

Course and complications

When asthmatic attacks do not respond to treatment with drugs, status asthmaticus exists and may last for many hours. This is a medical emergency requiring intensive steroid therapy which will be prescribed immediately. Salbutamol will be given via an oxygen driven nebulizer (Fig. 6.24) so that the drug will reach the bronchi and be effective as quickly as possible. Oxygen therapy will be prescribed by the doctor and the amount to be given is estimated after examination of oxygen levels in the arterial blood. Reassurance is essential for the patient in this stressful situation to allow effective treatment. Should the patient's condition fail to improve then assisted ventilation using an intermittent positive pressure ventilator (Fig. 6.24) will be necessary.

Figure 6.23
Nebulizer

Figure 6.24
Intermittent positive pressure ventilator

Rehabilitation and community care

Patients and those caring for young children with asthma should attend a clinic where counselling and a written programme of the individual's treatment can be given. Instruction should be given in the use of pressurized aerosols and inhalation techniques. An understanding and ability to recognize the first indication of an attack and to take the prescribed treatment will greatly improve the patient's life-style.

Carcinoma of the bronchus

The term lung cancer is often used to describe carcinoma of the bronchus. Common types of bronchial carcinoma are squamous cell, undifferentiated small cell carcinoma and adenocarcinoma. Small cell carcinoma spreads rapidly and produces metastases earlier than the other types. Carcinoma causes obstruction to the bronchus and can spread locally to the chest wall, pleura and mediastinum. The metastatic spread can be to the lymph nodes, brain, bones and liver. There is a higher incidence of the disease in men than in women, the age group being 40 to 70 years. The incidence is also higher in cigarette smokers and in those whose occupation exposes them to the inhalation of carcinogens such as asbestos and nickel.

Clinical features

The patient may present in the early stages with a history of weight loss, lassitude, cough and dyspnoea. Sputum can be bloodstained or there may be episodes of haemoptysis. In some instances the reason the patient seeks medical advice is due to symptoms arising from metastases.

Investigations

Chest X-ray normally includes postero-anterior and lateral views so that the whole lung area is examined. These areas can be examined in depth by tomography. Bronchoscopy will demonstrate vocal cords, trachea, main *carina* and bronchi. The surgeon may, by direct vision, assess the possibility of surgery and obtain a biopsy of any obvious tumour for histological examination.

Mediastinoscopy allows the surgeon to examine an area on both sides of the tracheal bifurcation and to obtain a biopsy from the lymph nodes situated there. These lymph nodes are frequently invaded by tumour cells and may be excised for histological confirmation of diagnosis.

A sputum specimen is sent for microbiological and cytological examination. Tests are carried out with the spirometer to estimate lung function and assess whether this will be adequate following surgery. Thoracotomy, an exploratory operation through the chest wall, may be necessary to assess the possibility of removing the tumour.

Treatment and nursing care

Adequate lung function and the localization of the disease should enable surgery to be considered, as excision of the affected lobe or lobes is the treatment of choice.

During the preoperative period smoking must be discouraged; intensive chest physiotherapy will help to prevent sputum retention and will encourage full lung expansion. It is also important to instruct the patient in effective breathing and coughing exercises, which will be necessary in the postoperative period. The operations which may be performed are **lobectomy**, the removal of a lobe or **pneumonectomy**, the removal of a whole lung. Postoperatively the usual care of a patient following major surgery will be carried out.

Following a lobectomy the patient will return to the ward with one or two chest drains, an upper one to remove air and a lower one to remove serous fluid, to prevent infection and promote lung expansion (Fig. 6.25). Care of the patient with underwater seal drainage is as discussed on page 221.

Following a pneumonectomy there will be no need for drainage tubes because there is no raw lung tissue remaining on that side to cause air leakage or serous oozing. Before leaving the operating theatre a negative pressure is introduced on the side of the pneumonectomy to draw the mediastinal contents slightly towards the space and allow full expansion of the remaining lung.

In the early postoperative period the patient may be sat up if his blood pressure is satisfactory. This will facilitate chest movement and pleural drainage. Observation

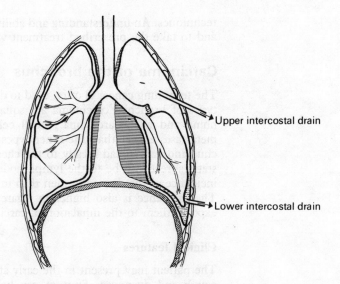

Upper intercostal drain

Lower intercostal drain

Figure 6.25
Lobectomy

and control of pain by the administration of analgesics will allow physiotherapy to be recommenced as soon as possible to prevent mucus remaining in the bronchi, which may cause atelectasis and require emergency bronchoscopy to remove the obstruction. Surgery is not appropriate when small cell tumour and metastases have been diagnosed or when the patient's general condition is poor. Radiotherapy or a combination of cytotoxic drugs and radiotherapy may be indicated to treat the primary tumour and metastases. Irradiation is of palliative value in the treatment of distressing symptoms such as bone pain, haemoptysis and obstruction of the superior vena cava. Relief can also be achieved by injecting cytotoxic drugs into the thoracic cavity when pleural effusion has become a problem. The patient may have treatment in a specialised unit or on an out-patient basis.

Course and complications

The complications are bronchial obstruction, causing atelectasis and leading to pneumonia and lung abscess. If there is pleural involvement the normal secretion and absorption of pleural fluid will be impaired, causing pleural effusion. Involvement of lymph nodes will cause venous congestion of the superior vena cava. A primary tumour in a bronchus may produce metastases in the brain, bone or liver. These deposits cause pain and debilitation and a variety of symptoms each requiring specific treatment.

Community care follow-up

The prognosis is generally poor, but following successful surgery 25% of patients survive for an average of 5 years. These patients and their families face a difficult future in which much support can be given by their general practitioner, nurse and medical social worker.

Cancer research has not yet discovered how carcinogens act nor has it produced any dramatic breakthrough in treatment. Therefore, prevention cannot be stressed enough. It is known, for example that cigarette smoking produces a high incidence of the disease, although this does not seem to have changed attitudes towards the habit.

Pulmonary tuberculosis

Pulmonary tuberculosis is caused by the micro-organism *Mycobacterium tuberculosis*. The route of infection is by inhalation of air containing tubercle bacilli which have been coughed and sneezed into the atmosphere by an infectious patient. When a large number of tubercle bacilli have entered the lung tissue the white blood cells surround the bacilli and invade the alveoli. This can result in a pneumonia-type condition, which may resolve after a period of time, or caseation may occur. Caseation means that the infected area has a cheesy consistency, which later becomes fibrosed, then calcified, with the formation of lung cavities. There will be extensive cavities in a severely affected lung and sputum culture will be strongly positive. Minimal or no cavities will be present in a mildly affected lung and the sputum may or may not produce a positive culture.

When infected with tubercle bacilli for the first time the lesion is known as primary and may heal spontaneously, providing the patient with an acquired immunity. A healed primary lesion may be reactivated in later life if the patient's general health deteriorates. Those susceptible to the disease are people who are in close contact with an infectious patient, those in poor general health or those whose social conditions are unfavourable and immigrants who have a low racial resistance to the disease.

Clinical features

Usually the onset is insidious, with tiredness, anorexia, loss of weight and a dry, irritating cough. If undiagnosed or untreated at this stage the patient will later present with dyspnoea, productive cough and elevation of temperature in the evening. The patient may also have enlarged glands in the axillae, neck or groin.

Nursing observations

Recording of temperature, pulse and respiration particularly in the evening.
Observation of sputum amount and colour, and whether it is bloodstained.
Side-effects of drug therapy are fairly common and may include gastrointestinal disturbance, skin rash, tinnitus and eye focusing problems. Any of these manifestations should be noted and reported.

Investigations

Diagnosis depends on the patient's history, clinical, radiological and laboratory examination. When the results suggest infection by tubercle bacilli, he will be asked to undergo further investigations. These include chest X-ray and tomography to demonstrate cavitation and the presence of enlarged lymph nodes. As bacilli may be scanty, sputum specimens are taken on 3 consecutive days to see if they are present. The tubercle bacilli are decribed as 'acid fast' because of the method used in the laboratory to demonstrate them. Sputum specimens will also be sent for concentration tests which demonstrate the virulence of the infection. Skin tests using purified tubercle protein are used to assess hypersensitivity to tubercle bacilli. This sensitivity is associated with previous infection that has resulted in an acquired immunity, or with effective artificial immunization against infection. Redness and swelling at the site of the skin test denote a positive reaction and show that the patient is immune to the disease.

Blood specimens will be taken to estimate the blood sedimentation rate, which is raised during infection (see Ch. 12). Once diagnosed the health authorities are notified and, through consultation with the patient, an attempt is made to trace the source of the infection and follow up contacts. The contacts will then attend a clinic for X-ray and investigation.

Course and complications

The disease will progess and cause increasing debility, haemoptysis and spontaneous pneumothorax. Pleurisy may develop with or without pleural effusion. An undiagnosed and untreated infectious patient becomes a risk to the community in which he lives and works.

Treatment and nursing care

The objectives of treatment are to return the patient well and safe to his or her family, to solve immediate medical, physical and social problems and to prevent the spread of infection to the community. Treatment depends on whether the patient is only infected or is both infected and infectious. An infected patient can be cared for in the community under the supervision of the health authorities, but if the patient is also infectious as shown by acid fast bacilli in his sputum he must be nursed in isolation until his sputum culture and concentration tests are negative. Initially the treatment is bed rest because of the patient's general debility and he will need a high protein diet with milk supplements. Rapid elimination of the bacilli can be achieved by the selection of a combination of drugs and the co-operation of the patient. A standard short course of chemotherapy is rifampicin, isoniazid and either streptomycin or ethambutal for 2 months followed by rifampicin and isoniazid for 7 months.

While nursing patients it is important to conform to the specific regulations regarding the disposal of sputum and infected material. Although there is no need to have separate crockery or special laundering arrangements, it is important to remember that the rules regarding the prevention of cross infection must be adhered to. The nurse must also be aware of the need to maintain her own general health and to protect her hands when administering injections of streptomycin, a drug which is known to produce skin rashes. When the infectious patient has a negative sputum concentration and culture he can be discharged from hospital and continue his drug therapy at home.

Community care

In the community the patient should be advised by the health authorities on drug therapy, diet, and rest for approximately 2 years or until the patient no longer requires treatment. It is important to stress the role that a nurse may assume in helping the patient to lead a healthy life.

SUGGESTED ASSIGNMENTS

1. Consider the measures which may be taken to detect, diagnose and control spread of pulmonary tuberculosis among and from:

   a. Vagrants.
   b. Immigrants.

2. The direct relationship between respiratory disease and air pollution from smoke and chemical agencies is undeniable. Discuss the means whereby prevention of disease and promotion of health can be achieved.

3. Discuss the problems which may confront both patient and family with regard to drug administration in the following circumstances:

   a. A man with chronic bronchitis going on holiday.
   b. A school-age girl with asthma.

4. Recognizing the psychological and physical problems of a person suffering from carcinoma of the bronchus, consider the role of the nurse when assisting the patient during complicated diagnostic tests and treatment.

FURTHER READING

Capra L G 1972 The care of the cancer patient. Heinemann, London

Crofton J, Douglas A 1975 Respiratory diseases, 2nd edn. Blackwell Scientific, Oxford

Grenville-Mathers R 1973 Thoracic medicine and surgery for nurses, 3rd edn. Sylviro Publications, London

Grenville-Mathers R 1983 The respiratory system, 2nd edn. Penguin Library of Nursing. Churchill Livingstone, Edinburgh

Lane D J, Storr A 1979 Asthma. Oxford University Press, Oxford

Roper N, Logan W, Tierney A J 1980 The elements of nursing. Churchill Livingstone, Edinburgh

Sykes M K, McNicholl M W A, Campbell E J M 1976 Respiratory failure, 2nd edn. Blackwell Scientific, Oxford

Tiffany R 1980 Cancer nursing — surgical. Faber & Faber, London

Chapter Seven
The cardiovascular system

Cardiac disease presents in many different ways and appearances can often be deceptive. Patients with severe heart disease may seem healthy and robust, but when they are examined and asked about their symptoms many are found to be badly disabled by breathlessness or pain on the slightest exertion and they may be unable to cope with normal daily activities. A patient with disturbance of heart rhythm and conduction may look well and have few symptoms, but because of the possibility of sudden fall in cardiac output he could be at risk of unexpected collapse at home, at work or even crossing the road. In contrast, a patient who develops infection of the endocardium might feel very unwell with fever and general malaise and a heart attack victim may look and feel extremely ill and be in severe pain.

As a result of the anxieties surrounding heart trouble, in particular heart attack, people who have been active and energetic can sometimes become 'cardiac invalids' and their relatives may become overprotective. It takes patience and skill to reassure patients and their families that a full and active life is possible despite cardiac disease. Those who do not understand their condition clearly or who are perhaps overanxious about it may need a great deal of encouragement to modify their life-styles in some way so that they can live happily and safely within the limits of their condition. The involvement of nurses in teaching and rehabilitation programmes and in giving psychological support is becoming more important as the impact of heart trouble on overall well-being becomes better understood. In helping with physical, social and emotional adjustment, nurses should try to think of the patient not only in the hospital setting, but also in his home and with his family, at work and in the community.

ANATOMY AND PHYSIOLOGY OF THE HEART

The heart has three layers:

The pericardium — a smooth membranous sac surrounding the heart, consisting of an outer fibrous and inner serous coat.
The myocardium — specialized muscle tissue.
The endocardium — an inner layer of endothelium which lines the chambers of the heart and the valve surfaces.

The heart is divided by a muscular septum into left and right sides which do not communicate with each other after birth (Fig. 7.1). Each side is subdivided into upper and lower chambers, the **atria** and the **ventricles**. Thus there is a right and left atrium and a right and left ventricle. Separating the atria from the ventricles are one-way valves, the **tricuspid** and **mitral valves**. At the outlet of the ventricles to the major vessels are the **pulmonary** and **aortic valves** which prevent backflow into the ventricles.

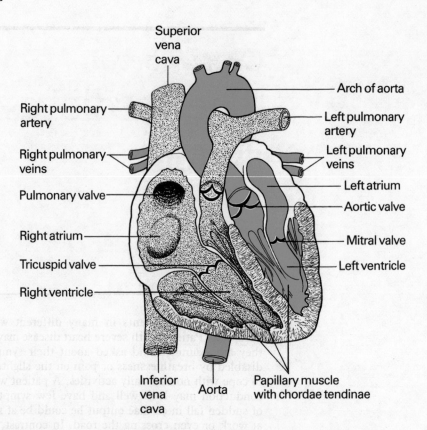

Figure 7.1
The anatomy of the heart

Pulmonary and systemic circulation (Fig. 7.2)

The heart pumps **venous blood** to the lungs, where carbon dioxide, a waste product of metabolism, is given off and oxygen is received, and **arterial blood**, carrying oxygen and nutrient materials to all body tissues.

Venous blood from the superior and inferior venae cavae passes into the right atrium, and then through the tricuspid valve to the right ventricle. As the right ventricle contracts, blood is pumped through the pulmonary valve to the pulmonary artery and lungs (**pulmonary circulation**). Arterialized blood from the four pulmonary veins passes into the left atrium and through the mitral valve to the left ventricle. As the left ventricle contracts, blood is pumped through the aortic valve to the aorta and the **systemic circulation**.

Figure 7.2
Pulmonary and systemic
circulations

Blood supply

The myocardium itself requires a blood supply. Arterialized blood is passed to the heart muscle by the right and left coronary arteries (Fig. 7.20A). Coronary venous blood is returned to the right atrium together with the venous return from the rest of the body.

Nerve control

Both sympathetic and parasympathetic nerves play a part in regulating heart action. **Parasympathetic nerves,** the vagi, decrease the rate and force of contraction and decrease blood flow through the coronary arteries supplying the myocardium. **Sympathetic nerves** have the opposite effect, increasing the heart rate and force of contraction and increasing blood flow to the myocardium, thus improving the oxygenation and nutrition of the myocardium. When a person is subjected to stress, sympathetic nerve stimulation allows the heart to cope by making it a more effective pump and improving blood flow through the circulatory system. While the body is resting, parasympathetic stimulation allows the heart to rest, thus preserving the heart's strength.

Conducting pathways

These are shown in Figure 7.3. Every heartbeat is initiated by an electrical impulse which passes along conducting pathways of specialized cells, some of which are grouped to form nodes.

Sinoatrial (SA) node or 'pacemaker'. The electrical impulse arises in this node and spreads in all directions across the walls of both atria causing them to contract (**atrial systole**).

Atrioventricular (AV) node and atrioventricular bundle. The impulse from the atria is conducted to the AV node situated in the right atrium close to the tricuspid valve. The AV node passes impulses to the specialized conducting muscle fibres of the AV bundle, which divides into right and left bundle branches. The impulse, spreading rapidly through these branches, causes the ventricles to contract (**ventricular systole**). After contraction, the atria and ventricles relax (**cardiac diastole**).

A block in the conducting pathways may occur, preventing the passage of impulses from atria and ventricles. This may follow acute myocardial infarction and can be corrected by the use of a temporary or permanent **artificial pacemaker** (p. 270).

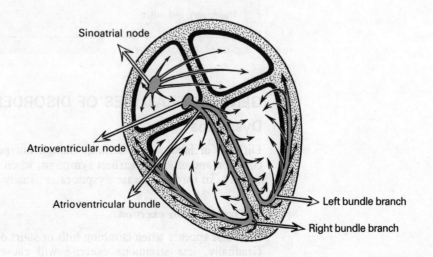

Figure 7.3
Conducting pathways

AETIOLOGY

Cardiovascular diseases are now the principal causes of death in the developed countries. Increasing attention is being paid to why these diseases develop and how they can be prevented. So far, however, the causes of many of them, especially of the modern epidemic of coronary artery disease and heart attack, are still not fully understood.

Cardiac diseases may occur singly or in association. The heart may be affected directly by **congenital defects** and **structural abnormalities**, such as atrial septal defect or pulmonary stenosis, or by **impaired blood supply** to its structure for example from diseased coronary arteries causing angina and myocardial infarction.

The heart may also be affected by **infection** both directly, as in diphtheria, syphilis, and a variety of bacterial and viral infections and indirectly, as in rheumatic fever.

Changes in cardiac function are associated with many other diseases, such as hypertension, thyrotoxicosis, myxoedema and anaemia, and the cardiovascular changes of pregnancy and childbirth may place such a circulatory strain on an already diseased heart that both the pregnancy and the mother's life may be in danger. Whether the structure and function of the heart are affected directly or indirectly, in time the heart muscle itself fails and cardiac failure results, precipitated by one or a combination of several of the factors mentioned above.

The main types of heart disease and the percentage mortality in the U.K. are shown in Table 7.1.

Table 7.1
Percentage mortality and age group for each type of heart disease in England, Wales and Scotland in 1980 (Source: WHO Annual Statistics 1982)

Type	Mortality (%)	Age group
Acute myocardial infarction	55	Middle and old age
Other ischaemic heart disease including angina	23	Middle and old age
Hypertensive disease	3	Middle and old age
Acute rheumatic fever	<0.1	Variable in U.K. (childhood and adolescence in developing countries)
Chronic rheumatic heart disease	1	Middle and old age
Congenital heart disease	<1	Infancy and childhood
Pulmonary and other heart diseases	17	Middle and old age

GENERAL FEATURES OF DISORDER

Dyspnoea

Difficult or laboured breathing, though not peculiar to heart disease, is the most common and often the earliest symptom; when severe it can cause great distress and anxiety. In cardiac disease dyspnoea is usually progressive.

1. Dyspnoea on exertion

This first appears when climbing hills or stairs or when doing heavy household work. Gradually, less strenuous exercise will cause shortness of breath, for example walking slowly on level ground (Fig. 7.4).

Figure 7.4
Dyspnoea on exertion

2. Dyspnoea at rest

Eventually breathlessness is present even when the patient is at rest, and finally **orthopnoea** occurs, that is the need to sit upright in order to breathe more easily. Many patients prefer to sleep using three or four pillows. Cardiac dyspnoea is usually due to pulmonary venous congestion. As left heart failure develops, back pressure of blood is transmitted to the pulmonary veins and capillaries. As the pressure rises, fluid exudes into the alveoli making the lungs less compliant and reducing the volume of air passing into and out of the lungs. As the lungs are stiffer, the work of breathing becomes more difficult.

3. Paroxysmal nocturnal dyspnoea (cardiac asthma)

Paroxysmal nocturnal dyspnoea is due to pulmonary venous congestion and it occurs in patients with left heart failure. After a few hours' sleep the patient wakens suddenly, gasping for breath, with a feeling of suffocation and intense anxiety as he struggles to breathe. He will quickly sit up on the edge of the bed and may go to an open window for fresh air to ease the distress. An unproductive cough and wheezing which resemble an asthmatic attack can occur, hence the term cardiac asthma.

Various mechanisms seem to contribute to the development of lung congestion, such as an increased venous return and an imbalance between the output of the two ventricles. Venous return to the right side of the heart and to the lungs can increase when lying flat or after slipping down in bed during sleep. The volume of venous blood may also be increased when fluid is reabsorbed from oedematous tissue in parts of the body previously dependent (Fig. 7.6A). If the left ventricle is failing, the left side of the heart will not be able to keep pace with the output of the right ventricle to the lungs and congestion develops in the lungs. Also, the vital capacity of the lungs is reduced by the elevation of the diaphragm when lying down.

Assuming the upright position makes it easier to use the accessory muscles of the shoulders to help breathing.

4. Acute pulmonary oedema

In advanced left heart failure, a profound and particularly anxiety-provoking form of dyspnoea occurs during attacks of acute pulmonary oedema. This is described on page 275.

Pain

Cardiac pain is experienced in myocardial ischaemia, myocardial infarction and pericarditis.

1. Myocardial ischaemia

When coronary arteries are narrowed, usually due to atherosclerosis, the supply of oxygenated blood to the myocardium is reduced. This gives rise to the chest pain known as *angina pectoris*.

Site of pain. Angina is usually a central chest pain, felt behind the sternum. It can radiate over the chest to the neck, the jaw and the arms, particularly the left arm and sometimes to the wrist and fingers.

Type of pain. Angina is described as a steady pressure or tightness in the chest, as a numbness or heaviness in the arms, as a choking in the throat or 'toothache' in the jaw.

Duration. Episodes of angina are usually brief, lasting only a few minutes and seldom more than 15 minutes.

Provoking factors. Angina occurs in circumstances where the myocardial need for oxygen increases. For example, it is associated with exertion such as walking upstairs or up a hill. In cold weather or after eating a heavy meal, rather less exercise than usual may provoke the angina. It can occur in situations of acute emotion, anxiety, anger or fear. It may also develop during sexual intercourse.

Relief of pain. When the oxygen demand of the myocardium falls, the pain eases. Angina is therefore relieved by rest. It is also relieved quickly by taking a glyceryl trinitrate tablet sublingually (p. 266).

2. Myocardial infarction

When a coronary artery becomes blocked by thrombus and atheroma, the part of the myocardium supplied by that artery becomes irreversibly damaged. Tissue death results because of the inadequate supply of oxygenated blood.

Site of pain. The distribution of heart attack pain is similar to that of angina, that is central chest pain with radiation to the jaw, shoulders and arms.

Type of pain. The pain is much more severe than angina and is described as a crushing or constricting pain.

Duration. It is usually a prolonged pain of increasing intensity. It lasts for more than 30 minutes and sometimes for several hours.

Provoking factors and relief of pain. Unlike angina, the pain generally comes on at rest and is unrelieved by rest or by glyceryl trinitrate. An opiate is needed to relieve this severe pain. Often angina has developed for the first time, or there has been a worsening of angina in the days or weeks before the heart attack.

3. Pericarditis

Inflammation of the pericardium may complicate rheumatic fever and acute myocardial infarction, often producing pain similar in distribution to the pain of myocardial infarction. It may be worsened by inspiration, swallowing and movement. Diagnosis is confirmed by the presence of a pericardial friction rub, which is heard as a scratching noise over the heart on auscultation. A chest radiograph may show a pericardial effusion — a collection of fluid in the pericardial sac — which is often serous but may be purulent in pyogenic pericarditis or bloodstained in malignant pericarditis. The effusion can cause compression of the heart and impair its action.

Palpitation

Palpitation is an awareness of the heart's action. It may be experienced by healthy people as well as those with cardiac disease.

The sensation is described in various ways: as a racing of the heart, as an awareness of irregular or missed beats and as a thumping in the chest.

In healthy people, emotion, excitement or anxiety and stimulants such as coffee and nicotine can be associated with a fast heart rate and extra beats, creating the sensation of palpitation.

Oedema

Accumulation of excess fluid in the tissues is often a feature of cardiovascular and other diseases. There are three types of mechanism which may be involved in the formation of oedema:

Physiological mechanisms.
Physical obstruction to circulation.
Impaired muscle action.

Physiological mechanisms

1. Retention of salt (sodium chloride) and water. In cardiac failure renal blood flow is reduced and the retention of water follows retention of sodium ions in the kidneys. The filtration of sodium ions by the glomeruli is reduced and the reabsorption of sodium ions from the tubules is increased.

2. Raised blood pressure in capillaries. Tissue fluid is formed at the arterial end and reabsorbed at the venous end of the capillary (Fig. 7.5). Normally balance is maintained by the following two pressures: first, blood pressure or hydrostatic pressure which forces fluid out through the capillary walls to the tissue spaces; second, osmotic pressure exerted by the plasma proteins, which draws fluid back into the capillary. At the arterial end, the blood pressure is greater and fluid exudes into the tissues. At the venous end the osmotic pressure is greater and fluid is reabsorbed from the tissues. When back pressure develops in veins and venous return is impaired, as in right heart failure (p. 276), engorgement at the venous end of the capillary will increase the blood pressure, and fluid will exude into the tissues and will not be adequately reabsorbed, that is, oedema develops.

Figure 7.5
The formation of tissue fluid

Physical obstruction to circulation

Back pressure on capillaries can also accompany localized blockage of veins, for example, when stockings, garters or constrictive clothing are worn. Venous return may also be impeded by pressure on the popliteal area, for example, when sitting with the legs crossed at the knee or with the bend of the knee at the edge of a chair. Below the point of pressure, venous capillary hydrostatic pressure will increase due to venous stasis, causing movement of fluid into the tissues.

Impaired muscle action

When there is little or no muscular activity in a limb, as occurs during prolonged sitting, or lying in bed, then venous return will not be assisted by the action of the 'muscle pump'. Lack of muscle contraction leads to pooling of blood in veins; venous stasis and oedema follow. Impaired lymphatic drainage also plays a part in oedema formation. Minute lymphatic capillaries in tissue spaces act as an extra system for the flow of fluid from tissues into the circulation. The oedema seen in a weak or paralysed limb following a cerebral vascular accident may be due to a combination of impaired lymphatic and impaired venous return. This occurs when the 'muscle pump', which acts on both lymphatic vessels and veins, fails to work effectively in the weak or paralysed muscles (p. 283).

Figure 7.6
Sites of oedema
(A) Dependent parts
(B) The effect of recumbency
(C) Total body oedema

Figure 7.7
Pitting oedema

Sites of oedema

Oedema accumulates first in the lowest parts of the body, that is, the site depends mainly on gravity (Fig. 7.6). Oedema which occurs in any part of the body lower than the heart is known as dependent oedema. The severity of the oedema will depend on the length of time the part remains dependent on the degree of slowing of venous return and on the extent of the loss of 'muscle pump' action. In the ambulant patient, or when sitting, oedema occurs first in the feet and ankles, then in the legs. When the patient is in bed, oedema gathers in the sacral areas and thighs. In left heart failure (p. 275), fluid accumulates in the lungs (**pulmonary oedema**). In right heart failure, oedema shows first in the lowest dependent parts. As the heart failure progresses and venous stasis increases, oedema increases. Fluid may accumulate in the peritoneal cavity (**ascites**) or in the pleural cavity (**hydrothorax**). In very advanced heart disease total body oedema may develop, (anasarca) affecting even the face.

Cardiac oedema is said to 'pit' on pressure. This means that if an oedematous area is pressed by the finger, an indentation remains when the finger is removed (Fig. 7.7).

Changes in the amount of fluid retention can best be assessed by daily weighing of the patient.

Effects of oedema

Oedema causes varying degrees of distress and discomfort and it impairs the function of vital organs and cells.

To some people, swollen feet and ankles particularly at the end of the day, are no more than an unsightly irritation. But to an elderly lady with cardiac failure, grossly oedematous feet and ankles might prevent her from wearing shoes and could eventually cause her to become housebound. In contrast, acute pulmonary oedema can severely impair the function of the lungs, producing sudden major discomfort and distress from severe shortness of breath (p. 275).

Oedema also impairs cell function and increases the possibility of cell death. In oedematous areas the distance between the cells and nutrient-bearing materials is increased. This has important implications for skin care and for potential to absorb medications. Pressure sores develop readily if there is impaired cell nutrition and oedematous tissue is especially vulnerable if damaged or subjected to pressure; for example, the dependent areas of sacrum and heels in a bedfast patient. All such areas should be regularly inspected and protected (p. 518). Where there is increased tissue fluid and reduced capacity of cells to absorb, oedematous sites should not be used for intramuscular injections.

Cyanosis

Cyanosis is observed as a blue discolouration of the skin or mucous membranes and is due to reduced haemoglobin in the blood of superficial vessels (Ch. 6).

Peripheral cyanosis

This is due to high oxygen extraction from the blood in the peripheral tissues, as in patients with a low cardiac output or with circulation impaired by vasoconstriction. A blue tinge appears in the lips and nails, and in the skin of the hands, feet, ears or cheeks. Peripheral cyanosis also develops in normal people when they are cold due to low blood flow through the skin, but it disappears when the skin is warmed.

Central cyanosis

This is due to inadequate oxygenation of the blood resulting from impaired gas exchange in the lungs, for example in pulmonary oedema. It also occurs in some forms of congenital heart disease when blood shunts through from the venous side of the heart, bypassing the lungs. Unlike peripheral cyanosis, central cyanosis affects the warm mucous membranes such as the tongue.

INVESTIGATIONS

History

When heart disease is being investigated, it is important to build up a picture of a person's past health, of his current illness and of any family history of cardiovascular problems. Nurses can contribute to this picture by using opportunities to learn about an individual's way of life and about his own and his family's worries and anxieties.

Observation should begin the moment the nurse meets the patient. How does he look? What does he say? Observe, for example, whether he is anxious, in pain, breathless, pale, flushed, cyanosed or sweating. Is he overweight? Is there evidence that he might be a cigarette smoker?

Discovering what a person knows and believes about heart disease and its causes is an essential first step in helping him to learn about and adjust to his condition and perhaps to alter his behaviour.

Clinical examination

In the diagnosis of cardiac disorders, **auscultation** is helpful, that is, listening to heart sounds with the aid of a stethoscope. Altered heart sounds and the presence of murmurs caused by abnormally turbulent blood flow can be assessed accurately in this way by an experienced physician. A quiet environment is an advantage during auscultation.

Inspection and **palpation** of the anterior chest wall will also be carried out for pulsations and vibrations.

Pulse

A pulse is the wave of expansion felt in an arterial wall when a superficial artery is compressed by the finger. As the left ventricle contracts, the blood ejected distends the aorta and the arteries, which contain elastic tissue in their walls. Some sites of the pulse are illustrated in Figures 7.8 and 7.9.

It takes practice to become skilled at assessing the rate, rhythm and volume of the arterial pulse. Accurate observation, recording and reporting of the features of the pulse of cardiac patients are essential. Accuracy requires concentration and every pulse feature must be assessed, not just the rate.

Figure 7.8
Arterial pulses in upper limb

Figure 7.9
Arterial pulses in head and neck

Rate

Pulse rate normally reflects heart rate. In a resting adult, the normal range is 60 to 100 beats per minute.

Bradycardia

This is the term for a slow pulse — that is less than 60. This is a normal rate in athletes but is also associated with excess vagal stimulation, for example due to raised intracranial pressure; with myxoedema when metabolic rate is decreased; with digitalis excess; and with 'heart block' where disease of the conducting system of the heart prevents normal conduction from atria to ventricles, thus allowing the ventricles to contract at their own intrinsic rate of 20 to 40 beats per minute.

Tachycardia

This denotes a rapid heart rate — that is greater than 100 beats per minute. It is normal in infants and young children, and in adults it is usual with exercise and anxiety. It also accompanies fever, shock, haemorrhage, thyrotoxicosis and cardiac failure.

Having recorded the patient's pulse rate on a graph, look at the trend of the recordings and assess if it is steady, or if there is a gradual or sudden increase or decrease. Any change over time should be reported, but sudden change should always be reported at once.

Rhythm

The normal heart rhythm is regular, but **sinus arrhythmia**, where the heart rate increases on inspiration and decreases on expiration, is common to children and young adults and is considered normal.

Extrasystoles or ectopic beats may appear as isolated irregularities in an otherwise regular pulse. These extra beats of the ventricles follow quickly upon the previous beat and are followed by a compensatory pause.

Pulsus bigeminus or bigeminy takes the form of coupled beats when normal and ectopic beats alternate. Extrasystoles and coupling may indicate digoxin toxicity.

Atrial fibrillation is an arrhythmia in which the electrical conduction in the atria is abnormal and the pulse is totally irregular. It is often associated with coronary artery disease, mitral stenosis and thyrotoxicosis.

In this arrhythmia, the SA node is replaced as pacemaker by irritable foci in the atrium. Impulses are discharged at a rate of over 300 per minute causing feeble, rapid twitching of the atria instead of strong regular contraction. At this rapid rate, only some impulses can be transmitted through the AV node to the ventricular conducting system and as a result the ventricles respond erratically and inefficiently.

When the left ventricle contracts irregularly and with variable force, not every contraction is strong enough to open the aortic valve and produce a palpable pulse wave of distension, and the pulse will be irregular in both time and force (rhythm and volume). This creates what is known as a **pulse deficit**, where the heart rate is greater than the pulse rate. The deficit is estimated by simultaneous recordings by two people, of heart rate by auscultation at the apex, and of pulse rate, by taking the radial pulse at the wrist. Rates should be counted for not less than one minute.

An irregularity of the pulse must be reported promptly, as it could indicate the onset of atrial fibrillation; this can be associated with serious complications (p. 259).

Volume

Pulse volume is reflected in the amount of movement of the finger caused by the pulse wave. Volume is related to the cardiac output.

Cardiac failure, shock and acute myocardial infarction are associated with low cardiac output and small volume pulse. In the elderly, calcification of the arterial wall reduces pulse volume. An incompetent or leaking aortic valve, severe anaemia and thyrotoxicosis are associated with high cardiac output and large volume pulse, but physiological factors such as emotion, exercise, heat and pregnancy will also increase pulse volume.

Respiration

Dyspnoea, or difficulty in breathing, is the commonest symptom of heart failure (p. 274). The normal respiratory rate for adults is 16 to 20 per minute, and for a child 20 to 40. Rate is assessed by observing chest wall expansions, or by touch, laying the hand gently on the patient's chest wall. Breathlessness of cardiac origin which indicates pulmonary venous congestion or pulmonary oedema may be observed both on exercise and at rest and especially when the patient lies flat. The nurse should use her eyes and her ears to be on the alert for changes in respiratory rate, rhythm or depth. Changes must be reported quickly, since acute pulmonary oedema may develop rapidly with a rate of 40 to 50 or more per minute, causing great distress and anxiety to the patient. **Cheyne-Stokes respiration** may indicate advanced left heart failure and is often a preterminal sign. The characteristic waxing and waning phases occur when the respiratory centre is affected by lack of oxygen from decreased cerebral blood flow.

Blood pressure

Blood pressure is the pressure exerted by the blood upon the walls of the blood vessels. It depends mainly on the cardiac output and the peripheral resistance in the arterioles. The normal blood pressure of a young adult is around 120 systolic and 80 diastolic, measured in millimetres of mercury (mmHg). Blood pressure rises with age, and also with anxiety and on exercise. It should be recorded when the patient is resting and relaxed.

Hypertension indicates high blood pressure with levels above 150 mmHg systolic and 90 mmHg diastolic (p. 271).

Hypotension indicates low blood pressure with levels below 100 mmHg systolic and 60 mmHg diastolic.

Blood pressure is assessed using a sphygmomanometer and by auscultation at the brachial artery. The inflatable cuff acts as a tourniquet, compressing the brachial artery until no pulse is discernible. The returning pulse can be heard with the aid of a stethoscope on gradual deflation of the cuff. The arterial sounds are at first faint and tapping, gradually becoming more intense, and then changing to an abrupt muffling before their final disappearance. **Systolic pressure** is that at which the sounds are first heard. **Diastolic pressure** may be taken either as the muffling or the disappearance of sounds, but it is important that one level be decided upon when a patient is being treated for hypertension, since consistency is needed to assess progress accurately.

Temperature

Body temperature is controlled by the heat-regulating centre in the hypothalamus. When the centre is affected by pyrogens from micro-organisms or broken-down tissue cells, pyrexia occurs. In cardiac disease, micro-organisms produce bacterial endocarditis and purulent pericarditis; rheumatic fever is also related to infection. Following myocardial infarction, a low grade fever begins within 24 to 48 hours and gradually subsides during the first week. This pyrexia is thought to be a reaction to myocardial necrosis. Nursing responsibility lies in the accurate recording and reporting of changes in temperature. A neat graph is vital for correct assessment of progress and response to treatment.

Weight

In the ward, patients with cardiac disease are weighed as often as daily, particularly if cardiac failure is present. Gradual weight gain might suggest the development of fluid retention. Gradual weight loss can indicate the success of diuretic and other drug therapy. Weight is also checked at each out-patient clinic visit.

Electrocardiography

The electrocardiogram (ECG) is a graphic representation of the electrical changes which initiate contraction of heart muscle. It is a means of recording the electrical activity of the heart from its different angles.

Cardiac cells are electrically charged. The discharge and recharging of these cells during each cardiac cycle can be detected at the body surface and measured by attaching electrodes to the chest and limbs at conventionally determined sites.

At rest, cardiac muscle cells are 'polarised', that is they are negatively charged inside and positively charged outside. When stimulated, the inside becomes positively charged, the outside negatively charged and the cells become 'depolarised'. It is this process of depolarisation and repolarisation which is detected by the ECG, depolarisation representing the periods of contraction, and repolarisation the periods of rest and recovery in the cardiac cycle.

The normal ECG deflections are shown in Figure 7.10. The P wave represents the spread of electrical activity across the atria; this activity arises in the SA node and initiates atrial contractions (Fig. 7.3). The QRS complex represents depolarisation of the ventricular muscles and ventricular contraction, as the electrical impulse passes through the branches of the AV bundle. The T wave represents the repolarisation or resting phase when the ventricles are relaxed.

The ECG is important for the diagnosis of cardiac disease. It is used for the detection of arrhythmias, for the diagnosis of injury to heart muscle from ischaemia and to confirm the exact site and extent of a myocardial infarction.

While the ECG is being recorded, the patient should be at rest, and asked to keep quite still and relaxed, to avoid distortion of the tracing by muscle activity. An ECG may be recorded at home, in the doctor's surgery or in an out-patient department to which the patient is referred for specialist opinion before hospital admission. Each patient's ECGs are kept on file, to allow assessment of any change in heart muscle activity over a period.

ATRIAL ACTIVITY

VENTRICULAR ACTIVITY

R

P

T

Q

S

The P wave
atrial
contraction

The T wave
ventricular
relaxation
(repolarisation)

The QRS complex
ventricular
contraction
(depolarisation)

Figure 7.10
Normal ECG deflections

Cardiac monitoring

Cardiac monitoring is a means of demonstrating continuously on a small screen the electrical activity of the heart. Monitoring is especially valuable when serious disturbance of heart rate and rhythm is present or suspected, for instance, following myocardial infarction or cardiac surgery. Serious arrhythmias can endanger life and careful observation for changes on the oscilloscope and prompt treatment may prevent sudden deterioration.

Particular skills and knowledge are required to use cardiac monitors and to interpret cardiac rhythms. Generally monitors are found in intensive and coronary care units where an individual bedside monitor can be linked to oscilloscopes and alarm systems at a central nursing area.

It should be remembered that monitoring is a valuable aid to, but not a substitute for skilled observation and care of patients.

24 hour monitoring

Sometimes arrhythmias are paroxysmal and they may be missed on a standard ECG. If the person is otherwise well, apart from perhaps occasional giddy spells and falls caused by an arrhythmia, and if hospital admission is not necessary, continuous cardiac monitoring can be carried out using a small portable recorder attached, for example, to a waist belt.

Chest X-ray

Enlargement of the chambers of the heart, displacement of vessels, calcification of valves and the diffuse congestion of lung fields in pulmonary oedema can be examined by X-ray.

Films are taken either in a radiography department or by a portable machine at the patient's bedside. A nurse should remember the patient's need for warmth, privacy and explanation of the procedure, and should ensure that it is carried out with minimal strain.

Echocardiography

Echocardiography is one of many applications of ultrasound. An echocardiogram is a record of the echoes of ultrasound (high frequency) waves transmitted into the chest and reflected back by heart structures. When the ultrasonic beam from the transducer meets a boundary between structures of different acoustic densities, for example, heart valve tissue and intracardiac blood, sound waves are reflected back and these can be amplified and displayed on an oscilloscope or graphically.

This is a non-invasive technique which produces no pain or damage to tissues. It is particularly useful in studying the function and disorders of the heart valves and in detecting pericardial effusion.

Exercise testing

Exercise testing is used to investigate chest pain and to diagnose angina. It is a way of observing directly a person's response to exercise, the amount of work he can do and the symptoms associated with exercise. In order to witness and investigate an attack of undiagnosed chest pain or angina, the patient is asked to exercise on steps, or a treadmill or a bicycle ergometer (Fig. 7.11) until chest pain is provoked. An ECG is recorded continuously during and after the exercise and examined for arrhythmias and certain characteristic changes which occur when coronary artery blood flow is poor.

A doctor must be present during and for some time after the test and full resuscitation equipment should be available.

Figure 7.11
Bicycle ergometer

Cardiac catheterization

Passing a small flexible tube into either side of the heart and the coronary arteries is now a widely practised technique to establish the exact cardiac diagnosis and to measure the severity of abnormalities, generally prior to surgical correction (Fig. 7.12).

Right heart catheterization

A radio-opaque catheter is passed into an arm or leg vein and advanced to the chambers of the right side of the heart, entering the right atrium and passing on as far as the pulmonary artery (Fig. 7.13).

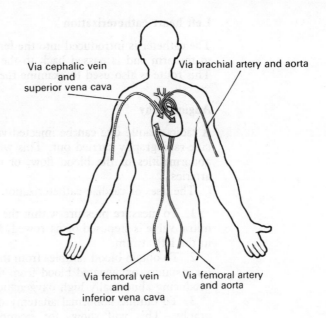

Figure 7.12
Cardiac catheterization routes

Figure 7.13
Right heart catheterization
The catheter has been passed
via the right subclavian vein,
superior vena cava and right
atrium to the right ventricle

Left heart catheterization

The catheter is introduced into the femoral artery in the groin or the brachial artery in the arm and is passed back to the left side of the heart, entering by the aorta. This route is also used to examine the coronary arteries which arise from the aorta.

Angiography

A radio-opaque dye can be injected via the catheters and simultaneous, high-speed cine-radiography carried out. This will demonstrate the anatomy of the heart, any abnormalities of the blood flow, or of the chambers, great arteries and coronary arteries.

The uses of cardiac catheterization are:

1. To measure pressure within the chambers and vessels of the heart. When the mitral valve is stenosed or narrowed, for example, pressure will be abnormally high in the left atrium.

2. To obtain blood samples from the chambers and vessels. In atrial septal defect, for instance, oxygenated blood from the left atrium may shunt to the right atrium, producing abnormally high oxygenation of the venous blood in the right atrium.

3. To outline abnormal anatomy or function by the injection of dye — angiography. This will show, for example, narrowed or blocked coronary arteries, abnormal blood flow through septal defects and backflow of blood through incompetent or leaking valves.

These procedures require great skill and involve risks to the patient of haemorrhage, arrhythmias and infection. Explanation of the procedure is best given by a person thoroughly familiar with it. The amount of detail provided will depend on the knowledge of the patient, the extent of his almost certain anxiety or fear and his desire or demand to know about the procedure. The test may involve lying on an X-ray table for an hour or more surrounded by seemingly threatening equipment and machinery. Administration of a mild sedative before the procedure, plus careful explanation and reassurance during it are helpful.

Precatheter preparation

A light meal may be given before the test. Local anaesthetic is injected at the site of introduction of the catheter.

Postcatheter care and observations

1. *The site.* Quarter hourly observations for haemorrhage are made for the first few hours. This is especially important after arterial puncture, since arterial bleeding may be brisk and heavy. Bruising or swelling around the pressure bandage may indicate formation of a haematoma (collection of blood). If bleeding occurs, firm pressure must be applied and help called immediately. The patient must have access to a bedside bell to call a nurse if bleeding occurs.

2. *Pulse.* Quarter hourly observations are made for the first 2 hours, or longer if necessary noting rate, rhythm and volume. Rising rate and weak volume may be due to haemorrhage. Irregularity of rhythm may indicate the onset of an arrhythmia. Changes should be reported immediately.

3. *Temperature.* Pyrexia may accompany infection.

4. *Pain.* Any complaint of pain whether at puncture site, limb, chest or abdomen should be considered abnormal and reported at once to the doctor.

Radionuclide studies

Nuclear imaging can also be used to detect abnormalities of myocardial blood flow in patients with coronary artery disease and suspected angina. This type of investigation has the advantage over coronary angiography of being a non-invasive technique, but it is relatively costly. It involves the injection intravenously of a small quantity of the patient's blood which has been labelled with radioactive material such as thallium-201 or technetium. When this passes through the heart it emits gamma radiation; the places where the gamma-emitting radioactive material has been deposited can be detected by a gamma camera outside the body. If the radioactive material is injected, for example, while the patient is undergoing exercise testing, ischaemic areas of heart muscle which are poorly perfused can be distinguished from the well perfused areas which take up the radioactive material.

CONGENITAL HEART DISEASE

Congenital abnormalities may be mild or severe, single or multiple. A person with a minimally malformed heart may go through life symptomless and completely unaware of the defect. Severe or multiple defects, on the other hand, will cause serious incapacity and may be incompatible with life, the child being born dead or dying soon after birth.

The cause may be genetic, or environmental. For example, if a woman contracts rubella (German measles) during the first 3 months of pregnancy, her child may have heart lesions as a result of arrested or faulty fetal development. Congenital defects are also often found in autosomal chromosome abnormalities such as Down's syndrome.

Examples of some clinical conditions are shown in Figure 7.14.

Higher pressure in aorta than in pulmonary arteries

Work load of right side is increased

Pulmonary blood flow is increased

Figure 7.14
Examples of congenital defect
Patent ductus arteriosus (PDA)
Atrial septal defect (ASD)
Ventricular septal defect (VSD)

Clinical features

In general, the larger the defect the earlier its presence becomes apparent, and if it permits the mixing of arterial and venous blood, as in ventricular septal defect, the child will be cyanosed. Cyanosis, dyspnoea, failure to thrive, clubbing of the fingers and heart murmurs are features common to many congenital heart diseases. A small defect may go unnoticed until the child or adult is much older and perhaps being examined at school, for employment or for insurance.

Treatment and nursing care

Many congenital abnormalities can be corrected by surgery. Prognosis depends largely on the severity of the defect, on the success of surgery and whether there have been associated problems such as chest infection, cardiac failure or infection of the endocardium (bacterial endocarditis).

Patients undergoing cardiac surgery are nursed at first in an intensive care unit by specially trained staff. Postoperative complications include haemorrhage, arrhythmias and infection, and close observation is essential during this period. Progress is assessed carefully after discharge at hospital out-patient clinic and by the general practitioner for at least a year.

RHEUMATIC HEART DISEASE

The incidence and severity of rheumatic fever, and of its sequel chronic rheumatic heart disease, have declined dramatically in the last 50 years in the Western world due to better social conditions, less overcrowding and risk of cross infection, the use of antibiotics and change in the virulence of streptococci.

In world terms, however, acute and chronic rheumatic heart disease is still a major problem for children and adults, especially in developing countries. In these parts of the world, where poverty and overcrowding continue, and where few people have access to expensive cardiac surgery, the hope is that control of the disease can be achieved through public health and preventive measures.

Acute rheumatic fever

Acute rheumatic fever is a febrile illness which follows infection with, and abnormal immunological response to, the Group A haemolytic streptococcus. Between the streptococcal infection, usually manifested as a sore throat, and the onset of rheumatic fever there is a latent period of 1 to 3 weeks. The effect of the disease may be widespread throughout the body, but especially involved are connective tissues, such as heart valves, heart muscle, joints and tendons.

Clinical features

Onset. Acute pharyngitis is followed after a few weeks by either a gradual onset of malaise, anorexia, low grade fever and weight loss, or a sudden onset of joint pain with high fever, sweating and tachycardia.

Polyarthritis. This is characterized by pain in joints. The joints most often affected are knees, ankles, elbows and wrists. They become swollen, painful, hot and tender, and the pain tends to be 'flitting' in nature, moving from one joint to another.

Rheumatic nodules. Painless, subcutaneous nodules appear, attached to tendons or over bony prominences such as the elbows, knees or back of the head.

Erythema marginatum. Reddish, crescent-shaped patches appear on the trunk.

Carditis. Heart involvement is the most serious feature of acute rheumatic fever. It takes three forms: endocarditis, myocarditis and pericarditis.

1. *Endocarditis*. Inflammation of the endocardium affects the valves. Characteristic minute warty vegetations form along the valve margins. Dilatation of the valve ring may result in the valve leaking.

2. *Myocarditis*. Inflammation of the myocardium is suggested by a rapid pulse rate. Often the pulse is faster than one would expect for the degree of fever present, and it may persist when the fever subsides. Irregularity of heart rhythm and pulse may occur. Cardiac failure may develop, and the heart may enlarge. Recording sleeping pulse rates can eliminate anxiety, activity and excitement as possible causes of tachycardia.

3. *Pericarditis*. Inflammation of the pericardium usually indicates severe infection (p. 246).

Investigations

Common findings in the blood are a raised white cell count, anaemia, a raised ESR and a high ASO (antistreptolysin 'O') titre giving evidence of a recent streptococcal infection. Episodes of sore throat are noted and a throat swab is sent for bacteriological investigation.

Treatment and nursing care

In this feverish debilitating illness, which carries a risk of cardiac failure, observations of temperature, pulse, blood pressure and respiration are important; fluid balance and weight should also be recorded.

In the active stage of the disease, when patients are feverish and sweating, and have malaise, joint pain and poor appetite, help will be needed with skin care and oral hygiene, nutrition and fluid intake. Nursing measures may be needed to reduce temperature, to relieve pain, to encourage limb circulation, to maintain bowel function and to promote rest and sleep.

A course of intramuscular penicillin is given to combat the streptococcal infection in the nose or throat. This will be followed by prophylactic oral therapy, lasting possibly for many years into adult life as a secondary preventive measure against further attacks of the disease.

Salicylates are used to reduce fever and pain. Steroids are given because of their anti-inflammatory properties where there is evidence of carditis.

Digitalis, diuretic therapy and salt restriction may be started if cardiac failure develops (p. 274).

Course and complications

The course of rheumatic fever may be short and acute or it may be prolonged for many months. Recurrent attacks are common with the risk of increasing cardiac damage and heart failure with each attack. The very young child rarely escapes cardiac damage, but risk diminishes with age. Most people affected live relatively normal lives until 40 or 50 years of age when the complications of chronic rheumatic heart disease become evident.

Chronic rheumatic heart disease

Following acute rheumatic fever and recurrences of the disease, rheumatic endocarditis may smoulder on for many years producing chronic rheumatic heart disease. This takes the form of valvular heart disease and presents sometimes in early adult life, but more often many years later, in middle or old age. Rheumatic endocarditis causes inflammation and distortion of the valve cusps and eventually fibrosis and calcification of the valve ring. This leads to different degrees of:

Stenosis or narrowing of the valves, causing obstruction to blood flow (Fig. 7.15).

Incompetence or imperfect closure of the valve, resulting in leakage and backflow of blood (regurgitation).

A valve may be stenosed or incompetent, or both. Patients may have disease of more than one valve.

Mitral valve disease

Mitral stenosis is more common than incompetence, but combined stenosis and incompetence often occur. As the mitral valve narrows, pressure in the left atrium rises and is transmitted back to the pulmonary veins and capillaries (p. 275). Lung congestion follows, making breathing more difficult, and the patient complains of progressive shortness of breath and tiredness. Dyspnoea appears first on exercise, but eventually less and less exercise is required to produce it. Orthopnoea, paroxysmal nocturnal dyspnoea and acute pulmonary oedema may result — that is the features of left heart failure occur.

Mitral valve disease also increases the risk of chest infection and chronic bronchitis, since either is more likely to develop when there is pulmonary congestion. Following left-sided heart failure and pulmonary congestion right heart failure gradually appears.

Echocardiography, cardiac catheterisation, ECG and X-ray are used to investigate valve disorders. In mitral valve disease, cardiac catheterisation is used to measure the pressures in the chambers of the left side of the heart and dye can be injected to assess whether backflow of blood is present, indicating mitral incompetence. High pressure in the left atrium eventually causes it to enlarge. This will show on X-ray and can best be seen when the patient has a barium swallow; the barium-filled oesophagus is displaced backwards by a bulging left atrium.

Atrial fibrillation

Atrial fibrillation is an important complication of mitral stenosis; weak and erratic contraction of the atria and the ventricles, altered blood flow and poor emptying of the chambers will result in stasis of blood, which in turn will allow thrombi to form. Sometimes the heart rhythm switches between normal sinus

Narrowed outlet

Fusion of adjacent cusps

Figure 7.15
Valve stenosis

rhythm (Fig. 7.30) and atrial fibrillation (Fig. 7.16A and B). If this occurs, turbulent blood flow can dislodge thrombi from the left side of the heart causing systemic embolism, which may block cerebral, limb, renal or mesenteric arteries (Fig. 7.39).

Normal sinus rhythm

Figure 7.16A
Normal sinus rhythm

Atrial fibrillation

Figure 7.16B
Atrial fibrillation

Aortic valve disease

Disease of the aortic valve is often due to rheumatic endocarditis, but it may also be caused by congenital malformation or syphilis. Stenosis and incompetence may occur singly or together.

Aortic stenosis

Stenosis causes an increased work load for the left ventricle, as it tries to overcome the obstruction of the narrowed valve. The left ventricle compensates by enlargement of individual muscle fibres (hypertrophy). Left ventricular hypertrophy increases as stenosis increases. Gradually, the coronary arteries become unable to meet the demands of the hypertrophied muscle for blood and angina is felt. While the heart compensates in this way fairly normal activities are possible, but eventually the heart fails. Heart failure is the most frequent complication requiring treatment (p. 275). The earliest symptoms of left heart failure are breathlessness and fatigue. Angina and syncope on exertion, for example fainting on climbing a hill, are both important features and sudden death may occur.

Cardiac surgery is carried out in severe cases where there is great risk of sudden death. Because of this risk, skill and patience are required from doctors and nurses to explain to the patient the need for major cardiac surgery, especially when the signs of the disease outweigh the symptoms and the patient does not perceive himself as being either severely disabled or at risk.

Aortic incompetence

Incompetence of the valve allows backflow of blood into the left ventricle during diastole. By increasing the volume of blood to be expelled, the work load of the left ventricle is increased, leading to left ventricular hypertrophy and eventual left heart failure.

Pulmonary and tricuspid valve disease

Pulmonary valve disease is uncommon; it is usually congenital in origin, and may be associated with a ventricular septal defect or Fallot's tetralogy.

Most patients with tricuspid disease will also have mitral and aortic disease, rheumatic in origin. Stenosis and incompetence give rise to right heart failure. Obstructed blood flow through the narrowed valve and backflow through the incompetent valve will cause, in the right atrium, a rise in pressure, which will be transmitted back to the venae cavae and systemic venous return.

Treatment of valvular heart disease

Cardiac surgery may greatly improve a patient's condition and increase life expectancy, but the risks of surgery itself and of subsequent complications are considerable. Surgery may be 'closed' or 'open'.

Closed heart surgery

In closed heart surgery, the circulation continues to flow through the heart during the operation. To relieve stenosis of the mitral valve, for example, a finger or dilator is introduced into the left atrium and positioned in the valve to stretch it, separating the cusps and thus relieving obstruction. This procedure is known as **mitral valvotomy**. Restenosis may occur several years after surgery and valvotomy may be repeated two or three times. As the valve becomes more rigid and calcified, replacement using artificial valves becomes necessary.

Open heart surgery

In open heart surgery or **cardiopulmonary bypass,** the heart and lungs are emptied of blood. Venous blood is drained from the superior and inferior venae cavae into an oxygenator. A pump recirculates the blood and returns it via the femoral artery or the aorta (Fig. 7.17). This technique is used for **replacement of valves** and for

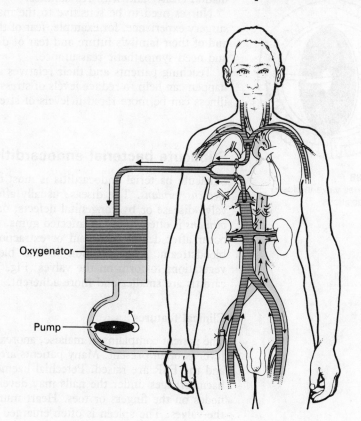

Oxygenator

Pump

Figure 7.17
Cardiopulmonary bypass

Figure 7.18A
Starr-Edwards aortic valve
prosthesis

Figure 7.18B
Medtronic-Hall valve in closed
and open positions

coronary artery bypass surgery (p. 261). There are several types of valve in use:

1. *Mechanical valves*. (a) Ball and socket type (Fig. 7.18A). (b) Disc occluder type (Fig. 7.18B). Because of the risk of thrombus formation on these valves, patients require anticoagulant therapy, sometimes for life; this may successfully prevent embolism, but it will add the risk of haemorrhage.

A tissue valve might be selected in preference to a mechanical valve, for example, for a patient with an existing peptic ulceration because of the risk of anticoagulant induced bleeding. A further problem with mechanical valves is turbulence of blood flow; the action of the valve destroys red blood cells (haemolysis) causing anaemia.

2. *Biological valves*. (a) Homografts — these are of human tissue; valves which are obtained within 12 hours of death and stored for a limited period. (b) Heterografts — these are of non-human tissue, usually of porcine (pig) origin. Anticoagulant therapy is not usually necessary with homograft and heterograft valves unless atrial fibrillation is present. Infection is a risk with all valve replacement.

Support and rehabilitation. Patients having cardiac surgery of any kind require skilled observation and a wide range of emotional, physical and technical care. In the immediate postoperative period, this care is given by a specially trained team of professionals in an intensive care unit.

It is important that patients know what will happen to them before and after surgery and what to expect in the period of recovery.

Most cardiac departments have specially prepared booklets giving information about different members of hospital staff, admission and convalescent wards and the intensive care area, the operation itself, drug regimes, the pattern of recovery in and out of hospital, and about appropriate levels of activity during convalescence.

Those who are about to undergo surgery may appreciate the chance to talk to someone who has already successfully undergone the same operation. Many such patients are members of special clubs or associations. However, some postoperative patients take delight in giving detailed accounts of their own experiences which, to the anxious preoperative patient, are very frightening. Nurses should be alert to this and should refer the patient to a member of staff who can give the necessary information clearly and with reassurance.

Nurses need to be sensitive to the many fears which patients undergoing heart surgery experience, for example, fear of the unknown, fear of pain, fear of their own and of their family's future and fear of death itself. Relatives, too, share these fears and need sympathetic reassurance.

Teaching patients and their relatives and helping them to understand what will happen can help to reduce levels of stress; and it has been shown that recovery from illness can be more rapid if levels of stress are reduced.

Subacute bacterial endocarditis

Subacute bacterial endocarditis is most often caused by the micro-organism *Streptococcus viridans*. The disease usually affects hearts already damaged by rheumatic valve disease or by congenital defects, or it may infect prosthetic valves. As *Strep. viridans* is often found in infected gums, teeth, or tonsils, bacterial endocarditis may occur after dental treatment or extraction when the bacteria are released into the bloodstream. The infection in the bloodstream causes large, loosely adherent vegetations to form on the valves (Fig. 7.19). The vegetations of rheumatic endocarditis are smaller and more adherent.

Clinical features

The patient complains of malaise, anorexia and tiredness. A prolonged, unexplained fever is often present. Many patients are anaemic, and the white cell count (Ch. 8) and the ESR are raised. Petechial haemorrhages into the skin (Ch. 8) and splinter haemorrhages under the nails may develop. Osler's nodes appear — raised, tender nodes on the fingers or toes. Heart murmurs develop, due to the inflammation of the valves. The spleen is often enlarged and haematuria may be present.

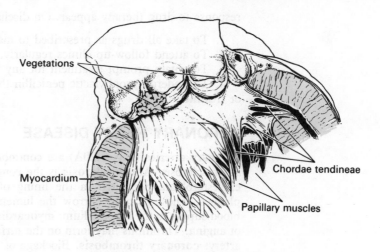

Figure 7.19
Vegetations of bacterial
endocarditis on valve

Labels on figure: Vegetations, Myocardium, Chordae tendineae, Papillary muscles

Investigations

The findings of unexplained pyrexia in patients with valvular or congenital heart disease, or in those who have undergone cardiac surgery, is significant. There may be a history of dental treatment or infection. The diagnosis is confirmed on obtaining a positive blood culture. Many specimens of blood are carefully taken under strict asepsis to eliminate the possibility of a false positive through contamination of the specimen. By examining the culture medium under the microscope, the infecting organism will be identified.

Nursing observations

Accurate recordings of temperature and of pulse rate and rhythm are vital to assess the course of fever and as an indication of effectiveness or abnormality of heart action. Weight gain or loss is assessed daily if cardiac failure is present, and observation of general appearance, appetite, vitality and mental state is important, particularly when the course of the disease is long and wearying.

Course and complications

The course of the disease may be long, and the length of treatment depends on the patient's response to antibiotics. Before antibiotic therapy was introduced, almost all patients died, and even today the disease is serious, especially if there is delay in starting antibiotics. The main danger is embolism from the vegetations on the endocardium of the valves. Emboli may lodge in the brain causing hemiplegia, in the kidneys causing renal damage, in the skin causing haemorrhages, in the retinae causing loss of vision, or in the spleen, limb or mesenteric vessels (Fig. 7.39). As a result of severe valve disease, heart failure develops.

Treatment and nursing care

The selection of antibiotic depends on sensitivity tests. Usually two or more antibiotics are given in combination. Over many days and possibly weeks, large doses given intramuscularly can cause severe discomfort to the patient, and careful observation of injection sites for local reaction is required, together with strict aseptic technique in the preparation and administration of injections. Continuous intravenous infusion of antibiotics may be necessary. Oral antibiotics will be given when the temperature falls, indicating a response to treatment.

As in rheumatic fever itself, while endocarditis persists bed rest may be prolonged. During the period of bed rest and fever, the same meticulous care of the skin, pressure areas and mouth, and the same observation of bladder and bowel function and sleep pattern will be necessary. Mobilization begins when signs of a response to drug therapy appear. On discharge from hospital, patients are advised:

1. To take all drugs as prescribed to maintain therapeutic blood levels.
2. To attend follow-up clinics regularly.
3. To obtain prompt treatment for any upper respiratory tract infection.
4. To undergo prophylactic penicillin therapy before and after dental extraction or treatment.

CORONARY HEART DISEASE

Coronary arteries (Fig. 7.20A) are commonly affected by the degenerative disease atherosclerosis. **Atherosclerosis** is the condition in which fatty substances such as cholesterol are deposited in the lining of arteries in the form of atheromatous plaques. These plaques narrow the lumen of the artery causing reduction in the blood supply to the myocardium: **myocardial ischaemia**. This may result in the pain of **angina**. Thrombus may form on the surface of the plaque eventually blocking the artery: **coronary thrombosis**. Blockage of blood supply to the myocardium causes necrosis or death of the area of muscle served by that artery: **myocardial infarction**. Patients and their relatives may be confused by the use of several terms for 'heart attack' and the meaning of words used should be explained.

Coronary artery disease (ischaemic heart disease) is the most common type of heart disease and the most frequent cause of death in middle and old age in developed countries. It is responsible for 1 in 4 deaths in the United Kingdom and the highest death rate in the world from the disease is now to be found in Scotland. In many countries, the incidence continues to rise but in others such as the United States, Canada and Australia there has been a sharp decline in heart disease deaths in the last 10 years. Exactly why this has happened is not clear. It has been suggested, for example, that people in the U.S.A. have been adapting their life-styles in response to health education. But coronary heart disease is complex and multi-factorial and the reasons for the changes in incidence are difficult to establish.

Incidence increases with age. In younger and middle age groups, coronary artery disease is much commoner in males than females. After the menopause, women become more likely to develop the disease and in older age groups it is equally common in both sexes.

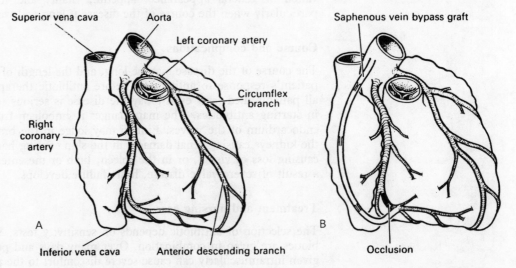

Figure 7.20
(A) Normal coronary arteries
(B) Coronary arteries showing blocked artery and bypass graft

Superior vena cava

Aorta

Left coronary artery

Circumflex branch

Right coronary artery

Saphenous vein bypass graft

A

B

Inferior vena cava

Anterior descending branch

Occlusion

Risk factors

Although the causes of coronary artery disease are not fully understood, certain risk factors have been shown to affect its development. Many of the factors are inter-related and some reflect 20th century life-styles.

1. **Smoking.** Atherosclerosis, heart attack and sudden death are far more prevalent in smokers than non-smokers. Figure 7.21 shows ischaemic heart disease as

Figure 7.21
Estimated deaths from
smoking, Scotland 1980
(Scottish Health Education
Co-ordinating Committee, 1983)

the major smoking related disease in Scotland, the others being lung cancer and chronic bronchitis (deaths from road accidents are shown for comparison).

Cigarette smoking is an important preventable cause of ill-health; giving up smoking will lessen considerably the risk of having a heart attack.

2. **Dietary fats and cholesterol.** A diet high in saturated (animal) fats (Ch. 4) is related to high blood cholesterol levels, and the higher the blood cholesterol level, the greater the risk of developing atheroma. Serum cholesterol levels can be lowered by substituting polyunsaturated fats (some margarine and vegetable cooking oils) for saturated (animal) fats in the diet. People at risk are therefore advised to reduce fat intake generally, and to increase the proportion of polyunsaturated fat in their diets in order to lower their serum cholesterol levels.

Although it has been shown that a high blood cholesterol is associated with a higher incidence of coronary heart disease, there is still a great deal of controversy about the overall advantages of changing dietary fat intake. People differ in the ways in which they manufacture cholesterol in the liver, and absorb and use cholesterol from the diet. Fats vary in type and complexity, and it seems that certain fats in the blood may have a protective function against the production of atheroma and against blood clotting. More research is needed to clarify the relationship between diet and heart disease.

3. **Hypertension.** Hypertension accelerates the development of atherosclerosis. The higher the blood pressure the greater the risk of developing coronary artery disease.

4. **Heredity.** Atherosclerosis is sometimes found in several members of one family and hereditary factors do seem to be involved in coronary artery disease. This might be related to the fact that high blood pressure and high serum cholesterol levels can also be inherited.

5. **Exercise.** Exercise is another controversial risk factor. Atheroma seems to occur more often in people with sedentary jobs. Many people today take little regular exercise and it has been shown that exercise can lower plasma cholesterol levels. Exercise may also encourage enlargement of the coronary arteries thus improving blood supply and protecting against heart attack.

6. **Obesity.** Due to the associations between being overweight and high blood pressure, little exercise and a high dietary intake of animal fat, obese people may be more often at risk.

7. **Diabetes.** Diabetics, particularly women, are more likely to have heart attacks than non-diabetics.

8. **Stress and tension**. There is no direct evidence to show that stress is a significant factor in death rates from heart attack; but it has been claimed that people who have a competitive nature and who experience high levels of emotional tension and stress are more likely to develop coronary artery disease.

Angina pectoris

The pain of angina is caused by inadequate blood supply to and oxygenation of the myocardium (myocardial ischaemia) generally as a result of narrowing of an artery or arteries by coronary atherosclerosis. Angina is also felt if coronary blood supply is inadequate to meet increased workload and therefore an increased oxygen need of the myocardium. This can occur in thyrotoxicosis; it also occurs in hypertension and aortic stenosis, conditions in which the left ventricular muscle enlarges. Angina may also be associated with anaemia; in this instance, the blood carries less oxygen for the myocardium.

Clinical features

The characteristics of anginal pain are described on page 246. Anxiety and a rapid pulse rate often accompany pain.

Investigations

1. History. Diagnosis can usually be made from the history of pain. Often all the major characteristics are present.

2. ECG. During an attack of angina, certain ECG changes occur and these can be provoked by an exercise test (p. 254). The ECG changes occur when the coronary arteries fail to supply the myocardium with enough oxygen to meet the extra demands made on it by exercise.

3. Cardiac catheterization — coronary angiography. The injection of dye outlines the vessels and shows the extent and severity of atheroma (p. 254).

4. Radionuclide studies (p. 256).

Nursing observations

It is important to observe patients for any sign of restlessness or anxiety which might indicate the onset of angina. Episodes of angina should be assessed and reported in terms of the major characteristics of pain already mentioned.

Course and complications

Most patients can live a fairly normal life with angina for many years. The prognosis depends on the underlying cause; the risk of heart attack and sudden death is probably related mainly to the anatomy and severity of the coronary artery stenosis.

Symptoms can lessen and eventually disappear in some people if **collateral circulation** develops; small branches of arteries can enlarge and new vessels can grow to improve the blood supply to the myocardium.

Treatment and nursing care

Rest is encouraged, but unnecessary restrictions can make the person consider himself an invalid, and an optimistic attitude will help to overcome or adjust to angina. Generally it is enough to use common sense to modify activity, avoid overwork, worry or anxiety and live within the limits of the pain.

Obesity should be corrected, large meals avoided and a diet low in saturated fat may be recommended. Cigarette smoking should be stopped. Exercise is encouraged, provided it does not provoke pain, as it can promote the development of collateral circulation.

Drugs

1. Glyceryl trinitrate. Angina may be prevented and relieved by taking a tablet of glyceryl trinitrate sublingually. The drug is not addictive and as many tablets as are necessary to relieve the pain may be taken; patients should always carry their tablets with them and should be taught to use them prophylactically before exertion. The drug causes lowering of blood pressure and hence a reduction in the work of the heart and, in some cases, dilatation of the coronary arteries. It can induce an unpleasant headache or pounding sensation and a half tablet at a time may be advised. A fresh supply of tablets should be obtained regularly as glyceryl trinitrate loses its strength over time. Oral long-acting nitrates are also available and a skin patch containing a drug reservoir of glyceryl trinitrate has been developed to give a 24 hour controlled release form of treatment.

2. Beta receptor blocking drugs, so-called 'beta blockers', propranolol, meto-prolol, oxprenolol. These drugs block the stimulant effect of the sympathetic nervous system, which increases the rate and force of the heart beat. By reducing these, they reduce the oxygen demands of the myocardium. Angina is thus prevented by reduction of oxygen demand.

3. Calcium antagonists. The exact action of these drugs such as verapamil and nifedipine is not fully understood, but calcium is involved in the electrical activity of the heart and its conducting system and in the contraction of the coronary arteries. By influencing the electrical activity, calcium antagonists can reduce tachycardia, slowing the heart and reducing the oxygen demand of the myocardium thus easing the angina. By dilating the coronary arteries, they improve myocardial blood supply.

Surgery

In recent years, open heart surgery has been used for severe angina. It is carried out by grafting blood vessels to bypass blocked arteries, for example by using a saphenous vein from the patient's leg to provide a bypass from aorta to peripheral coronary artery (Fig. 7.20B).

Myocardial infarction

Irreversible damage to an area of myocardium occurs when the coronary artery serving that area is blocked by thrombus or atheroma (p. 264). The site of infarction depends on the vessel blocked; the size of infarction varies, and the area of muscle involved may be small or very extensive.

Clinical features

Pain is the major symptom. Note carefully its features and how it compares with anginal pain (p. 246). The sudden onset of severe, prolonged pain is associated with distress, sweating, pallor, nausea and vomiting. Many patients will describe having had a worsening of angina or a vague feeling of ill-health for some weeks before the acute attack.

Investigations

1. Clinical examination and history of the characteristic features of the pain.
2. ECG changes — daily recordings of ECG are taken, as infarction produces a recognizable series of changes over several days in most patients.
3. Levels of serum enzymes — when heart muscle is damaged, enzymes present in the muscles are released into the bloodstream and their levels are measured daily over several days. Creatine phosphokinase (CPK) — this enzyme can be detected quickly, within 6 hours of infarction. After 2 to 3 days the level returns to normal. Serum glutamic oxaloacetic transaminase (SGOT) — peak level is reached after 24 hours and returns to normal in 3 to 5 days. Lactic dehydrogenase (LDH) — peak level is reached more slowly and levels are elevated for up to 2 or 3 weeks.

Nursing observations

Relief of pain and anxiety is vital, and nurses must observe for and report any sign of pallor, sweating, anxiety or restlessness which might indicate returning pain.

Temperature. Fever occurs during the first few days. The temperature is usually recorded 4 hourly during this period.

Pulse. Recordings are made hourly at first, noting rate, rhythm and volume. When cardiac monitoring ends, usually after 48 hours, and there is no longer a visual image of the heart beat, it becomes all the more important to report any change in the pulse so that an ECG can be taken to establish the exact nature of the change.

Blood pressure. Hourly recordings are taken initially; changes will indicate altered cardiac output.

Respirations. Dyspnoea may indicate the onset of left heart failure.

Fluid balance. When cardiac output is impaired and renal blood flow is reduced, fluid intake and output must be accurately measured.

Complications

The risk of sudden death is great, and it occurs within minutes of onset in 25% of cases. Complications and a deterioration in condition are common within the first few hours after heart attack and for this reason mobile coronary care units carrying equipment for immediate treatment or for resuscitation are being used in several centres. They enable help to reach patients who survive the first critical hours by providing treatment at home. By stabilizing the condition, and by keeping the patient under continuous cardiac monitoring, the journey to an intensive care unit can be undertaken safely. The overall risk of heart attack will depend on the patient's age, the size of infarction and whether there has been previous infarction; after the first 48 hours, the risk quickly lessens.

There are several important complications following myocardial infarction:

Arrhythmias

Most patients have an alteration in heart rate, rhythm or conduction during the first 48 hours. Nursing and medical staff of coronary care units are specially trained in the use of cardiac monitors to observe, interpret and treat arrhythmias as they occur, thus preventing cardiac failure and cardiac arrest. Ventricular fibrillation (in which the ventricles do not contract but rather 'twitch' so that cardiac output ceases) is the most serious arrhythmia. Death will occur unless ventricular fibrillation is treated by using the emergency technique of defibrillation (p. 282).

Cardiac failure

After infarction, the effectiveness of the pumping action of the myocardium may be reduced to varying degrees. Left-sided heart failure can develop suddenly causing acute pulmonary oedema. Right-sided heart failure may eventually follow (p. 276).

Cardiogenic shock

In extensive infarction, the condition may deteriorate very quickly due to a fall in cardiac output and blood pressure. The heart becomes unable to provide enough circulation to oxygenate vital organs and tissues and the patient will be cynased, pale, cold, sweating and often has mental confusion.

Other complications

These include:

Systemic arterial embolism. Blood clots ('mural thrombi') can form on the infarcted wall of the left ventricle (Fig. 7.39). If these clots break loose and travel as emboli in the arterial system, they may block cerebral, mesenteric, renal or peripheral arteries.

Pulmonary embolism following deep venous thrombosis in the legs.
Ventricular aneurysm and rupture of the heart wall causing sudden death.

Treatment and nursing care

Relief of pain. This is urgent. An opiate, usually morphine, is given immediately intramuscularly, together with an anti-emetic such as cyclizine, since morphine causes vomiting. This is repeated until the acute pain has eased. To relieve fear and anxiety, a tranquilliser, for example diazepam, is given for several days or longer if anxiety persists despite reassurance. Other drugs are started as necessary such as a night sedative to aid sleep, drugs to control arrhythmias or anticoagulants to reduce the risk of thromboembolism.

Rest. Complete bed rest is essential at first. If shocked and hypotensive, the patient lies flat in bed and everything is done for him. All movement should be gentle and double lifting techniques should be used. Exercises will be essential to improve venous return and to help prevent the formation of deep venous thrombosis. The nurse should try to anticipate the patient's needs in order to prevent him having to strain and become tired. The bedside locker must be within reach and he must have some means, such as a bell, of calling a nurse.

Personal hygiene. While bed rest continues the following are necessary: daily bedbath, frequent observation and care of pressure areas and observation of the mouth. Oxygen is given while there is pain, dyspnoea or cardiac failure; even when humidified, oxygen therapy may dry the mouth, and frequent mouthwashes can be refreshing. Once pain has eased or if the infarction is not too severe, increasing involvement in self care should be encouraged as this can help to restore confidence.

Most patients worry about bowel function and will find using a commode less stressful than using a bed-pan. Straining at stool should be avoided; constipation for 2 or 3 days is not harmful provided the patient is reassured that normal function can easily be restored by giving a mild oral aperient or suppositories.

Diet. If the patient is obese, a low calorie diet is started. Restriction of animal fat may be advised. Meals should be light initially. Salt restriction is necessary only if severe cardiac failure develops (p. 274).

Mobilization. Early ambulation is now encouraged. The patient may be allowed to sit out of bed from the second or third day and to walk from the fifth or sixth day. The length of time out of bed and the distance walked are gradually increased, but both may be delayed or restricted if the patient becomes tired, if the infarction is extensive or if complications develop. After 2 or 3 weeks in hospital the patient is discharged home. The family doctor then supervises convalescence.

Rehabilitation

After a heart attack, and after various forms of heart surgery such as coronary artery bypass, patients and their families are often anxious about the future and about the possibility that this sudden and life-threatening event will alter their lives radically. A nurse can help to relieve anxiety by calmly explaining with reassurance and optimism what these events mean and by indicating that a full and active life is possible despite them.

Since the 1970s cardiac rehabilitation programmes have been developed. They aim to help patients to return to a life-style of their own choice and to slow the development of existing coronary artery disease by correcting risk factors. The rehabilitation scheme might include such things as a programme of gradually increasing physical activity, teaching about prevention and risk factors, and psychological and social counselling for the patient and the family. For example, there is often anxiety about how much exercise and strenuous activity is possible and safe after a heart attack. There will be uncertainty and a need for advice about exactly what has happened to the heart, about when to return to work and start driving, about weight and what to eat, and when to resume sexual activity.

It is often possible to return to many activities within 6 to 8 weeks, but life-styles and levels of anxiety differ and each patient and his family will need opportunities to ask questions and to discuss their own circumstances and worries with experienced staff. Patients themselves can experience a variety of reactions after heart attack, for example, tiredness, irritability, depression, denial, boredom, poor concentration or loss of confidence. Often the anxieties of the spouse and other members of the patient's family can be equally or even more severe than the patient's, creating overprotectiveness and preventing the patient from setting his own goals and limits.

Rehabilitation will include community colleagues. In many areas liaison schemes are being developed in which a community nurse visits the patient and his family while he is in hospital and continues to give support after discharge. Booklets have been compiled to give advice and to answer some of the commonest questions. An example of a cardiac rehabilitation programme is given by Jillian Howard and Helga Erlanger in *Patient Teaching* (1983). They describe the nurse's role in the programme and the way in which its effectiveness was tested.

Cardiac pacemakers

Normally the SA node acts as the pacemaker, initiating the events in the cardiac cycle. Following a heart attack, there may be damage to the conducting pathways and the arrhythmia known as heart block may develop. In this arrhythmia, some or all of the impulses from the SA node become blocked on the conducting pathways, usually at the AV node. When this happens, the atria and ventricles contract independently; the ventricles may contract at a half, third or quarter of the atrial rate, possibly as slowly as 20 to 40 beats per minute. As a result, cardiac output drops and the heartbeat cannot be stepped up to meet the demands of exercise.

In the most severe form of heart block, brief periods of ventricular standstill can occur. A sudden drop in cardiac output leads to reduced cerebral blood flow and cerebral ischaemia which presents as temporary but alarming attacks of fainting and convulsions known as **Stokes-Adams attacks**.

To correct the various degrees of heart block, artificial pacemakers are used. Pacemakers consist of a pulse generator which acts as the power source, and a lead or insulated pacing wire which carries the impulse to the heart. Artificial pacemakers can be temporary or permanent. **Temporary pacemakers** are used in emergencies or as a stopgap measure for short term disturbance after a heart attack, or while waiting for the insertion of a permanent pacemaker. In temporary pacing, the battery box is external and portable; the pacing wire is inserted usually via the subclavian vein or external jugular vein and advanced to the tip of the right ventricle.

Permanent, implanted pacemakers are used if the heart block is likely to be severe and long term. In this case, the pulse generator is inserted in subcutaneous tissue in the chest wall and the pacing wire inserted via the cephalic or external jugular vein (Fig. 7.22A, B).

The pulse generators can be set at a fixed rate or they can be 'on demand'. The demand type is useful if heart block is intermittent as it can be set to cut in when

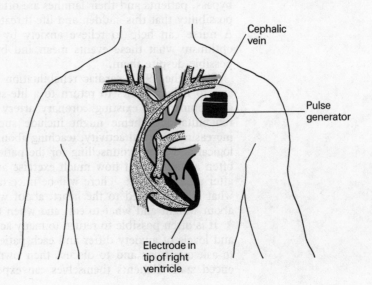

Cephalic vein

Pulse generator

Electrode in tip of right ventricle

Figure 7.22A
Implanted cardiac pacemaker

the patient's own conduction system alters and his ventricular rate drops. Fixed rate pacemakers deliver impulses at a pre-set rate; they are used in severe, chronic heart block but not in intermittent block when there might be a risk of the pacing impulse and the patient's own impulses competing.

Insertion of a pacemaker

This can be a stressful event, as the idea of a wire being inserted into the heart can seem strange and threatening. Careful explanation of what will happen can relieve some of the anxiety and calm support during the procedure can help the patient to relax.

Patients are usually conscious throughout the procedure, but intravenous diazepam is given just before the insertion of the pacemaker. Local anaesthetic is used at the insertion sites and strict asepsis is vital because of the risk of introducing infection. Continuous cardiac monitoring is carried out, since the insertion of the wire can irritate the myocardium and trigger arrhythmias. Monitoring is also necessary after pacemaker insertion to assess the pacing stimuli.

In temporary pacing, a firm dressing is applied where the wire emerges from the vein. In permanent pacing, a pocket for the pulse generator is made in the subcutaneous tissues. The insertion sites should be inspected daily for signs of infection and the temperature observed. Pyrexia should be reported at once. Bed rest is necessary for up to 2 days to prevent displacement of the pacing wire.

Aftercare

In permanent pacing, the pulse generator can last for as long as 6 to 10 years but eventually batteries need to be replaced. Regular out-patient checks are carried out at first and the patient is taught to check the rate and rhythm of his own pulse daily for one minute. Bradycardia would suggest a failing battery.

If necessary, the rate and duration of the pacing pulse in most modern pacemakers can be altered externally, by using a small programmer held over the patient's skin above the implanted pacemaker box.

A phone check system has also been devised in which a telephone signal from a patient transmitter can be converted, at a clinic, to a digital readout of pacemaker function including an ECG record. This is particularly valuable for elderly, disabled pacemaker wearers or for those who would otherwise need to travel long distances to clinics.

Booklets are available giving advice to patients about various aspects of life with an implanted pacemaker. For example, certain electrical equipment such as microwave ovens and some library security systems can affect their function and warning signs are displayed where these are in use.

In addition to their use in heart block, pacemakers may also be necessary after heart surgery, after cardiac arrest or in other diseases of the heart which affect the conducting system.

ABNORMALITIES OF BLOOD PRESSURE

Blood pressure varies widely from person to person and, within one individual, it varies throughout the day; therefore, it is difficult to define normality.

The cardiac output and the peripheral vascular resistance are the two main factors which determine arterial blood pressure. Peripheral resistance is determined by arteriolar tone. If the arterioles are narrowed by vasoconstriction the pressure in the arterioles rises and hypertension results.

Hypertension

Blood pressure is considered abnormally high if it consistently exceeds 150/90 mmHg in a person who is resting quietly.

When high blood pressure is secondary to a recognizable disease it is called **secondary hypertension**. In the younger patient, hypertension is more often 'secondary' and successful treatment is more likely through correction of the cause.

Figure 7.22B
Cardiac pacemaker — pulse generator (actual size)

The most important conditions to which hypertension can be secondary are:

1. Renal diseases, such as glomerulonephritis and chronic pyelonephritis.
2. Endocrine diseases, for example tumour of the adrenal gland.
3. Coarctation (narrowing) of the aorta.
4. Toxaemia of pregnancy.
5. Some drugs such as oral contraceptives.
6. Some cerebral lesions such as brain tumours.

In some forms of kidney disease the enzyme renin is liberated into the blood-stream from the damaged kidney. Renin activates angiotensin, a polypeptide which causes vasoconstriction, thus raising the arterial pressure and causing hypertension. Angiotensin also activates the aldosterone mechanism; increased aldosterone excretion produces sodium and water retention and increased blood pressure.

In most middle-aged persons no definite cause can be found; this type is called **essential hypertension**. It is the commonest form, affecting men and women equally, usually between the ages of 40 and 60 years.

Essential hypertension can be further divided into two groups, benign and malignant. Benign hypertension is mild and may even be symptomless. Malignant hypertension, on the other hand, is a severe form of the disease characterized by papilloedema (p. 273), a very high diastolic pressure and renal failure. Usually the onset is rapid and the course brief, although it is possible for a person known to have benign essential hypertension to move into the malignant phase after a number of years. Younger people are more often affected, typically between the ages of 30 to 40 years. The prognosis is poor and few patients survive more than a year without treatment.

Associated factors

In normal individuals, a transient increase in blood pressure occurs with anxiety, cold and exercise. Pressure also rises with age. Obesity and emotional stress are contributory factors and there is definite evidence of an hereditary factor and strong familial tendency to hypertension.

Clinical features

These are extremely variable and there may be no symptoms for many years. The disease affects coronary, renal and cerebral vessels and the myocardium; it should also be remembered that hypertension accelerates the development of atherosclerosis in coronary, renal and cerebral vessels (p. 286).

Level of blood pressure

Severity of hypertension is not judged by level of blood pressure alone. The course of the disease may vary in patients with similar heights of blood pressure. At first the blood pressure is 'labile', that is, it becomes abnormally high in response to emotion, anxiety or exercise. Eventually hypertension is found at rest, and in the later stages the clinical features indicate cardiac, renal and cerebral involvement.

Cerebral features

Dizziness, vertigo and memory impairment with cerebral deterioration may occur. Raised pressure and atherosclerotic changes in cerebral arteries may lead to cerebral haemorrhage or thrombosis (p. 111).

Hypertensive encephalopathy is a rare but severe condition characterized by paroxysms of very high blood pressure and associated with disturbance of vision or speech, vomiting, paralysis, fits or loss of consciousness. It may occur in malignant hypertension and is due to acute localized cerebral ischaemia.

Renal features

Raised pressure and atherosclerotic changes in renal arteries cause thickening and narrowing of the vessels. Diminished renal blood flow causes impaired renal function and proteinuria appears. Eventually renal failure develops and in malignant hypertension death often occurs from uraemia (p. 337).

Cardiac features

High arterial pressure increases the work load of the myocardium, particularly that of the left ventricle. As a result, the left ventricle hypertrophies and eventually left heart failure develops (p. 275). Dyspnoea is the first symptom of left heart failure. As the disease progresses, the features of right heart failure appear.

Hypertrophied myocardium demands increased coronary blood supply. If atherosclerotic coronary artery disease, which tends to be aggravated or accelerated by hypertension, is present, then angina and myocardial infarction may occur (p. 267).

Eye features

Changes in the eyes, particularly the retinae, are assessed using an ophthalmoscope. Such changes are significant and directly proportional to the severity of the disease. In severe hypertension — especially malignant hypertension — papilloedema, that is, oedema of the optic disc, occurs.

Investigations

The priorities are to establish the cause and to assess the effect of raised blood pressure on the heart and the kidneys. The following are necessary:

Detailed history and physical examination.
Urinalysis for blood and protein.
Serum urea levels.
Creatinine clearance test and possibly intravenous pyelogram (IVP) to assess renal function.
A series of midstream specimens of urine to exclude urinary tract infection.
Chest X-ray to show heart enlargement.
ECG.
Echocardiography to assess the severity of left ventricular hypertrophy.
Assessment of blood pressure must be accurate. The patient should be relaxed, with his arm bare to allow smooth application of the cuff and to prevent constriction from the sleeve. The nurse should know whether the doctor wishes diastolic pressure to be recorded as the muffling or as the disappearance of sounds. Recordings may be as frequent as quarter hourly if pressure is very high and if treatment is being given to lower the pressure. Casual recordings may be preferred to regular 4-hourly recordings, but once daily is the minimum. Results should be charted neatly and any marked rise or fall in blood pressure should be reported at once and reassessed.

Course and complications

Hypertension can often be present for many years, remaining undetected until a routine health check perhaps for life insurance purposes. Many people with high blood pressure live to old age in good health and with few symptoms. In general, however, the higher the blood pressure, the greater the risk of cardiac, renal or cerebral complications, in particular, heart attack and stroke.

Treatment and nursing care

Mild hypertension may not require any treatment, and often to avoid unnecessary anxiety patients are not told that the blood pressure is raised or, if told, they are carefully reassured. There is increasing interest among doctors in the possibility of assessing hypertension outside a hospital ward or clinic. If the stress of hospital visits can be avoided then patient anxiety may be reduced and more reliable recordings of blood pressure obtained, for example by the general practitioner. Many other investigations can also be made by the general practitioner or at an out-patient clinic.

Rest and relaxation are advised in cases of severe hypertension. If serious complications develop, such as cardiac failure, then rest in bed is essential.

Diet. Restriction of animal fat may be advised, and if the patient is obese a low calorie diet is required. The hospital dietitian will discuss diet content with the patient and his family if a restricted diet has to be continued at home.

Smoking should be stopped.

Drug therapy

Hypotensive drugs act by reducing cardiac output or by reducing peripheral vascular resistance. Beta receptor blockage, using propranolol, decreases heart rate and cardiac output. Sympathetic blocking drugs such as debrisoquine and methyldopa reduce vasoconstriction. Treatment is started by giving a small dose. Dosage is gradually increased until the blood pressure is controlled or side-effects appear, for instance **postural hypotension** due to pooling of blood in the lower body. This is assessed by taking lying and standing blood pressures; a marked fall in pressure on standing, or any complaint of dizziness on rising from bed should be reported.

Oral diuretics which reduce blood volume and are mildly antihypertensive are often given with hypotensive agents.

Other drugs frequently used are tranquillisers and sedatives to ease anxiety, tension and insomnia; analgesics and antiemetics are given for symptomatic relief of headache or nausea.

Hypertensive patients may look well but are often at considerable risk and may be anxious, particularly if they have heard of the association of high blood pressure with stroke. The nurse's contribution toward their care is considerable. Careful recording of blood pressure, teaching the patient about the disease and the importance of drug therapy, reacting with understanding, and relieving anxiety through reassurance are all essential responsibilities which nurses share with other members of the health team.

Hypotension

Hypotension or low blood pressure may cause **syncope** or **fainting** — a transient loss of consciousness due to decreased cerebral blood flow.

Fainting may occur due to postural hypotension when there is some loss of vasomotor tone, for example during antihypertensive drug therapy or after a long illness requiring prolonged bed rest. When the patient stands up suddenly, poor vasomotor tone results in a rapid fall in blood pressure due to widening of the arterioles by peripheral vasodilatation.

A faint or vasovagal attack may also be psychogenic, that is associated with emotional upset such as fear and sudden anxiety, or it may be caused by a stuffy atmosphere or pain.

Treatment

The recumbent position, keeping the head low, improves the venous return to the heart and consequently the cerebral blood flow. Fresh air and a cold drink will help the patient to recover quickly.

To distinguish between a syncopal attack and cardiac arrest, check the pulse of the patient. The syncopal patient has a palpable pulse, but following cardiac arrest the patient is pulseless.

CARDIAC FAILURE

Cardiac failure or 'pump failure' is present when the ventricles become unable to empty completely and when the cardiac output is insufficient for the needs of the tissues. Left and right heart failure can best be understood by considering the heart as two pumping systems; the left heart being the pump for the systemic circulation and the right heart being the pump for the pulmonary circulation. Normally, during diastole, the ventricles fill with blood from veins (venae cavae and pulmonary) and during systole the ventricles expel blood to arteries (pulmonary and aorta). If the ventricles do not empty completely and blood remains at each contraction, there will

If L. ventricle fails, ventricle empties poorly, and output falls

↓

Pressure rises in L. atrium

↓

Pressure rises in pulmonary veins and capillaries

↓

Features of left heart failure

↓

Eventually pressure rises in pulmonary artery

↓

R. ventricle empties poorly

↓

R. atrial pressure rises and output falls

↓

Systemic venous pressure rises

↓

Features of right heart failure

Figure 7.23
Sequence of events in cardiac failure

be a gradual build up of back pressure via the atria to the venous systems, pulmonary and systemic (Fig. 7.23).

Causes of cardiac failure

The heart will fail if it has to cope with an increased workload or if there is damaged and poorly functioning heart muscle.

Disease of the myocardium makes the pump less effective, for example, in myocardial infarction where there is irreversible damage to some muscle tissue or in the myocarditis of rheumatic fever when there is poor contractility.

Thyrotoxicosis increases the metabolic rate thus increasing tissue demands for blood and oxygen, while in anaemia the blood carries less oxygen. In both instances an extra load is put on the heart to supply sufficient blood to the tissues. A stenosed valve causes increased resistance to the outflow of blood as does hypertension, where there is increased resistance from peripheral arterioles. An incompetent valve increases the volume of blood to be expelled from a chamber of the heart, as regurgitated blood is added to the normal volume in the chamber.

Several of these factors may be combined, one or both sides of the heart may be affected, and the degree of failure may be small or great. There are also other precipitating factors: pregnancy, which causes an increase in blood volume and cardiac output; excessive sodium intake, which causes water retention; infections and excessive exertion, which add to the myocardial workload.

Left heart failure

Its causes are associated with (1) **outflow obstruction** as in mitral stenosis and (2) **left ventricular failure** due to hypertension, aortic valve disease, mitral incompetence, ischaemic heart disease and myocardial infarction. The left ventricle is the most common site for heart attack.

Clinical features

These are due to rising pressure in the lungs and pulmonary venous congestion. When the left ventricle fails to empty completely, back pressure develops in the left atrium and the pulmonary veins. The increased venous pressure forces fluid from the lung capillary system into lung tissues causing pulmonary oedema. Symptoms are at first mild, for example, dyspnoea on exertion. In time dyspnoea at rest, orthopnoea and paroxysmal nocturnal dyspnoea occur (p. 245) and in advanced left heart failure acute pulmonary oedema may develop.

Acute pulmonary oedema

The onset may be sudden, requiring immediate medical and nursing attention. Fluid accumulating in the alveoli of the lungs causes intense dyspnoea, which is extremely frightening for the patient. Breathing is noisy, cyanosis develops rapidly, the skin is moist and cold and a cough develops with copious, frothy, blood-tinged sputum. Secretions can often be heard rattling in the larynx and trachea, and on auscultation, crepitations are heard throughout the chest. The patient may also be agitated and confused due to cerebral hypoxia.

Treatment of acute attack

Relief is dramatic with the following treatment:

1. Morphine intravenously, to calm the patient and relieve anxiety; the nurse must not leave the patient until the acute dyspnoea and fear begin to ease.
2. A rapid-acting diuretic intravenously, such as frusemide, to get rid of excess fluid and relieve breathing.
3. Aminophylline given very slowly intravenously, to ease bronchospasm.
4. Upright position in bed to increase the vital capacity of the lungs.
5. High concentration of oxygen to relieve cyanosis.

If these measures are successful, the patient's fear and breathlessness should subside quickly. Frequent recordings of respiratory rate, rhythm and depth and of blood pressure will be required at first. Arterial blood gases will be checked and the extent of lung congestion assessed by chest X-ray.

As acute pulmonary oedema is such an anxiety-provoking event, prompt action, a calm and reassuring approach during the attack and careful explanation afterwards about the cause of the problem and the treatment will all be important.

Right heart failure

This may be due to disease of the right side of the heart itself, but it is usually secondary to left heart failure. Eventually, back pressure is transmitted from the lungs to the pulmonary artery, right ventricle, right atrium and venae cavae. When venous blood returning to the venae cavae meets resistance, back pressure spreads throughout the peripheral venous system causing widespread congestion. Right heart failure is often referred to as 'congestive' heart failure.

The causes are therefore (1) those of left heart failure, (2) pulmonary disease such as chronic bronchitis and emphysema, (3) pulmonary and tricuspid valve disease, (4) septal defects and (5) myocardial infarction affecting the right ventricle.

Clinical features

These are due to rising pressure in the systemic veins and retention of sodium and water in the body. Oedema is the principal sign, varying in degree from mild ankle oedema to generalised oedema, including ascites and pleural effusion (pp. 246–247).

Hepatic vein engorgement and liver congestion develop causing enlargement of the liver with mild jaundice.

Loss of appetite, nausea and vomiting appear, due to portal vein engorgement and congestion of the stomach and bowel.

Engorgement of the jugular veins (Fig. 7.24) can be seen by examining the sides of the neck when the patient is reclining. The height of the pulsation wave in the jugular veins is related to the degree of failure; when severe the pulsation may be seen at the level of the ear lobes.

Mental confusion occurs when the cardiac output is insufficient for cerebral tissue needs.

Kidney congestion causes a reduction in secretion of urine (oliguria).

When the right heart failure is secondary to left heart failure, dyspnoea is also present.

The course of the disease is variable; it is long if associated with chronic rheumatic heart disease, and short if associated with acute myocardial infarction.

Investigations

Clinical examination and history will reveal the underlying cause.

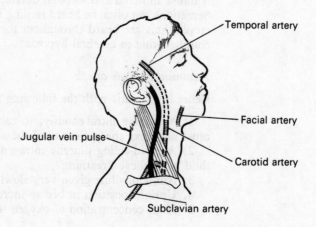

Figure 7.24
Jugular vein
Venous pulsation is seen but not
felt; arterial pulsations are
readily felt

Temporal artery

Facial artery

Jugular vein pulse

Carotid artery

Subclavian artery

Nursing observations

The observations required will depend upon the precipitating cardiac disease, but those of temperature, pulse, respiratory rate and blood pressure will always be necessary.

Changes in pulse rate, rhythm and volume should be reported promptly, as abnormalities of heart rate and rhythm are common and can aggravate existing levels of heart failure. The respiratory rate should also be observed regularly, noting particularly any increase in breathlessness; a change in position, restlessness, cough, a disturbed sleep pattern or an anxious, tense facial expression might all indicate breathing difficulty.

Accurate assessment of fluid balance is necessary because of the risk of impaired renal function due to lowered cardiac output. Whenever possible, the patient is weighed daily to assess the development of fluid retention, or response to diuretic therapy. Nurses must look regularly for and assess changes in the amount of oedema present remembering to observe all possible sites.

Treatment and nursing care

The first principle of treatment is to correct medically or surgically the underlying cause. Weakness, tiredness, breathing difficulties and fluid retention are major problems in congestive cardiac failure and the following aspects of care are important.

Rest

Complete rest is essential at first to reduce the demands on the heart. The amount of restriction will depend on the severity of the failure. When the symptoms such as dyspnoea are relieved, and when the signs, say, of oedema diminish, the patient is allowed to increase activity very gradually.

While the patient is weak and tired, help with personal hygiene will be needed. Strain should be avoided by ensuring that anything required is within reach and a call-bell should be at hand.

The upright position, well supported by pillows and a bed table to lean on will improve chest expansion and the ability to breathe (Fig. 7.25). The pressure areas and oedematous tissue will be at risk and pressure should be relieved and the vulnerable areas inspected regularly. A rubber ring may be comfortable to sit on and this may help to maintain position by preventing the patient from slipping down in bed, which could worsen dyspnoea. A bed cradle can be used to take the weight of bed clothes off the legs.

Sitting in an arm chair is sometimes more comfortable than lying in bed, and being out of bed even for a short time may improve morale.

Whenever possible, a bedside commode or sanichair should be used in preference to a bedpan.

Figure 7.25
Upright position in bed

Oxygen

While the patient is acutely breathless, oxygen is given. Mouth washes should be offered regularly and oral hygiene checked. If the patient is restless and uncomfortable, he may need help and encouragement to keep the oxygen mask or cannulae in place. If he is confused, his safety should be observed; for instance, he may be at risk if he tries to get out of bed or if he wants to light a cigarette while oxygen is being used.

Physiotherapy

Physiotherapy to improve leg circulation and lung expansion will be given, and nursing staff can help by encouraging leg exercises and deep breathing. Impaired venous return greatly increases the risk of venous thrombosis, and lung hypostasis increases the risk of pneumonia; prolonged bed rest is therefore usually avoided.

Diet

The diet must be light, easily eaten and easily digested; a tired, dyspnoeic patient may have neither energy nor inclination to cut up or chew food or peel an orange. The appetite may be poor and nausea and vomiting are features of stomach congestion. For all these reasons, the nurse should check that the quantity of food is not too great, the food is appetizingly presented and the tray and utensils are easily reached.

Kilojoule restriction will be necessary if the patient is obese, as obesity increases the work load of the heart.

Salt restriction is effective in controlling the retention of fluid, but with the development of oral diuretics, severe restriction is now rarely necessary. Generally the patient is first advised not to add salt at table. This will reduce the daily intake of salt from 10 g to 5 g. Salt may also be withheld from the cooking, reducing intake to 3 g. When cooking for a family, this need not pose difficulties if the other members are prepared to add extra salt to their own food, but some patients prefer to prepare their own food separately. Salty foods such as bacon, meat extracts, sauces, salty fish, tinned food except fruit and baking powder should be avoided. Sodium-free salt can be bought. A 'salt-free diet' is very unpalatable and seldom recommended. It involves obtaining salt-free bread and butter and taking little milk, in addition to the other restrictions.

Fresh fruit juices which are high in potassium are useful dietary supplements; low serum potassium levels can be a problem if large doses of diuretics are being given.

Drugs

Digitalis is most often used in the form of digoxin. Digoxin slows the heart by depression of the conducting pathways and by vagal stimulation. It improves the efficiency of the action of the myocardium by strengthening contraction, thus improving the cardiac output. Improved cardiac output will lead to improved renal blood flow and an increase in glomerular filtration; consequently digoxin has a diuretic action and will help to relieve oedema. Anorexia, nausea and vomiting are the most common side-effects. The pulse rate may become very slow, and the development of coupled beats (pulsus bigeminus) will indicate digoxin toxicity.

Diuretics. A diuretic is a substance which increases the excretion of sodium and water by the kidneys. The most commonly used diuretics are the thiazides such as bendrofluazide and chlorothiazide, and the loop diuretics such as frusemide, bumetanide and ethacrynic acid, all of which inhibit the reabsorption of sodium and water by the kidney, thus promoting a diuresis. Many diuretics act quickly, and nurses should know their speed of action in order to warn the patient what to expect after taking the drug. Frequent requests for bedpans may be embarrassing for the patient and inconvenient during tests or examinations or during visiting times. When at home, patients will decide the most suitable time to take a diuretic according to the daily pattern of activity. A long-acting diuretic may be more suitable for an elderly person.

Potassium. Potassium chloride supplements are given with most diuretics, since potassium is lost in large quantities in the urine. This is important when digitalis is being given, because potassium depletion causes increased sensitivity to digitalis and dangerous arrhythmias may develop. A potassium conserving diuretic such as spironolactone may be used together with or in preference to a thiazide or loop diuretic if there is a risk of potassium depletion.

Mechanical measures

Intractable oedema may be removed by mechanical means: pleural aspiration to drain a hydrothorax; abdominal paracentesis to drain ascites.

Pulmonary heart disease (cor pulmonale)

This is the name given to right heart failure secondary to disease of the lungs. Chronic bronchitis, emphysema or pneumoconiosis will increase the work load of the right heart, and cause chronic cor pulmonale. The incidence of this form of heart disease is greater in industrial areas. Acute cor pulmonale will follow massive pulmonary embolism (p. 291), since a major blockage of the pulmonary artery or one of its branches will put great strain on the right ventricle, causing right heart failure.

Cardiac arrest

Cardiac arrest is sudden failure of the heart to supply adequate circulation. The brain is the organ of the body most sensitive to lack of blood and oxygen, and effective circulation must be restored within 3 minutes to prevent irreversible brain damage. The commonest causes of cardiac arrest are myocardial infarction, anaesthesia, electrolyte imbalance, drowning and electrocution.

The nurse must know:

1. How to diagnose cardiac arrest quickly.
2. How to summon the emergency team promptly.
3. How to initiate resuscitation effectively.
4. Where to find the necessary equipment.

Cardiac arrest is diagnosed and treatment initiated on finding a patient **unconscious and pulseless** (absence of carotid or femoral pulse). Other signs include pallor, cyanosis, gasping, apnoea and, after a short interval, dilated pupils. Remember that the patient who has fainted has a palpable pulse.

The main objective of treatment is to restore an oxygenated blood supply to the brain by means of **cardiopulmonary resuscitation**.

Restarting the heart

The heart will sometimes be restarted by a sharp blow with a clenched fist (as one would thump a table) over the lower third of the sternum. External cardiac massage restores heart action and cardiac output by compression of the heart between the sternum and the spine. The compression, which empties the blood from the ventricles, is effective only when the patient is on a firm surface. For this reason, the patient should be lying flat and a cardiac arrest board should be placed under his chest. The heel of one hand is placed on the lower third of the sternum and the heel of the other hand is placed over the first (Fig. 7.26). The sternum is depressed forcefully and rhythmically by about 3 to 5 cm 60 times per minute in an adult. Rhythmic compression with the appropriate force will be easier to sustain if the arms are kept straight. It is important not to compress too quickly otherwise the ventricles will not have enough time to refill with blood. Some find it helpful to establish the rhythm by saying, 'one, one thousand: two, one thousand: three, one thousand'. The hands must be carefully positioned and should not lose contact with the point of compression in order to maintain the correct position. If too low, pressure on the xiphoid process may cause internal injury. The fingers should be raised: pressure by the fingers or the hand on the ribs may cause rib fractures.

In infants the procedure is different. The hands encircle the chest. Much less

Figure 7.26
External cardiac massage —
position of hands

pressure is applied by the thumbs, at mid-sternal level, at a rapid rate of 100 times per minute.

If external cardiac massage is effective, a carotid or femoral pulse will be felt.

Ventilating the lungs

To oxygenate the blood supply restored by external cardiac massage, lung ventilation must be started. First, the airway must be cleared. False teeth are removed and put in a safe place. Attention to this important detail only takes seconds and is vital, since dentures are easily lost or damaged during an emergency procedure. The neck is extended and the jaw pulled forward to stop the tongue falling back. A plastic oral airway is inserted. Direct mouth to mouth breathing at a rate of 12 respirations per minute will provide adequate ventilation (Fig. 7.27 A and B). The ratio should be one inflation of the lungs to 5 cardiac compressions.

The nurse should become familiar with aids to ventilation and their use (Fig. 7.28) — the Guedel airway, the Brook's airway, and the Ambu bag and endotracheal tubes which can be connected directly to oxygen supply.

To be of maximum help to the emergency team, the nurse should also try to become familiar with the location and use of equipment and drugs on the emergency trolley, such as the defibrillator and suction apparatus. ECG electrodes will be re-

Figure 7.27A–C
Cardiopulmonary resuscitation

A Head hyperextended
and chin raised to
clear airway

B Nose held. Mouth
to mouth breathing

C External cardiac massage
at lower end of sternum

Figure 7.28A
Guedel airway

Figure 7.28B
Brook's airway

Figure 7.28C
Ambubag

Figure 7.28D
Ventilation endotracheal tube

quired and applied at once to record heart rate and rhythm, and sodium bicarbonate will be used to correct the quickly developing, severe acidosis.

Cardiac arrest is due to **ventricular asystole** (a — without, systole — contraction of the heart), or **ventricular fibrillation**. In ventricular asystole or 'standstill', the ventricles cease to contract. Atrial activity may continue, therefore P waves can remain on the electrocardiograph (Fig. 7.29); but because there is no conduction from the atria to the ventricles, the ventricles stop functioning. The sudden appearance of a completely straight line on a monitor may be alarming, but it could indicate simply that an electrode had become disconnected. Always check the patient first before calling the emergency team. In ventricular fibrillation, the ventricles 'twitch' or contract in an unco-ordinated way due to chaotic electrical disturbance, and the electrocardiogram shows an irregular, bizarre pattern (Fig. 7.30). Cardiac output stops because the ventricles cannot fill or empty properly.

Ventricular
asystole

Figure 7.29
Ventricular asytole

Ventricular
fibrillation

Figure 7.30
Ventricular fibrillation

Ventricular fibrillation can be corrected by **electrical defibrillation**. The defibrillator machine delivers an electric shock to the heart muscle in order to stop the chaotic electrical activity, and to allow normal electrical conduction and normal heart rhythm to resume. The defibrillator paddles are first covered with electrode jelly, or gel pads are placed on the skin below the paddles to prevent skin burns. The paddles are placed at the upper chest and the left axilla so that the electric current will pass across the chest through the cardiac muscle (Fig. 7.31). To avoid getting an electric shock, everyone should stand well clear of the patient and the bed when the defibrillator is operated.

Figure 7.31
Defibrillation: position of paddles

Aorta

Large arteries

Small arteries

Arterioles

Capillaries

Venules

Small veins

Large veins

Vena cava

Figure 7.32
Components of the vascular bed

ANATOMY AND PHYSIOLOGY OF THE BLOOD VESSELS

The **systemic** or **peripheral circulation** includes the whole vascular bed (Fig. 7.32) excluding the heart and pulmonary circulation. Arteries and veins have the same structure:

Outer layer of fibrous tissue — **tunica adventitia**.
Middle layer of muscle and elastic tissue — **tunica media**.
Inner layer of endothelium — **tunica intima**.

Arteries differ from veins by having a smaller lumen, more muscle and elastic fibres in the middle layer, and thicker walls. Most veins have valves, which consist of a fold of endothelium with the concave surface towards the heart, permitting flow only towards the heart (Fig. 7.33).

Arteries distribute the cardiac output, transporting oxygen and nutrient materials to the body tissues and cells according to their needs. Arteries also help maintain an adequate blood pressure by offering resistance to blood flow. The small vessels, arterioles, act as the main regulators of blood flow. By contraction and relaxation of their smooth muscle walls, the diameter of arterioles can change markedly, causing change in the resistance to blood flow through the vessels, that is change in **peripheral resistance**.

The vasomotor centre in the medulla is responsible for maintaining the arteriolar muscle in a partial state of contraction by continuous sympathetic action. Increased vasomotor centre activity causes **vasoconstriction** and increased peripheral resistance; decreased activity allows parasympathetic stimulation causing **vasodilatation** and decreased peripheral resistance.

The capillaries play an important part in cell respiration and nutrition by bringing blood into close relationship with all body cells. A capillary wall, composed of a single thin layer of cells, forms a semipermeable membrane. This allows the passage of water, oxygen and low molecular weight substances from the blood in the capillaries to the interstitial fluid, then to the cells, by the process of **diffusion**. At the arterial end of the capillary, oxygen diffuses through the capillary wall to the tissue fluid and cells; at the venous end, carbon dioxide diffuses from the cells to the tissue fluid and blood. By this same process of diffusion nutrient materials in solution in the blood pass through the semipermeable membrane to the cells.

Veins return deoxygenated blood from the body tissues to the heart. They act as a store of blood and return it at the rate required to maintain cardiac output. The action of the valves in the veins of the legs is of particular importance during exercise. When the veins are compressed by the contracted leg muscles the valves ensure that blood flows in the direction of the heart. This 'muscle pump' action is shown in Figure 7.34.

Valves which do not function properly subject the veins in the legs to high pressures, causing them to become tortuous and dilated (see varicose veins, p. 290).

Figure 7.33
Valves in vein

TO HEART

MUSCULAR CONTRACTION

FROM PERIPHERY

Figure 7.34
Action of the 'muscle pump'

AETIOLOGY

A blood vessel may be diseased in several ways, and causes of disease may occur singly or in association.

Arteries are affected by degenerative disease such as arteriosclerosis and atherosclerosis, and by thrombosis and embolism. Thrombosis is seen less often in arteries than veins, as arterial circulation is more rapid. Coronary artery thrombosis (p. 264) and cerebral artery thrombosis (p. 111) are considered elsewhere. Thrombosis and its association with degenerative disease in peripheral limb arteries will be considered here in more detail, as will the effect of embolism in limb arteries.

Arterial embolism is a complication of three cardiac diseases already discussed: mitral stenosis associated with atrial fibrillation, subacute bacterial endocarditis, and myocardial infarction.

Veins are affected by inflammation (phlebitis), by thrombosis (phlebothrombosis) or by combined inflammation and thrombosis (thrombophlebitis).

Varicosities are common. The term **varicose veins** describes the abnormal dilatation of leg veins caused by defective valve structure. Varicosities are also found as haemorrhoids (p. 200) and in the oesophagus as oesophageal varices due to obstructed portal venous return.

GENERAL FEATURES OF DISORDER

It is important to be able to differentiate between the effects of impaired arterial supply to, and impaired venous drainage from, a limb.

Arteries

Impaired arterial supply causes pain and cold extremities.

Intermittent claudication

This is the term for pain felt in a limb on exercise and relieved by rest. Usually the cramping pain is felt in the calf muscles or the foot when walking. As the arterial obstruction increases, the distance walked before claudication occurs shortens and the resting time required before the pain disappears lengthens. Eventually the degree of ischaemia is such that pain occurs at rest. These features can be compared with those of angina (p. 246). A similar pain can be reproduced if one raises an arm and rapidly clenches and unclenches the fist. Pain develops as the arterial supply fails to meet the exercised muscles' demands for oxygen and as waste products of muscle metabolism accumulate in the tissues.

Impaired arterial supply is associated with arteriosclerosis and atherosclerosis. In the early stages, symptoms may not appear if there is adequate **collateral circulation**, that is vessels arising behind and ahead of the affected vessel providing the necessary blood.

Distinction should be made between the features arising from impaired arterial supply and complete occlusion of an artery. When a limb artery is suddenly occluded by thrombosis or embolism there is not only pain and coldness but also pallor, numbness, absence of pulses distal to the block, and eventually tissue necrosis and gangrene. Alternative blood supply via collateral circulation may delay tissue death, but ultimately gangrene occurs.

Veins

Impaired venous flow is associated with inflammation and the formation of thrombus. These two processes cause local pain, tenderness, redness of the overlying skin if a superficial vessel is affected, dilated veins, increased warmth in the affected limb and oedema. When a vein is obstructed pressure in the vein distal to the obstruction is raised. This raises the blood pressure in the venous end of the capillaries causing oedema (p. 245). An adequate collateral circulation may prevent undue back pressure and oedema, but when a major vessel is blocked considerable swelling occurs.

Figure 7.35
Arterial pulses in the lower limb

A Femoral pulse
B Popliteal pulse
C Posterior tibial pulse
D Dorsalis pedis pulse

INVESTIGATIONS

Pulse

Limb pulses are observed to assess the adequacy of blood supply when arterial vessel disease is present (Fig. 7.35 A–D).

Limb temperature

Feeling and comparing the warmth of limbs is a useful measure of the adequacy of circulation.

Arteriography

Femoral arteriography is performed under local anaesthesia to investigate lower limb arteries. Children or very anxious adults may require general anaesthesia. Following the injection of a radio-opaque contrast medium, a series of films is taken in quick succession down the length of the limb, demonstrating filling of the leg vessels and narrowing or obstruction of vessels.

Preparation

The procedure may be long and the injection of dye causes a feeling of heat. Information about the length of the examination should be given together with warning about discomfort, since sudden pain or discomfort will alarm the patient and make him think that something has gone wrong.

The groins are shaved and the bladder emptied before examination. A mild sedative may be given.

Aftercare

A pad of gauze is firmly strapped over the puncture site to prevent arterial haemorrhage. Movement from trolley to bed may dislodge the pressure pad and a haematoma may form rapidly. The following care is advisable: bed rest for 24 hours; quarter-hourly recording for 4 hours of pulse, blood pressure and of foot pulse for development of arterial occlusion; inspection of wound site for haemorrhage; then 4-hourly recordings including temperature and respiratory rate. After-effects should involve no more than local groin stiffness or bruising.

Venography

Peripheral venography or phlebography is the radiographic examination of the venous system of the limb following injection of a radio-opaque contrast medium. The procedure is carried out under local anaesthesia, usually on a lower limb. It demonstrates the patency of deep veins, areas of non-filling or irregular filling indicating past or present thrombosis and the competence of valves. It is also used to investigate cases of acute or recurrent pulmonary embolism where venous thrombosis is likely and venous ligation necessary.

Preparation

The examination may be carried out on an out-patient basis. Preparation is as for arteriography with the exception of the groin shave. In this case, the contrast medium is injected either directly into a vein on the dorsum of the foot or via a small cannula after venous cut-down under local anaesthetic. The flow of the contrast is watched and a series of films taken as it enters and fills the venous system.

Aftercare

The patient may walk about at once or as soon as the effects of sedation have worn off. Cut-down sutures are removed after 5 days.

Ultrasonography

Ultrasonography is a diagnostic procedure employing high frequency sound waves. The ultrasound waves pass as a beam through body tissues and are partially reflected at junctions between various structures in the path of the beam. The Döppler effect, which depends on the echo from a moving surface, is used to demonstrate the presence or absence of pulsation in peripheral vessels. The sound reflected from a moving column of blood alters in frequency and the audible signal is monitored.

Apart from explanation of the procedure to the patient, no special preparation or after care is necessary.

DISORDERS OF THE ARTERIES

Arteriosclerosis

This disease, which may affect any artery, causes shrinking of the intima, loss of elasticity and atrophy of the muscle fibres of the media, as a result of which the lumen of the vessel gradually narrows. This is often called 'hardening' of the arteries.

Many middle-aged and elderly people are unaware of the presence of arteriosclerosis until vessel narrowing causes symptoms due to ischaemia (impaired blood supply to the tissues supplied by those vessels).

Atherosclerosis

Atherosclerosis affects mainly the aorta, large arteries, coronary and cerebral arteries. Although it becomes more common with age, it can develop at any age and may be present in seemingly healthy people.

Normal artery

Plaque of atheroma in subintimal layer

Occluded artery

Figure 7.36
Arterial atherosclerosis

Figure 7.37
Some effects of impaired blood supply

As noted earlier atherosclerosis results from the deposition of fatty plaques in the intima causing reduced blood flow to tissues or a blockage to blood flow following associated formation of thrombus (Fig. 7.36). In coronary arteries this process causes angina and myocardial infarction (p. 267). Atherosclerosis in leg vessels causes intermittent claudication; in cerebral vessels mental changes may result from an impaired blood supply. When thrombosis follows in leg or cerebral vessels, gangrene of the limb or stroke may occur (Fig. 7.37).

Arterial degenerative disease may result in intracerebral haemorrhage when it occurs in hypertensive patients due to the high pressure of blood in diseased, weakened vessels.

The management of these two degenerative diseases is considered below, under peripheral vascular disease.

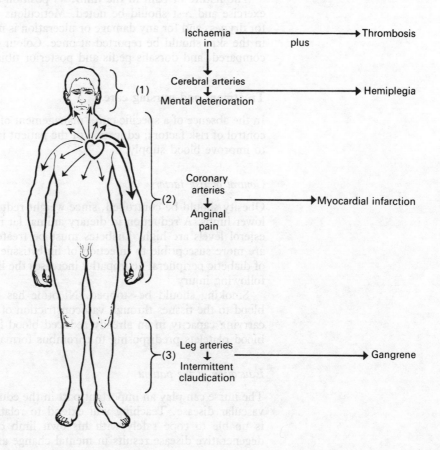

Peripheral vascular disease

This term describes the condition in which there is impaired blood supply to the limbs resulting in lack of oxygen and nutrients for the tissues. The main cause is degenerative disease, principally atherosclerosis. The disease is more common after the age of 50, and as the proportion of elderly people in the population increases, the incidence of these degenerative diseases rises. It affects men more often than women. It rarely affects upper limbs, and is associated with diabetes.

Clinical features

Early symptoms are cold extremities and the characteristic pain, known as intermittent claudication, which appears on exercise and is relieved by rest. The course of the disease is usually progressive with the development in time of severe ischaemia and pain at rest. Eventually ulceration and gangrene may occur.

Investigations

Full clinical examination and medical history are taken, noting particularly the presence of risk factors of atherosclerosis. It is important to note whether limb pulses are absent or present. Arteriography will show the extent and severity of vessel occlusion and impaired blood supply, and it is necessary for determining whether reconstructive surgery is possible.

Nursing observations

Unless the nurse examines the state of the limbs and compares them in detail initially subsequent changes may not be noticed or accurately assessed.

The nature of pain in the limb, its position and intensity and its relationship to exercise and rest should be noted. Meticulous observation of the state of the skin for dryness and for any damage or ulceration is necessary. The first sign of any break in the skin should be reported at once. Colour and warmth of the limbs should be compared, and dorsalis pedis and posterior tibial pulses checked.

Treatment and nursing care

In the absence of a specific cure, management of peripheral vascular disease includes control of risk factors, education of the patient in the care of the limbs and measures to improve blood supply.

Control of risk factors

Obesity should be controlled, since weight reduction can ease the work load on the lower limbs. A reduction in dietary animal fat intake may be advised if blood cholesterol levels are high. Diabetes must be treated and stabilized. Diabetic patients are more susceptible to infection of limb tissue and to gangrene, and the presence of diabetic peripheral neuropathy increases the likelihood of ulceration and gangrene following injury.

Smoking should be stopped. Nicotine has three harmful effects: reduction of blood to the tissues through vasoconstriction of blood vessels, reduction of oxygen-carrying capacity in an already reduced blood flow and an increase in stickiness of blood platelets predisposing to thrombus formation.

Education of the patient

The nurse can play an important part in the education of the patient with peripheral vascular disease. Teaching will extend to relatives and other carers if the patient is unable to cope safely with his own limb care, for instance when generalized degenerative disease results in mental change and impaired cerebral function.

Since minor injury may precipitate gangrene, great care should be taken of the skin of the limb. Poorly nourished tissue heals badly, therefore all trauma, even minor trauma such as cut skin when trimming toenails or corns should be avoided. Regular attention to feet by a chiropodist is essential. Pressure from badly fitting shoes or stockings, or prolonged pressure of heels on a mattress can also lead to skin damage. Shoes should be checked for protruding nails and seams, lumps or torn linings, and new shoes should be broken in gradually by alternating their use with an old pair. Stockings, preferably seamless, must fit correctly. Pressure areas should be carefully inspected and treated. Patients with peripheral vascular disease should also be advised never to walk barefoot, and to avoid crowded areas where foot injuries are likely, such as supermarkets or football matches. A doctor should be told of any injury or infection. Fungal infection of the feet must be treated and the skin kept clean and dry.

Limb temperature is important. Direct heat increases tissue demands for oxygen and nutrients. In ischaemic areas these needs may not be met adequately by impaired blood supply. Therefore patients should be taught how to avoid increasing local tissue metabolism in their limbs. The limbs should be kept warm, but extremes of heat and cold must be avoided, for example, from fires or radiators, hot water bottles, sun-bathing, or wading in cold water.

Analgesia and sedation may be required, especially when continuous rest pain occurs.

Measures to improve blood supply

Blood supply to the limb may be improved by **reflex dilatation**. An electric heat pad is placed on the body trunk. Warmed blood stimulates the vasomotor centre in the brain causing vasodilatation of the vessels in the affected limb.

A physiotherapist may teach the patient **Buerger-Allen exercises** (Fig. 7.38). Several times in succession, the legs are alternately raised 45 degrees above the level of the bed for 1 minute then lowered for one minute and the feet exercised.

If the claudication seems to be stable, and if the condition has not reached the chronic, severe stage, patients may be encouraged to take regular exercise as this can promote the development of collateral blood supply.

Several surgical measures are possible. In milder cases, lumbar **sympathectomy** is performed. Revascularization techniques are used for severe ischaemia with rest pain and early gangrene. There are two commonly used methods of direct reconstructive surgery: **endarterectomy**, in which the thickened, diseased, inner layer of the artery is cored out, and **bypass grafting**, in which synthetic material such as Dacron, or the patient's own long saphenous vein is used. Because of the presence of valves, the length of vein is reversed before insertion to prevent blood flow being impeded. Such techniques often prevent the need for amputation and allow many elderly people to retain their independence; but despite success in retaining limb function, it must be remembered that many such patients will also suffer from generalized degenerative disease.

Figure 7.38
Buerger-Allen exercises

Acute arterial occlusion

In addition to progressive atherosclerotic narrowing of vessels, thrombosis and embolism may occur in a limb artery causing complete occlusion of the vessel. Sudden occlusion will require prompt action and possible emergency surgery — embolectomy — to save a limb, especially if a major artery is affected.

A nurse must report immediately to the doctor the occurrence of the following limb features which indicate sudden arterial blockage: rapid onset of pain, coldness, numbness, pallor and absence of pulses distal to the block.

If this occurs, the limb should be rested and overheating avoided by keeping the limb at room temperature; a bed cradle should be used to permit air to circulate freely. This also allows the limb to be observed easily, but care should be taken to avoid overexposing the patient. Reflex dilatation is used, analgesia given and anticoagulation started. If surgery is required (embolectomy) it should be remembered that the combination of pain and haste in preparing for surgery will be alarming for the patient, and the reasons for carrying out emergency surgery must be calmly but carefully explained with reassurance to the patient and his family.

Rehabilitation

The community health team is vital for the continued and successful care at home of patients with peripheral vascular disease, many of whom are elderly and without family help. Careful assessment of the impact of the disease upon the person's ability to carry out his or her usual range of daily activities will be needed.

As the disease progresses and exercise tolerance lessens, some patients may have to change to lighter, more sedentary work. Social service workers will help the patient find new employment. For the housebound, the general practitioner, community nurse and chiropodist may all give support, and visits to a day centre can be valuable in providing the stimulation of change of environment, interest and friendship.

DISORDERS OF THE VEINS

Superficial phlebitis

Superficial phlebitis, or inflammation of superficial veins, is a common condition caused usually by injury to vessels following surgery, childbirth or intravenous infusion. As veins have thinner walls than arteries they are more subject to endothelial damage. The intima thickens and narrows, and thrombus may form causing superficial thrombophlebitis — a condition often seen after prolonged infusion of intravenous fluids. Phlebitis of leg veins is frequently associated with varicosities.

The affected area becomes swollen, red and tender. Such inflammation may be seen tracking along a length of affected vein from the site of intravenous infusion. Pain is relieved by giving analgesia, and the application of local heat in the form of a kaolin poultice may be soothing. Careful observation of infusion sites is important and early signs or symptoms must be reported promptly, especially when life is being maintained by intravenous infusion and when progressive occlusion of veins from frequent change of site has occurred.

Varicose veins

Varicosities are the commonest vein lesions. The presence of valves in veins and the action of the muscle pump are responsible for maintaining venous return from the legs. When the valves are defective or incompetent, the veins dilate causing back pressure and stasis of blood which further dilates the veins. Superficial phlebitis often occurs, and stasis of blood predisposes to thrombus formation and oedema. Varicose eczema is common and a break in the skin may lead to varicose ulceration (p. 520).

The long and short saphenous veins are most often affected, and early symptoms are pain and fatigue in the leg on standing. Nurses will often care for patients who have varicose veins in addition to other diseases, and varicosities must not be overlooked, particularly as there is always the additional risk of the development of deep venous thrombosis. The legs must be observed carefully and handled gently to avoid trauma or rupturing a vein. A bed cradle should be provided and any abrasion or skin break reported. When out of bed, prolonged standing should be avoided and support elastic bandages or stockings should be worn.

Surgical treatment includes injection, ligation or stripping of the vessels. In some centres, day surgery for varicose veins is available; the patient is discharged directly home on the day of operation, to the care of the community nursing sister and general practitioner.

Venous thrombosis

Thrombosis is the process of coagulation of circulating blood in the vessels.
Thrombus is the solid substance formed from blood constituents. A thrombus which becomes detached is termed an **embolus**. Atheromatous plaque, micro-organisms, fat cells or air may also be carried in the bloodstream as emboli and may become lodged in a blood vessel some distance from their original site.

Several factors may precipitate venous thrombosis:

1. Injury to endothelial lining. Intravenous infusion or injections, accidents, operations and inflammation may damage the inner lining to which platelets then adhere.
2. Increased blood coagulation. Dehydration causes the blood to become more

viscous, as does polycythaemia where there is an excess of red blood cells. Blood clotting is also affected by tissue damage for example after operations, myocardial infarction or childbirth. There is also a small but significant increase in risk in women using oral contraceptives.

3. Slowing of venous circulation. This is the most important factor in the formation of venous thrombosis and any condition which produces slowing of venous circulation will predispose to thrombus formation in veins. Rest in bed, especially prolonged rest and immobility after an operation and the reluctance to move in bed which is characteristic of some elderly people, causes circulatory stasis. A pillow under the knees will compress the calves and slow the circulation, as will cardiac failure which causes impaired venous return.

Deep venous thrombosis

Deep venous thrombosis or phlebothrombosis is mainly a hazard of immobilization, with slowing of the rate of blood flow being the principal factor. Risk is particularly high after prolonged rest, limb paralysis or major surgery. Following surgery, the plasma becomes more viscous and there is an increase in the number and stickiness of platelets, which tend to adhere. Around the tenth postoperative day this aggregation of platelets is at its maximum, making this the most crucial period for the occurrence of the dangerous and often fatal complication, pulmonary embolus (Fig. 7.39).

Thrombosis often starts in the deep veins of the gastrocnemius muscles.

+ = venous source
X = arterial source
⇨ = arterial movement
➡ = venous movement

STROKE
↑
BRAIN

ARTERIAL EMBOLI

Atrial thrombus associated with mitral stenosis and atrial fibrillation

Valve thrombus associated with bacterial endocarditis

Mural thrombus associated with myocardial infarction

PULMONARY EMBOLUS

KIDNEYS
↓
HAEMATURIA

+ LIMB
Deep vein thrombosis

LIMB
↓
GANGRENE

Figure 7.39
Sources and movement of emboli

Clinical features

The following may be present: slight calf pain or heaviness; limb oedema which may be gross if a large vessel is blocked and collateral drainage is poor; increased warmth in the affected limb; dilatation of veins; low grade fever.

Often the diagnosis is missed, either because there are no signs, as in about 50% of cases, or because the signs, though present, are overlooked. When the thrombus is only loosely adherent to the vessel wall, the first indication may be sudden collapse or the onset of the clinical features of pulmonary embolus, the thrombus having loosened from the vessel wall and travelled in the venous return flow to lodge in the pulmonary artery or one of its branches.

Prevention

Active measures can be taken to prevent deep venous thrombosis. To avoid slowing of venous return, prolonged bed rest should be avoided and early ambulation encouraged with active walking rather than just sitting in a chair. If bed rest is necessary, immobilization of the body or limbs must be prevented and the patient should not lie in one position for long periods of time. Leg exercises, either active or passive, must be carried out to include both ankle and knee joints. The patient should dorsiflex and plantarflex the foot against resistance, or the nurse should put the patient's ankle and knee joints through their full range of movement.

Deep breathing exercises, which promote venous return, should be taught and encouraged.

Leg vein compression or injury can be avoided by careful handling and positioning of the limbs during and after surgery. Any position in which pressure is exerted on veins should be avoided. For example, sitting or lying with pillows under the knee or calf, crossing the legs at the knee, or sitting in chairs which compress the popliteal space. Many patients are accustomed to these practices at home and should be advised about their dangers.

Anticoagulant therapy, using small doses of heparin, may be given subcutaneously to high risk patients.

Whether the patient is at home or in hospital, the nurse must share the responsibility with others in the health care team for taking measures to prevent deep venous thrombosis.

Nursing observations

The nurse also has a major part to play in the prevention of pulmonary embolus by early detection of deep venous thrombosis through meticulous observation and prompt reporting of warning signs such as a slight temperature rise, slight pulse rate increase, ankle oedema or any complaint of calf pain or tenderness. While the legs are being examined, the opportunity for encouraging the patient to exercise the limbs should always be taken.

Treatment and nursing care

The patient is nursed in bed for a few days, by which time the pain and swelling should be resolved. The limb is elevated to promote venous drainage by raising the foot of the bed, and a bed cradle is used to keep the weight of the bed clothes off the limb. During this time, careful attention to the care of the patient's skin, pressure areas and mouth, and observation of dietary intake, bladder and bowel function and sleep pattern are necessary. In particular, dehydration must be avoided to prevent an increase in blood viscosity. Constipation should be prevented, since straining at stool is associated with the complication of sudden pulmonary embolus. The addition of bran to the diet, additional fluids, and a mild aperient or suppositories may be necessary. Deep breathing exercises should be encouraged.

When the patient is allowed up, the full length of the affected limb should be supported by applying an elastic bandage or stocking before getting out of bed. Elastic stockings increase the velocity of blood flow in veins, but the fit and application are important. The stockings should be smooth and wrinkle-free. If too slack they will not be effective and if too tight they may cause local constriction and impair blood flow. High risk patients may have full length anti-embolism stockings applied to the legs as soon as bed rest begins on admission to hospital.

Anticoagulant therapy is started immediately. Intravenous heparin is given initially.

Heparin is a powerful anticoagulant which works by preventing the conversion of prothrombin to thrombin. It has a rapid action but is short lasting; therefore oral anticoagulation using warfarin is started 24 to 48 hours before heparin is stopped to allow uninterrupted therapeutic action, since warfarin is not fully effective for 24 hours. Warfarin has no direct effect on the blood but works on the liver by reducing the formation of prothrombin. The nurse must remember that anticoagulant therapy involves the danger of haemorrhage. Any sign of bleeding must be reported. Analgesia and night sedation may be necessary and congestive cardiac failure will be carefully controlled.

Venography may be carried out, and if there is major risk, for instance when thrombus is known to be present and when several minor embolic episodes have occurred, it may be necessary to ligate or partially constrict the inferior vena cava to prevent further emboli passing to the pulmonary circulation.

SUGGESTED ASSIGNMENTS

1. How would you explain to a patient or relative of a patient in your ward the meaning of the terms 'pacemaker' and 'heart attack'?

2. Consider the anxieties a patient might experience following a coronary thrombosis. How can the hospital nurse and the community nurse help to relieve these anxieties?

3. If you were working in the community what dietary advice would you give to:
   a. A family with a history of atherosclerosis?
   b. A mother with cardiac failure?
How would you explain the reasons for the advice you offer, and how would you try to make your suggestions acceptable?

4. How well do you observe your patients? Much nursing care is planned on the basis of skilled observation of patients using all the senses. Your eyes, ears, nose and hands can tell you that a patient has suffered an acute myocardial infarction. Describe what you discover through sight, hearing, smell and touch.

5. Does advertising affect you? What influence, if any, has publicity about risk factors and about ways of preventing heart disease had upon your way of life?

FURTHER READING

Hampton J R 1980 The ECG made easy, 2nd edn. Churchill Livingstone, Edinburgh

Hampton J R 1981 All about heart attacks. Patient Handbook Series. Churchill Livingstone, Edinburgh

Housley E 1982 Peripheral vascular disease. Medicine International 18: 844–847

Howard J A, Erlanger H 1983 Teaching methods for coronary patients. In: Wilson-Barnett J (ed) Patient teaching. Recent Advances in Nursing Series. Churchill Livingstone, Edinburgh

Maclean U 1981 Heart attack. Granada, London

Mayberry J, Kent S V 1983 Recent progress in cardiac nursing and rehabilitation programmes. Journal of Advanced Nursing 8: 329–333

Ross A 1981 Cardiac surgery in infants with congenital disorders. Nursing 32: 1412–1415

Scottish Health Education Co-ordinating Committee 1983 Health education in the prevention of smoking-related disease. Scottish Health Education Unit, Edinburgh

Wilson-Barnett J, Fordham M 1982 Recovery from illness. Developments in Nursing Research Series. Wiley, Chichester

Chapter Eight
The blood

Blood disorders are diverse; they may affect any age group and their treatments demand a wide variety of skills from doctors and nurses. Some conditions are common to all mankind while a few are found in more localised communities such as sickle cell anaemia in black people. The ease with which individuals can move from one part of the world to another means that nowadays a nurse may help to care for people with blood disorders which she would have been unlikely to encounter in the past. A few blood diseases, notably some types of anaemia, respond very quickly to treatment, and although this is rewarding it may not present a particular nursing challenge. On the other hand, highly skilled nursing care is vital for a person with acute leukaemia, for example, and thoughtful support from all members of the health team is necessary for the relatives as much as for the patient.

ANATOMY AND PHYSIOLOGY

Blood is red in colour, sticky to the touch and salty to the taste. In health it is slightly alkaline (ph 7.4) and the normal volume is 3.5 to 6 litres. The main constituents are plasma, an aqueous solution of proteins, and, suspended in it, blood cells (Fig. 8.1).

Plasma

Plasma is a yellowish fluid containing 91% water. Of the remaining 9%, approximately 7% are the plasma proteins — albumin, fibrinogen and globulins, which include the coagulation proteins.

Many other substances, including electrolytes (notably sodium chloride, potassium and calcium), hormones, enzymes, nutrients and waste products are to be found in small amounts in plasma. Collectively these substances make up the remaining 2%.

The cellular components

At birth blood cell formation (haemopoiesis) takes place in the marrow of all bones. As the child grows, his red haemopoietic marrow gradually becomes restricted to flat bones such as the ribs, sternum and skull bones, irregular bones, for example the vertebrae and pelvis, and the ends of the long bones. All blood cells originate from stem cells in the bone marrow.

Red blood cells (erythrocytes)

Red cells are small, biconcave, non-nucleated discs (Fig. 8.2). As there is no nucleus each cell has a short life span of about 120 days. In consequence constant replace-

Figure 8.1
Blood proportions

Plasma 55%

Cells 45%

Figure 8.2
Red blood cells

ment of red cells is necessary: normally the red bone marrow makes about 3 million every second. The normal red cell count varies between men and women as shown in Table 8.1.

Table 8.1
Normal range of blood cell values

Type of cell	Number of cells per litre	Percentage of total
Red cells		
men	$4.5-6.5 \times 10^{12}$	
women	$3.8-5.8 \times 10^{12}$	
Total white cell count	$4.0-11.0 \times 10^{9}$	
Differential white cell count		
neutrophils	$2.0-7.5 \times 10^{9}$	40-75
lymphocytes	$1.5-4.0 \times 10^{9}$	20-45
monocytes	$0.2-0.8 \times 10^{9}$	2-10
eosinophils	$0.04-0.4 \times 10^{9}$	1- 6
basophils	$0.01-0.1 \times 10^{9}$	0- 1
Platelets	$150-400 \times 10^{9}$	

Red blood cells contain a high concentration of **haemoglobin**, the molecules of which are composed of protein (globin) and an iron-containing pigment (haem). It enables oxygen to be carried from the lungs to the tissues and carbon dioxide to be transported back from the tissues to the lungs. For the proper development of red cells (erythropoiesis, Fig. 8.3) various nutrients are essential; these include iron, vitamin B complex (in particular vitamin B_{12} and folic acid), vitamin C and protein. Certain hormones are also needed including thyroxin and androgens. The formation of haemoglobin is shown in Figure 4.9, page 155.

A phase of proliferation takes place from proerythroblast to normoblast during which the required number of cells is formed. One of the factors which is thought to stop this cell division is the level of haemoglobin. A lack of iron will lead to continued division of cells which become increasingly smaller and paler (**microcytic and hypochromic**) until division eventually stops. Maturation of cells is also taking place in the bone marrow and continues until the nucleus is eventually extruded leaving fully developed erythrocytes circulating in the bloodstream. The reticulo-

Figure 8.3
Erythropoiesis

Vitamin B_{12} (& intrinsic factor) Folic acid   Iron

Stem cell   Proerythroblast (megaloblast)   Normoblast (Hb appears)   Reticulocyte (nucleus extruded)   Erythrocyte cytes, with a total life-span of approximately 3 days, spend about half of this time in the bone marrow and the other half in the bloodstream. They normally make up less than 2% (Table 8.1) of the circulating red cells. An increase in this percentage indicates that the bone marrow is producing more red cells than normal.

Platelets (thrombocytes)

Platelets, also non-nucleated and formed in the red bone marrow from fragments of megakaryocyte cytoplasm, are much smaller than red blood cells. They have a life-span of 9 to 11 days and play a vital role in the clotting of blood. The normal platelet count is shown in Table 8.1.

White blood cells (leucocytes)

White cells are larger than red cells; they are nucleated and there are two main types (Fig. 8.4):

1. **Polymorphonuclear leucocytes**, which are the most-numerous, form up to 75% of the total white cell count (Table 8.1). There are three subgroups distinguished by the type of stain taken up by the granules of the cells. This stain can be either neutral, acid (eosinophil) or alkaline (basophil).

2. **Mononuclear leucocytes** have two main subgroups of monocytes and lymphocytes. Lymphocytes can be subdivided into B and T varieties.

Like other blood cells, all leucocytes originate from stem cells in the bone marrow and go through stages of proliferation and maturation from primitive blast cells to fully developed white blood cells (Fig. 8.5). Lymphocytes take a different course from other white cells by entering the lymph nodes and spleen where they can proliferate and recirculate in the bloodstream. B lymphocytes move to the lymph nodes while other lymphocytes travel to the thymus gland, become T lymphocytes and then migrate to different areas of the body including other parts of the lymph nodes. All other white blood cells, once they enter the tissues from the bloodstream will function briefly and then die after a life-span of a few days. Lymphocytes may live for very long periods of time.

The normal white cell count is variable (Table 8.1) and is related to the amount of activity as the cells increase in number in response to certain changes in the body. In some disorders the number of cells may fall below the normal range.

Each type of white cell contributes in its own way to the protection of the body against micro-organisms and other foreign substances. Neutrophils have the ability to increase rapidly in number before engulfing and destroying micro-organisms. This process is known as **phagocytosis**. Many neutrophils may die in the process and their dead bodies can be found in collections of pus. Eosinophils increase in number in allergic conditions and have some phagocytic action. The function of basophils is unclear but they are known to contain heparin, an anticoagulant. B lymphocytes are changed into plasma cells and produce antibodies in response to the presence of antigens. They may need the presence of T lymphocytes to recognize antigens. T lymphocytes are sensitized before moving to an area where their immune function

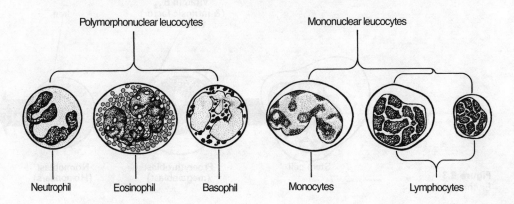

Figure 8.4
White blood cells found in circulating blood

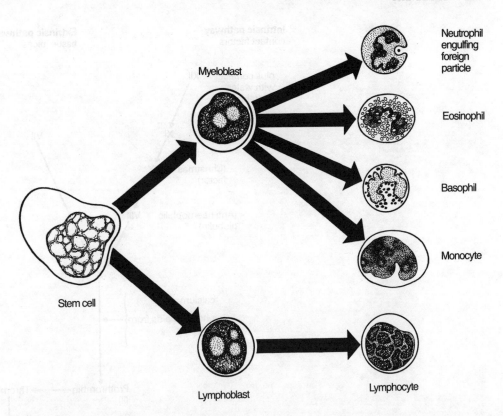

Neutrophil
engulfing
foreign
particle

Eosinophil

Basophil

Monocyte

Myeloblast

Stem cell

Lymphoblast

Lymphocyte

Figure 8.5
Leucopoiesis

(see p. 12) is needed. They are described as providing cell-mediated immunity and can destroy foreign cells as occurs in the rejection of grafted tissue following transplant operations. Monocytes (macrophages) help in the immune response by capturing and processing foreign (antigenic) material before presenting it to the B and T lymphocytes. In this way the monocytes and lymphocytes work cooperatively.

Physiological arrest of haemorrhage (physiological haemostasis)

The phenomenon of natural haemostasis which includes clotting or coagulation of blood is important because without it even slight injury could result in a person bleeding to death. In health blood is kept fluid within the vessels because of a delicate balance between the tendency of the blood to clot and its ability to breakdown any clot (**fibrinolysis**) which does form. The lining of the blood vessels (endothelium) is described as non-water wettable and does very little to stimulate the formation of blood clots. Natural anticoagulant (**heparin**) is also present in blood. As soon as a vessel is damaged, blood comes into contact with surfaces which stimulate an intense clotting reaction, so upsetting the balance and causing the blood to clot.

For coagulation to take place, several **factors** (chemical substances) are needed. These come via two pathways:

1. Extrinsic — blood vessel and body cells are damaged releasing **tissue juices**.
2. Intrinsic — platelets come into contact with and stick to damaged endothelium releasing **contact factors**. These increase platelet stickiness and encourage them to form a loose plug for the damaged vessel. A sequence or cascade of changes is set off as one factor activates another (Fig. 8.6).

When an artery or vein is cut, the walls contract, especially if the cut is clean rather than ragged. This helps to slow down blood flow and reduce blood loss. A loose platelet plug forms out of which fibrin grows, trapping red and white blood cells and tying down the damaged tissues. The clot retracts, if there are adequate

Intrinsic pathway
contact factors

Extrinsic pathway
tissue juices

plus contact
with water
wettable
surface

XII

XI

IX

VII

(Christmas
factor)

VIII

(Anti-haemophilic
globulin)

X

calcium
phospholipids from
platelets
V

Prothrombin ──→ Thrombin
(II)

XIII (Fibrin
stabilising
factor)

Fibrinogen ──→ Fibrin
(soluble)   (insoluble)

Figure 8.6
Coagulation of blood

numbers of platelets present, then gradually hardens and dries as serum oozes out. Underneath this the whole process of repair of the tissues gets under way almost immediately and is well advanced within a few days.

Clotting may be accelerated by warmth which speeds up the chemical changes. Conversely, the process of clotting in shed blood may be slowed down by cooling. It is possible to prevent clotting within the human body by giving substances which will either actively interfere with the coagulation process or passively reduce the quantities of coagulation proteins. Heparin, which must be given by injection, interferes with the thrombin-fibrinogen reaction and so prevents the formation of fibrin. The coagulation proteins, factors II (prothrombin), VII, IX and X, need vitamin K for their manufacture in the liver. Warfarin, an oral anticoagulant and vitamin K antagonist, can be given to reduce the quantities of these proteins. When blood is removed from the body to be collected and stored for various purposes, it is possible to make the calcium in the blood inactive and so prevent coagulation. This knowledge is used clinically in:

1. Transfusion. As blood is removed from a donor it is added to citrate solution with dextrose which is both anticoagulant and nutritive. Calcium is bound to the citrate and is no longer available for coagulation. This ensures that blood remains fluid. Dextrose provides nourishment for the survival of red cells.

2. Examination of samples of peripheral blood. Various specimen bottles are issued by the haematology laboratory containing different types of anticoagulant, for example EDTA (ethylene diamine tetra-acetic acid), or sodium citrate, particularly when the coagulation mechanism is being studied. The nurse should be familiar with the types of bottles and anticoagulants used in her own hospital so that she may select the appropriate ones when needed by the doctor.

Blood groups

It is always essential that the blood of a patient requiring a transfusion is cross-matched with the donor blood he is about to receive. The reason for this precaution is that individuals differ in the blood groups to which they belong. A person's blood group is identified by his red blood cells and his plasma. There are a number of blood grouping systems, although only the two most important in medical practice will be considered here. Other systems are of considerable importance from the point of view of neonatal jaundice and transfusion reactions and are also of interest in criminology and paternity disputes.

A B O blood groups

An individual's blood is classified A, B, AB or O according to the chemical substances called agglutinogens carried by his red blood cells. Blood group O is so named because of the absence of agglutinogens on the red cells. The agglutinogens can be identified according to the way in which they react with antibodies or agglutinins, designated anti-A and anti-B, found in the plasma (Table 8.2).

Table 8.2
Blood groups and their distribution in Western Europeans

Blood group	Antibodies in plasma	Population (%)
A	anti-B only	42%
B	anti-A only	9%
AB	no antibodies	3%
O	anti-A and anti-B	46%

For transfusion purposes it is **the effect that the plasma of the recipient will have on the red cells of the donor blood that must be considered**. If, for example, a patient of Group A was to be transfused with Group B blood the relatively large volume of the patient's plasma containing anti-B agglutinins would cause the tranfused Group B red cells to come together in clumps, that is to agglutinate. In some instances the red cells would break down (haemolyse, p. 303). Table 8.3 shows the blood groups which, in theory, safely 'mix', but since there are subgroups, direct cross-matching is the only means by which compatibility of blood groups can be ensured.

Table 8.3
Compatible blood groups

Red cells of donor	Blood group of recipient			
	A (anti-B)	B (anti-A)	AB (neither anti-B nor anti-A)	O (anti-A & anti-B)
A	compatible		compatible	
B		compatible	compatible	
AB			compatible	
O	compatible	compatible	compatible	compatible

The Rhesus factor

About 85% of the people in Western populations carry a Rhesus factor in their red blood cells and are therefore classified as being Rhesus positive (Rh +ve). Those who lack this factor are called Rhesus negative (Rh −ve).

Haemolysis of
fetal red cells

Rh +ve
fetus

Blood cells
via placenta

Rh antibodies
produced

Rh −ve
mother

Figure 8.7
Rhesus antibody production in
pregnancy

Although there is no naturally occurring Rhesus antibody, if a Rh −ve person is exposed to Rh +ve red cells, then antibodies may be formed, and once formed they stay in the blood. Exposure may occur through:

1. Transfusion of Rh +ve blood.
2. Pregnancy (Fig. 8.7), when the mother is Rh −ve and the fetus is Rh +ve.

In this situation the mother may form Rhesus antibodies in her blood which then pass back via the placenta to the fetus. This results in destruction of the baby's red blood cells (haemolysis) giving rise to haemolytic disease of the newborn. If very seriously affected, the baby may be born dead; he may survive if given an immediate exchange transfusion of Rh −ve blood at birth. Subsequent pregnancies are always at greater risk because there is a progressive build-up of antibodies.

Investigations

History

From an accurate history, the doctor may elicit symptoms which could suggest a cause of a blood disorder, for example, frequent use of aspirin by the patient causing gastric irritation and blood loss.

General physical examination

This may reveal signs of disease of which the patient may be quite unaware but which are of crucial importance in indicating the type of blood disorder, for example, purpura or splenomegaly may not have been noticed by the patient.

Examination of circulating blood

Venepuncture is the withdrawal of venous blood for diagnostic purposes. Samples of venous blood are taken by a doctor from a peripheral vein, usually a vein in the antecubital fossa. Laboratory findings often enable an accurate diagnosis to be made of comparatively simple blood disorders such as iron deficiency anaemia.

The correct bottles containing the appropriate anticoagulant should be available. Whenever possible, a nurse should be with a child and with an apprehensive adult during venepuncture. No special preparation is necessary. A haematoma may form at the puncture site, but this can be avoided by the application of digital pressure to the site. Where bleeding is liable to occur elevation of the limb is also very useful.

The most common investigation is a blood count. It is usually done by sophisticated electronic apparatus which estimates such things as the haemoglobin level, white cell count and platelet count.

Cell count

The number of circulating blood cells of each type is determined (Table 8.1) and their size, shape and other characteristics are noted.

Haemoglobin

To estimate haemoglobin level, a small quantity of blood is obtained in a tube containing an anticoagulant called EDTA (sequestrene). Normal levels are:

Men: 13.0–18.0 g/dl
Women: 11.5–16.5 g/dl

Investigations appropriate to the underlying conditions

While examination of the blood itself may give an answer to the type of disorder, the cause may have to be sought in other systems such as the gastrointestinal, urinary or female reproductive systems where chronic blood loss (p. 303) can produce iron deficiency anaemia. Investigations may include isotope scanning of bone, passage of a Crosby capsule (p. 183), or a staging laparotomy as in suspected Hodgkin's disease (p. 314).

Examination of bone marrow

The procedure known as marrow puncture involves the removal of a specimen of red bone marrow by aspiration using a stout needle with an adjustable guard such as the Salah needle (Fig. 8.8). In adults, the sternum and the iliac crest are the most accessible sites. The tibia or iliac crest is preferred for very young children and on rare occasions the vertebral spines are used for the obese patient.

Laboratory examination of red bone marrow provides a useful aid to diagnosis in blood disorders such as pernicious anaemia and the leukaemias. It is also important when the diagnosis of a blood disorder is not clear following examination of the peripheral blood. During the course of the disease, repeated examination of bone marrow may be required to assess the effect of treatment.

The procedure is performed under local anaesthesia by a doctor using an aseptic technique. Nursing responsibilities are to ensure patient comfort before and after the procedure and to prepare the equipment. A technician from the haematology department may be present to collect the bone marrow, having brought with him the appropriate specimen container. Adults will require careful explanation of the procedure, and light sedation may be given. Children are generally sedated beforehand, both to allay fear and to prevent excessive movement during the procedure. In this case two nurses will be required, one to assist the doctor and one to hold and comfort the child. In some instances it may be preferable for a parent to do this. The patient will be positioned according to the site being used.

The actual removal of bone marrow is painful. Following the procedure, some patients may require mild analgesia as the effect of the local anaesthetic wears off. Patients who have been sedated should not be allowed up for 2 to 3 hours. Complications are rare, but infection could result from poor aseptic technique. When using the sternal site, the possibility of inadvertently inserting the puncture needle right through the sternum causing damage to the organs in the mediastinum is always present. This risk can be virtually eliminated by correct positioning of the guard on the needle.

Figure 8.8
Salah needle

Schilling test

This is a method of assessing the body's ability to absorb vitamin B_{12}, a vitamin essential for formation of red blood cells.

Following a fasting period of not less than 6 hours, an oral dose of vitamin B_{12} 'labelled' with radioactive cobalt is given. An intramuscular flushing dose of non-radioactive vitamin B_{12} is also given immediately afterwards, in the form of 1000 micrograms of cyanocobalamin. A 24-hour urine collection is then started, from which laboratory staff can estimate the amount of radioactive vitamin excreted. The intramuscular 'flushing' dose of vitamin B_{12} totally saturates the binding capacity for this vitamin in the plasma. Any excess is lost in the urine. As the oral dose of radioactive vitamin B_{12} is then absorbed from the terminal ileum, it is unable to be bound in the plasma and is also lost in the urine. Thus virtually all of the vitamin absorbed from the intestine will appear in the urine giving a fairly accurate measure of the amount of absorption.

A healthy person stores and requires a comparatively small amount of vitamin B_{12} and would therefore excrete most of a given dose. However, people with disorders of intestinal absorption and those in whom a compound of gastric secretion known as the intrinsic factor is absent cannot absorb vitamin B_{12}. In these instances, the amount of vitamin B_{12} found in the urine would be negligible, thus proving a deficiency in absorption. The test can be repeated exactly as before, after an interval of at least 7 days, giving a capsule of Hog intrinsic factor along with the capsule of radioactive vitamin B_{12} to see whether or not this will correct the problem. Where the results then show a normal level of vitamin B_{12} in the urine this would indicate that there is a lack of intrinsic factor which is virtually diagnostic of pernicious anaemia (p. 306). The nurse must ensure that the patient fasts and then has at least 1500 ml of fluid during the 24 hours of the collection, that the correct dose of vitamin B_{12} is given at the appropriate time and that all urine is collected over an exact 24-hour period otherwise the test will be invalid.

DISORDERS OF THE RED CELLS

Diseases affecting the red blood cells are common in all parts of the world. There may be overproduction or underproduction of cells or abnormality of the cells themselves.

An increase in the number of circulating red cells is called **erythrocytosis**. This will occur in response to hypoxaemia (p. 219) and can be found among people living at high altitudes. The same compensatory mechanism operates in some disorders, for example congenital heart conditions and chronic pulmonary disease. In these circumstances the erythrocytosis can be beneficial to the individual as it increases the oxygen-carrying power of the blood. However, erythrocytosis also increases the viscosity of blood and this can be a disadvantage for people with chronic pulmonary disease. These patients may benefit from withdrawal of a quantity of blood (**venesection**) to reduce the number of red cells. Treatment will of course be needed for the underlying condition.

Erythrocytosis also characterizes a rare condition of unknown origin called **polycythaemia vera**. In this relatively mild malignant disease of adults there is an extension of red marrow throughout the long bones producing a very high haemoglobin level and a plethoric appearance. Platelets also increase in number. Treatment is usually by venesection, repeated as necessary and as tolerated by the patient, with the withdrawal of not more than half a litre of blood on any one occasion. The main disadvantage of venesection is that prolonged use can lead to iron deficiency. Unless symptoms are produced by the deficiency, replacement iron is not given as the deficiency curbs erythropoiesis. Other forms of treatment are the use of radioactive phosphorus or the giving of cytotoxic drugs such as busulphan.

The most common and the most important group of diseases affecting the red cells is the anaemias.

Anaemia

Anaemia may be defined as a level of circulating haemoglobin which is below normal for the person's age and sex. A reduction for any reason in the number of red cells or their haemoglobin content or both will cause anaemia.

Causes of anaemia

Blood loss (posthaemorrhagic anaemia)

The seriousness of haemorrhage depends on both the amount and the speed with which blood is lost; for example, a sudden rapid loss of 1.5 litres or more in an adult will result in collapse and shock. The same amount lost over a period of several days would be less harmful, although the reduction in haemoglobin will be similar.

Acute blood loss. Haemodilution, whereby fluid is drawn from the tissues into the circulation, follows rapid haemorrhage. The degree of anaemia which results is not measurable until the circulating volume is fully restored, and this can take from 24 to 36 hours. Immediately after the haemorrhage the haemoglobin level is the same as before, if not higher.

Chronic blood loss (Fig. 8.9). Repeated small losses of blood usually occurring internally, for example from a peptic ulcer or haemorrhoids, cause a progressive fall in haemoglobin. Small amounts of blood loss can be made up by increased erythropoiesis and anaemia does not appear until the stores of iron have been depleted.

Excessive destruction of red cells (haemolytic anaemia)

Whenever red cells are destroyed more rapidly than they are being formed anaemia will result. This may occur in one of two ways:

1. The red blood cells are abnormal and are therefore destroyed more easily, as in pernicious anaemia and some hereditary diseases such as sickle cell anaemia and thalassaemia.

2. The red cells are normal but their environment is abnormal as when the presence of infection, such as malaria, toxins or the undesirable side-effects of certain drugs, causes them to be destroyed. Antibodies can also produce haemolysis as in haemolytic disease of the newborn (p. 300), where antibodies come from the mother, or autoimmune haemolytic anaemia where the body raises antibodies against some part of its own red cell structure.

Diminished production of red cells (hypoplastic or aplastic anaemia)

Hypoplastic anaemia, in which blood formation is inadequate, is most likely to be caused by lack of important nutrients such as iron, vitamin B_{12} or folic acid. Other factors which may be lacking are intrinsic factor from the stomach, thyroxine or androgens. Much less commonly failure of production may result from treatment of other disorders, such as cancer with cytotoxic drugs and irradiation, exposure to toxins in kidney or liver failure or an idiosyncratic reaction to a drug such as chloramphenicol. Very rarely the cause is unknown (**idiopathic**). Aplastic anaemia, in which no red cells are produced, is likely to be fatal and is fortunately rare.

Regardless of the cause all anaemias have certain clinical features in common.

Clinical features of anaemia

General symptoms and signs of anaemia whatever its origin are due to a lowered haemoglobin which results in a decreased supply of oxygen to the body tissues. Both the severity of the anaemia and the rapidity of its onset will affect the degree to which the patient will experience the following:

1. Increasing tiredness and lassitude, particularly at the end of the day when the body is finding progressive difficulty in coping with a poor oxygen supply.

2. Pallor of the skin and mucous membranes: a reduced pigmentation of the blood results from a lowered haemoglobin level. However, this is a very unreliable

Figure 8.9
Types of chronic bleeding causing iron deficiency anaemia

Epistaxis

Haematemesis

Melaena

Abnormal menstrual loss

Rectal bleeding

sign as some people look extremely pale but are not anaemic or an anaemic person may have a good skin colour.

3. Anorexia and dyspepsia which are often accompanied by some weight loss.

4. Breathlessness on exertion which occurs as the respiratory system tries to compensate for the reduced oxygen supply (Chap. 6). The oxygen-carrying power of the blood cannot, however, be improved until the anaemia is corrected and there is enough haemoglobin to carry the oxygen to meet the body's needs.

5. Tachycardia and possibly heart failure. As with breathlessness, the increase in heart rate is a direct result of the body trying to compensate for the reduced amount of oxygen available. In addition, since anaemia makes the blood less viscous or sticky, it flows much more rapidly than normal through the peripheral circulation. These two factors increase the workload of the heart and the heart may then fail, particularly if the patient is elderly or weak. The patient may also complain of hearing the pulse pounding in the ears at night.

6. Dizziness, fainting attacks, irritability and deterioration in memory may be present due to the reduced oxygen supply to the brain.

7. Tingling felt in the extremities (paraesthesiae) when neurological involvement occurs.

Iron deficiency anaemia

This is the most common type of anaemia in every country in the world. Women of child-bearing age are the most susceptible because of the increased demand for iron during pregnancy and following each menstrual loss. Insufficient dietary intake of iron and lack of hydrochloric acid necessary for the absorption of iron are other important factors. Haemorrhage as referred to previously results in an iron deficiency type of anaemia.

Clinical features

The condition has a gradual onset and the level of haemoglobin may be very low (7 g per dl) before the patient seeks medical advice. Typically, the patient waits until he has become incapacitated before consulting his doctor. By this time he may have developed all the general symptoms and signs of anaemia due to diminished oxygen supply. In addition he may display those features specific to the nutritional deficiency of iron. These are:

1. Glossitis: the tongue appears red and raw.
2. Angular stomatitis: inflammation at the corners of the mouth.
3. Brittleness of nails which may occasionally progress to koilonychia where the nails become concave and are therefore described as spoon-shaped (Fig. 8.10). The blood examination shows a hypochromic, microcytic anaemia.

Figure 8.10
Koilonychia

As iron deficiency anaemia is really a symptom of some other disorder, there are likely to be clinical features of this as well.

Investigations

Examination of peripheral blood samples for haemoglobin estimation and a cell count is carried out. A variety of investigations may be necessary to elicit the cause; for example, a suspected carcinoma of stomach will call for endoscopy and a barium meal.

Treatment and nursing care

Treatment depends on the severity of the patient's clinical condition.

Rest. If the haemoglobin is below 5 g per dl it may be necessary to let the patient rest in bed but he should be helped to remain in the upright position. This reduces the work load on the heart. When a person lies flat, the blood return to the heart is increased and in a severely anaemic patient this extra work could lead to the development of cardiac failure.

Correction of anaemia. Oral preparations of iron, for example ferrous sulphate

(200 mg) given three times daily after meals, is effective for the majority of patients. Gastrointestinal upsets may occur if the iron is not given after main meals. Occasionally a patient will have difficulty in swallowing pills, in which case a liquid preparation, usually in the form of a syrup such as Fersamal, will be prescribed.

If none of the oral preparations can be tolerated or if the anaemia is not responding, then intramuscular iron, for example Imferon or Jectofer, may be ordered by the doctor, the dosage being calculated according to the patient's body weight. Unless these preparations are injected very carefully and deeply into the muscle they will cause irritation and staining of the tissues. Some physicians prefer to give Imferon intravenously in which case a test dose is given first as a severe anaphylactic reaction can occur. The patient must be observed carefully both during and for 1 hour after completion of the total dose infusion. Any sign of pyrexia, flushing, metallic taste, dyspnoea, nausea and vomiting, or fall in blood pressure must be reported immediately. Antihistamines must be available.

Blood transfusion is reserved as initial treatment for the severely ill patient. Concentrated red cells are always used and the blood is usually given slowly with diuretic cover. This prevents the development of cardiac failure and allows the anaemia to be corrected quite quickly.

Mouth care. Oral hygiene is very important and mouth care is often necessary 4-hourly. Gentle swabbing and frequent rinsing are usually effective.

Treatment of underlying and associated conditions. Cardiac symptoms should improve with iron therapy but the physician may prescribe digoxin to control tachycardia.

When the anaemia is due to haemorrhage the cause must be found and treated.

Dietary deficiency must be corrected by encouraging the patient to eat iron-rich foods (Ch. 4). The best sources of iron are found in red meats, including liver and kidney, and red wine. Contrary to popular belief, spinach is a very poor source as the iron is in an inabsorbable form.

If adequately treated, and in the absence of other serious problems such as renal disease, the patient's haemoglobin will rise by 1% per day, which means that the normal level will be reached in 4 to 8 weeks.

Community care

Preventive care

Health education is important and the community nurse should advise on suitable diet, giving special attention to those whose sex or age group places them at particular risk. Medicinal iron should be administered to women during pregnancy and lactation and if menstruation is heavy. Infants, particularly if of low birth weight, should have iron-containing foods introduced into their diet by the age of 3 months. Elderly patients (Ch. 20) living alone often need a good deal of persuasion to eat suitable meals that contain adequate amounts of iron.

Follow-up

After immediate treatment for iron deficiency anaemia, continued iron therapy is necessary for a further year. This is to ensure that the patient's depleted body stores of iron are replenished. Iron absorption in the non-anaemic patient is poor and the establishment of a stock will take a long time. Regular check-ups will also be necessary.

A common reason for failure of treatment is when the patient does not take the iron because of gastrointestinal disturbance such as nausea, diarrhoea or constipation. Part of this may be due to suggestion where a patient has been told by some other person that the tablets will upset her.

Megaloblastic anaemias

There are two main types producing very similar clinical pictures. **Folic acid deficiency anaemia** is more common than **vitamin B$_{12}$ deficiency anaemia** but lack of either vitamin will affect all dividing cell systems in the body due to disturbance of

DNA synthesis. Megaloblasts are abnormal red cell precursors found in bone marrow.

Body stores of folic acid are very small and deficiency can arise within a few weeks. Deficiency commonly occurs when a person eats very little fresh fruit and vegetables, or has too many foods cooked for a long time so destroying the folic acid. The elderly and those living alone can be particularly at risk as are pregnant women who have a high rate of normal cell proliferation with an increased need for folic acid. The vitamin may also be deficient in coeliac disease and other malabsorption disorders. Absorption of folic acid can also be upset when a person is taking certain drugs such as primidone or barbiturates.

Pernicious anaemia (Addisonian anaemia)

This condition is much less common than iron deficiency anaemia, but when it does occur it is most prevalent in the middle-aged group and affects women more often than men. It is very rare in younger people. The condition is the result of the inability of the stomach to produce the intrinsic factor which in health ensures the absorption of vitamin B_{12} from the terminal ileum. Body stores of vitamin B_{12} last for 2 years or more and dietary lack is unlikely unless the person is a true vegan eating no animal products of any kind.

The effects of the disease are particularly destructive and, if untreated, the patient will die — hence the adjective 'pernicious'.

Clinical features

The disease has a gradual onset and early symptoms are often unnoticed or ignored by the patient so that the anaemia may be well advanced by the time he visits his doctor.

The general symptoms and signs of anaemia will be present, and in addition the following features, which are specific to the lack of vitamin B_{12} will occur:

1. Achlorhydria, absence of hydrochloric acid in the stomach.
2. The skin, as well as being pale, has a slight lemon tint. This is due to the presence of bilirubin resulting from the excessive breakdown of red cells. Urobilinogen will then be found in the urine (Ch. 5).
3. The tongue may be sore, but very often is not and is classically smooth and atrophic having lost its papillae. There may be a loss of taste and a dislike of certain foods.
4. Intermittent diarrhoea may occur.
5. A feeling of numbness and 'pins and needles' (paraesthesiae) in the fingers and toes is present in advanced cases, particularly if a relapse occurs in the disease. It indicates involvement of the nervous system.

Blood examination shows a *macrocytic anaemia* with considerable evidence of disordered red cell protection.

Course and complications

Degenerative changes may appear in the spinal cord if treatment is delayed or inadequate. Sometimes they precede the development of anaemia. As both the ascending and the descending tracts are involved, the term subacute combined degeneration of the cord is used.

The disease will run a progressive course with increasing anaemia and further damage to the nervous system if it is untreated. The patient may die either from anaemia or from infection, to which he becomes increasingly susceptible.

Investigations

Examination of samples of peripheral blood.
Marrow puncture to reveal the presence of megaloblasts.
Schilling test (p. 302).
Gastric analysis is done occasionally when there are diagnostic problems. In

pernicious anaemia there is no hydrochloric acid in the gastric juice even after the injection of pentagastrin (p. 180) which will stimulate its secretion.

Treatment and nursing care

As with other types of anaemia this varies according to the severity of the disease. The majority of people are investigated as out-patients and only come into hospital if they are very ill when nursing care would be similar to that for a patient with iron deficiency anaemia (p. 304).

Correction of anaemia. A blood transfusion of concentrated red cells will be given with diuretic cover if the haemoglobin is dangerously low (below 4 g per dl). Replacement of vitamin B_{12} (cobalamin) must be by intramuscular injection for all patients since they are unable to absorb the vitamin if it is given by mouth. The preparation of cobalamin most commonly prescribed is hydroxocobalamin. The dosage is 1000 micrograms given twice in the first week and then 1000 micrograms once a week until the blood is normal. The nurse will find it very rewarding to see that after the first injection the patient begins to feel and look much better. As the bone marrow responds by producing normal red cells very rapidly there is a much greater need for iron. For this reason ferrous sulphate may also be prescribed.

A light nourishing diet, rich in iron, protein and vitamin C, will also aid the production of normal cells.

Community care

The patient will need a maintenance dose of hydroxocobalamin for life. Dosage is regulated so that haemoglobin and blood count are kept within normal limits. Most patients require 1000 micrograms once every 3 months unless there is a neurological complication when a monthly dose is given.

If the patient is elderly and living alone the community nurse may be asked to give the injections. At this time she will advise the patient about diet.

Anaemia secondary to other conditions

The treatment must first be directed at the underlying cause. If, for example, there is a hypoplastic type of anaemia in which the bone marrow is failing to produce blood cells due to some toxic factor, then the toxic factor must be removed if possible. This may mean treating an infection or discontinuing administration of a drug. When the toxins result from liver failure or from cancer then blood transfusion may be the only means of supporting life. Sometimes the androgen oxymethalone is prescribed in order to stimulate the bone marrow to produce more blood cells.

Intractable anaemia

Patients with intractable anaemia may need to be given a blood transfusion every 3 to 4 weeks, possibly on a day-patient basis. To minimise the risk of reactions (p. 317) either washed or filtered red cells may be given along with the intravenous injection of hydrocortisone and chlorpheniramine. A diuretic such as frusemide is also given to prevent cardiac failure. These patients are easily tired and can be quite demanding to look after, so the nurse needs to show considerable understanding and empathy towards them.

DISORDERS OF HAEMOSTASIS

Absence of one of the substances in the blood necessary for clotting or disorder of the normal physiological process whereby haemorrhage is arrested (p. 297) will result in an abnormal tendency to bleed. Conditions in which this occurs are known collectively as the haemorrhagic disorders.

Bleeding due to defects in the clotting mechanism

A defect in the production of factor VIII causes haemophilia A and of factor IX Christmas disease (haemophilia B). A slightly different defect in factor VIII production will cause von Willebrand's disease. All of these disorders are inherited. Factor VIII is a product of two genes, one of which is part of the X sex chromosome and the other is autosomal (p. 377). In haemophilia A the sex chromosome is affected, as is the case in Christmas disease, and so both diseases are found only in males while females act as carriers. Von Willebrand's disease is due to an autosomal defect and so can be found in both males and females.

Haemophilia A

The main clinical feature is persistent and excessive bleeding. The blood clot which forms will break down easily and so bleeding is likely to recur. In moderate cases excessive bleeding may develop following treatment, such as dental extraction, or minor injury. In more severe forms, spontaneous bleeding can take place into areas such as the gastrointestinal or urinary systems or into joints (haemarthrosis). Recurrent haemarthrosis will cause gradual destruction of the joint with resultant deformity.

Treatment and nursing care

In very mild forms the person may not even be aware of the condition and does not require treatment. In moderate to severe forms it is now possible to give the missing factor which can be extracted from fresh frozen plasma, stored as freeze dried powder until required when it is easily dissolved in distilled water, and then given by intravenous injection. The size and number of doses required will depend on the severity of the bleeding and the patient's own natural amount of factor VIII. Other treatment will also be needed appropriate to the cause of the bleeding, such as aspiration of a joint or insertion of sutures.

Centres are available in different parts of the country which provide a 24-hour emergency treatment service for treatment of haemophilia. Home therapy is also possible where the child is treated by his parents, or an older child by himself. This is of particular benefit in more severe forms of haemophilia as treatment can be started earlier, so reducing the amount of pain and distress involved for the patient and his family, especially where the home is some distance from a centre or bleeds occur at night when tiredness and irritability are likely to aggravate the situation. Regional haemophilia centres also provide laboratory and advisory services, including genetic counselling.

Advice must be given on how to avoid situations likely to produce bleeding. Good oral hygiene and dental care are essential to preserve the natural teeth and the dentist must be told about the haemophilia. Products containing aspirin should not be taken as aspirin interferes with normal platelet function and can irritate the gastrointestinal mucosa, possibly leading to severe bleeding. In moderate to severe forms of haemophilia the patient must try to avoid situations likely to produce injury, especially to joints. It is also recommended that some form of identification is worn, such as a Medic Alert bracelet, in the event of illness or injury.

Christmas disease

This is much less common than haemophilia A and tends to be less severe. However, treatment and nursing care are the same except that factor IX must be given instead of factor VIII.

Von Willebrand's disease

This resembles mild haemophilia. Along with a defect in factor VIII production, there is also a defect in the function of platelets and capillaries. This means that the patient is more likely to bleed from small cuts than the haemophiliac patient but rarely has bleeding into deeper structures such as joints and muscles. Treatment is very similar to that required in haemophilia A.

Deficiency of prothrombin factors (Hypoprothrombinaemia)

This can result from any process which interferes with the absorption or utilisation of vitamin K (p. 298) needed by the liver to make the prothrombin factors II, VII, IX and X. Hypoprothrombinaemia can occur in the first few days of life, especially in a preterm baby (p. 622) where the liver cells are immature, and is the cause of **haemorrhagic disease of the newborn**. It may also complicate obstructive jaundice and some forms of malabsorption due to failure of the intestine to absorb vitamin K. Administration of vitamin K by injection will correct the hypoprothrombinaemia unless liver cell function is impaired when the missing factor may have to be given. Hypoprothrombinaemia can also be produced artificially in people who are at risk of developing thrombi and emboli as in deep venous thrombosis (p. 291) and after cardiac surgery where mechanical valves (p. 262) are inserted. Heparin (p. 293) can be given initially to produce a prompt response with each dose being effective for up to 6 hours. Warfarin is started at the same time but takes 36 to 48 hours to produce its effect of blocking prothrombin formation. The dose of warfarin is adjusted to prolong the prothrombin time by two to four times the normal value.

Anticoagulant therapy

Patients who have to take anticoagulants over a long period of time, as after cardiac valve surgery, need to be given specific advice to ensure maximum effectiveness of the anticoagulant while recognizing that there will also be a risk of haemorrhage. The patient must attend regularly at the clinic for prothrombin checks and remember to take the correct dose at the correct time. It may be useful to mark off each dose on a calendar or in a diary. A repeat prescription should be obtained when at least 7 days supply of tablets remains. A normal diet should be taken avoiding marked changes, especially in fat content. Alcohol should be taken only in moderation. Other medicines are best avoided, if possible, because of the risk of potentially dangerous interactions (Table 8.4), and aspirin (acetylsalicylic acid) preparations must never be taken. In the event of other illness, bleeding or severe bruising, medical advice should be sought immediately. When another doctor or dentist is consulted, who may not know about the anticoagulant therapy, this must always be mentioned.

Table 8.4
Medicines which interact with warfarin

By increasing anticoagulant effect	By decreasing anticoagulant effect
acetylsalicylic acid	barbiturates
clofibrate	carbamazepine
mefenamic acid	dichloralphenazone
liquid paraffin	glutethimide
phenylbutazone	oral contraceptives

Bleeding due to defects of the capillary walls or a diminished number of platelets

Defects in the capillary walls may occur as a manifestation of some other (usually serious) disease or infection during the course of which the endothelium becomes damaged thus allowing blood to escape. Meningococcal meningitis, septicaemia, malignant disease and scurvy are a few examples of conditions which will cause this to happen. Occasionally some drugs have toxic side-effects with the same result, aspirin, phenobarbitone, phenytoin and phenylbutazone being among the culprits.

A diminished number of platelets (thrombocytopaenia) may accompany other conditions, for example leukaemia, or may arise spontaneously.

Figure 8.11
Petechiae

In all these conditions there is bleeding into the skin or mucous membranes appearing as haemorrhagic spots called **purpura**. If the haemorrhages are only small they are termed **petechiae** (Fig. 8.11); larger purpuric spots are called **ecchymoses**. Bleeding may also take place in the eyes and is very distressing because of the disturbance of vision and time taken for it to clear.

DISORDERS OF THE WHITE CELLS

White cells are seen in the blood as they migrate from the bone marrow to the tissues. The numbers that are found generally reflect the demand for white cells and the types of white cell seen vary with age, lymphocytes being more common in young children than they are in adults.

An increase in the number of circulating white blood cells is called **leucocytosis**. This is the normal body response to bacterial invasion and will resolve when the infection has subsided. Too few white cells is termed **leucopenia**; this may occur in response to certain specific infections such as tuberculosis and enteric fever, or it can be the result of a very severe infection to which the body has no resistance.

Agranulocytosis

This is an extremely rare, but very serious illness, where few or no granulocytes are present in the bloodstream. It can be due to the side-effects of drugs such as chloramphenicol, phenylbutazone and thiouracil. Any patient taking such drugs should tell his doctor as soon as possible if he is feeling unwell or has a sore throat.

Treatment includes the withdrawal of any drug which could be responsible and otherwise the management is the same as for acute leukaemia.

The leukaemias

Leukaemia is the malignant overproduction of white cells and their precursors. The type of cell involved, whether myeloid or lymphoid, is important because of differences in treatment and prognosis. The disease is also classified as acute or chronic. In the acute form, cells do not mature and so accumulate in the marrow leaving insufficient room for other types of cell to develop normally. As a result, the patient will develop anaemia and a tendency to bleed, in addition to having a reduced resistance to infection. Chronic types of leukaemia produce cells which are mature and able to function normally but which proliferate abnormally as in chronic myeloid leukaemia. Chronic lymphatic leukaemia shows a combination of proliferation and maturation problems.

In the majority of cases a cause cannot be found, but there is increasing evidence that viruses may be responsible in some types of leukaemia. Other causes include irradiation, cytotoxic drugs and exposure to the chemical substance benzene.

Acute leukaemia

Acute leukaemia can occur at any age. In adults, nine out of every ten cases are myeloid in type, which unfortunately responds poorly to treatment. Acute lymphoblastic leukaemia is more common in children between the ages of 2 and 5 years and this has the possibility of being cured.

Clinical features

These are extremely variable. In some patients the symptoms are quite trivial and may include those of a recent flu-like illness and a general deterioration in health. At the other extreme the onset may be abrupt and obviously serious.

The patient has a raised temperature and looks and feels very unwell. Epistaxis, bleeding gums and purpura (see above) soon appear. There is sore throat and ulcers in the mouth because of the lowered resistance to infection. The symptoms and signs of severe anaemia are also present, and muscular and joint pains add to the patient's misery.

Diagnosis is established after examination of the blood which shows anaemia, thrombocytopaenia and either a raised, normal or even severely reduced white cell count. When no white cells are found in the blood, this is described as **aleukaemic leukaemia** and diagnosis depends on examination of the marrow which will show large numbers of very primitive leukaemic 'blast' cells (Fig. 8.5) with a reduced number of other cell precursors.

Course and complications

Untreated, the patient will die within a few weeks from anaemia, haemorrhage or severe infection, either bacterial or viral.

Treatment and nursing care

Modern treatment has induced encouraging, and sometimes prolonged, remissions of the disease even in the acute myeloblastic variety. Some children, and a smaller number of adults, with acute lymphoblastic leukaemia will be cured.

Drug therapy. Cytotoxic agents, such as daunorubicin, vincristine and cyclophosphamide, interfere with cell division, but resistance to therapy often develops and side-effects appear (Table 8.5). Normal cells in the bone marrow may be suppressed, especially white cells and platelets, increasing the risk of haemorrhage and infection. Damage to the epithelium of the gastrointestinal tract may occur. Mouth ulceration, nausea, vomiting and diarrhoea may be troublesome. Alopecia often follows cyclophosphamide therapy, and although this may be temporary, many patients will be saved anxiety and embarrassment if fitted with a wig before therapy is started. As the long term effects of exposure to even low levels of these drugs are not

Table 8.5
Some commonly used cytotoxic drugs

Drug	Principal side-effects	Notes on administration
Adriamycin	Nausea and vomiting 6–36 hours later. Alopecia. Urine becomes red for 24 hours after administration. Bone marrow depression. Mucosal ulcers.	Avoid extravasation because of irritant effect on tissues. Explain to patient that red discolouration of urine is to be expected but also check that bleeding is not taking place.
Cyclophosphamide	Nausea and vomiting. Haemorrhagic cystitis. Bone marrow depression. Alopecia.	To minimise cystitis ensure that patient has a high fluid intake and is given drug early in day to avoid it lying in bladder overnight.
Cytosine arabinoside	Nausea and vomiting. Bone marrow depression. Mucositis and diarrhoea.	Can be given intrathecally. Ensure adequate fluid intake to replace loss from dehydration.
Mustine hydrocholoride	Bone marrow depression and nausea even after small doses.	Give in fast running intravenous infusion and avoid extravasation as it is highly irritant. Give at night after anti-emetic and hypnotic to minimise nausea.
Procarbazine	Nausea and vomiting. Anorexia.	Avoid alcohol and cheese (see p. 563) as drug is a monoamine oxidase inhibitor.
6-Thioguanine	Bone marrow depression. Uric acid crystal formation.	Ensure that patient has a high fluid intake to aid excretion of uric acid.
Vincristine	Peripheral neuropathy. Constipation. Abdominal pain. Paralytic ileus.	Report any numbness or tingling of fingers and toes and any muscle weakness. Check for and correct constipation before therapy is started and try to prevent constipation from developing during therapy. Avoid extravasation as it is very irritant.

fully known, extreme care is needed in their preparation and administration to avoid contamination of either people or the environment.

Singly, drugs are of little use, but the more aggressive use of combinations of drugs has proved effective. These combinations are given in varying cycles to reduce the development of resistance to treatment. The first stage is to induce remission of the disease. In acute lymphoblastic leukaemia the aim is to destroy the leukaemic cells while the marrow continues to work normally. However, in the myeloblastic type, the aim is to wipe out almost completely all blood cell production then hopefully the normal cells will develop at a faster rate than the leukaemic cells. Treatment is then altered during a period of consolidation. For lymphoblastic leukaemia in particular, this involves cranial irradiation and the intrathecal administration of cytotoxic drugs to destroy any leukaemic cells which are using the central nervous system as a sanctuary site. The third phase is a maintenance period of 2 to 3 years when other drugs may be used. After this time, if the patient is still in remission, the drugs will be stopped. For some patients a less aggressive regime is used just to palliate and provide reasonable control of the disease without being designed to cure.

Potent antibiotics are given intravenously when septicaemia is thought to be present even though no actual evidence of an infection is found.

Red cell and platelet transfusions. These are given at intervals as supportive therapy to keep the haemoglobin above 10 g per dl and to control problems of bleeding due to thrombocytopenia. Gentle handling and movement of patients is particularly important to prevent bruising. Intramuscular and subcutaneous injections are best avoided if possible and the use of an electric razor is advisable for shaving to reduce the risk of bleeding. The skin and oral mucous membranes should be inspected for bleeding when personal hygiene is being attended to, and urine and stools may also need to be examined for blood.

Rest. Rest in bed will be required while the patient is acutely ill. Careful attention should be given to the relief of pressure. The patient who is comfortable will be less restless and this will reduce oxygen demand in a person who is already anaemic.

Prevention of infection. As there exists the possibility of infective complications which can be fatal, a high standard of observation is essential and any sign of pyrexia should be reported promptly. The normal signs and symptoms of infection may not be as noticeable in a patient who is receiving cytotoxic drugs or a corticosteroid, such as prednisolone. These patients are also very susceptible to moniliasis (p. 184).

To prevent the development of infection while the patient is at a low level of resistance, protective isolation units have been set up allowing each patient to be nursed in a single room. Alternatively, if a laminar flow unit is available (Fig. 8.12) the patient can be nursed in a ward beside other patients. This helps to prevent the psychological problems of being nursed in a single room. The patient is now protected by an invisible barrier of positive pressure air which prevents air-borne organisms from coming in to the patient. However, all items which are taken into the unit must be either sterile or scrupulously clean. This method of care is unsuitable if the patient is infected.

Figure 8.12
Laminar flow isolation unit

Careful attention to personal hygiene on the part of both patient and nurse is imporant.

Mouth care. The problems of bleeding gums and mouth ulcers and the risk of superimposed candida infection as a result of antibiotic or corticosteroid therapy make regular inspection of the mouth essential. Gentle swabbing may be needed and the patient should be encouraged to rinse his mouth frequently using a non-irritant fluid such as isotonic saline. Chlorhexidine gluconate as a mouthwash prevents the formation of plaque. Dentures, if worn, must be removed and cleaned regularly. A toothbrush should not be used by the neutropenic patient and when one is used it needs to be very soft. Soaking the brush in hot water before use will increase the softness. The patient may also need to avoid very hot or cold foods and fruit juice when the mouth is sore.

Psychological care. The needs and conditions of patients vary and each patient must be considered individually. Some patients will want to know very little while others will expect to be fully involved in discussions about their illness and its management.

The decision on whether — and how — to tell an adult patient about his condition requires careful discussion among nursing and medical staff and the patient's relatives. The hospital chaplain or family minister and the family doctor can be of great help in such a situation.

Nursing staff may be faced with difficult questions from the patient, for example on prognosis, and it is important that ways of handling these situations should be discussed. Although junior staff may not feel they have the necessary experience or knowledge to help the patient, they can ensure that questions are not ignored by getting assistance promptly from more senior nursing or medical staff. By explaining the problems to be expected, such as certain side-effects of drugs and that these do not mean that anything has gone wrong, a feeling of trust can be developed and anxiety may be eased.

The parents of a child suffering from acute leukaemia should be told the prognosis and should be given continued support from the health team at home or in hospital. Every effort is made to enable children to be looked after in their own homes.

Chronic myeloid leukaemia

Chronic myeloid leukaemia affects men slightly more frequently than women, usually between the ages of 35 and 60 years.

The onset is gradual and the patient presents with the features of progressive anaemia. Tiredness and weakness may have been present for many months. Abdominal pain may occur and the patient may have noticed swelling in the left flank due to massive enlargement of the spleen.

The blood will show a very high cell count with a combination of immature and mature cells, the latter being able to function reasonably normally. The platelet count may also be raised. The majority of these patients will have a unique chromosome abnormality known as the Philadelphia chromosome and its presence indicates a better prognosis than would otherwise be the case.

Treatment of chronic leukaemia is often less rigorous than treatment of acute leukaemia. Cytotoxic drugs such as busulphan or hydroxyurea may control the cellular proliferation for about 3 years, or occasionally for very much longer, in those patients who have the Philadelphia chromosome. Where this is absent survival is likely for only 1 year. Blood transfusion is used to correct anaemia, which is assessed by frequent blood examinations. Radiotherapy, by localized irradiation, will reduce the size of the spleen. The final outcome will probably be the development of acute leukaemia which is usually very resistant to treatment. A cure is not possible unless a successful bone marrow transplant can be performed.

Chronic lymphatic leukaemia

Chronic lymphatic leukaemia is more common than chronic myeloid leukaemia. This is a disease mainly of B lymphocytes. T lymphocytes are rarely affected. It occurs more often in men than women and affects an older age group, usually between 45 and 75 years.

The onset is very gradual, with a very slowly developing anaemia. The disease may go unnoticed until enlarged lymph nodes are found, often in the cervical, axillary or inguinal areas. The liver and spleen enlarge, but the splenic enlargement is not as great as that found in chronic myeloid leukaemia. The combination of mild anaemia, a moderately raised white cell count, although not to as great an extent as in chronic myeloid leukaemia, a slightly reduced platelet count and enlarged lymph nodes will confirm the diagnosis.

There is an increased susceptibility to viral infections, especially of the respiratory system. In some patients the disease is discovered accidentally during a medical check or treatment for some other condition such as an infection.

Many patients, especially the more elderly, may be able to lead a normal active life for many years and their life expectancy may not be reduced by the disease. As the disease progresses, treatment becomes necessary. A cytotoxic drug such as chlorambucil is given, and radiotherapy is used to treat enlarged lymph nodes.

Whenever possible, the treatment of patients with chronic forms of leukaemia is supervised by the family doctor. However, as the bone marrow progressively fails, the risks of anaemia, haemorrhage and infection increase, and hospital admission becomes necessary to allow steps to be taken to correct anaemia, control haemorrhage or treat infection.

DISORDERS INVOLVING LYMPH NODES

Lymph nodes play an important part in the immune mechanism (Ch. 1) and are widely distributed around the body. As a result of this, any disorder present can produce a wide variety of signs and symptoms and the patient's resistance to infection will be much lower than normal.

Disorders of the nodes may be either inflammatory or neoplastic. Inflammation develops as a response to either infection, as in glandular fever, or as a reactive phenomenon, as in rheumatoid arthritis. The neoplastic disorders, or lymphomas, affect both lymph nodes and other body tissues and are very similar to leukaemia, particularly lymphatic leukaemia. Lymphomas are divided into two groups, Hodgkin's disease and non-Hodgkin lymphomas, according to their histological appearance.

Hodgkin's disease

This group of malignant disorders mainly occurs in the 15 to 40 year age range but can occur at any age. The cause is unknown.

Clinical features

In the early stages the disease usually presents with painless enlargement of lymph nodes, especially in the cervical region. On occasion the patient may first present with a pyrexia of unknown origin. As the disease progresses, with other sites being involved, the signs and symptoms may include tiredness, general malaise, anaemia, dyspnoea, night sweats, fever and weight loss. Resistance to infection is also reduced.

Course and complications

The disease is slowly progressive and eventually fatal with some cases progressing very slowly and others quite rapidly. Those patients who have heavy night sweating, fever and weight loss greater than 10% of their body weight in the previous 6 months are regarded as having B symptoms. This makes the prognosis worse. However, with present day treatment cure is now possible for many patients where the disease is localized and there are no B symptoms.

Investigations

Very intensive staging procedures are carried out to determine the extent of the disease as this has an important bearing on the way in which treatment is given.

There are four stages from stage one, where the disease is confined to a single site, to stage four with widespread involvement of different parts of the body. The absence or presence of generalised symptoms is described as category A or category B. The actual investigations may include a full blood count, marrow puncture, lung tomography, lymph node biopsy, lymphangiography and a staging laparotomy.

The patient and his family will need a considerable amount of support and encouragement during this period to help them to cope with the intensity of the investigations as well as the probable diagnosis.

Treatment and nursing care

Radiotherapy is now used only when the disease is relatively localized and the patient has no category B symptoms. Cytotoxic drugs are the treatment of choice when the disease is more extensive and B symptoms are present. To minimize resistance, a combination of drugs is usually given such as mustine hydrochloride, vincristine, procarbazine and the corticosteroid, prednisolone. Sometimes both radiotherapy and chemotherapy are used. The nursing problems encountered are similar to those of patients with leukaemia (p. 311).

Non-Hodgkin lymphomas

This is another group of progressive malignant disorders of lymphoid tissue which are more numerous than the Hodgkin lymphomas. They occur most commonly in the 50 to 60 year age range but can be found at all ages. The cause is unknown but there may be a viral connection.

Signs and symptoms vary depending upon the sites involved, but in many respects the non-Hodgkin lymphomas are similar to Hodgkin's disease although their effects are often more widespread at the time of diagnosis. For this reason chemotherapy is the treatment of choice although radiotherapy is sometimes used. Some types of non-Hodgkin lymphoma will respond well to treatment and the patient is cured but in the majority of patients, resistance to treatment will eventually develop with a fatal outcome. Young patients have a poorer prognosis than older patients. Treatment and nursing care are similar to that of Hodgkin's disease.

Other malignant disorders related to the blood

Myeloma

This is a malignant disease of the plasma cells (p. 295) in the bone marrow found in the over 50 years age range, mainly in men. The tumour in the marrow erodes the bone and may eventually lead to a pathological fracture. Large amounts of immunoglobulins are also produced which cannot function normally and so the patient has a reduced resistance to infection.

The most common presenting symptoms are bone pain, often in the back and due to fracture of a vertebra, or infection, of the respiratory system in particular. The patient will be feeling generally unwell with signs of anaemia, neutropenia and thrombocytopenia due to marrow changes. This combination of clinical features can produce considerable disability especially where severe bone pain is present and fractures have developed. Hypercalcaemia is likely to develop as calcium ions are released into the bloodstream following erosion of bone. Severe renal damage may result from the high level of abnormal immunoglobulins in the blood. Both of these complications may prove fatal.

Investigations

1. Bone X-ray or scan will show changes in structure where tumours are present. More than one area may be affected.

2. Marrow puncture will show excessive numbers of abnormal plasma cells.

3. Examination of urine for presence of Bence-Jones protein, which comes from the abnormal immunoglobulins, and is excreted in urine.

Treatment and nursing care

The majority of patients will show improvement from chemotherapy using melphalan and severe bone pain can be eased very considerably by localized radiotherapy.

During the more severe stages of the illness a high degree of nursing skill is required to move and position such a patient without causing further pain, or even fractures. Regular attention is required to pressure areas, including changes of position. A bed cradle is essential. While the patient will need adequate amounts of rest, he should be encouraged and helped to move about within his limitations. This will help to minimize further loss of calcium from bone which can occur during prolonged periods of immobility. The patient also needs to be encouraged to have a good fluid intake each day to help in the excretion of calcium and so minimize the risks of renal damage.

Careful observation and reporting are needed to detect complications such as infection or hypercalcaemia quickly and treat them promptly. Early signs of hypercalcaemia are lethargy and constipation followed by vomiting, dehydration and signs of renal failure. The patient with myeloma also needs to be kept free from infection and, while protective isolation may not be needed, he should be kept away from other people who have infections, especially of the respiratory system. Relatives and friends should be advised not to visit if they have colds or sore throats. A considerable amount of help and encouragement will be needed until he begins to make progress but there is a good chance that he will improve to the extent where he will become reasonably fit and active, possibly for a number of years although the disease is normally fatal eventually.

Myelofibrosis

This is a relatively uncommon chronic progressive disorder of the blood forming tissues in the marrow. It usually occurs in the middle aged. Increasingly extensive fibrous tissue formation takes place in the bone marrow along with considerable enlargement of the spleen and liver in which blood formation takes place. The disease is eventually fatal as the result of a chronic wasting process.

Essential thrombocythaemia

This is a malignant disorder of platelet production usually found in the elderly. It is associated with a tendency both to thrombose and to bleed and is very easily treated with radioactive phosphorus. This brings the platelet count back to normal and the patient may then have many years of life.

CARE OF THE PATIENT HAVING A BLOOD TRANSFUSION

Human blood may be transfused in several forms: as whole blood or as a derivative of it, such as plasma, concentrated red cells, platelets or factor concentrates.

Plasma is given most commonly in the form of plasma protein fraction (P.P.F.). This is a useful substitute for whole blood when blood volume has to be restored quickly. However, if a coagulation defect is present or massive transfusion is necessary, then fresh frozen plasma (F.F.P.) is more suitable as it contains all the labile coagulation factors. Concentrated red cells are used when the haemoglobin level is to be raised without greatly increasing blood volume. Before transfusion, compatibility of blood must be established, that is whether the donor blood will mix with the recipient's blood without causing agglutination. The recipient's blood group is determined and, whenever possible, blood of the same group as his own is given (see Table 8.3, p. 299). The donor blood is always cross-matched by mixing it with a little of the recipient's serum to ensure that there is no agglutination. If this is not done and incompatible blood is given, serious transfusion reactions will occur. The early signs and symptoms are fever, rigors, headache, backache, urticarial rashes, vomiting and diarrhoea. Jaundice may follow haemolysis, and in severe reactions oliguria, anuria and uraemia are found.

Blood from volunteer donors is stored in 'blood banks', in special refrigerators maintained at a temperature of 4°C. The domestic ward refrigerator is not suitable for this purpose as its temperature varies. During collection, storage and administration of blood, its sterility must be maintained. Containers of whole blood or blood cells also need to be handled carefully to avoid breakdown of the cells.

It must be remembered that whole blood, as used in transfusion, is a rather different substance from the original because of the addition of the anticoagulant and nutritive solution (p. 298) needed to keep the blood in a suitable state to transfuse. Also, white blood cells and platelets are lost when the blood is stored for more than 24 hours. Whole blood can be stored for up to 4 weeks. If blood has been obtained and is not to be used for a patient it should be returned to the blood bank as quickly as possible. If this is not done the blood is wasted as once it has warmed up it cannot be reused. It is a very expensive form of treatment, especially where specific parts such as platelets or factor concentrates are required.

Complications of blood transfusion

Haemolytic reaction

Most of these reactions, in which there is an increased rate of destruction of red cells, are due to blood group incompatibility. This results from either incorrect grouping or cross-matching, or from an error in identification of the blood. The cross matching procedure is now very sophisticated and it is very unlikely that this will lead to incompatibility. Haemolytic reactions are most likely to occur because of clerical or identification errors. Failure to check the labels on the blood or confusion of identity of patients with the same or similar names may result in the wrong blood being given. The following must therefore be checked carefully by two nurses before transfusion is started: the patient's identity, the number of the unit of blood, its group, and whether it has been cross-matched and found to be compatible. If there is any discrepancy the blood must not be given. All clinical features of transfusion reaction may be present.

Allergic reaction

Mild reactions cause slight elevation of temperature and urticarial rashes. Severe reactions may lead to anaphylactic shock and are best controlled by the administration of antihistamines.

Febrile reaction

Most reactions are due to pyrogens, but haemolytic and allergic reactions and reactions due to infected blood will also cause pyrexia. The degree of elevation of temperature varies from a slight transient rise to severe rigors with hyperpyrexia or a fever prolonged over several days. The majority of these reactions are harmless to the patient, although unpleasant, and are best treated by an antipyretic such as aspirin unless this is contra-indicated.

Circulatory overload

Infusion of too much fluid over too short a period may lead to pulmonary oedema and acute heart failure because of the increased work load for the heart brought on by the increase in blood volume. For this reason, concentrated red cells are used in preference to whole blood.

Nurses should be alert to this danger when giving blood to patients with existing heart failure and should ensure that blood is given at the prescribed rate.

Increased pulse rate and sudden dyspnoea are warning features. To compensate for the increased blood volume, the doctor may prescribe a diuretic to cover the transfusion.

BLOODBANK　　**HAEMATOLOGY**

Surname		
	Ward	**Unit No.**
Forename(s)		
	D.O.B./Age	**BLOOD GROUP (if known)**
Address		ABO ǀ Rh
	Reason for request	

TRANSFUSION HISTORY			
	Yes	No	Unknown
1. Previously Transfused	☐	☐	☐
2. Transfusion Reaction	☐	☐	☐
3. Previous Pregnancy	☐	☐	☐
4. Irregular Antibodies	☐	☐	☐
5. History of Hepatitis	☐	☐	☐
DETAILS			

WHEN REQUIRED

Date　　　　　　　Time

NO. OF UNITS REQUIRED

Red Cell Conc.	Whole Blood

Group and Hold Serum ☐

Doctor's Signature

EMERGENCY TRANSFUSION REQUEST PLEASE INDICATE ☐

LAB REF. No.　　　　　**SPECIMEN RECEIVED: Date**　　　　Time

PATIENTS BLOOD GROUP		X MATCH DETAILS		
ABO	Rh			
		TIME SET UP		**READ**
UNITS X MATCHED				
ABO	Rh	UNIT No.	EXPIRY DATE	ISSUE DETAILS OF BLOOD

COMMENTS	Signed

WARD USE ONLY — To be completed by staff giving transfusion

Unit No.	Set Up By	Checked By	Date	Time Started	Finished

COMMENTS

Figure 8.13
Blood transfusion request form

Specific infections

Blood may be infected due to poor asepsis during collection, storage or transfusion. Septicaemia, profound collapse and shock, or death within hours may follow transfusion of infected blood.

A disease carried by a blood donor may be transmitted by transfusion, for example serum hepatitis, malaria or syphilis. This is prevented by careful screening of blood donors. All blood is checked for hepatitis positivity after it has been donated and before anything else is done with it and, if found to be positive, is discarded.

Due to the possibility of transfusion reactions, the form (Fig. 8.13) used to request blood from the bank is also used in the ward to check the details of every unit of blood before it is given to a patient.

The nurse has several responsibilities in the prevention of complications:

1. Ensuring that the correct blood is given to the correct patient at the prescribed rate.

2. Observing the patient carefully.

3. Recording temperature and pulse quarter hourly for the first hour of each unit and then hourly until completion of the unit.

4. Recording of fluid balance during the time of the transfusion. Should reaction be suspected, the transfusion must be slowed or stopped and the doctor informed immediately.

SUGGESTED ASSIGNMENTS

Projects

1. Compare the cost of a 2-month supply of drugs for the following patients:
   a. An elderly man with pernicious anaemia (maintenance dose).
   b. A 5-year-old child with acute leukaemia.
   c. A middle-aged housewife with mild iron deficiency anaemia (note cost of different preparations of the same drug).

2. How is blood for transfusion purposes collected, prepared and stored? If possible find this out from a visit to your nearest centre.

3. Consider what it means in practical terms to be a schoolboy with haemophilia. What facilities are provided by the government to help such a child? What advice and encouragement can be given during the periods that the boy is in hospital?

Discussion topic

To what extent should the formal education of a sick child be pursued if it is known that her prognosis is poor? Consider the implications for the education and health care teams as well as for the child and her family.

FURTHER READING

Borley D 1984 Overcoming the fears. Nursing Mirror 158 (11 January): 38–40
Bourbonnais F, Bedard J 1982 Total nursing care for the bone marrow transplant patient. The Canadian Nurse 78 (11): 17–21
DHSS Committee of Regional Transfusion Directors 1975 Notes on transfusion, 6th edn. D.H.S.S., London
Hagan S J 1983 Bring help and hope to the patient with Hodgkin's disease. Nursing 83(13): 58–63
Jones P 1974 Living with haemophilia. Medical and Technical Publishers, Lancaster
Sickle Cell Society A hand book on sickle cell disease — a guide for families.
Speechley V 1984 Administration of cytotoxic drugs. Nursing Mirror 158 (11 January): 22–25
Woodliff H J, Hermann R P 1979 Concise haematology, 2nd edn. Edward Arnold, London

Chapter Nine
The urogenital system

In keeping with tradition, the male genital and urinary tracts will be considered together in this chapter. It should however be noted that, although some structures are common to both, they are two quite separate systems. Female urinary disturbances associated with disorders of the reproductive tract are discussed in Chapter 10; those female urinary disturbances *not* associated with the reproductive tract are included in this chapter.

As many of the disorders mentioned here are unrelated to each other, a common core of symptoms and signs is not evident; for this reason there is no section dealing with the general features of disease. Some disorders of the urinary tract are found with equal frequency in both sexes and others are not; bladder infection, for example, occurs more often in women than men.

ANATOMY AND PHYSIOLOGY
The kidneys

The two kidneys flank the aorta and the inferior vena cava to which they are joined by stout blood vessels. Figure 9.1 shows the right kidney in section. The most important function of the kidneys is to **maintain constant composition and volume of the body fluids.** This control comprises:

1. Regulation of water content.
2. Regulation of electrolyte content (particularly sodium, chloride and potassium).
3. Maintenance of acid-base balance (pH of the blood).
4. Excretion of waste products of metabolism, drugs and toxic substances.

The kidneys have other functions including the production of the hormone erythropoietin, which stimulates the manufacture of red blood cells, and the hormone renin, which plays a part in vasoconstriction (Ch. 7).

Table 9.1
Normal plasma concentrations of substances referred to in text

Urea	3.3 – 6.6 mmol/l
Creatinine	44 – 150 μmol/l
K^+	3.5 – 5.0 mmol/l
Na^+	135 – 147 mmol/l
Cl^-	95 – 105 mmol/l
Bicarbonate	21 – 28 mmol/l
Ca^{++}	2.1 – 2.5 mmol/l
PO_4	0.85 – 1.55 mmol/l
Protein	65 – 80 g/l (6–9 g/dl)

Figure 9.1
Vertical section of kidney
showing normal macroscopic
appearance

Capsule

Cortex

Medulla

Renal artery

Renal vein ⎫ Hilum

Ureter

Pelvis of kidney

Glomerular capsule (endothelial cells)

Proximal convoluted tubule

Distal convoluted tubule

Efferent capillary

Afferent capillary

Glomerulus

Cubical epithelium

Squamous epithelium

Second capillary network

Collecting duct

Cubical epithelium

Position of a nephron
within the substance
of the kidney

Loop of Henle

Figure 9.2
A nephron

Maintenance of constant composition and volume of body fluids

In health the kidneys carry out this function by the formation of urine, the composition of which can be varied to suit the body's needs. For example, the end-products of protein metabolism are highly acidic, so the urine of a person taking a protein-rich diet would be more acidic than that of a vegetarian; the composition of the blood of the two individuals, on the other hand, would show only very minor differences, if any.

Each kidney is composed of approximately 1 million nephrons (Fig. 9.2), which are the basic functional units responsible for the formation of urine. Urine is derived from the blood by two important processes:

1. **Filtration,** which occurs in the glomerulus of each nephron. Because the diameter of the blood vessel entering the glomerulus is larger than that of the blood vessel leaving it, the blood pressure within the glomerular capillaries is higher than in tissue capillaries elsewhere in the body. For this reason a larger quantity of water and substances dissolved in water pass through into the glomerulus. In a normally functioning kidney substances with large molecules, for instance plasma proteins and the blood cells, are retained within the bloodstream by the capillary basement membrane (Fig. 9.3). In disease, however, protein and red cells may escape into the urine (p. 332). The kidneys have a very rich blood supply and it is estimated that around 170 litres of fluid per day are filtered through the glomeruli.

Figure 9.3
Relationship of the glomerulus to Bowman's capsule showing capillary basement membrane

2. **Selective reabsorption,** which occurs in the renal tubules. Fortunately, under the influence of ADH (Ch. 11), most of the water passed into the glomeruli is reabsorbed leaving only 1.5 litres to be passed out of the body as urine.

Production of ADH is increased during sleep and in consequence the amount of urine produced overnight is reduced. Damage to the distal portion of the tubule on which ADH acts, as in chronic renal failure, leads to a large amount of dilute urine being produced.

Substances of importance in the nutrition of the body, such as glucose and amino acids, are completely reabsorbed.

Salts, for example sodium, chloride, potassium and calcium, are removed from the filtrate according to the body's needs. Sodium reabsorption is partly controlled by the adrenal cortical hormones (Ch. 11).

Waste substances such as urea and creatinine are not reabsorbed; therefore all appear in the urine.

There is some secretion through the distal parts of the tubule of, for example, drugs and toxic substances. The filtrate continues its passage out of the nephrons and through the collecting tubules where it has the same composition as voided urine.

Healthy kidneys are so efficient that minor variations in the composition of blood plasma are corrected immediately and the proper balance is restored.

From the foregoing it becomes evident that disease of the kidneys may have far-reaching effects and, as the power to eliminate fails, waste substances begin to build up in the blood.

GLOMERULAR FILTRATION RATE

(GFR) 120 ml/min

Amino acids, glucose, lipids, Na^+, K^+, Cl^- $HCO_3^-H^+$

Vitamins, waste products and salts, acids etc.

DISTAL TUBULE
ALDOSTERONE ACTIVITY

Na^+ reabsorbed

H_2O reabsorbed into bloodstream

STRAIGHT
COLLECTING DUCT

ZONE OF
ADH ACTIVITY

Na^+ K^+ H^+ NH^+ secreted or absorbed depending on body needs— controlled by aldosterone

H_2O reabsorbed amount depends on 'body needs' —controlled by antidiuretic hormone (ADH)

PAPILLAE

BLOOD

45% Cells

55% Plasma

10% Dissolved solids

90% H_2O

Proteins 6–8 g/dl lipids

Glucose amino acids

Hormones enzymes

Salts—Na^+ K^+ Cl^- Ca^{++} etc

$HCO_3^-H^+$

Urea, uric acid creatinine

Renal blood flow (RBF)

1200 ml/min

(1.2 l/min)

PROXIMAL TUBULE
REABSORPTION

65% H_2O and Na^+

All of the glucose, amino acids, lipids, vitamins reabsorbed.

Also urea, bicarbonate, phosphate, potassium mainly by means of active transportation

K^+ and Urea secreted

H^+ secreted

NH_3^+ secreted into filtrate

The counter current mechanism by which the kidneys concentrate urine

Na^+

LOOP OF HENLE

$H_2O + Na^+$ reabsorbed ascending limb. Osmotic pressure differences between the loop of Henle and blood in the capillaries

VASA RECTA
(Capillary blood vessel)

URINE 1 ml/min

H_2O—96%

solids

organic
2%

urea

creatinine

uric acid

etc.

inorganic
2%

Na^+ Cl^-

K^+ Po_4

etc.

specific gravity 1002–1030

pH 4.5–8.2

Figure 9.4
Dynamics of kidney function

One of the earliest and most important signs of disorder is the inability of the kidneys to concentrate urine, and in the more serious of the chronic disorders the specific gravity becomes fixed at 1010. The measurement of specific gravity of urine is sometimes regarded as a chore by busy nurses who may overlook its significance: it is actually very important.

Many of the investigations listed (Table 9.2, p. 329) are concerned with the estimation of renal function.

The ureters

The ureters are two muscular tubes which convey urine from the kidneys to the urinary bladder (Fig. 9.5). Each is continuous with the renal pelvis, which itself is continuous with the hilum of the kidney. The ureters are about 25 cm long and pass down the posterior abdominal wall behind the peritoneum. They pass over the brim of the pelvis and enter the lower posterior surface of the bladder at an oblique angle. The mucous lining of the ureter is of transitional epithelium. Urine is funnelled into the ureter via the renal pelvis and is conveyed to the bladder by peristaltic-like action. The oblique entry of the ureters into the bladder and the arrangement of the bladder muscle normally prevent reflux of urine.

Figure 9.5
Kidneys, ureters and bladder:
relationships

The urinary bladder

The urinary bladder is a hollow, muscular organ which lies in the anterior part of the pelvic cavity immediately behind the symphysis pubis (Fig. 9.6). The upper surface is covered by peritoneum in the male (For details of the pelvic anatomy in the female, see Chapter 10.)

The muscle is chiefly made up of interlacing bundles of involuntary muscle tissue. The inner lining consists of several layers of transitional epithelium which allows expansion as the bladder fills with urine. The urethra leaves the bladder at its lowest point. The triangle formed by the openings of the ureters and the urethra is called the trigone. This area does not expand as the bladder fills (see incontinence, p. 327).

Figure 9.6
Sagittal section of male pelvis
showing bladder only partially
sectioned

The urethra and the penis

The urethra is the passage which conveys urine from the bladder to the outside of the body. In the male it can be divided into three main parts:

1. Prostatic.
2. Membranous.
3. Penile.

The prostatic urethra is about 2.5 cm long and is closely surrounded by the prostate gland. The membranous urethra passes through several layers of membranes and muscles which form the external urethral sphincter. The bulbourethral glands, which secrete a lubricating fluid, lie between these membranes. Their ducts enter the membranous urethra. The penile urethra traverses the length of the corpus spongiosum, which is one of the three cylinders of cavernous erectile tissue comprising the penis (Fig. 9.7). The urethral meatus opens on to the bulbous anterior part of the penis — the glans penis. The glans is covered by a movable cuff of skin called the prepuce or foreskin.

The urethra in the female is very short and for this reason micro-organisms gain access to the bladder more readily than in the male (see cystitis, p. 326).

The prostate gland

The prostate gland completely encloses the urethra as it leaves the bladder. It is about the size of a chestnut and produces a watery fluid which is added to the secretions of the testes and seminal vesicles. Also entering the prostate gland are the ejaculatory ducts from the seminal vesicles. The seminal vesicles are, in turn, linked to the testes by the vas deferens, which conveys the spermatozoa from the testes.

The seminal vesicles

These are two small hollow organs; they produce a 'sticky fluid' which is added to that produced by the testes and prostate gland. Spermatozoa are stored in the ampulla of the vas deferens.

Figure 9.7
Transverse section of penis

Corpus cavernosum

Urethra

Corpus spongiosum

Epididymis

Vas deferens

Tunica vaginalis

Tunica albuginea and septa

Seminiferous tubules

Figure 9.8
Section of testis

Spermatozoa

Interstitial cells

Figure 9.9
Microscopic appearance of seminiferous tubule

The testes

The two testes lie in a small, muscular sac called the scrotum. Each testis is a solid organ and is about 4 cm long. It is surrounded by a serous membrane, the tunica vaginalis, and once this is removed a tough fibrous coat of a whitish appearance, the tunica albuginea, is exposed. The fibrous coat gives rise to septa which divide the testis into about 250 lobules (Fig. 9.8). Each lobule contains from one to four seminiferous tubules. The lining of the seminiferous tubules generates the spermatozoa (Fig. 9.9), which are wafted towards the epididymis and on to the vas deferens. Under the influence of a hormone from the anterior lobe of the pituitary gland the interstitial cells, which lie between the seminiferous tubules, produce testosterone. Testosterone helps maintain the secondary sexual characteristics.

INVESTIGATIONS

An array of tests and examinations may be carried out, particularly in renal disorder, either to pinpoint a diagnosis or to monitor the patient's progress. Table 9.2 shows those most often used.

Minor variations in practice are common so the nurse should be quite certain of local procedure before embarking upon any test. Failure to do so may mean that an entire investigation has to be repeated which will cause the patient inconvenience and will prolong his stay in hospital.

DISORDERS OF THE URINARY TRACT

Urinary tract infections

Urine provides an excellent medium for the growth of micro-organisms so that infections of the urinary tract are very common, especially in women. The infection may be a complication of some anatomical abnormality but more often than not the urinary tract is quite normal. There is little doubt that most of the urinary tract infections gain access to the urinary bladder by ascending the urethra. In the female the urethra is only about 3 cm long and appears to offer little resistance to invasion by micro-organisms found in and around the entrance to the vagina. Once in the bladder these normally commensal bacteria for example *E. coli* become pathogenic. In males, not only is the urethra longer but the seminal chord and prostatic secretions are thought to be bactericidal and so create an additional barrier to invading micro-organisms. No similar secretion has been identified as yet in females.

In the past few years doctors have become increasingly aware of the problem of vesicoureteric reflux especially in young girls; in this condition some of the urine passes back into the ureters during micturition. If the urine is already infected the kidney also quickly becomes infected. Often this type of infection is asymptomatic and attempts are now being made to establish screening procedures for girls, when they start school or earlier, so that the problem can be dealt with. It is also becoming increasingly obvious that it is this group of individuals, who have established urinary tract infection by the age of 10 or so, who go on to develop chronic renal disease in adult life. A woman who develops an upper urinary tract infection for the first time in adult life, and whose infection is adequately treated and followed up, rarely develops chronic pyelonephritis. It still remains a fact however, that among women who develop chronic renal failure pyelonephritis is one of the more common causes.

Cystitis and urethritis

Some infections of the urinary tract are confined to the urethra and bladder; in adult women one predisposing factor to recurring bladder infection is sexual intercourse causing mechanical irritation or bruising of the urethra. In this group of patients it is important, when establishing a diagnosis, to enquire about the relationship of symptoms to sexual intercourse.

Clinical features

The features of systemic illness are slight: the patient complains of frequency of micturition which is accompanied by pain in the region of the urethra on voiding urine. In cystitis, although the bladder is empty, there may be an intense desire to pass more urine (strangury) due to spasm of the inflamed wall. In some patients with symptoms suggestive of urethritis and cystitis no organisms can be cultured from the urine.

Treatment

Treatment of urethritis and cystitis is the same as that of infection elsewhere in the urinary tract, namely, the use of antibacterial drugs, for example sulphonamides. The choice of drug should be governed by the sensitivity of the organisms.

Normally a midstream specimen of urine is obtained for culture, and treatment is started immediately with the drug that is most likely to be effective. When the laboratory report is available drug therapy is reconsidered in the light of the organisms found.

Even well-selected drugs, however, cannot be effective if there is an anatomical deformity or obstructive lesion of the urinary tract, so the underlying cause must be sought when infection is persistent or recurrent.

It is common practice to give a 2-week course of drugs followed by a repeat urine culture when treatment is completed. A high urine output is an advantage because frequent emptying of a full bladder voids many organisms and so discourages their multiplication; therefore, the patient should be encouraged to take plenty of fluids.

Doctors exercise care when using some of the antibacterial drugs useful in treating urinary infections because, in patients with impaired renal function, they accumulate in the blood and this may lead to permanent nerve deafness and vestibular damage.

Pyelonephritis

Pyelonephritis is a condition in which there is bacterial infection of the kidney substance and renal pelvis. Of the many predisposing factors obstruction of the urinary tract, diabetes mellitus, pregnancy, ureteric reflux, sexual activity and, in the hospital setting, the introduction of instruments into the renal tract are perhaps the most common. As many as 50% of women will develop a urinary tract infection at some time in their lives. Clinically pyelonephritis may be acute or chronic. The term pyelitis is best avoided as it suggests that the condition is confined to the renal pelvis.

Acute pyelonephritis

This is an acute inflammatory infection of the kidney parenchyma. It nearly always occurs as a result of ascending infection. The most common infecting micro-organism is *E. coli*, 85% of cases, whilst enterobacter, klebsiella, proteus, pseudomonas and enterococci account for the other 15%. The micro-organisms have several major hurdles to overcome before reaching the kidney but once in the kidney the medulla region is very susceptible to infection and the cortex only slightly less so.

Clinical features

All the features of cystitis and urethritis (p. 326) are present. In addition there is pain and tenderness in both loin regions. There will be pyrexia or hyperpyrexia depending on the severity of the infection. Nausea, vomiting, sweating and on occasion rigors are all indicative of considerable systemic involvement. The urine may look cloudy and usually has an unpleasant smell; a 'fishy' odour is associated with infections caused by *E. coli*.

The diagnosis is confirmed by obtaining a midstream specimen (MSU) for culture and sensitivity. A colony count of 10^5 indicates significant bacteriuria, counts of 10^4–10^5 are uncertain and counts of 10^4 or below suggest contamination. If the results are in doubt, then the MSU is repeated.

Treatment and nursing care

The medical treatment is to give antibiotics. These are started when a presumptive diagnosis is made and may have to be changed once the results of the culture and sensitivity tests become available. The most common antibiotics used are cotrimoxazole, ampicillin, cephalexin, kanamycin, nalidixic acid, carbenicillin, gentamycin and doxycycline. These patients are often very ill and must be confined to bed during the acute phase until the temperature falls. They will not usually feel like doing much else anyway. The patient will require all the nursing care of a febrile patient. A liberal fluid intake is ensured. A fluid intake and output chart is maintained and the urinary output observed carefully. Any evidence of a decrease in urine output may indicate the beginning of renal failure, as also may a rise in blood pressure.

Four hourly TPR and BP should be recorded and any changes reported to the medical staff. The midstream specimens of urine are obtained at intervals to find out whether or not the infection has cleared. If the infection is recurrent a full urinary tract investigation is necessary. A micturating cystogram (Table 9.2) may show evidence of vesicoureteric reflux. Sometimes in the case of a child, this may right itself spontaneously as the child grows older, but in other cases the urologist may have to operate on the faulty valve. Failure to treat acute episodes of pyelonephritis adequately may very well lead to the development of chronic pyelonephritis.

Chronic pyelonephritis

As the term implies this is a continuing pyogenic infection of the kidneys. It is usually rather patchy in distribution and ultimately causes distortion of the kidneys due to fibrosis or scarring (Fig. 9.10B.) The disease may follow an attack of acute pyelonephritis which has been treated inadequately. It may also be caused by infection occurring above an obstruction in the urinary tract, such as stones, urethral stricture or prostatic enlargement.

Clinical features

Often the symptoms are non-specific and the patient may approach the doctor because of lassitude and vague ill health. Symptoms from the urinary tract may, however, be present and include frequency of micturition, dysuria and occasionally loin pain.

The clearest way of demonstrating chronic pyelonephritis is by an intravenous urogram, which may reveal a decrease in thickness of kidney cortex, irregularity of the renal outline and differences in the size of the two kidneys.

Figure 9.10
Kidney diseases

A Normal kidney

B Chronic pyelonephritis

C Chronic glomerulonephritis

D Polycystic

E Hydronephrosis

F Papillary necrosis

Table 9.2
Investigations

Procedure	Purpose and method	Preprocedure, care of patient and notable points	Special postprocedure care	Complications	When used
History and clinical examination	To establish main features of disorder and make provisional diagnosis. To establish base lines	No special care. Examination performed by doctor	Nil	Nil	All patients
Urine testing	To detect abnormal constituents, e.g. sugar, albumin, bile, urobilinogen (follow reagent manufacturer's instructions). Observe colour, odour, deposits, specific gravity, osmolality and measure amount	Explain need for specimen of urine. Provide suitable receptacle labelled with patient's name. Specimens should be tested when fresh.	Record results and report to nurse in charge	Nil	All patients as part of routine screening
Midstream specimen of urine (MSU)	To obtain specimens of urine not contaminated with micro-organisms from outside the urinary tract. Specimen is tested in laboratory for presence of micro-organisms and their sensitivity to antimicrobial drugs	Explain procedure to patient. Cleanse genital area around urethra as per hospital policy. Ask patient to start passing urine. Collect specimen in a sterile container before flow ceases. (N.B. Not the first urine passed.)	Send specimen immediately to laboratory in sterile universal container with relevant forms	Nil	When urinary tract infection (UTI) is suspected or as a screening procedure
Catheter specimen of urine (CSU)	As MSU	See care of self-retaining catheter	As MSU	Nil	As MSU
24-hour urine collection	To measure amount of certain substances excreted in 24-hour period. Results compared with known normal values	Explain procedure to patient. Collect labelled container provided by laboratory (may have preservative depending on test). Start test at 8 a.m. Ask patient to empty bladder and discard specimen. Collect all urine passed during next 24 hours. The last specimen is obtained at 8 a.m.	As in MSU/CSU, above	Nil	In kidney function tests, hormone gland studies, investigation of blood disorders, etc.
Concentration dilution tests	To assess kidney function and posterior pituitary function	For details of these tests consult local procedure manuals, as practices vary considerably	Some patients require close observation to ensure that dehydration does not occur, especially in pituitary studies.	Dehydration	Kidney and pituitary disease
Urea and creatinine clearance tests	Index of kidney damage. Designed to show how much blood is cleared of a substance per minute. (Creatinine once filtered into the tubule is not reabsorbed.)	As for 24-hour urine collection. Blood specimens are taken concurrently	Specimens are sent to laboratory in appropriate containers with request forms.	Nil	Kidney disease

Table 9.2
Investigations (*contd*)

Procedure	Purpose and method	Preprocedure, care of patient and notable points	Special postprocedure care	Complications	When used
Straight X-ray	To show up tissues of different density	Explanation of procedure	Nil	Nil but caution in pregnancy	Initial screening. Assess kidney size, calculi, suspected chest secondaries
Blood chemistry tests	To measure kidneys' ability to excrete metabolic wastes, e.g. urea, creatinine and electrolytes	No special care	Nil	Rare if properly executed	Routine screening procedure and indicator of direction of disease process
Intravenous pyelogram (IVP) (urogram)	To show an outline of the whole urinary tract on X-ray and indicate kidney function. A radio-opaque compound is introduced intravenously which is then excreted by the kidney	Explain procedure to patient. Consult local instruction manual. Preparation usually includes giving light diet day before and laxative evening before to clear stomach and intestines of gas. Food and fluids are restricted for 6–8 hours before procedure	A cup of tea and toast will be appreciated	May have a reaction to contrast media during the procedure. Patient needs special care if in renal failure	Any suspected kidney disease. Not normally used during pregnancy
Retrograde pyelography	Used to outline detail of pelvis, calyces, ureter. Contrast media is injected into the kidney via a ureteric catheter inserted through a cystoscope	As for anaesthetic. See cystoscopy below	Observe urinary output and test for blood. Other care as for postanaesthesia.	Haematuria, infection, trauma to the urethra, bladder and ureter	When detail has not been obtained from IVP as in non-functioning kidney. Renal calculi.
Voiding cystogram or micturating urethrogram	To show outline of bladder on X-ray, contrast media is introduced into the bladder through a catheter. Patient asked to empty bladder and serial X-ray pictures will show behaviour of lower urinary tract	Explain procedure, patient is catheterized. See catheterization	Observe urinary output. Test for blood. High fluid intake	Urinary tract-infection, haemorrhage, damage to urethra or bladder	Bladder tumours, diverticulitis, incontinence, vesico-ureteric reflux
Isotope renography	To give an indication of renal blood flow. (Hippuric acid labelled with I^{131} is injected i.v.) A Geiger counter placed over the kidneys records the appearance and disappearance of radioactivity	Explain procedure	Nil	Very rarely reaction to the isotope	Suspected obstruction in kidney. Renal transplant
Isotope scanning of kidney	A radioactive isotope of mercury or technetium is given i.v. This is taken up by the kidney tubules and a sensor device is passed to and fro over the kidney and a picture of the isotope concentration can be built up	Explain procedure	Nil	None	Renal tumours and cysts

Table 9.2
Investigations (contd)

Procedure	Purpose and method	Preprocedure, care of patient and notable points	Special postprocedure care	Complications	When used
Renal biopsy	To remove a small section of the kidney substance for pathological examination. Light, electron and immunofluorescent microscopy techniques are used	Explain procedure. Assess patient and gain co-operation. Obtain written consent. Other care as for any minor operation under local anaesthetic. Kidney is localized by X-ray and surface anatomical landmarks. Blood must be available for transfusion if necessary	Patient must be nursed in bed at complete rest for first 4 hours. Observations of BP and pulse $\frac{1}{4}$ hourly initially. If condition remains satisfactory the frequency of observations can be reduced. All urine is observed for haematuria — bed rest until urine is clear, at least 24 hours of bed rest is advisable	Haemorrhage, shock, infection, pain	Diagnosis of diffuse renal disease, e.g. differentiation of glomerulonephritis. Contraindication perinephric abscess and renal tumour
Cystoscopy and biopsy	To inspect the interior of the bladder, diagnose and treat urethral and bladder disorders by means of an endoscope introduced through the urethra	Explain procedure. As for general anaesthetic (may on occasion be done under local anaesthetic)	As for general anaesthetic depending on whether procedure is for diagnosis or treatment (see postoperative care). Observation of vital signs, and urine for blood	Haemorrhage. Trauma of urethra and bladder. Complications of general anaesthetic. Urinary tract infection	Diagnosis of bladder and urethral disorders. Treatment of bladder tumours. Transurethral prostatectomy. Taking biopsies for pathology (see retrograde pyelogram)
Renal angiogram	To obtain details of the renal blood supply using X-ray and fluoroscopy techniques. A contrast medium is introduced via a catheter inserted into a major artery, e.g. femoral	As for IVP (see above)	Bed rest 8 hours. Pressure dressing over puncture wound. Observations of vital signs and pulses distal to puncture site.	Haemorrhage from puncture site. Haematuria.	Diagnosis of suspected renal artery stenosis. Renal neoplasms. Abnormal renal vessels
Cystometrogram	To assess the response of the detrusor muscle to filling	As for cytoscopy above	As for cystoscopy above	As for cystoscopy above	Urinary incontinence

Treatment

If treatment is to be really effective it must be started before serious renal damage has occurred. The principles of treatment are the same as for acute pyelonephritis: isolation and efficient eradication of the infecting organism and investigation of the urinary tract for any abnormalities of structure. Where the damage to the kidney tissue is substantial the management is similar to that of chronic renal failure.

Tuberculosis

Tuberculosis of the kidney is always secondary to a primary infection elsewhere in the body and, reflecting the overall pattern of tuberculosis, has diminished in incidence in the United Kingdom over the past few decades.

Clinical features

The patient is often relatively fit, the chief complaint being that of increasing urinary frequency which may become so severe as to be intolerable. Pain in the loin due to obstructive lesions may also be a feature. Diagnosis is confirmed by culturing the tubercle bacilli from specimens of early morning concentrated urine, but as these organisms can take anything up to 12 weeks to culture radiological confirmation of the disease may be sought.

Treatment

Once the diagnosis has been established conservative treatment with the proven antituberculous drugs is commenced. Drugs are used in combination and include the following: sodium aminosalicylate (PAS), isonazid, ethambutol, rifampicin and streptomycin. Two or three of these drugs are given at any one time, the combinations being changed at intervals to avoid bacterial resistance. The treatment is continued for up to 2 years. Surgery is only indicated if the disease is very advanced on one side — provided the other kidney is functioning satisfactorily.

DISORDERS OF THE KIDNEYS

A number of pathological disorders may involve the kidneys, among them the group of diseases known to the layman as Bright's disease or nephritis. Nephritis is classified variously by different authorities and the terminology is changed as new discoveries regarding the complex functions of the kidneys and disease processes are made.

The following classification is generally accepted in the Western world:

Acute proliferative glomerulonephritis.
Minimal lesion glomerulonephritis.
Membranous glomerulonephritis.
Chronic glomerulonephritis.
Chronic renal failure may be a sequel to any of these conditions and nephrotic syndrome may follow minimal lesion or membranous glomerulonephritis.
Acute renal failure more commonly arises from some sudden severe disturbance of the circulation than from disease within the kidney itself.

In health the products of metabolism are excreted by the kidneys but in disease of the kidneys their function is impaired allowing urea, creatinine and anions such as phosphate and sulphate to build up in the blood. The concentration of blood urea gives useful indications of the degree of failure; the level only rising when function is reduced by 50% or more. It is for this reason that urea levels are monitored so closely, not because the rise in the amount of urea itself is more harmful than accumulations of other end products of metabolism.

It follows that the clinical features of nephritis and renal failure mostly result from abnormalities in chemical composition of the body or from hypertension and not locally from the site of the diseased kidneys.

The protein in urine when it is present is albumin rather than globulin because albumin is of smaller molecular size and can therefore penetrate the diseased glomerular membrane in larger amounts.

Acute proliferative glomerulonephritis

This is an acute inflammatory disease of the glomeruli. There is often a history of streptococcal infection of the throat or occasionally of the skin some 10 to 14 days before the onset of the renal illness. It can affect any age group but is most likely to happen in childhood.

Clinical features

As a result of glomerular damage there is reduced filtration and increased reabsorption of water and salt by the tubules causing the patient to develop generalized oedema. This is most noticeable in the face, which looks pale and puffy. Urinary output is low (oliguria), about 500 ml daily, and small amounts of blood (haematuria) give the urine a smoky appearance. Proteinuria is also present. The patient usually shows features of an acute infection, including malaise, fever and anorexia.

Hypertension, dyspnoea, and pulmonary oedema are often prominent features. Headaches, papilloedema, convulsions and loss of consciousness may follow.

Investigations to confirm the diagnosis include urinalysis, blood chemistry, fluid balance charting and weighing. The antistreptolysin titre may be raised and a throat swab may show the presence of haemolytic streptococci.

Treatment and nursing care

Bed rest and warmth are important during the acute phase and should be continued until haematuria, proteinuria, oedema and hypertension have disappeared. Reduction of protein intake to 20–40 g/day controls the degree of uraemia (that is, when the blood level of urea rises above 6.6 mmol/l). Fluids are restricted to half a litre plus the equivalent of the volume of the previous day's output while the oedema is present and until a diuresis occurs.

A 'no added salt' diet is prescribed in which no salt is used in cooking and no table salt is added to meals; if the oedema is severe a very low salt diet may be given (Ch. 7). The nursing staff should appreciate that this is an extremely unpalatable diet and should do everything possible to tempt the patient to eat. It is important that meals are served attractively.

The original infection, if still present, is treated with an antibiotic. If the hypertension is not controlled by salt and fluid restrictions, drug therapy will be required especially if the dangerous complications of hypertensive encephalopathy (Ch. 7) develops. Pulmonary oedema and acute renal failure (see p. 335) are other complications.

The prognosis for children suffering from this type of glomerulonephritis is good, the majority recovering completely. Recovery is less complete when it occurs in adults, acute renal failure is more common and may progress to chronic glomerulonephritis.

Minimal lesion glomerulonephritis and membranous glomerulonephritis

In minimal lesion glomerulonephritis, as the name suggests, there is very little change in the microscopic appearance of the kidneys but serious functional disorder. In membranous glomerulonephritis histological examination of a biopsy specimen shows thickening of the capillary basement membrane. Some authorities attribute this to an antigen-antibody reaction which results in an allergic response.

The two conditions are described together because they are clinically indistinguishable at the outset. Minimal lesion glomerulonephritis, however, usually occurs in the 5 to 15-year-old age group while membranous glomerulonephritis more commonly occurs in those approaching middle age.

Clinical features

The conditions are associated with an increase in the permeability of the basement membrane leading to proteinuria; it may be only slight and therefore may persist undetected for some time. As the proteinuria increases in severity generalized oedema occurs, which is often the first presenting sign. As much as 30 g of protein per day may be excreted in the urine causing the total plasma content to become greatly depleted.

Diagnosis is established by renal biopsy and histological examination of a specimen of renal tissue.

Treatment

Where minimal lesion glomerulonephritis occurs in children a course of steroid treatment is given.

The prognosis for patients with membranous glomerulonephritis is less favourable and at present there is no form of drug treatment for this condition. One-third of sufferers will recover to complete health but the remainder are liable to develop arterial hypertension (Ch. 7) and progressive renal destruction leading to gradual impairment of renal function and chronic glomerulonephritis.

Chronic glomerulonephritis

This condition may follow either acute proliferative glomerulonephritis or membranous glomerulonephritis. The glomeruli are progressively destroyed and replaced by fibrous tissue. Kidneys so affected are much smaller than normal and have a granular appearance (Fig. 9.10C).

Often, however, no history of either disease is obtained and the pathological changes in the kidney seem to develop insidiously over many years. The end result is the same, however — chronic failure of renal function.

Nephrotic syndrome

Any patient with heavy proteinuria (more than 5 g/24 h), gross oedema and a low serum albumin is described as having nephrotic syndrome; this is regardless of his age and the cause of his condition.

Causes

The main causes of nephrotic syndrome are glomerulonephritis, renal vein thrombosis, diabetes mellitis, amyloidosis, certain drugs, malaria, connective tissue (collagen) diseases and new growths.

Clinical features

The most striking feature of this syndrome is very heavy proteinuria. Such a loss of protein in the urine is more than can be met by the dietary intake and the result is a low serum albumin (hypoalbuminaemia) which in turn results in a low osmotic pressure and a reduced volume. The low osmotic pressure is responsible for the generalized oedema (anasarca) which is so distressing for the patient. The liver, in an attempt to synthesize enough albumin, manufactures an excess of cholesterol and lipids so that hyperlipidaemia is another characteristic of the syndrome.

Patients with nephrotic syndrome are very prone to infection and premature atheroma.

A variety of other clinical features related to the underlying cause may of course also be present.

Investigations

In addition to investigating the predisposing condition a full urinary tract investigation (Table 9.2) is carried out.

Treatment and nursing care

Treatment is directed towards the relief of oedema and the control of proteinuria. Nursing care of the oedematous patient is described in Chapter 7.

A protein intake of 90–100 g per day is desirable to make good the urinary loss of protein as long as the blood urea is not elevated. Salt intake is restricted by prohibiting salty foods, cooking and table salt. Diuretics may also be used to control oedema.

Corticosteroids such as prednisolone are often effective in young patients whose condition has resulted from glomerulonephritis.

The course of the disease is unpredictable and just occasionally it resolves spontaneously.

Renal failure (uraemia)

Renal failure is a state in which kidney function is no longer able to maintain the body chemistry within normal limits. It can be acute, acute on chronic or chronic.

Figure 9.11
Acute renal failure

Acute renal failure (acute uraemia)

A wide range of disorders may cause this condition and it is convenient to classify these as prerenal, renal and postrenal (Table 9.3). The effects produced are similar regardless of cause and even with all the resources currently available there is still a very high mortality rate. Acute tubular necrosis (severe damage to the renal tubules due to ischaemia) is a feature of around a third of patients with acute renal failure.

The possible outcomes of acute renal failure are shown in Figure 9.11.

Clinical features

The onset is sudden, the first sign being a marked reduction in urinary output (oliguria) which may progress to complete anuria. The blood urea level rises rapidly especially in patients who are hypercatabolic and using up body proteins for instance following burns. There is also serious disturbance of electrolytes with a dangerous accumulation of potassium (K^+) which in turn produces changes in the electrical conductivity of the heart leading to life threatening arrhythmias. Changes in rhythm may be seen on an ECG.

Investigations

Tests are carried out to establish baselines and to record the response (or lack of response) to treatment. The role of the nurse in monitoring the patient's condition is crucial.

Urinalysis is essential and all urine passed, however small the amount, must be saved and kept in separate containers. Urine volume is often less than 500 ml in 24 hours. In addition to volume, specific gravity (often fixed at 1010) and osmolality measurements are carried out. The urine is tested for blood and other abnormal constituents in the ward whilst specimens are also sent to the laboratory for estimates of myoglobin, sodium and urea. Serial measurements of blood urea, creatinine and electrolytes together with the urine volumes are an essential guide to treatment. The patient should be weighed daily on sensitive bed scales.

Four hourly records of TPR and BP are obligatory.

If a postrenal cause is suspected (Table 9.3) a plain abdominal X-ray may show the presence of calculi (see p. 347) and intravenous urography and/or retrograde pyelography may be necessary to establish the level of obstruction.

Treatment and nursing care

As these patients are very ill the general nursing care must be of the very highest standard. Treatment is aimed at reducing or minimizing the disturbances due to the renal failure, preventing infection and maintaining nutrition.

Prerenal	*Impaired blood supply to the kidneys*
	Severe haemorrhage
	Shock, burns, dehydration, crush injuries
	Incompatible blood transfusion
	Myocardial infarction
	Disseminated intravascular clotting
	Nephrotoxic poisons such as:
	    carbon tetrachloride, paraquat, phenindione,
	    cephaloridine and gentamycin
	Overwhelming infection

Renal	Diseases of the renal parenchyma Acute glomerular nephritis Acute tubular necrosis Acute pyelonephritis Connective tissue disorders
Postrenal	*Obstruction to the outflow of urine* Stones: ureter/urethra Strictures: ureter/urethra Tumours: kidney/bladder Crystalluria Prostatic hypertrophy

Table 9.3
Causes of acute renal failure

Following the initial assessment of fluid and electrolyte balance a planned intake of fluid is given to replace fluids lost as urine and as insensible loss, i.e. 400–500 ml plus an amount equivalent to the previous day's urine volume. It is vital therefore that accurate fluid balance charts are maintained. Because of the low urinary output, very little salt is excreted in the urine so that dietary salt must be limited strictly to 1.5 g/day (24 mEq). Dietary potassium must be restricted for the same reason and if plasma potassium levels cannot be controlled in this way, an ion exchange resin such as Calcium Resonium 15 g three times a day may be prescribed. This substance is rather unpalatable so it may be necessary to administer it via a nasogastric tube or per rectum. If the rise is very rapid and the level goes above 6 mmol/l then other measures such as glucose 20–50 g and soluble insulin 10–20 units via an intravenous infusion may be given. The insulin promotes the transfer of K^+ ions into the cells and so lowers the serum potassium levels. Calcium gluconate 1–2 g i.v. may be given to protect the heart from the toxic effects of hyperkalaemia.

The restrictions in the amount of fluids, salts and proteins which can be given may make it difficult to ensure an adequate Kilojoule intake. However these patients must receive sufficient kilojoules (11.8 MJ–14.7 MJ) with just enough protein (30–40 g) to meet the body's needs and to prevent the breakdown of tissue protein which would cause the serum urea and potassium levels to rise rapidly. Concentrated glucose solutions such as Hycal and Caloreen which are fairly palatable are often used to boost Calorie intake. They are free of electrolytes. If the patient cannot take food orally or if this route is contraindicated for some other reason, then parenteral nutrition may be necessary. Lipids, carbohydrates and amino acid preparations can all be given intravenously.

One of the most serious complications is infection; indeed it is infection that is the cause of the high mortality rate which is still a feature of this disorder.

Nursing measures to prevent the spread of infection (Ch. 1) must be followed carefully. Procedures such as catheterization should be avoided if possible. If nutritional needs are being met parenterally, diligence is required in caring for the infusion site and equipment as infection is often a sequel to this procedure.

Specific nursing measures to prevent pressure sores (Ch. 14), stomatis (Ch. 5), chest infections (Ch. 6) and deep venous thrombosis (Ch. 7) are essential. Antibiotics are not usually prescribed prophylactically but will, of course, be ordered if needed. In general drugs which are excreted by the kidneys are avoided. Nurses need to be watchful for the side effects of drugs and report any such occurrence promptly.

Patients suffering from acute renal failure who are in a hypercatabolic state and those where the measures outlined above have not been successful in keeping the blood urea below 34 mmol/l will require either peritoneal or haemodialysis (see pp. 341–346).

Following the phase of oliguria lasting several weeks the urinary output increases dramatically as the nephrons begin to heal. This second stage is called the diuretic phase but this does not mean that the kidneys have made a complete recovery. It is several weeks or months before the kidneys are able to maintain homeostasis. Therefore during this phase dietary and other measures, even dialysis must continue until there is a definite spontaneous improvement. Some doctors prescribe diuretics such as frusemide during the oliguric phase and it is claimed this shortens this phase.

Chronic renal failure (chronic uraemia)

Chronic failure occurs when the kidneys are progressively and irreversibly destroyed over a period of time.

The renal diseases which most commonly lead to chronic renal failure are glomerulonephritis, pyelonephritis and polycystic disease (see p. 340) of the kidneys. It may also arise as a complication of hypertension, diabetes mellitus and many other diseases. Infections, nephrotoxic drugs and chronic obstruction of the urinary tract are additional causes. In most patients the disorder runs a slow insidious course and is often missed initially.

Clinical features

The clinical picture is seldom clear cut. The early symptoms of lassitude, anaemia, mild depression and so on are all too vague to warrant very active investigations. Other more specific symptoms such as polyuria and nocturia have often become so much a part of the patient's accepted routine that they are not mentioned to the doctor. For these reasons the disease is often well advanced by the time the patient is referred for a full renal investigation.

As the disease progresses to severe renal failure every system and part of the body is affected in some way (Table 9.4). Anaemia caused by lack of erythropoietin, which normally stimulates production of red blood cells by the bone marrow, is responsible for the lethargy. Polyuria develops because of the impaired concentrating ability of the kidneys and the excess sodium secreted by the diseased tubules. Anorexia, nausea and vomiting are common.

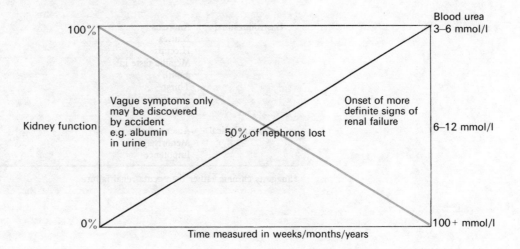

Figure 9.12
Chronic renal failure

Table 9.4
Severe renal failure (After Curtis J R 1978 Chronic renal failure. Practitioner 220:909 June 1978)

	Symptoms		Signs
Neurological	Poor memory Lack of concentration Drowsiness Fits Paraesthesiae in feet Restless legs	Uraemic encephalopathy	Tremor Twitching Asterixis Coma Hyperreflexia Signs of peripheral neuropathy*
Muscular	Cramps Weakness		Signs of proximal myopathy* especially of pelvic girdle musculature in renal osteomalacia
Psychiatric	Hallucinations Depression Delusions Mania Anxiety		
Ocular	Sore eyes		Corneal and conjunctival calcification* 'Red eyes' Hypertensive retinopathy Detached retina
Haematological	Fatigue Dyspnoea Bruising Nose-bleeds		Anaemia* Purpura Bruises
Cutaneous	Itching		Scratch marks Pigmentation* Purpura Dry skin
Skeletal	Bone pains		'Renal rickets' in children*
Joints	'Arthritis'		Gout and pseudogout*
Cardiovascular	Dyspnoea Chest pain Orthopnoea Swelling of the legs		Hypertension Left ventricular failure Raised jugular venous pressure Oedema Left ventricular hypertrophy* Pericardial effusion Pericardial rub* Saline depletion and hypotension
Gastrointestinal	Anorexia Nausea Hiccups Metallic taste in mouth Thirst Vomiting Diarrhoea		Oral ulceration Foetor (ammoniacal) Parotitis
Endocrinological	Amenorrhoea Menorrhagia Impotence		Gynaecomastia*

*Suggests chronic rather than acute renal failure

Continuing deterioration in renal function results in an increasing build-up of urea and acid waste products of metabolism. This relative acidity of the blood — in fact the pH indicates that it is still slightly alkaline — is called **acidosis.** Deep, sighing respirations are characteristic of severe renal failure; so too is the almost ammoniacal smell of the patient's breath and sweat. There are other associated features such as hypertension, which may in turn lead to left and then right-sided heart failure.

Distressing hiccups, muscle twitchings and increasing drowsiness precede terminal coma and death.

Figure 9.12 shows the effect of diminishing kidney function over a period of time.

Treatment and nursing care

It is important to realise that the different syndromes described above may occur in succession during the course of a single disease. Some patients may have symptomatic proteinuria when they first come to attention, but later may become nephrotic before eventually succumbing to chronic renal failure. The patient therefore needs to be assessed frequently. This is vital so that the nursing care given is what is needed. Patients, when feeling well, may be reluctant to comply with dietary and drug regimes and need help and encouragement. Each patient should be involved in planning his own care. His dietary dislikes and likes must be considered, so that a diet he is likely to comply with is planned. This sort of reasoning applies to all aspects of care. As the condition deteriorates over many years, changes need to be made which will enable him to remain independent for as long as possible. Any treatable underlying cause of the renal dysfunction such as infection and obstruction must be dealt with. This may arrest the disease process and lead to a marked improvement in the individual's health. In many, however, there are no specific treatments though some measure of control by drugs and diet will help. All such regimes are restricting and to the individual who feels constantly miserable and unwell compliance may seem hardly worthwhile.

Diet

Protein is usually restricted to 40 or 60 g/day but with no attempt made to exclude second class proteins. The aim is to conserve the patient's own proteins and to keep the production of urea down so that the kidneys can excrete what is produced. If this measure is not successful a much stricter diet of the Giovanetti style may be prescribed. (For details of this diet the student should consult a textbook on dietetics.) It is important to provide sufficient kilojoules in the diet to meet the patient's needs because if not the patient will burn up his own proteins and the object of the exercise is defeated. Glucose supplements are useful in chronic failure. Additional iron and vitamin supplements will usually be required to combat anaemia.

Electrolytes. Each patient is an individual and while some who have chronic renal failure retain sodium, most lose it to excess. Salt, then, is restricted or supplemented accordingly. Potassium may be retained so that restriction becomes necessary. The patient must be instructed to avoid foods rich in potassium which otherwise would be permitted in his diet.

Water. Most patients will not need to have their water intake restricted. If, however, the glomerular filtration rate is very low, the kidneys may not be able to excrete extra water. If too much water is taken, this will lead to water intoxication resulting in headaches and possibly fits. It is a fallacy therefore, to instruct the patient to consume large amounts of fluid to 'flush out his kidneys' when he is in renal failure.

Control of acidosis. As the kidney in failure cannot regulate the pH of the blood a metabolic acidosis develops. This is treated by giving sodium bicarbonate or lactate. If the conservative treatment outlined above is not successful haemodialysis and/or kidney transplant is the patient's only hope.

Complications

The complications of chronic renal failure are many. Two of these, anaemia and bone disease, are so prevalent as to warrant more detailed consideration:

Anaemia. This is usually a hypochromic normocytic anaemia and is almost invariably a feature of chronic renal failure. The diseased kidneys fail to produce enough of the hormone erythropoietin which stimulates the bone marrow to produce the red blood corpuscles. Also it is thought that the high blood urea levels depress bone marrow function. Patients may have haemoglobin levels as low as 6 to 9 g/dl but have adapted to this and even when requiring dialysis are not invariably given blood transfusions. Blood transfusions in these circumstances reduce the bone marrow's response to the anaemia.

Bone disease. Calcium and phosphorus metabolism are seriously disturbed in renal failure and the development of bone disease is common. The kidney plays an essential role in the metabolism of vitamin D (Ch. 4) converting the biologically inactive 25-hydroxycholecalciferol to the active 125-dihydroxycholecalciferol. This latter substance acts in the gut to promote the absorption of calcium and phosphorus and on bone to increase reabsorption and to mineralize uncalcified osteoid. Children develop rickets whilst adults develop its counterpart osteomalacia (Ch. 4). In renal failure this complication is treated by giving 125-dihydroxycholecalciferol (vitamin D_3) — or a synthetic preparation $1\propto5$ — hydroxy vitamin D_3.

Plasma phosphate levels increase in renal failure, because the kidney is unable to excrete the absorbed dietary phosphorus. The plasma calcium levels, on the other hand, become low partly because of the vitamin deficiency and partly because of the hyperphosphataemia. The fall in calcium levels causes a secondary hyperparathyroidism which is responsible for the increased reabsorption of calcium from bone resulting in renal osteodystrophy (see also Ch. 11). One way of countering the hyperphosphataemia is to reduce the absorption of phosphorus by giving aluminium hydroxide which binds with the phosphorus in the diet.

Nursing care, like medical treatment, is largely symptomatic. Frequent mouthwashes and mouthcare are essential for the patient with a dry, brown, furred tongue and will help to relieve him of the bitter taste of which he so often complains. A piece of fresh pineapple gently applied to the tongue will usually remove obstinate fur and freshen the mouth. Regular bed-baths help to keep the skin free from sweat, which may cause irritation in chronic renal failure.

Very careful recordings of fluid intake and output must be made and the prescribed diet must be followed unless the patient is unable to tolerate it; this fact must then be reported. Hiccups, restlessness, muscular twitchings and vomiting must also be reported to the doctor since even in the terminal stages it is possible to keep the patient relatively comfortable with correct medication.

Polycystic disease

This is the commonest of the hereditary disorders of the kidney. Most of the patients are well into adult life — 40 years or more — before obvious symptoms appear. They may have hypertension, a history of haematuria and renal pain and may already have evidence of renal failure. Both kidneys are enlarged and grossly abnormal with multiple cysts which cause anatomical distortions (Fig. 9.10D). The onset of renal failure is usually slow so many patients are able to lead useful lives for some years after the diagnosis has been made. Anaemia is often less marked in these patients than in other forms of renal disease. Progression to complete renal failure is however almost inevitable.

Treatment and nursing care are as for patients with chronic renal failure.

Management and nursing care of patients undergoing dialysis

Dialysis is the transfer of solutes across a semipermeable membrane from a solution of high concentration, in this case the blood, to one of low concentration, the dialysate. This process is used to remove waste products, for example urea and creatinine,

Figure 9.13
Diffusion

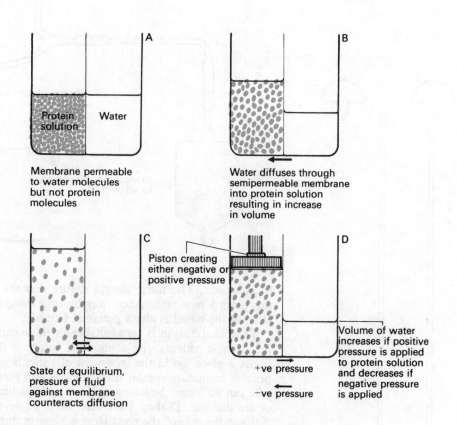

Figure 9.14
Osmosis

excess salts and fluid from the blood when the kidneys are failing to do so for some reason. As an 'aide memoire', the principles of diffusion and osmosis are illustrated in Figures 9.13 and 9.14 respectively. There are two types of dialysis namely peritoneal and haemodialysis.

Peritoneal dialysis

Here the patient's peritoneum is used to provide over two square metres of semipermeable membrane. The dialysing fluid is run into the peritoneal cavity (Fig. 9.15) by means of a semirigid plastic catheter such as the McGaw 'Trocath' (Fig. 9.16). The catheter is introduced through the abdominal wall under local anaesthesia and positioned in either the left or right iliac fossa. The catheter is then secured in position by means of a 'purse string' suture. Strict attention to aseptic technique is essential as the patients who require this form of dialysis are very prone

Figure 9.15
Peritoneal dialysis

Dialysis solution

Peritoneal catheter

Graduated collecting bag
for effluent

Stilette

Catheter

A   B

Figure 9.16
Trocath peritoneal dialysis
catheter
(A) Stilette in catheter
(B) Stilette and catheter
separated (Note curve of the
catheter) (McGaw Laboratories)

to infections. The nurse should ensure that the patient's bladder is empty before this procedure is undertaken to reduce the danger of perforation. Accidental perforation of the bowel is also a potential hazard.

Peritoneal dialysis is very suitable for those patients who require dialysis urgently, for example patients with acute renal failure or those suffering from self poisoning. It has a place too in the treatment of patients suffering from chronic renal failure prior to beginning regular dialysis. It is also used on a long-term basis for patients who can no longer be haemodialysed perhaps because they have no accessible veins or are diabetic. Diabetics are very liable to develop retinal bleeding when haemodialysed because of the need to give heparin during the procedure.

After the peritoneal catheter has been secured it is attached to the giving set and two litres of dialysate solution (Table 9.5) are run into the peritoneal cavity. The dialysate must be warmed up to body temperature (38°C) in a hot air oven or lotion cabinet set to that temperature, or passed through a special warming coil. On no account should the dialysate bags be warmed in buckets of hot water because of the risk of introducing infection.

The dialysate is left in the peritoneal cavity for ½ to 2 hours to allow the waste products and salts to diffuse into it. It is then drained out into a collecting bag. It may on some occasions prove difficult to get all of the fluid returned but changing the patient's position, for example by sitting him up, will usually be effective. When a volume of fluid, equal to that which was run in, is returned the procedure is repeated. It may be necessary to continue this every hour or 2 hours as prescribed for 2 or perhaps 3 days until the patient's condition is stable. Thereafter dialysis for a period daily or on alternate days may be all that is required. If the patient is overhydrated, the stronger dialysate solution will be used. The increased osmotic effect of this solution means fluids will leave the bloodstream and enter the peritoneal

Table 9.5
Typical peritoneal dialysis solutions

Anhydrous dextrose B.P.	1.36% w/v	6.36% w/v
Sodium lactate	0.5% w/v	0.5% w/v
Sodium chloride B.P.	0.56% w/v	0.56% w/v
Calcium chloride	0.039% w/v	0.039% w/v
Magnesium chloride	0.015% w/v	0.015% w/v
Sodium metabisulphite B.P.	0.005% w/v	0.012% w/v
Water to 100%		

cavity so that the amount of fluid returned will be greater than that run in. Regular weighing of the patient will also help keep a check on the effectiveness of dialysis. Most doctors add a small amount of heparin to the dialysate as this prevents fibrin deposition on the catheter tip. During dialysis observations of blood pressure are necessary in case excessive fluids are being lost in which case the patient may become hypotensive. In the longer term specimens of the returned dialysate should be sent regularly for culture and sensitivity. Should infection become evident gentamycin can be added to the dialysate. Systemic antibiotics may also be necessary.

The amount of general nursing care the patient will require during peritoneal dialysis will vary. In acute renal failure very intensive care will be required while long-term patients will be almost self sufficient. Indeed a recent development in this country is the introduction of *continuous ambulatory peritoneal dialysis*. In this type of programme the patient has a permanent silastic peritoneal dialysis catheter implanted in the abdominal wall and is trained to connect up the dialysate bags himself. Dialysis continues around the clock and is very successful in maintaining a stable body chemistry. Patients have a full check up once a month in the out-patient department. Not everyone is able to carry out the prescribed routines safely and a patient is assessed carefully for his suitability for this form of dialysis.

The introduction of the automatic peritoneal dialysing machines in recent years has made the work of the nurse very much easier. The machine, though not yet widely available, will become more so in the next few years. One of its several advantages is that by providing a closed system it reduces the risk of infection very considerably: the machine automatically warms the fluid, controls rate, measures the peritoneal fluid balance and has a built-in alarm should any malfunction arise.

Haemodialysis

Modern management of renal failure would not be possible without the use of the artificial kidney. Artificial kidneys are used in two main ways:

1. For temporary support of patients with acute reversible renal failure whose blood urea cannot be controlled adequately by the use of peritoneal dialysis, or in situations where peritoneal dialysis for such patients would be impracticable, for example the presence of an abdominal wound.

2. For regular treatment of patients with end-stage renal failure for whom the ultimate goal in most cases is a successful renal transplant.

In order to dialyse a patient repeatedly a method must be available for regular and convenient access to his blood circulation.

One method is a Scribner shunt (Fig. 9.17), which basically consists of a loop of Silastic tubing connecting an artery and a vein. When not in use for dialysis, blood

Figure 9.17
External arteriovenous (Scribner) shunt

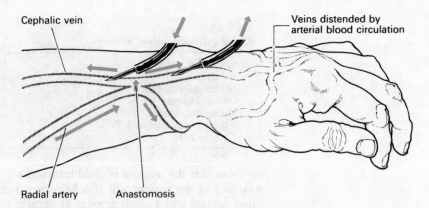

Figure 9.18
Internal (subcutaneous)
arteriovenous shunt

Figure 9.19
Butterfly 14 A.V. fistula set
(Abbot Laboratories)

flows continuously through the shunt from artery to vein. To carry out a dialysis the shunt is clamped and taken apart in the middle. The arterial end is connected to the arterial tube of the kidney machine and the venous end is connected to the venous tube of the kidney machine.

Regular care of shunts and connections are nursing responsibilities and it is vitally important that they should be handled skilfully. Shunts should never be tugged, jerked or twisted, and the area of skin around the site of insertion should be kept covered with a sterile dressing. When not being used for dialysis the shunt should be examined at frequent intervals for patency as revealed by a 'thrill' and the temperature of the tubing.

Because of the disadvantages of clotting and infection the Scribner shunt is used mainly in short-term dialysis. For long-term dialysis the surgical construction of a subcutaneous arteriovenous fistula (Fig. 9.18) is an alternative. The fistula has to be left for about 6 weeks before it is ready for use. During this period the veins become distended and thickened and the blood flow is greatly increased. Once established a thin walled silicon coated needle such as in the Abbot Butterfly A.V. Fistula Set (Fig. 9.19) is used. This set allows easy connection to the artificial kidney.

Table 9.6
Typical haemodialysis solution

Sodium	135–138 mmol/l
Calcium	1.25 mmol/l
Potassium	1.3 mmol/l
Chloride	108.8 mmol/l
Acetate	40 mmol/l
Dextrose	2 g/l

During dialysis blood is taken from the patient's artery (or arterialized vein), passed between layers of cuprophane which are sterile on the blood side and returned to the circulation (Fig. 9.20). The outside of the membrane is bathed by a fast-moving stream of dialysis fluid. The concentration of salts within this fluid is carefully calculated and, since it contains no end-products of metabolism such as urea, uric acid and creatinine, these substances diffuse from the blood into the dialysis fluid. Excess body fluids are removed during haemodialysis by means of ultra-filtration in which a negative pressure is created in the system. Blood is prevented from clotting in the tubes and between the layers of cuprophane by the use of heparin which is given as a continuous infusion or as intermittent injections into the tubing of the machine.

During dialysis the patient must be carefully observed. Nurses should always be readily available to deal with any emergency or fault which may arise. A patient protection system is incorporated into all dialysis machines which monitors for faults such as leaks or air bubbles. Patients on long-term dialysis who have been trained

Figure 9.20
The principles of haemodialysis

Blood from patient

Waste products

Excess water

Excess salts

Return to patient

Semipermeable membrane

Ideal salt solution from tank

To waste

Figure 9.21
Haemodialysis machine. Note small size of exchange unit
(A) IV pump
(B) Central console
(C) Exchange unit.

or are being trained towards independence and who are familiar with the machines will be able to make minor adjustments themselves. In the case of a more serious malfunction the machine must be switched off, the blood lines secured and assistance summoned from staff able to deal with the problem.

The frequency of pulse and blood pressure recordings depends on the circumstances. If the patient is very ill, frequent recordings are necessary. In the case of regular long-term dialysis, hourly blood pressure recordings are sufficient. The patient is carefully weighed before starting the dialysis and immediately on finishing.

Ever since haemodialysis became common practice there have been sporadic outbreaks of viral hepatitis among patients and staff. This infection is probably carried and transmitted via the blood and can be a serious and even fatal illness, so care should be taken to reduce the risks by regarding all blood as a potential source of hepatitis. Avoidance of blood spillage and the use of gloves when handling blood are some of the precautions necessary. The incidence of hepatitis in haemodialysis units is now rare because of the very high standard of care in these units and an awareness of the danger. Another important factor has been the reduction in the number of blood transfusions given. Blood transfusions are not given unless absolutely necessary and all blood which is given is of course screened for viral hepatitis antigens. The introduction of small compact disposable dialysis packs has also been a factor in reducing cross infection as well as making the work in these units much easier.

Community care

As the number of patients requiring dialysis far exceeds the facilities available for them in hospital, it has become necessary for patients to learn to carry out dialysis in their own homes.

Training for home dialysis usually takes 6 to 8 weeks in hospital. If technical problems subsequently prevent the patient carrying out dialysis successfully at home, provision must be made to admit him to hospital whenever the need arises.

Financial outlay for home dialysis is quite considerable, both for the equipment and for alterations to the home. If kidney transplantation is contemplated it is not worth spending a lot of money to establish the patient on dialysis in his own house. Regular haemodialysis in hospital or home has meant that many people continue to lead useful lives who would otherwise be dead, but the degree of rehabilitation achieved is variable and sometimes disappointing.

The nurse must be prepared to give emotional support to the patient and his family, and this she may find psychologically demanding. The dialysis machine, besides being very expensive, imposes restrictions which are often a continuing source of frustration and anxiety; for such a patient a successful kidney transplant offers a chance to lead an almost normal life: within weeks of operation he will notice a dramatic return of his old strength and vigour.

Unfortunately enthusiasm for transplantation must be tempered by the realization that mortality is still significantly higher than mortality on regular dialysis; survival rates are between 70 and 80% at 1 year, compared with over 90% at 1 year on dialysis.

Kidney transplant

This consists of removing a kidney from either a living identical twin, sibling or parent or a human cadaver donor and inserting it into a recipient. Usually the patient's kidney which is non-functioning has been removed and he is maintained on a dialysis programme until a kidney from a suitable donor becomes available (see p. 347).

Inferior vena cava   Abdominal aorta

Renal artery
sutured to
iliac artery

Renal vein
sutured
to iliac vein

Inguinal ligament

Figure 9.22
Kidney transplant

The donor kidney is transplanted retroperitoneally in either iliac fossa (Fig. 9.22). The ureter of the newly transplanted kidney is transplanted into the bladder or anastomosed to the ureter of the recipient.

The major limiting factor in this procedure is the body's immunological response that leads it to reject the transplanted kidney. The recipient's body recognizes the new kidney as foreign protein and attempts to destroy it. Rejection or threatened rejection of the kidney can occur several hours or several years after the transplant.

Thus the survival of the transplanted kidney depends upon the success of techniques that suppress these immune reactions. In order to minimize or overcome the body's defence mechanism, immunosuppressive drugs such as Imuran and prednisolone are given and continued indefinitely. As these drugs suppress the immune response of the body's reaction to foreign protein, the patient is more susceptible to infection, making infection a major complication of renal transplant. Therefore, postoperative care should include very strict sterile techniques and aseptic procedures. The nurse must be alert to signs of threatened rejection: fever, swelling and tenderness at the site of transplant, decrease in urinary volume, rise in blood urea and hypertension. Anorexia, malaise and vague feeling of uneasiness may also be experienced by the patient.

Obviously, one of the most important aspects of kidney transplant is the availability of suitable kidneys. In Great Britain, a nationwide scheme has been developed to ensure that each available kidney is matched to the most suitable recipient. The National Organ Matching Service based at Bristol receives and stores data (including tissue type) about all prospective recipients. When a kidney becomes available the donor details are supplied and the matching process is set in action. The most suitable recipient is selected and prepared and arrangements are made to transport the kidney to the recipient's hospital.

Calculi

The reason for the formation of calculi or stones in the urinary tract is poorly understood. Several conditions are known to predispose a person to calculi formation, and these are:

1. Excessive loss of water by sweating, for example in hot climates or under certain occupational conditions.
2. Urinary tract infection or stagnation.
3. Hypercalciuria.
4. Prolonged bed rest when calcium is mobilized from the bones.
5. Increased excretion of uric acid as in gout or leukaemia.
6. Dietary factors.
7. Some congenital abnormalities.

Calculi are made up of various combinations of calcium, phosphate, oxalate, ammonia, magnesium and other trace elements and metabolites. The calculi which form vary in size from small particles like sand, to round stones, to staghorn calculi — so named because of their characteristic shape (Fig. 9.23).

Renal calculi are becoming more common in developed countries, while bladder calculi (Fig. 9.24) are becoming less common. This is thought to be due to changes in the standard of living.

Clinical features

The clinical features vary according to the site of the calculi and may be largely asymptomatic in the early years. The patient often complains of a dull pain in the loin area and of being below par. Recurrent kidney infections and haematuria are the main presenting features and always need to be investigated thoroughly.

Treatment

Various operations have been devised for removing calculi depending on where the stone is lodged. Figures 9.25–9.31 summarize the various operations. The pre-and

Figure 9.23
Staghorn calculus

Figure 9.24
Large bladder calculus showing rough spiky surface

postoperative care of patients undergoing kidney, ureter and bladder operations is further described below.

Some types of calculi, namely uric acid stones can be prevented from recurring by giving the drug allopurinal. Abnormal serum levels of uric acid are a feature of gout and also of leukaemia. There are no drugs available which will effectively dissolve calculi in the urinary tract once they have formed. Treatment of known underlying causes for example hormone disorder may prevent calculi forming.

Figure 9.25

Disorder
Staghorn calculus in calyces of the kidney

Operation
Nephrolithotomy

Description
Calculus is removed from the body of the kidney

Special complications
Haemorrhage (especially secondary), infection, urinary leakage, renal fistula, renal failure — anuria, UTI

Drains
See nephrostomy (Fig. 9.29)

Management
See nephrostomy (Fig. 9.29)

Figure 9.26

Disorder
Dilated renal pelvis due to obstruction — hydronephrosis

Operation
Pyeloplasty

Description
Excess tissue is removed and the renal pelvis refashioned — the obstruction which gave rise to the disorder is treated first

Special complications
Haemorrhage, leakage of urine from the renal pelvis wound, UTI, renal failure

Drains
Precautionary drain in renal bed retained until urine leak has ceased. Doctor will advise when to remove

Management
Monitor urinary output; test urine for blood; 4 hourly TPR & blood pressure CSU or MSU. Liberal fluid intake 3000 ml+

Figure 9.27

Disorder
Large stone lodged in renal pelvis

Operation
Pyelolithotomy

Description
The stone is removed via an incision in the renal pelvis

Special complications
Haemorrhage, leakage of urine from incision, UTI

Drain
Precautionary drain in renal bed — keep in situ until urinary leak has ceased

Complications
Haemorrhage, urinary leakage, ureteric obstruction, UTI, renal failure, urinary fistula

Drains
Cautionary drain in the renal bed plus a nephrostomy drain for drainage and possible irrigation of renal pelvis. Doctor will advise

Management
Monitor urinary output; test urine for blood; report any loin pain to doctor and/or any increase in nephrostomy drainage; MSU/CSU 4 hourly observations of vital signs

Instrument passed up ureter beyond impacted stone

'Basket' opened

Instrument withdrawn trapping stone which can then be removed

Figure 9.28
Basketing a stone in ureter

Disorder
Stone impacted in ureter

Operation
Removal of stone using a 'wire' basket

Possible complications
Haematuria — observe urine frequently for 48 hr

Drains
No drains. May have urethral catheter in situ for 24–48 hr

Management
Liberal fluid intake; analgesia as required; 4 hourly TPR & blood pressure

Figure 9.29

Disorder
Urinary tract obstruction e.g. ureteric stricture, calculi, bladder tumours

Operation
Nephrostomy — an opening into the kidney for drainage and irrigation purposes

Complications
Haemorrhage, urinary leakage or fistula, UTI, renal failure

Drains
Possible precautionary drain in renal bed, usually removed in 48 hr. Catheters — syphon or straight — attached to bladder drainage bottle. Doctor will advise re irrigation etc.

Management
Monitor urinary output; test urine for blood; observe vital signs; 4 hourly report any loin pain

Figure 9.30

Pyeloplasty for hydronephrosis with stricture of the ureter

Disorder
Gross hydronephrosis due to long-standing urinary tract obstruction, often concurrent UTI

Operation
Pyeloplasty

Description
Remodelling of the renal pelvis by removal of excessive renal tissue

Figure 9.31

Disorder
Stone impacted in ureter

Operation
Ureterolithotomy

Description
Removal of stone via an incision in the ureter

Special complications
Haemorrhage, leakage of urine, stricture of ureter

Management
Monitor urinary output; test urine for blood; report any complaints of loin pain to doctor; MSU; 4 hourly TPR & BP

Stricture of ureter

Tumours of the kidney

Some renal tumours are relatively benign, others highly malignant. Two of the latter group are hypernephroma and Wilms' tumour.

Hypernephroma (renal carcinoma)

Hypernephroma is an adenocarcinoma which develops in the kidney tissue.

Clinical features

There may be few signs in the early stages. Later, pain in the loin, a palpable mass in the flank and painless haematuria indicate this serious disorder. A full urinary tract investigation (see Table 9.2) is carried out as painless haematuria is always an ominous sign. Blood-borne metastases occur, giving rise to the so-called 'cannon ball' secondary tumour deposits in the lungs. In some patients the tumour produces an excess of erythropoietin and these patients are found to have polycythaemia. Should this be the case, after removal of the tumour it is likely that there are secondary deposits. Prognosis depends on the degree of malignancy. Not all kidney tumours are equally malignant.

Treatment

After a thorough investigation of the urinary tract the diseased kidney is removed (nephrectomy). A course of X-ray therapy is sometimes given postoperatively depending on the malignancy.

Wilms' tumour (nephroblastoma)

This rare but usually very malignant tumour is one of the few that develops in children. Usually it is discovered in the first 3 years of life. It grows rapidly and gives rise to secondaries, especially in the lungs.

Clinical features

The child is noted to have a large abdomen and to be failing to thrive.

Treatment

In recent years the prognosis for a child with a Wilms' tumour has improved considerably. As with other tumours the earlier it is discovered the better the chances of cure. Treatment consists of surgery and if the tumour is unilateral this usually means removal of the offending kidney. Even if the tumour is bilateral, judicious surgery is assisted by radiotherapy and the use of the cytotoxic drugs — actinomycin D and vincristine — and the outlook is not as bleak as it used to be.

The parents of these children require considerable emotional support to help them and help the child through the difficult strenuous treatment regimen.

Nursing care of patients undergoing renal surgery

The pre- and postoperative regimen is essentially the same for most kidney and ureter operations with changes in some details only.

Preoperative care

Before any operation on the kidney, and in particular when removal of the kidney is performed, a thorough investigation must be made of both kidneys (Table 9.2). Increasingly the preliminary investigations are being carried out in the out-patient department or in day bed areas, the patient being admitted only a few days before operation for final tests and preparation.

The general care is the same as for any major abdominal surgery including:

1. Skin preparation. The surgeon will indicate whether he intends to use a lumbar or abdominal approach. The appropriate area **and side** will be marked **by the surgeon** using a skin marker which is not easily rubbed off and does not cause sensitivity reactions.
2. Urine testing.
3. Chest X-ray.
4. Blood transfusion if necessary to correct anaemia.
5. Bowel preparation by evacuant suppositories or enema.
6. Breathing exercises.
7. Consent for operation.

Postoperative care

The postoperative care of the patient following nephrectomy is similar to that required for other abdominal operations. Particular attention is paid to fluid balance and urinary output.

On return from theatre the patient is usually placed in a lateral position but local practice may vary.

Adynamic ileus occurs in many patients who have had retroperitoneal operations and the surgeon will indicate when oral fluids can be given and the amount. Oral fluids may be withheld for 24 to 48 hours. Adynamic ileus is treated by giving intravenous fluids and by gastric aspiration (p. 215). To prevent chest infections the patient is sat up in bed well supported by pillows and tilted towards the side of the operation to assist in the drainage of the kidney bed. The physiotherapist will continue to assist the patient with breathing exercises and expectoration to keep his lungs clear.

The vacuum drains are maintained for 2 to 3 days, after which time the haemoserous discharge from the kidney bed will become less and the surgeon will indicate when they may be shortened or removed. The dressing should not be changed unless it becomes soaked. In some kidney operations when removal has not taken place a nephrostomy drain may be left in place. This must be managed strictly according to the surgeon's wishes. Great care must be taken to avoid infection gaining entry into the kidney via this form of drain which is inserted into the renal pelvis.

If the patient's condition is satisfactory he is allowed up the day after operation, early ambulation being encouraged as it helps to prevent postoperative complications. All urine should be measured and carefully observed for blood. The kidney is a very vascular organ and following operation haemorrhage is a very likely occurrence. There will always be blood in the urine initially but this should become less over the first 24 to 48 hours. Any obvious continuation of haemorrhage or any reappearance of blood in the urine must be reported immediately. A fall in the urinary output will be evidence that kidney function is becoming impaired. Some simple kidney function tests may be carried out before discharge to ensure that all is well and the patient should be ready for discharge 2 weeks after operation. Some patients may be given a course of radiotherapy.

DISORDERS OF THE URETERS AND BLADDER

Anything which impedes the flow of urine from the kidneys to the outside of the body is likely, sooner or later, to require removal or to be bypassed. Within the genitourinary tract the main causes of obstruction are calculi, tumours, strictures and, in particular, an enlarged prostate gland (p. 366). Outside the urinary tract the most common causes of obstruction are masses within the abdominal and pelvic cavities, for example intestinal tumours, aberrant vessels, ovarian cysts and uterine enlargement. Various disorders of the central nervous system can also cause urinary tract dysfunction. Prolonged back pressure on the kidney eventually leads to impaired kidney function and renal failure. In addition, stagnation of urine almost inevitably leads to infection and to calculi formation.

Ureteric (renal) colic

Sometimes small calculi migrate from the kidney into the ureter and an attack of ureteric colic develops.

Clinical features

In this condition pain is of sudden onset and very severe, reaching a peak 10 to 30 minutes after it begins. The patient is restless and may assume all sorts of positions or may pace up and down the room in agony. Many vomit. Urinary symptoms include frequency and haematuria. The diagnosis is usually made on the basis of the history. If facilities are available an intravenous urogram during an attack will confirm the cause and is useful in the differential diagnosis.

Treatment and nursing care

The patient is confined to bed and an analgesic such as pethidine or morphine is given in addition to an antispasmodic such as atropine. Some surgeons request that all urine passed by the patient be sieved to see if any calculi are passed. This is mainly to confirm the diagnosis. Usually no calculi are observed as they are often very small and difficult to detect. Observations of the patient's temperature, pulse and blood pressure are carried out every half hour. All urine is tested for blood and if this is positive it will tend to confirm the diagnosis.

Bladder calculi

The clinical features are recurrent infections, dysuria, strangury, scalding on micturition and haematuria. The calculi may migrate and block the urethra causing acute retention of urine (p. 355).

Tumours of the bladder

The cause of cancer of the bladder remains elusive but many diverse factors have been implicated, both by observation in animal experiments and by clinical observations of patients. The following are the most common associated factors:

Chemicals used in the manufacture of rubber, plastics, insecticides, cables and dyes.
Cigarette smoking.
Calculi.
Chronic inflammation and diverticulum.
Schistosomiasis.

It is now fairly well established that it is the metabolic products of the various chemicals that cause the cancer, the exact mechanism, as indicated above, being unknown.

The tumours develop in the epithelial lining of the bladder and quite often start as papillary growths. They are relatively benign at this stage and with adequate treatment remain so. Without treatment the tumours become malignant and invade by stages into the superficial muscle layer, the deep muscle, and eventually into the surrounding tissues (Fig. 9.32). Metastasis, especially to bone, is also common. The tumours are often at an advanced stage before discovery.

Figure 9.32
Bladder tumours
(A) Pedunculated papillomata
(B) Stages of bladder tumours showing extension through the bladder wall and invasion of the neighbouring structures

Clinical features

The first evidence of a bladder tumour is often painless haematuria, the blood being bright red. Clot retention may develop. Some patients also have cystitis, frequency of micturition and dysuria. As the tumour spreads it invades the surrounding organs causing relative dysfunction. Involvement of the sacral nerves often results in intractable pain.

Investigations

Diagnosis is usually confirmed by cystoscopy and biopsy. Bimanual examination will give the surgeon some indication of the tumour's stage of development. Other urinary tract investigations include intravenous urogram, micturating cystogram and MSUs (see Table 9.2). Chest X-rays and skeletal surveys along with examination of the blood will also be required.

Treatment

In the early stages when the tumour is seen waving around like a sea anenome when viewed through the cystoscope (Fig. 9.2) the treatment is by diathermy. This procedure has to be repeated at regular intervals as the papillomata have a tendency to recur.

Malignant tumours are treated in various ways depending on the site, degree of malignancy and extent of the tumour.

Tumours which have not invaded deeply into the muscle layer can be treated by radiotherapy. Other more advanced tumours require surgery and several ingenious operations have been devised to cope with this problem. Partial cystectomy is of limited value only, because it reduces bladder capacity and the surgeon cannot be sure he has removed all of the tumour, especially a tumour which has multiple foci.

Figure 9.33A
Ileal conduit showing three different methods of inserting the ureter into the conduit

Stoma

Kidneys

Blood vessels

Large intestine

Small intestine

Appendix

Ileal anastomosis

Figure 9.33B
Position of the stoma on the anterior abdominal wall

Usually more radical procedures are called for. One procedure is to remove the bladder and transplant the ureters into the rectum, which then acts as a reservoir for the urine. This operation is only suitable if the anal sphincter is intact. The risks of infection are enormous, as can be imagined. Also, reabsorption of urinary products can give rise to serious electrolyte imbalance.

Another procedure is to isolate a section of ileum and bring it to the surface of the abdomen as a stoma. The ureters are transplanted into the isolated loop of ileum which acts as a conduit (ileal conduit) (Fig. 9.33) for the urine. It is not in any way a storage vessel for urine and a stoma bag has to be worn (see Ch. 5 for care of stoma). The ureters cannot be brought to the surface of the abdomen directly because in this position they become stenosed and within a short while cease to function, hence the need for the ileal loop. Following this operation it is necessary to rest the bowel for a few days until bowel sounds return. In addition to tumours this type of procedure is often carried out where there is lack of bladder function, for example in spina bifida.

Anticancerous drugs

A number of drugs have been discovered which can be used in the treatment of tumours. They act in various ways but, like radiotherapy, they are all designed to disrupt the metabolism and function of tumour cells to a greater extent than normal cells. With bladder tumours a few of these drugs can be used locally and are introduced via a catheter into the bladder; one such drug is ethoglucid (Epodyl). Others can also be given either orally or by injection. They are now widely used in the treatment of many forms of cancer.

Important features of disordered bladder function

Retention and incontinence of urine are conditions occurring alone or in conjunction with other diseases; for the patient they are distressing and embarrassing.

Acute retention of urine

Acute retention of urine exists when a person is unable to empty his bladder even when it is socially convenient for him to do so.

Clinical features

Palpation

Percussion

Figure 9.34
Assessing for retention of urine

The onset is sudden, as the name suggests. The patient complains of severe pain in the flank and loin regions. His temperature may be raised and he may be sweating and anxious. If treatment is delayed the patient will become shocked, with a low blood pressure, rapid pulse and a cold, clammy skin. The bladder can usually be palpated and may extend as high as the umbilicus or higher. Figure 9.34 shows the method of palpating and percussing the distended bladder.

Treatment and nursing care

The patient requires catheterization (see p. 360) in most instances except in postoperative retention, which is usually less acute and of psychological origin. Privacy, getting the patient up to the side of the bed, if allowed, running taps in the vicinity and a calm, confident manner in the nurse usually will help the patient to empty his bladder naturally.

If catheterization is required great care must be taken not to precipitate acute renal or cardiac failure by too rapid decompression of the bladder. The sudden release of pressure does produce this effect in some patients. The surgeon will indicate whether he wishes the bladder decompressed over a few hours.

Chronic retention of urine

In this condition the retention is incomplete. The patient may have a distended bladder with overflow incontinence or be unable to empty the bladder completely so that, on voiding, there is a residue of urine left in the bladder.

Causes

1. Prostatic disease.
2. Urethral stricture.
3. Bladder tumours.
4. Bladder calculi.
5. Central nervous system disease.
6. Gynaecological disorder.

Clinical features

The patient feels unwell and is usually aware of having progressive difficulty in passing urine. Urinary stagnation gives rise to infection of the urinary tract. The constant high pressures in the bladder cause changes in the bladder wall in which trabeculae and diverticulae form (Fig. 9.35). In some patients the bladder becomes

Figure 9.35
Prostate gland
(A) Normal structure during bladder filling
(B) Normal bladder emptying (Note funnelling of bladder neck into prostatic urethra)
(C) Hypertrophy of the prostate gland showing the changes resulting from chronic urinary tract obstruction:
1. hypertrophied bladder wall
2. trabeculae
3. diverticulum
4. hydroureter
5. residual urine
6. urinary tract obstruction

thin-walled and grossly distended. In addition to increased bladder pressure distortion of the ureters as they enter the bladder causes urine to dam back, resulting in hydroureters and hydronephroses. (Fig. 9.10E). These latter conditions give rise to loin pain and repeated kidney infections. The back pressure on the kidney impairs its function. The blood urea level rises and there is an electrolyte imbalance. It is this and the infection which cause the patient to feel unwell. Many patients, especially the elderly, become confused and disorientated. A full urinary tract investigation is required (Table 9.2).

Treatment and nursing care

Initially catheterization is required and, as in acute retention, if the bladder is grossly distended slow decompression is necessary. It is usually necessary to drain the bladder by catheter for a few days until the blood urea and electrolytes return to normal. This correction of the composition of body fluids often brings about a dramatic improvement in the patient's mental state. (See the section on care of the in-dwelling catheter (p. 360), for management during this period.)

As soon as the patient's condition allows and when the investigations are completed the underlying condition (see below) is treated.

Incontinence of urine

Incontinence of urine is one of the most distressing and troublesome features of a wide variety of disorders. It is a very intricate disorder in which physical, psychological, social and economic factors all play a part, either directly or indirectly. One definition of this complex problem is: any involuntary voiding of urine, per urethra, after the age at which control of bladder fuction is usually established.

Applied physiology

The urinary bladder has the function of storing the urine and, by its powerful detrusor muscles, expelling the urine. Urine is retained in the bladder by the sphincter mechanism (Fig. 9.36), which prevents urine from escaping when it should not. This is a passive action most of the time, only becoming active when it is not convenient for micturition to take place.

Detrusor muscles (expelling force which raises the pressure in the bladder)

Urethral sphincters (retaining force)

Figure 9.36
Balance of forces between detrusor muscle and urethral sphincters (schematic)

Figure 9.37
Nervous control of bladder
(schematic)

Brain

Frontal lobe

Upper pathways giving cortical control
of micturition

Bladder

Sacral spinal cord

Lower reflex pathways

Acquisition of bladder control

Babies and young children up to the age of 18 to 24 months pass urine quite involuntarily, as a purely reflex action. This automatic bladder action is present in every normal child at birth. As the bladder fills up with urine, sensory nerve endings in the bladder wall respond to stretching and pressure and relay the information to the 2nd, 3rd and 4th sacral segments in the spinal cord (Fig. 9.37). This triggers off a motor stimulus which causes relaxation of the sphincter mechanism and contraction of the bladder muscle, and micturition takes place.

This state of affairs prevails in babies and young children because the central nervous system has not developed to a stage where voluntary inhibition of micturition can be established. Voluntary inhibition is a learned activity which centres in the frontal lobe, the hypothalamus and the medulla oblongata interact in a complex manner. They enable the external urethral sphincter to be constricted and the reflex response inhibited. Once control is established, the bladder is emptied only when it is socially convenient. For some, however, this 'freedom' is never acquired; for others the system breaks down and control is lost.

Causes

As shown in Table 9.7, a variety of local and generalized conditions may give rise to incontinence of urine.

Investigations

Before any treatment can be started it is important to investigate the problem very thoroughly. Attempts to establish a pattern of voiding are the first steps towards control.

Often the incontinence does not seem to fit readily into any particular category and no one single cause can be isolated. However, unless the disorder is properly investigated and diagnosed, the correct treatment will not be given and the patient may well be labelled 'incontinent' and relegated to a life-style largely determined by his incontinence.

Nurses are often involved in charting patterns of incontinence (Ch. 20) and in observing the patient's behaviour for clues which will help in the diagnosis. Also, various urinary tract investigations may be carried out (see Table 9.2) as suggested by the history and clinical features.

Table 9.7
Causes of incontinence (After L E Edwards 1975 Incontinence. The Practitioner 214: 46–55)

Sphincter incompetence	Detrusor abnormalities	Spurious causes
Congenital urethral defects	Neurological lesions of any kind and at any level	Iatrogenic, perhaps following administration of sedatives or diuretics
Urethral trauma, as for instance in fractures of the pelvis	Acute infections	Constipation
Stress incontinence following multiple pregnancy	Chronic infections such as tuberculosis	Locomotor disorder
Bladder neck operations	Postradiation contractures	
Damage at prostatectomy:	Interstitial bladder cystitis	
— damage to sphincter		
— incomplete removal of prostate preventing sphincter closure	Bladder tumours	
— stricture preventing sphincter closure	Psychological enuresis	
Carcinoma of prostate involving sphincter		

Treatment and nursing care

The treatment will depend on the cause of the incontinence. Any underlying conditions are treated, such as urinary tract infections which so commonly afflict elderly women. Obstruction of the urethra is treated, and gynaecological conditions may also be discovered and, if possible, remedied. Various operations have been devised to improve sphincter function when sphincter weakness is the cause of incontinence. One such operation is vesico-urethral suspension in which the bladder and urethra are supported in a better anatomical position (Fig. 9.38). These and other operations are not always successful but improvements in assessment and new operative techniques are being devised which will benefit those whose lives are made a misery by incontinence. The distressing problem of stress incontinence experienced by so many older women is one such condition for which surgery may bring relief.

Figure 9.38
Vesico-urethral suspension ('sling' operation)

Treatment of detrusor muscle abnormality

In some patients the cause of the incontinence is a detrusor abnormality (p. 357). If the bladder is atonic some patients will be helped by cholinergic drugs such as carbachol and pyridostigmine bromide. Where bladder function is unstable and uninhibited anticholinergic drugs such as propantheline bromide and emepronium bromide are of benefit. The latter is fairly free of side-effects. Sometimes surgical intervention, in which the bladder above the trigone is denervated, is worthwhile to relieve severe symptoms of urgency, frequency and incontinence. Urinary diversion, where the ureters are transplanted into the sigmoid colon or into an isolated loop of ileum or colon, which is brought to the surface of the abdomen as a urinary stoma, may be the operation of choice (Fig. 9.33, p. 354). These last-mentioned procedures are used where there is a neurological deficit involving sphincter mechanisms of both urinary and faecal outlets.

For many patients, however, the incontinence problem is not readily amenable to any of the treatments described above and other more traditional methods of management have to be used (Ch. 20).

Treatment of non-urethral urinary incontinence

Some patients have non-urethral incontinence via a fistula, for example vesicovaginal or vesicorectal. Very often these patients have urinary tract infections in addition to other pathological conditions. Any such fistula requires surgical repair with treatment of any underlying condition. A full urinary tract investigation will be necessary.

Catheterization

In this procedure a catheter is introduced into the urinary bladder for purposes of:

1. Relieving retention of urine.
2. Emptying the bladder before and after operations on the bladder, prostate or urethra; before some gynaecological operations; and before and after operations on the rectum.
3. Facilitating bladder irrigation.
4. Introducing agents which will dissolve calculi (cysteine and uric acid calculi are soluble).
5. Introducing anticancer drugs for bladder carcinoma.
6. Enabling bladder function tests to be done.

It may also be necessary to measure residual urine or urinary output very accurately in some circumstances, for example in patients who have extensive burns. From the above list, which is not exhaustive, it will be appreciated that catheterization is a fairly commonly performed procedure. However, a catheter should not be introduced into a patient's bladder unless a careful consideration of its necessity has been made. The dangers of introducing infection into the urinary tract and of causing injury to the urethra or bladder cannot be stressed too strongly.

A wide variety of catheter types are in use, made from many different materials. The choice of catheter depends on why the patient is being catheterized. Most catheters are packed individually, sterilized and ready for use. Catheters are generally disposable and should be used once only. The best policy is to follow the manufacturer's instructions.

No one should attempt to pass a catheter without having first observed a skilled operator or without having acquired a sound knowledge of the anatomy of the lower urinary tract. The equipment used is usually prepacked and sealed before sterilization in a way which is convenient for use and which lowers the risk of contamination.

If the reason for catheterization does not warrant leaving the catheter in situ, the procedure for which it was passed is completed and the catheter is removed. If it is to be retained the appropriate amount of sterile water is injected into the balloon (Fig. 9.41). The catheter is then connected to a sterile, closed drainage system preferably with a non-return valve to help minimize the risk of infection.

The catheter should be secured to the thigh or abdomen to prevent the catheter dragging on the urethra.

Occasionally urine by-passing the catheter may be a problem. This is usually due to bladder spasm which may be secondary to irritation of the mucosal lining. Too large a catheter or too much water in the balloon may be contributing factors. There is a temptation to pass an even bigger catheter when by-pass is a problem which often makes the condition worse. Changing to a catheter made of a different material may help as will giving drugs to relieve bladder spasm.

Care of in-dwelling catheters

The main problems involved with in-dwelling catheters are the risk of ascending infection and damage to the urethra and bladder.

Infection can get into the urinary tract at various stages in the procedure. These are:

1. By inadequate skin preparation before passing the catheter.
2. By faulty aseptic technique.
3. By injury during passage of the catheter, especially if it is the wrong size.

4. By breaking the closed system of drainage.

5. By lifting the bag above bladder level so that urine flows from the bag or tubing back to the bladder.

The drainage system should be kept closed; the use of spigots, sterile or otherwise, is to be condemned. Bags which can be drained without disconnecting the catheter should be used. Some people advocate putting antiseptic lotion in the drainage bag each time it is drained. The bag must be emptied every 8 hours and strict attention to hand washing is necessary as infection is easily transferred from one bag to the next. The patient must also be warned not to raise the bag above the level of his bladder. The urethral meatal area should be washed twice daily with soap and water. Some surgeons also prescribe the use of an antiseptic cream such as chlorhexidine.

The patient should be provided with plenty of fluids, if there are no contraindications. The aim is to drink at least 2 litres per day — more if possible.

Urine specimens

Patients with in-dwelling catheters all too frequently develop urinary tract infections. The infection often starts off insidiously with few if any clinical features. The patient's urine may have a foul odour or he may have a rise in temperature for a day or two, but little else; hence taking regular catheter specimens of urine (CSU) for culture is advisable. Specimens can be obtained from the catheter using a needle and syringe so that the closed system is not broken. The site on the tubing is cleaned using an isopropyl alcohol swab (Fig. 9.39).

Changing the catheter

If a rubber Foley catheter is used it is recommended that it be changed once a month. However, one of the new silicone, elastomer-type catheters can be left in situ for up to 3 months or longer. It should be changed if it becomes encrusted with calcific and other debris or if the urinary tract becomes infected. These complications are much less frequent when a Silastic catheter is used.

Bladder irrigation

There are several ways in which bladder irrigation may be performed.

1. By a **bladder syringe** which holds 50 ml of fluid. Specially prepared antiseptic lotion is introduced into the bladder via a catheter. There is a very high risk of introducing infection using this method of irrigation. It is useful when local bladder antiseptics such as Noxyflex have been prescribed.

Figure 9.39
Technique of obtaining a urine sample without breaking the closed drainage system

Figure 9.40
Methods of bladder irrigation
(A) Three-way Foley catheter
(B) Irrigating fluid entering the bladder via a Foley catheter and leaving via a suprapubic catheter to which suction may be applied
(C) Irrigation via a suprapubic catheter with drainage via a Foley catheter in the urethra

A   B   C

2. By **continuous closed irrigation**. This entails the use of three-way Foley self-retaining catheter through which a large amount of sterile water for irrigation is passed into the bladder and, after irrigation of the bladder, is allowed to flow out through the other channel into a closed drainage system (Fig. 9.40A). This form of irrigation is used following prostatectomy and in some bladder operations. The aim is to keep the bladder free of blood clots. The specific regimen and duration will be determined by the surgeon.

3. By **suprapubic cystostomy**. When it is not possible to pass a catheter via the urethra, in order to drain the bladder or for irrigation purposes, the surgeon may have no choice but to perform a suprapubic cystostomy. A catheter is introduced through the stoma (Fig. 9.40B and C). Either a Foley, Malecote or a de Pezzer catheter is used (Fig. 9.41A, B and C). The bladder and abdominal muscles constrict down on to the catheter so that leakage does not occur. The stoma is kept scrupulously clean and dressed as a surgical wound.

Unidirectional valve

Balloon not inflated — Balloon inflated

Figure 9.41
Three types of self-retaining catheter
(A) de Pezzer
(B) Malecote
(C) Foley

DISORDERS OF THE MALE GENITALIA

Disturbance of structure and function may be congenital in origin or may result from trauma, infection or neoplasm. Only the more common disorders will be described.

Congenital disorders of the urethra and penis

Malformation of the urethra from congenital defects will be seen on neonatal examination (Ch. 17).

Hypospadias

In this condition the urethral meatus does not open on to the anterior tip of the glans but on to the lower surface. Most commonly the abnormal opening is on the undersurface of the glans and is known as glandular hypospadias (Fig. 9.42A). This is fairly easily treated by plastic surgery, as a result of which the urethral meatus is enlarged. Usually the patient experiences no further difficulties either in passing urine or in sexual function (Fig. 9.42B).

Occasionally the openings are further back along the lower surface and, as can be imagined, are much more difficult to treat. Several operations may be required and the urine has often to be bypassed via a temporary perineal urethrostomy. This diversion allows healing to take place following surgery.

Figure 9.42
(A) Glandular hypospadias
(B) Various sites of urethral opening in hypospadias (schematic)

Figure 9.43
Epispadias

Epispadias

In this condition the urethra opens on to the dorsal surface of the penis (Fig. 9.43). As in hypospadias the urethral meatus can be at any point along the penis. It is often associated with another very serious congenital abnormality, namely ectopia vesicae, in which the anterior parts of the bladder and the abdominal wall are imperfectly formed.

These conditions require extensive plastic surgery, quite often with transplantation of the ureters (Fig. 9.33, p. 354). For a discussion of these procedures a more specialized text should be consulted.

Traumatic conditions

Urethral stricture

In modern times urethral stricture is usually a result of trauma, more rarely it is a sequel to gonococcal urethritis. The same sequence of events follows as in obstruction of the urinary flow, but for other reasons. The treatment is dilatation of the urethra using *bougies* and graduated metal sounds. Usually, several treatments are required to dilate the scarred portion of the urethra. An antibiotic drug is often given to prevent infection, which is made likely because of repeated instrumentation and especially if there has been a degree of urinary stasis.

Rupture of the urethra

Occasionally, the urethra is ruptured as a result of trauma, or it may rupture spontaneously because of stricture. This is very troublesome and several operations may be necessary before satisfactory urethral function is established.

Phimosis

The condition of phimosis, which is a narrowing of the foreskin (Fig. 9.44), is usually acquired. It comes about as a result of attempts to retract the foreskin back over the glans before complete separation of the foreskin from the glans has taken place and before the foreskin is big enough to be retracted. The separation is usually complete at about 2 years of age. Retraction before separation is complete splits the adherent areas leaving raw surfaces which cause scar formation and narrowing of the foreskin. This later gives rise to difficulty in retracting the foreskin with consequent problems of hygiene. Infection of the glans (balanitis) is then more common. The operation of circumcision is required. This operation is also done for religious and social reasons.

Phimosis may on occasion be a congenital abnormality.

Figure 9.44
Phimosis

Figure 9.45
Paraphimosis

Paraphimosis

Paraphimosis is a condition where the foreskin has been retracted back over the glans and the patient is unable to replace it. The tight foreskin interrupts the circulation and the glans becomes tense and swollen. (Fig. 9.45).

The condition can usually be treated without anaesthesia by manipulating the glans under the rolled-up foreskin. Cold compresses applied to the penis may help to reduce the swelling and make manipulation easier. Occasionally, a dorsal slit is made under anaesthesia. A follow-up circumcision may be called for to prevent a recurrence.

Carcinoma of the penis

This is a squamous-celled carcinoma caused by long-standing irritation. It is very rarely, if ever, found in men who have been circumcised before the age of 5 years. It is not a common condition. There is no pain initially and the patient is often late in seeking help. Metastases in the inguinal region are common.

Treatment

The treatment is radiotherapy and/or partial or total amputation of the penis, with block dissection of the inguinal glands. There is no specific preoperative care other than skin preparation. Urine is required for culture and sensitivity. Any urinary tract infection must be treated. The surgeon will give the patient a careful explanation of what is involved and of the need for such radical treatment — if amputation is decided upon.

Postoperatively, attention to hygiene and micturition is important. If surgery is refused one of the cytotoxic drugs such as bleomycin can be used.

Maldescent of the testes

This is a condition in which **one or both** testes fail to pass down the inguinal canal into the scrotum before birth (Fig. 9.46A and B). The embryo testes begin life in the upper coelomic cavity and usually descend around the seventh month of intra-uterine life. It is a fairly common disorder, occurring in 30 to 40 per 1000 full-term male births. The reason for the descent of the testes into the scrotum is to keep the testes cooler than would be possible in the abdominal cavity, where the higher temperature would cause germ cell degeneration.

There are three different orders of maldescent:

1. **Retractile testicle,** a normal gonad which has been drawn up into the super-ficial inguinal pouch.

Figure 9.46
Maldescent of testes
(A) Normal scrotum
(B) Left side of scrotum empty

Testicle still in abdomen

Testicle in inguinal canal

Testicle in upper scrotum

A   B

2. **Ectopic testicle,** where the testicle is prevented from entering the scrotum by a fascial barrier.

3. **Undescended testicle** (also called cryptorchid), where the testicle, which is often abnormal, either partially or completely fails to pass down the inguinal canal to the scrotum.

Treatment

The aim of treatment is to produce a normally functioning testicle. Because the testicle starts to function by the eighth to tenth year of life treatment should be complete by that age at the latest. Two main forms of treatment are used. First, hormones may be given in an attempt to get the testicle to migrate naturally. Some do migrate spontaneously even without treatment, especially in the retractile group. The second form of treatment is surgical. Surgery is always required for an ectopic testicle; an operation called an orchidopexy is performed in which the testicle is brought down and embedded in a pocket of skin in the thigh or anchored by means of a suture to the thigh. In the former operation a second operation is required in 3 months to free the testicle, while in the latter procedure the suture is removed in 7 to 10 days.

In true undescended testes more extensive surgery is often required including removal of the testes and repair of the inguinal hernia which is often present in these patients. There is a high risk of malignancy if the testes are left in the abdominal cavity.

Hydrocele

This is a collection of watery fluid in the tunica vaginalis. There are two types:

1. **Primary hydrocele,** which can occur at any age without obvious cause.
2. **Secondary hydrocele,** which accompanies acute or chronic inflammation of the testes or epididymis, for example gonorrhoea.

A hydrocele is always translucent unless there has been injury or previous tapping when blood in the vaginal space may render it opaque. They can grow to quite an outrageous size but this is uncommon. Other occasions when scrotal swelling may be extensive include severe oedematous states, for example nephrotic syndrome and congestive heart failure, elephantiasis and inguinal herniation. The latter is the only condition which may be easily reducible though this is not always the case.

Treatment

Most hydroceles, even when quite large, will usually reabsorb. If any persist an operation on the tunica vaginalis is necessary. For elderly patients unable to withstand an operation the hydrocele can be tapped using a fine trocar and cannula introduced into a translucent area. It is not without risk: haemorrhage and infection are common complications.

Varicocele

This is a disorder of the blood vessels draining the testes. The veins from the testes are dilated causing enlargement of the spermatic cord in the upper part of the scrotum and in the groin. It may cause discomfort and an aching pain. In addition, the temperature of the testes is raised which may cause testicular dysfunction in the form of oligospermia. This is a cause of infertility where the wife is normal. Usually no treatment is required; however, in cases of infertility and where discomfort is persistent a small operation to remove a portion of the vein is required. This is not always successful in increasing fertility.

Epididymo-orchitis

Acute epididymo-orchitis is a fairly common cause of acute testicular swelling. It is associated with urinary tract infections so it is necessary to obtain a specimen of urine for microbiological investigation. There is considerable pain and discomfort. The patient will be febrile and should therefore be confined to bed. A scrotal support is necessary. He should have all the care of the febrile patient. A liberal supply of fluids should be provided, and an antibiotic will be prescribed. It is usual, once the acute episode has been treated, to investigate the urinary tract more fully (Table 9.2) so that any underlying disease process can be treated.

New growths of the testes

There are several new growths which arise in the testes; the large majority, however, are either teratomas or seminomas. The former are remarkably complex tumours which arise from embryonic tissues and have areas of tissue of variable origin. The seminomas are more homogeneous tumours and are believed to be derived from spermatocytes. They are less highly malignant than teratomas.

Clinical features

The onset is often gradual, most of the patients being young men. There is a firm, expanding, palpable mass felt in the scrotum. Any young man who presents with a non-translucent mass in the scrotum deserves careful investigation.

Treatment

The scrotum is explored using an inguinal incision and, once the diagnosis is confirmed, the testis, epididymis and cord up to the inguinal ring is removed. A course of radiotherapy is then given as the seminomas are radiosensitive, the teratomas less so. In recent years various cytotoxic drugs have been given in the treatment of testicular tumours. The Einhorn regime in which a combination of cisplatinum, vinblastine and bleomycin are given has been found to be the most successful. Serum levels of alphafetoproteins (AFP) and human gonadotrophin (HCG) are monitored to assess this treatment.

Nursing care of patients undergoing testicular surgery

The general pre- and postoperative care is the same as for any major surgery. Because of the area's close proximity to the anal region, particular care must be taken with hygiene and skin preparation, as infection is often a troublesome problem. Pain can be quite severe following some operations and analgesics must be given. The area should be closely observed for haemorrhage and swelling. Psychological problems following removal of the testes must be met with understanding and sympathy.

Diseases of the prostate gland

As the prostate gland closely surrounds the urethra as it leaves the bladder (see Fig. 9.35, p. 356), changes in the size, shape or form of the gland may cause disturbance of bladder and urethral function. Changes in the gland are very common after the age of 50 and surgery on the prostate gland makes up much of the work of most surgical urology units. Many — indeed most — of the patients are elderly, so this condition presents more interesting problems in surgical and nursing management.

Changes in the gland are known collectively as **prostatism**. The changes may be benign or malignant.

Benign growths of the prostate gland

In the benign change a nodular hyperplasia develops. The nodules of glandular and fibrous tissue coalesce to form a large mass which compresses the outer, normal glandular tissue into a false capsule. As the mass grows it compresses and elongates the prostatic urethra making catheterization difficult in some cases. The enlarging gland also pushes up the floor of the bladder causing distortion of the ureters

Figure 9.47
Sagittal section showing
enlarged prostate gland

(Fig. 9.35). A complication of the hypertrophy is chronic prostatitis in which the gland substance undergoes inflammatory changes. Acute prostatitis is more usually a complication of gonorrhoea. The malignant changes are described on page 369.

Clinical features

The patient has a history of not feeling well for some time, hesitancy and difficulty in starting to pass urine, a slow stream of urine and dribbling at the end of micturition (see chronic retention, p. 356). Many patients present with acute retention (p. 355).

Investigations

Most of the patients are elderly and a thorough assessment of their physical condition is necessary. A full urinary tract investigation is required (see Table 9.2). A rectal examination is essential in the diagnosis of prostate disease. The urine is tested and a specimen is sent for microbiological investigation.

Figure 9.48
Four routes for removal of
prostate gland

Surgical treatment and nursing care

The general preoperative care is the same as for any major surgery.

Several routes to the prostate gland are available (Fig. 9.48). The route chosen will depend on the surgeon and on the patient's circumstances. Once the gland is exposed the nodular hyperplastic area is shelled out, including the prostatic urethra, leaving the false capsule. This leaves a raw area which has a tendency to bleed and which later becomes covered with epithelial tissue.

Figure 9.49
Transurethral prostatectomy
(A) Hypertrophied prostate gland
(B & C) Resectoscope cutting away abnormal tissue which can be flushed out via the operator cystoscope

Description
Removal of prostate gland via an operating resectoscope

Disorder
Benign hyperplasia of the prostate

Special complications
Haemorrhage

Management
Remove catheter 48 hr; fluids ++; bladder training regime

Figure 9.50
Disorder
Benign hypertrophy of the prostate gland

Operation
Retropubic prostatectomy

Description
The prostate gland is removed via the retropubic space

Special complications
Haemorrhage, infection, incontinence (usually temporary)

Mangement
Wound drain out on 48 hr; bladder irrigation catheter in situ for 3–5 days — doctor will advise. Fluid balance chart. ½ hourly observation vital signs (see main text)

Drains
Wound drain in the retropubic space. Three self-retaining catheters for irrigation of bladder.

Figure 9.51
Disorder
Benign hypertrophy of the prostate gland

Operation
Transvesical prostatectomy

Description
The bladder is opened via a suprapubic wound and the prostate gland is removed

Special complications
Haemorrhage, infection, incontinence (usually temporary)

Management
Drains out 48 hr; irrigate bladder 24–48 hr; catheter out 3–7 days — doctor will advise; monitor fluid intake and output; initially ½ hourly BP & pulse, later 4 hourly BP & TPR (see also main text)

Drains and catheters
Wound drain to remove haemoserous fluid and 3-way Foley catheter in situ for irrigation of the bladder

Postoperative nursing care

The general postoperative care is the same as for any patient undergoing major surgery. The more specific care relating to these patients will depend on the type of operation performed and on the preference of the individual surgeon.

On return from the operating theatre an intravenous infusion will be in progress and, if the patient has lost more than 500 ml of blood, a transfusion may be given. Care must be taken not to overload the circulatory system and so precipitate heart failure.

Provided there are no complications and the patient can take oral fluids in adequate amounts, that is about 3 litres per day, the infusion can be discontinued after 24 hours.

Most patients will have an in-dwelling catheter, which may be a Foley three-way self-retaining type, which facilitates bladder irrigation. Bladder irrigation will reduce the likelihood of clot formation. Even so some patients will develop clots, and this causes severe pain and shock. Clot retention is most likely to occur during the first few hours and most surgeons will prescribe a bladder irrigation regimen.

Clot retention causes severe pain and shock which is not entirely due to blood loss as removal of the clot brings about an immediate improvement in the patient's condition. Sometimes clots form in spite of irrigation.

The catheter is usually removed 2 days after a transurethral resection of the prostate and 3 to 5 days after retropubic resection. It may be left in for up to 7 days if a transvesical approach has been used; practice, however, does vary widely. Bleeding continues longer in some patients and therefore, removal may have to be delayed. On removal of the catheter the patient may not have good control of his bladder initially. He will probably experience frequency of, and considerable discomfort on micturition and will need reassurance that this is only a temporary disturbance. The patient is instructed to do stop-start exercises when micturating to strengthen the external urethral sphincters. Some patients will experience much more serious problems and not regain continence. They will need to be given a Cunningham clamp or condom sheath, which is attached to a collection bag. In about 1% incontinence will be permanent whilst in the majority full control is regained in about 6 weeks though up to a year may pass before some men regain continence.

If there has been a drain in the retropubic space this is removed after 2 to 3 days. The sutures are removed 8 to 10 days later.

Early ambulation is advisable and, if he is able, the patient will be allowed up the day after operation for a short time. This, along with leg exercises, will help to prevent deep venous thrombosis.

The patient is usually fit for discharge in about 2 weeks. He will frequently admit to feeling better than he has for years. He should, however, be advised to take things easy for a time, gradually increasing his activity back to what for him is normal. Before discharge a specimen of urine is sent for culture and sensitivity tests are made to ensure there is no residual infection.

Carcinoma of the prostate gland

Carcinoma of the prostate is the most common form of neoplasm found in men over 65 years. The tumour is known to be hormone-dependent.

Clinical features

Like many other cancers found elsewhere in the body it seldom gives rise to symptoms while in a curable stage. Often, the symptoms are indistinguishable from those of prostatic hypertrophy. Dysuria and bed-wetting, flank pain, sciatic pain due to secondaries, anaemia and impotence are the most common presenting features. Many patients present with more wide-ranging symptoms because of secondary deposits.

Investigations

Diagnosis is based on the history, rectal examination, skeletal surveys and blood tests. The latter are not always positive. A biopsy is essential to corroborate the evidence.

Treatment and nursing care

The treatment is removal of the prostate gland and the use of anticancerous drugs and female hormones. Sometimes the prostatic urethra is simply widened a little to allow free passage of urine. The transurethral approach is also used. Some surgeons remove the testes as the tumour is hormone-dependent and this reduces malignant activity. The female hormones used (stilboestrol and its derivatives) also have the effect of damping down malignant activity. They do not bring about a cure. The pre- and postoperative regimen is the same as that for prostatectomy performed for other reasons.

CONTRACEPTION

Because of the permanency of sterilization as a means of contraception, not all males are willing to undergo such a procedure. There are, however, other methods of contraception, namely coitus interruptus, sheaths and spermicidal agents, although none is as reliable as vasectomy (see p. 386).

Coitus interruptus

This is a widely practised means of trying to prevent conception. In this method the man withdraws his penis from the woman's vagina just before ejaculation in an effort to prevent spermatozoa from entering. The method is not reliable, partly because it requires very careful timing and also because a very large percentage of the spermatozoa are in the first two-thirds of the ejaculation. Due to the uncertainty this is a very unsatisfactory method of contraception. It gives rise to tension between the couple and the fear of unwanted pregnancy is real enough as the failure rate is very high.

Sheaths and spermicidal agents

The use of a sheath (or condom), usually made of rubber, is a commonly used means of contraception. The sheath is placed over the penis and acts as a barrier to the spermatozoa entering the vagina. As a method of contraception it is fairly reliable if used properly. Some agencies recommend the use of spermicidal cream or foam in addition to the sheath as an added protection. The spermicidal agents, which can also be used on their own, are introduced into the vagina directly from their containers via special applicators.

Sheaths and spermicidal agents are available from family planning centres and chemists.

The use of sheaths is thought to help in limiting the spread of sexually transmitted diseases, for example gonorrhoea.

Male sterilization

The most common method of rendering the male sterile at present is by removing a short length of each vas deferens. The procedure is called a vasectomy (Fig. 9.52), and is one of the most effective means of sterilization. It is easier to perform, more free from complications than female sterilization (Ch. 10) and is now becoming an accepted procedure in this country.

Preoperative preparation

A careful explanation of what is involved should be given to both husband and wife, and the wife should also give her consent. The operation is usually performed under

Figure 9.52
Vasectomy
(A) Isolation and section of the vas deferens
(B) One method ligating the sectioned vas deferens

a local anaesthetic but a general anaesthetic is given on some occasions. The patient is asked to shave his pubic area and to wash thoroughly.

The operation involves making a small opening into the neck of the scrotum on each side and isolating the vas deferens. A small section is removed and various operations, for example folding ends of the vasa back, have been devised to overcome the problem of recanalization of the vasa. The wound is closed usually with a single silk suture and sprayed with Nobecutane.

Postoperative care and follow-up

The scrotum must be supported and must be observed closely for 15 to 30 minutes in case of haemorrhage. On discharge the patient is advised to seek help if any swelling or haematoma should form. Some pain may be experienced in the testes for a few days. The main complications are haemorrhage, infection and psychological problems.

The man's semen is examined for spermatozoa at regular intervals for 3 months. He must be warned to use some other form of contraception until at least three negative specimens have been obtained. Usually about 3 months has to elapse before the seminal vesicles are completely empty of spermatozoa. The operation does not cause impotence and seems to give rise to very few psychological problems.

SUGGESTED ASSIGNMENTS

1. 'Often the incontinence does not seem to fit readily into any particular category and no one single cause can be isolated.' (p. 359).
Over a specified period of clinical experience in more than one area, do a survey of all the patients whom you nurse who are incontinent and see whether this statement stands up to close examination.

2. Discuss the advantages and disadvantages
   a. to the patient
   b. to the health service
of home dialysis versus hospital-based heamodialysis.

3. Using the nursing process model, devise a home nursing care plan for the parents of a child who is about to be discharged from hospital having had an ileal conduit constructed. How best may the parents be helped to contribute to such a plan and put it into action? What sort of problems would you anticipate?

Discussion topic

Discuss the merits of different methods of bladder irrigation from the nursing point of view.

FURTHER READING

Blandy J 1982 Lecture notes on urology, 3rd edn. Blackwell Scientific, Oxford
Lerner J, Khan Z 1982 Manual of urologic nursing. Mosby, St Louis
Scott R, Deane R F, Callander R 1982 Urology illustrated, 2nd edn. Churchill Livingstone, Edinburgh

Chapter Ten

The female reproductive system

THE FEMALE REPRODUCTIVE TRACT

The organs of the reproductive tract are described collectively as the **genitalia** (L. genitalis, to beget). These organs are inactive until the onset of puberty, which usually occurs between the ages of 12 and 17 years.

The female child is prepared for puberty by the increase in the amount of hormones produced by the pituitary gland, resulting in the secretion of oestrogen from the ovaries and adrenal cortex. At puberty the girl begins to develop the secondary sex characteristics which stamp her as a woman. These are the development of breasts, the enlargement of the genitalia, the growth of pubic and axillary hair and the appearance of deposits of fat on the breasts and hips, resulting in the rounded contours of the body that distinguish the female from the male. This change reaches its climax with the onset of the menarche, the first menstrual period. The girl is now physically able to bear a child.

During the childbearing years most women have a regular menstrual cycle, broken only by pregnancy, until the menopause is reached — between the ages of 45 and 52 years. At this time menstruation ceases and the woman is no longer able to bear children. Thereafter, because of the decreasing production of the female hormones oestrogen and progesterone, the genitalia and breasts shrink and pubic and axillary hair becomes scanty.

Both puberty and the menopause may be accompanied by psychological changes.

ANATOMY AND PHYSIOLOGY

For purposes of description the genitalia are divided into external and internal organs.

The internal genitalia are housed in the abdominal cavity and are protected by the pelvic girdle, which forms a basin-shaped structure with an outlet in its base. This is known as the **true pelvis** and is important in obstetrics.

The outlet of the pelvis is spanned by muscles and ligaments which form a sling to support the pelvic organs. There are three perforations or openings, permitting the passage of the urethra in front, the vagina in the middle, and the rectum at the back. They are all sites of potential weakness in the pelvic floor.

A wedge of muscle between the vagina and rectum is known as the **perineal body**. It has attachments to eight muscles and is the corner-stone of the pelvic floor. If it is damaged in childbirth or weakened by slackening of the muscles in old age, the whole pelvic floor ceases to function adequately. The skin covering this area is known as the perineum.

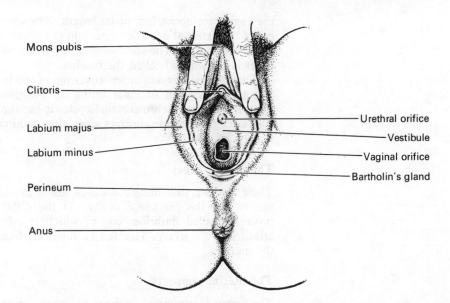

Figure 10.1
The external genitalia

Figure 10.2
The internal genitalia

External genitalia

The external genitalia are shown in Figure 10.1.

Internal genitalia

These organs are illustrated in Figure 10.2.

The vagina

The vagina is the link between the internal and external organs. It is a muscular canal which begins at the introitus, passes upwards and backwards and ends at the uterus. Its lining is in folds allowing it to expand easily. The vaginal walls secrete a cleaning and lubricating fluid which is acidic during the childbearing years and alkaline before puberty and usually after the menopause.

The uterus

The uterus is a hollow, muscular, pear-shaped organ lying almost at right angles to the vagina and bent over the urinary bladder. Its lower end, the cervix, projects into the vagina for about half of its length. The opening of this part into the vagina is called the **external os**. The upper end of the cervix opens into the body of the uterus at the **internal os**. The area between the points of entrance of the uterine (Fallopian) tubes is domed and called the **fundus**.

The uterus has an outer covering of peritoneum, a middle muscular layer (myometrium), and an inner lining of epithelium (endometrium), which alters in thickness during each menstrual cycle. It has the ability to expand to accommodate a 40-week fetus and to contract again after childbirth to its normal length of approximately 7.5 cm.

The uterine tubes

These are two thin muscular tubes which provide a passageway directly from the uterus into the peritoneal cavity. At the distal end of each tube are finger-like processes called **fimbriae**, one of which is a little longer than the others and is attached to the ovary. The uterine tubes are like long arms flopping at the sides of the uterus.

The uterine supports

The uterus is supported in the pelvic cavity by the surrounding organs, the muscles of the pelvic floor — particularly the levator ani muscles — and ligaments, which are derived from folds of peritoneum and connective tissue.

The **broad ligaments** are formed by double folds of peritoneum on either side of the uterus. They hang down over the uterine tubes and are attached to the sides of the pelvis. They contain the round and ovarian ligaments.

The two cardinal ligaments are attached to the sides of the cervix and extend laterally to the walls of the pelvis.

The two uterosacral ligaments are attached to the posterior wall of the cervix and extend backwards, on either side of the rectum, to the sacrum.

A deep depression between the vagina and rectum formed by peritoneum is known as the **pouch of Douglas**.

The ovaries

The ovaries are the female gonads (sex glands) which secrete the hormones oestrogen and progesterone.

They are approximately 3 cm long and 1.5 cm wide and lie in the peritoneal cavity on the back of the broad ligament near the fimbriated ends of the uterine tubes.

The medulla or central part of the ovary is composed of fibrous tissue and contains blood vessels, lymphatic vessels and nerves.

The cortex or outer layer is composed of connective tissue called stroma which contains follicles in various stages of development. The appearance of the cortex depends on the age of the individual and the stage of the menstrual cycle.

Before puberty the surface of the ovary is smooth. The follicles in the stroma, called primordial follicles, are small and immature. During the childbearing years at each menstrual cycle, one or more follicles are stimulated to grow. Each follicle contains a maturing ovum and, during each cycle, one of these follicles matures, rises to the surface of the ovary, ruptures and releases the ovum into the uterine tube. This process is known as ovulation. The remainder of the follicle develops as the corpus luteum.

If the ovum is not fertilized, towards the end of the cycle the corpus luteum degenerates into a scar-like white body called the corpus albicans.

After the menopause there is a gradual disappearance of the follicles but there are numerous white bodies throughout the stroma.

The menstrual cycle

Menstruation and the events leading up to it are termed the menstrual cycle (Fig. 10.3) and are under the control of hormones.

Figure 10.3
The menstrual cycle

The anterior pituitary gland secretes the follicle stimulating hormone (FSH) which stimulates a primordial follicle to grow and mature.

As the follicle develops it secretes oestrogen which eventually inhibits the secretion of FSH and stimulates the release of the luteinising hormone (LH), also from the anterior pituitary. Oestrogen causes the endometrium to begin to thicken.

When it is sufficiently mature the follicle ruptures and releases an ovum which is then carried slowly along the uterine tube towards the cavity of the uterus. Ovulation has now taken place.

The remainder of the ruptured follicle develops into the corpus luteum which secretes progesterone. Progesterone prepares the breast and uterus for *gestation* and is only present in the circulation after ovulation, unlike oestrogen which is secreted throughout the cycle.

If the ovum is not fertilized, about 12 days after ovulation the corpus luteum degenerates and the secretion of progesterone and oestrogen ceases. Lack of progesterone causes the endometrium to break down giving rise to the menstrual flow which normally lasts from 3 to 5 days.

This entire process is under the control of the hypothalamus.

Related structures lying in close proximity to the reproductive organs are shown in Figure 10.4.

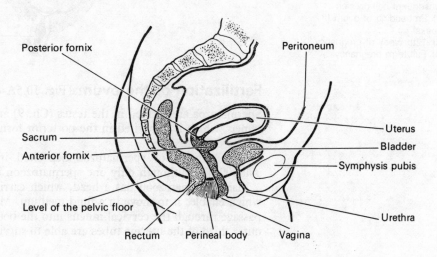

Figure 10.4
Sagittal section of pelvis

A
1. Primordial follicle
2. Graafian follicle
3. Ovulation
4. Fertilization of the ovum
5, 6, 7, 8. Cell division
   of morula as it goes
   along the Fallopian
   tube

B   3 weeks
Chorionic villi forming placenta

Embryo

Decidua

C   12 weeks
Amnion

Chorion (fused)

Fetus

Placenta

Amniotic fluid

D

Placenta

Cervix

Figure 10.5
(A) Fertilization of ovum and subsequent cell division
(B) Embedding of ovum (3 weeks)
(C) 12th week of pregnancy
(D) Full term pregnancy

Fertilization of the ovum (Fig. 10.5A–D)

Spermatozoa are formed in the testes (Ch. 9) and are contained in a fluid known as semen, which is deposited in the posterior fornix of the vagina during sexual intercourse or coitus.

The number of spermatozoa deposited in one act of intercourse is about 300 000 000, although only one spermatozoon is needed to fertilize the ovum.

Each spermatozoon has a head, which carries genetic material, and a long tail, which enables it to move in a fluid medium. Many spermatozoa perish during their passage through the cervical mucus into the body of the uterus; those that reach the outer third of the uterine tubes are able to survive there for approximately 36 hours.

Fertilization occurs when the head of a spermatozoon penetrates an ovum and the genetic material of both mix. The fertilized ovum is propelled along the uterine tube by gentle peristaltic movements; during this time it begins to divide; it finally reaches the uterine cavity as a small mass of cells. About 6 to 8 days after fertilization this mass becomes embedded in the endometrium, which has been specially prepared to receive the fertilized ovum. The endometrium is now known as the decidua.

Chromosomes

Each cell in the body contains 46 chromosomes **arranged in pairs**. Two of these are the sex chromosomes; the remaining 44 are called autosomes. At fertilization the reproductive cells — the ovum and the spermatozoon — each contains 23 chromosomes, so that when they unite the resulting embryo has 46 chromosomes. The new individual is different from both parents but has some characteristics of both.

Genetic abnormalities

Some abnormalities seen in babies at birth or in later life are caused by chromosomal abnormalities. The diagnosis is made by examining cells from the body under a microscope. An example of such a disorder is Down's syndrome (Ch. 15).

Genetic counselling

Couples can now have genetic counselling when there is a history of hereditary disease in the family. They will be told the chances of recurrence of the abnormality before embarking on a pregnancy. Alternatively, a pregnant woman can be investigated and counselled at an early stage in gestation.

It must be remembered, however, that many congenital abnormalities in the newborn are caused by viral infection and by the effects of drugs taken by the mother before the 12th week of pregnancy. At this time the placental barrier, which protects the growing embryo, is not fully developed. The rubella virus is particularly dangerous. Care must be taken to ensure that the mother avoids all drugs except those prescribed by her doctor.

Preconception clinics

These clinics have been set up to meet the needs of couples with certain medical and/or obstetric problems in order to ascertain whether pregnancy is advisable for them or not.

In many instances with a carefully structured plan of antenatal care backed up with the appropriate specialist skills and resources, a happy outcome of pregnancy can be predicted.

Signs and symptoms of pregnancy

1. Amenorrhoea occurring when hitherto the cycle has been regular. The expected date of delivery (EDD) should always be estimated from the first day of the last normal period, to which 9 months and 7 days are added. For instance:

Last menstrual period (LMP)   —1st March
Expected date of delivery (EDD)   —8th December

The immunological pregnancy diagnosis test may be carried out 14 days following the missed expected menstrual period. Pregnancy can therefore be diagnosed at about 6 weeks gestation.

2. Breast changes. The breasts become enlarged, tense and tender. The veins around the areolar area of the breast become prominent and pigmentation of this area occurs. The Montgomery follicles enlarge (Fig. 10.6).

3. There may be nausea and occasionally vomiting, which can be troublesome during the early months.

4. Frequency of micturition may also occur. This is principally due to displace-

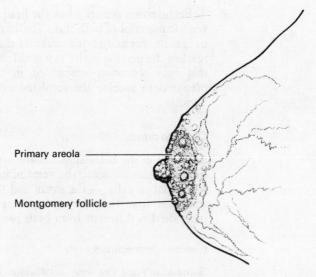

Primary areola

Montgomery follicle

Figure 10.6
Enlargement of the breast in
pregnancy

Figure 10.7
Growth of uterus showing the
fundal heights at the 12th, 18th
24th, 30th, 36th and 40th week

ment of the bladder and subsequent reduction of the bladder capacity by the growing
uterus.

5. The uterus is palpable per abdomen by the 12th week of pregnancy
(Fig. 10.7). *Quickening* or 'feeling life' is experienced about the 18th week of pregnancy — earlier in *multipara*.

The fetal heart may be heard by using an *ultrasonic* device called the *Doptone* after
12 to 14 weeks of pregnancy and by using an ordinary fetal heart stethoscope from
the 20th week. Fetal parts can be palpated at 26 to 28 weeks.

Antenatal care

As antenatal care has improved throughout the years so have the chances of survival
for the mother and the baby.

Antenatal care from the beginning of pregnancy is essential and all babies should
be born in hospital where expert care can be given by obstetricians, paediatricians
and midwives, who have available all the sophisticated equipment and facilities of
a modern obstetric hospital. It is essential to include instruction on parentcraft
during the antenatal period and to prepare both parents for labour and the subsequent care of the baby.

Antenatal screening for congenital abnormalities

Recent research has evolved a method of detecting neural tube defects, such as major
degrees of spina bifida, by estimating the *alpha-feto* protein level in the blood at the
16th week of pregnancy. If the level is raised above normal limits the test is repeated
and, if still raised, a specimen of amniotic fluid is withdrawn (amniocentesis)
(Fig. 10.8). From this specimen the diagnosis is made and termination of pregnancy
is offered to the patient and her husband. Amniocentesis may also be offered, in an
increasing number of centres, to patients who are over 35 years of age to exclude
Down's syndrome (Ch. 15). This is carried out at the 16th week of pregnancy. Other
genetic abnormalities may be diagnosed in this way (see p. 377).

Ultrasonography

Ultrasonography is used in all fields of medicine as a diagnostic aid. In obstetrics
the ultrasonic scan (Fig. 10.9), which has no radiation hazards, has almost totally
replaced the X-ray examination (Fig. 10.10).

Scans are particularly useful for:

1. Diagnosis of pregnancy as early as 6 weeks.
2. Estimating fetal growth and maturity by measuring the fetal biparietal
diameters.

Figure 10.8
(A) Amniocentesis being carried out in the scan room. Scan result is shown on the screen (left) to locate the placental site.
(B) Amniocentesis detail.
(Bv courtesy of Dr J. B. Scrimgeour, Consultant Obstetrician and Gynaecologist. Western General Hospital, Edinburgh)

3. Locating the placental site prior to amniocentesis and in antepartum haemorrhage.
4. Diagnosis of multiple pregnancy in the early weeks of pregnancy.
5. Diagnosis of breech presentation.

To carry out this procedure olive oil is applied to the abdomen and the probe which is connected to the ultrasonic machine is 'run over' the abdomen (Fig. 10.9). The uterine contents show up on the screen (Fig. 10.9B). This result is photographed by a polaroid camera and the photograph is placed in the patient's records.

Figure 10.9
(A) Ultrasonic scan in process
showing probe passing over
abdominal wall.
(B) Scan result at 16 weeks of
pregnancy — P: placenta; B:
body; H: head.
(By courtesy of Dr J. B.
Scrimgeour, Consultant
Obstetrician and Gynaecologist,
Western General Hospital,
Edinburgh)

Labour

This is the process by which the baby is born.

Signs of onset of labour

1. Rupture of the membranes (Fig. 10.11).
2. Appearance of a blood-stained mucus discharge. During pregnancy the cervical canal contains a plug of mucus which is discharged at the onset of labour and is known as *show*.
3. Onset of painful uterine contractions which may begin with general abdominal discomfort and backache. The contractions of true labour can be timed by the clock and occur at 15–20 minute intervals, gradually becoming more frequent and of longer duration.

Labour may begin with any of the above signs in any order or all signs may be present.

Figure 10.10
X-ray of unusual breech
presentation

The onset of labour occurs spontaneously but where there are certain medical
disorders or obstetric complications such as diabetes or pre-eclampsia labour may
be induced (*induction of labour*). The mother-to-be requires sympathetic encouragement and support especially from the midwives in attendance. Labour is divided into
three stages.

The **first stage** (Fig. 10.11) is from the beginning of dilatation of the external
cervical os until its full dilatation. The membranes or bag of *forewaters* may rupture
at any time before the onset of labour, during the first stage or at the beginning of
the second stage of labour. This is the longest stage of labour but its duration has
been reduced by modern obstetric practice, such as using intravenous syntocinon.
Drugs such as pethidine and diamorphine may be prescribed by the doctor for the
relief of pain.

Fetal head
Cervical canal opening
Bag of forewaters (membranes)
Vagina

Figure 10.11
First stage of labour

Figure 10.12
Second stage of labour

In the **second stage** (Fig. 10.12), during which the baby is born, the mother 'bears down', assisting the action of the uterus in expediting the birth of the baby. (The care of the baby is described in Ch. 17.)

The **third stage** (Fig. 10.13) is concerned with the expulsion of the placenta and membranes. The contraction during which the shoulders and body of the baby are born detaches the placenta from the wall of the uterus and the uterus contracts and retracts, causing a reduction in its size. The placenta is pushed into the lower part of the uterus and during the next contraction it appears at the vulva and is expelled.

Haemorrhage is a grave risk at this stage and *ergometrine* or *syntometrine* is used to prevent and control haemorrhage if it occurs.

False labour

False labour may occur towards the end of pregnancy. The uterine contractions, though painful, are irregular and there are no other signs of labour present. The doctor or midwife may carry out an examination per vaginam to differentiate. If the patient is in true labour the cervix will be dilated and in false labour no dilation will have occurred.

Figure 10.13
Third stage of labour

Puerperium

The puerperium begins when the placenta is expelled and ends 6 weeks later. During this time the uterus, ligaments, pelvic floor and vagina return to their pregravid state. Lactation is initiated (p. 409) and the mother recovers from the physical and emotional stress of childbirth.

Great patience and tact are required at this time in handling the new mother and her baby. The mother may have frequent spells of weeping over apparently trivial incidents, particularly in association with her baby. This emotional instability is part of the normal pattern of the puerperium and an experienced midwife and health visitor can give invaluable support.

Planned early discharge

This may be requested by a mother who wishes to return to her home and family as soon as possible or who would have preferred a home confinement but is willing to come into hospital for delivery only. The duration of stay could be as short as 6 hours or it may last 2 or 3 days depending on the condition of mother and baby. Agreement to this request must be reached between the consultant obstetrician and general practitioner and the domiciliary midwife who will make an assessment of the home conditions.

Domiciliary midwifery

Although Scotland has a 99.52% hospital delivery rate (1981 figure) the option still remains open for a home confinement.

There are women who prefer to remain at home but maternal and perinatal statistics have indicated that the hospital provides the maximum safety for the mother and baby. Serious complications may arise in labour which cannot be forecast such as postpartum haemorrhage endangering the mother's life or an asphyxiated baby who may not survive or survive with a risk of brain damage.

Emergency flying squad (emergency obstetric service)

This service is based at a hospital providing cover for the surrounding area and is available to the medical practitioner and midwife to deal with obstetric emergencies at home. The service provides resuscitation for the mother and baby if necessary and may transport them to hospital for further treatment. It is equipped however to carry out forceps deliveries in the home. Although the Emergency Flying Squad service is very effective, there could be considerable delay in reaching the patient and this might prove fatal; because such a service is necessary it lays emphasis on the dangers of confinement in the home.

Figure 10.14
Emergency delivery

Emergency delivery

Delivery of a baby in the street or in an ambulance, private car or aircraft, perhaps en route to the hospital usually hits the newspaper headlines. Although this does not occur frequently, the nurse may be faced with this emergency. Occasionally the expectant mother experiences no discomfort or pain and reaches the second stage of labour without being aware of what is happening. The second stage can progress to delivery of the baby very rapidly, especially in a multiparous patient.

Dealing with emergency delivery

1. The nurse should ask a responsible person to dial 999, explain that an ambulance is required urgently and what it is required for.
2. As the mother-to-be will be very upset and afraid, the nurse must comfort her and endeavour to promote confidence and keep calm.
3. It is essential to ensure as much privacy as possible and all onlookers must be sent away firmly.
4. The mother should be placed flat on her back lying on newspaper, a coat or anything clean to protect her from cold and contamination from the ground or floor. Clothing from the lower part of her body should be removed and she must be encouraged to keep her legs widely open. The baby will be expelled and the nurse should gently hold him head down by supporting the head and shoulders with one hand and with the other grasping the ankles to allow mucus to drain away from the nasopharynx so that he can breathe. A clean tissue or handkerchief, if available, could be used to wipe the eyes, nose and mouth. The baby's colour is blue at birth but when respiration is established it becomes pink. If the baby fails to breathe, gentle skin stimulus by flicking the soles of the feet may initiate respiration. A newborn baby loses heat very quickly and should be placed against the mother's body so that heat will be transmitted, lying on its side to promote drainage of mucus. Clothing can be tucked around mother and baby. If the cord is long enough the mother may hold the baby in her arms. It is much safer to leave the baby attached to the placenta as sterile materials will not be available to cut the umbilical cord. If the placenta appears at the vulva it should be gently lifted out and placed in close proximity to the baby. It is essential that no traction is put on the cord or any effort made to hasten the delivery of the placenta as severe haemorrhage could occur. If however there is excessive bleeding from the vagina the fundus of the uterus should be palpated and gently massaged with a circular movement of the hand which will stimulate uterine contractions and thus control bleeding.

The mother and baby should be transported to hospital accompanied by the nurse as soon as possible.

CONTRACEPTION

The best method of preventing unwanted births is to prevent pregnancy from occurring by the judicious use of contraception. Advice and literature on this subject are readily available from family planning services.

Methods

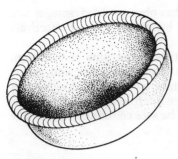

Figure 10.15
Vaginal diaphragm

Various methods are available:

1. Mechanical methods, the vaginal diaphragm (Fig. 10.15) and the condom (see Ch. 9) are commonly used. Neither is completely effective.

The vaginal diaphragm is a dome made of fine latex or plastic and attached to a circular wire spring giving the appearance of a cap hence its other name, cervical cap. It fits across the upper vagina to provide a barrier preventing the ejaculated spermatozoa from reaching the cervix. It is made in various sizes and every woman using it is individually fitted.

Women using this method of contraception are advised to insert the diaphragm routinely every night after cleaning it and smearing the rim and the dome with a spermicidal cream.

It should be left in position for at least 6 hours after coitus.

2. Intrauterine devices (IUDs, Fig. 10.16) in a variety of shapes are also widely used. They are made of inert radio-opaque plastic and must be fitted into the uterus by a skilled practitioner. Threads are attached to them so that the woman can check regularly that her IUD is in place.

IUDs are simply foreign bodies in the uterus. They have a contraceptive effect but are not completely reliable. They have recently been modified to include copper or zinc which allows smaller devices to be used without loss of effectiveness.

Figure 10.16
Intrauterine devices (A) Lippes loop (B) Dalkon shield (C) Saf-t-coil (D) Copper 7

Another device, the Progesterat (Fig. 10.17) is T shaped and releases a small amount of progesterone daily which increases the efficiency of the method. This particular device must be replaced once a year.

3. The most effective method, if used correctly, is oral contraception. The contraceptive pill usually contains some form of oestrogen and progestogen. It works mainly by inhibiting ovulation but also has an effect on the endometrium and the cervical mucosa which can prevent implantation occurring. Clear instructions for use are given with each packet.

Oral contraceptives regulate the menstrual cycle and shorten the length of flow of each menstrual period. Initial side effects sometimes experienced by women are:
Nausea.
Sore and swollen breasts.
Slight weight gain.

These are of short duration. More serious complications, such as deep venous thrombosis, are comparatively rare, but all women who take the pill should have regular medical examinations every 3 to 6 months.

4. Natural forms of contraception such as coitus interruptus (see Ch. 9) and those which make use of the 'safe period' are the forms recommended to people who are opposed to artificial means of contraception. The life-spans of spermatozoa and ova are short and fertilization occurs near the time that the ovum is released. Both these methods are based on calculating the time of ovulation and avoiding intercourse during the fertile period, that is for approximately 10 days. The remaining days of the cycle are termed the 'safe period'. Special calendars and the calculation of body temperature are used to determine the time of ovulation.

Figure 10.17
Progesterat

This method known also as the 'rhythm method' has obvious disadvantages and is not recommended to women with irregular cycles, but it can be used effectively by those determined to do so.

The Billings method is also based on the calculation of the time of ovulation. According to Billings every woman has a mucus loss from the cervix and vagina whenever she ovulates. Billings maintains that by teaching a woman to recognize her own cervical mucus pattern she can then calculate her infertile and possibly fertile days by daily charting of her cervical mucus loss. To be safe coitus should not take place for 3 'dry' days following mucus loss.

Sterilization

The ultimate resort in contraception is sterilization. Both male and female sterilization should be regarded as irreversible.

Male sterilization

The operation of vasectomy is not effective immediately. Only after 3 months can the couple dispense with alternative forms of contraception (see Ch. 9).

Female sterilization

Female sterilization is effective immediately but involves an operation under general anaesthesia and normally a short stay in hospital. Usually the uterine tubes can be cauterized through the laparoscope. Failing this, laparotomy, involving an 8 to 10 day stay in hospital, is performed to cut and tie the uterine tubes.

Following sterilization intercourse can be enjoyed normally by both sexes.

INFERTILITY

The term 'infertility' is preferred to 'sterility'. Infertility is the state in which a couple who desire conception are unable to achieve it. During the early years of marriage many couples practise contraception; therefore a marriage cannot be considered infertile until the couple have performed regular coitus without the use of contraceptives for a period of 2 years.

Infertility may be either primary, when the wife has never conceived, or secondary, when there has been either one child or an aborted conception of the marriage.

Initially, when a couple decide to have their infertile marriage investigated, they should be seen as a unit by one person such as the family doctor. Often during these preliminary discussions erroneous ideas are corrected and the couple can be instructed in techniques of sexual intercourse and in the most suitable time for coitus in relation to conception. In many cases this 'treatment' is sufficient and pregnancy soon follows. If it does not then ideally the couple should be investigated at the same time, the husband by a urologist and the wife by a gynaecologist.

Infertility in the female is commonly caused either by some factor preventing the spermatozoa from having free passage to the uterine tubes where the ovum is fertilized or by the woman failing to ovulate so there is no ovum to be fertilized.

Investigations

Vaginal examination.
Laparoscopy with insufflation of the uterine tubes.
Hysterosalpingogram.
These investigations should confirm or eliminate anatomical deformities of the tract and patency of the tubes.
If one or both uterine tubes are found to be obstructed, further tests may be performed to exclude tuberculosis.
Ovulation is confirmed by:
Charting daily basal body temperature.

Vaginal cytology.

Ferning of cervical mucus.

Endocrine assays for progesterone.

Endometrial biopsy performed during the second half of the menstrual cycle.

In some couples it may be possible to perform a postcoital test. An hour or two following coitus a specimen of mucus from the cervical canal is examined under a microscope for the presence of motile spermatozoa. If large numbers of live and active sperms are present the husband is considered normal and intercourse satisfactory. It may be that some secretion in the vagina is killing the sperm.

Most of these investigations involve only a short stay in hospital or may be performed on an out-patient basis. The nurse has a valuable role to play. She can offer reassurance and guidance to the patient and should have sufficient knowledge of the subject to be able to answer questions intelligently.

Investigations of husband and wife may be ineffective and no cause may be found for the couple's infertility. Psychiatric assessment may then be necessary. This may, for example, disclose that the wife has an abnormal fear of pregnancy itself or of the responsibilities of motherhood.

New hope has been given to many childless couples by the recent successes of artificial insemination of the husband's semen (AIH), artificial insemination of an unknown donor's semen (AID), fertility drugs, and the 'test tube babies'.

AETIOLOGY OF DISORDERS

There are four main groups of causes of disease of the female reproductive tract:

1. Anatomical deformity.
2. New growths.
3. Hormone imbalance.
4. Infection.

Anatomical deformity may be congenital, for example malformation or absence of one or more organs, or it may be acquired by trauma to organs, muscles, ligaments or other structures. This trauma may be associated with childbirth, surgery, obesity, old age or disordered bladder and bowel functions.

New growths may be either benign or malignant and may involve the reproductive organs or the pituitary gland.

Hormone imbalance may be due to disordered function of the ovary or the pituitary, or disturbance of the hypothalamus, which is the nerve centre controlling the pituitary gland. Hormone imbalance is common at the onset of puberty and at the menopause.

Infection in the pelvic area may follow childbirth or abortion. It is usually associated with ignorance regarding personal hygiene or it may be transmitted from the sexual partner. During the childbearing years when the woman is more exposed to infection she is afforded some protection by the acidic vaginal secretion. After the menopause this safeguard no longer exists because the vaginal secretions become considerably less acidic.

GENERAL FEATURES OF DISORDER

Vaginal discharge

In health there is a white mucoid discharge from the vagina which increases in amount and thickens in consistency immediately before and after a menstrual period, at ovulation and during sexual excitement.

Abnormal or excessive vaginal discharge takes various forms. It may be merely an excess of the normal secretion or it may contain micro-organisms that cause it to become mucopurulent or purulent. Discharge containing pus is greenish-yellow in colour, offensive and accompanied by itching.

Other causes of vaginal discharge are the presence of foreign bodies in the vagina, such as radium implants and occasionally tampons which have been left in place more than 48 hours. These produce a foul-smelling discharge and vaginal toilet is essential following their removal.

Carcinoma of the cervix in its later stages causes a bloodstained, fetid discharge. Frequent baths and the use of bidets should be encouraged. The patient will need sensitive management because she may feel extremely embarrassed by the constant foul smell which surrounds her.

Advice on the use and disposal of sanitary napkins is essential, especially in the prevention of spread of infection.

Pruritus vulvae

Itchiness of the vulva is commonly associated with vaginal discharges, particularly those produced by the organisms *Candida albicans* and *Trichomonas vaginalis*. It may also be a feature of skin diseases, allergies, diabetes and psychosomatic disorders. It disturbs sleep and is both a distressing and socially embarrassing condition.

Menstrual disturbances

Menorrhagia

This term is used to describe a menstrual period occurring at the normal cyclical time but accompanied by heavy and prolonged bleeding.

Metrorrhagia

This is intermenstrual bleeding — that is bleeding which occurs between the normal menstrual periods and in addition to them.

Polymenorrhoea

This term refers to unusually frequent menstruation.

Oligomenorrhoea

This defines infrequent menstruation.

Amenorrhoea

The absence of menstruation is known as amenorrhoea. It may be either primary or secondary.

Primary amenorrhoea is the term used when menstruation has never occurred. It may be described as 'real amenorrhoea', in which case there is usually some endocrine abnormality, or 'apparent amenorrhoea' because, although the girl has developed all the secondary sex characteristics and experienced the symptoms of menstruation, she has never had a menstrual flow. This is because the membrane occluding the vaginal opening has no perforation and therefore the flow cannot escape. It is simply treated by making a hole in the hymen with the patient under general anaesthesia.

Secondary amenorrhoea may be defined as the absence of menstruation for a period which is twice that of the normal menstrual cycle of a woman who has menstruated previously. This state is normal during pregnancy.

Dysmenorrhoea

This is the word used to describe pain associated with menstruation. There are two recognized types of dysmenorrhoea.

Primary or spasmodic dysmenorrhoea is colicky pain experienced on the first day of menstruation. There is usually no organic cause and it is common in young girls.

Secondary dysmenorrhoea occurs in older women and is secondary to pelvic abnormality such as pelvic congestion, uterine colic or endometriosis.

Premenstrual tension

Irritation and lability of emotions are experienced to a lesser or greater extent by most women in the days prior to menstruation.

Bleeding per vaginam

Dysfunctional uterine bleeding

This is the term used to describe abnormal bleeding following any of the above patterns for which no organic cause can be found.

Postmenopausal bleeding (PMB)

This is vaginal bleeding which occurs in women who have stopped menstruating. Such bleeding is only called PMB when it has been established that the woman has not had a menstrual period for approximately 1 year.

Postcoital bleeding

This is bleeding after sexual intercourse.

Pain

Low back pain and low abdominal pain are common features of disorder in the pelvic area. Referred pain is a feature when nerve pathways are disturbed.

Dyspareunia

This is pain during or after sexual intercourse.

Urinary symptoms

These are commonly associated with gynaecological disease because of the close proximity of the bladder and urethra to the uterus and vagina.

Urinary incontinence is very distressing. A particular symptom of gynaecological disease is stress incontinence. Increased abdominal pressure such as coughing, laughing and sneezing causes a small amount of urine to escape involuntarily from the bladder. It is common in pregnancy and uterovaginal prolapse and is associated with a congenital weakness of the internal sphincter of the bladder.

Large bowel symptoms

These include, for example, constipation, which may occur as a result of pressure on the bowel due to retroverted or prolapsed uterus or the presence of a fistula.

Abdominal swelling

The presence of tumours or ascites in the abdominal cavity may give rise to an increase in the size of the abdomen.

Anaemia

Iron deficiency anaemia is a common accompanying feature of disorders of the female reproductive tract.

INVESTIGATIONS

History

History taking is an important preliminary to diagnosis of gynaecological diseases, particularly in relation to menstrual bleeding, vaginal discharge and urinary symptoms.

Figure 10.18A
Dorsal position

Figure 10.18B
Sims' position

Figure 10.18C
Lithotomy position

General physical examination

General physical examination is essential prior to surgery, particular attention being paid to the patient's blood picture.

Pelvic examination

Examination of the pelvic organs via the vagina enables the gynaecologist to detect any obvious disorder, such as the presence of polyps, tumours or uterine displacements, and to estimate the gestation of a pregnancy.

Figure 10.18A, B and C show the positions which are commonly used and referred to in gynaecology.

Figure 10.19
Bimanual examination

Figure 10.20
Sims' speculum

Figure 10.21
Cusco's bivalve speculum

Vaginal examination

Vaginal examination may be performed in a variety of ways:

1. **Bimanual examination.** Two fingers of one hand are inserted into the vagina while the other hand is used to palpate the abdomen (Fig. 10.19).
2. **Speculum examination.** Insertion of a vaginal speculum such as a Sims' speculum (Fig. 10.20) or more commonly Cusco's speculum (Fig. 10.21), allows the cervix to be inspected visually.

Rectal examination

It is possible but more difficult to palpate the cervix, uterus and appendages via the rectum. Rectal examination may be used in conjunction with vaginal examination to determine the presence or to assess the extent of a lesion.

During vaginal and rectal examination the nurse plays a vital role. She preserves the patient's modesty by ensuring that she is correctly positioned and adequately draped. She reassures the patient by her presence, by guiding her into the positions required by the doctor and by her repeated exhortations to relax. The muscles of the abdomen and pelvic floor must be relaxed if the doctor is to gain any information from the examination.

Examination under anaesthesia

A diagnosis can sometimes be confirmed by vaginal examination under anaesthesia and by dilatation and currettage whereby scrapings are obtained from the cervix and lining of the uterus. Biopsy may also be performed by this route.

Laparoscopy

Laparoscopy is performed under general anaesthesia. Approximately 4 litres of gas (carbon dioxide or nitrous oxide and air are used) are injected either through the abdomen or via the cervix to inflate the peritoneal cavity, giving the surgeon a wider area in which to work. A large trocar and cannula are inserted into the abdominal cavity through a small incision made just below the umbilicus. A special endoscope, called a laparoscope, which has a fibreoptic lighting system is passed through this cannula allowing the pelvic organs to be examined visually. Using forceps attached to the cervix the uterus can be manipulated during the procedure.

There are a variety of attachments available which allow biopsies to be taken from the ovaries, dye to be inserted to test the patency of the uterine tubes, and diathermy to cauterize the tubes.

This procedure has largely superseded laparotomy as a means of investigation and tubal ligation as a means of sterilization.

Nursing care

Preparation of a patient for this procedure may include abdominal and pubic shave, administration of suppositories or disposable enema and the usual preparation prior to general anaesthesia.

One or two clips are used to close the abdominal incision; they are usually removed within 48 hours. Following this procedure many patients experience shoulder tip pain which is pain referred from the diaphragm due to the distension of the abdomen by CO_2. Oral analgesics and reassurance are normally all that is required.

Hysterosalpingogram

A hysterosalpingogram is an X-ray of the genital tract following the injection, through the cervix, of a radio-opaque fluid to demonstrate intrauterine abnormalities and to test the patency of the uterine tubes.

Cervical smear

A cervical smear is an aid to the diagnosis of cancer. To take a cervical smear a Cusco's bivalve speculum (Fig. 10.21) is inserted into the vagina. An Ayre's spatula (Fig. 10.22) is passed through the speculum to take scrapings from the neck of the cervix. The scrapings are deposited on a glass slide, fixed with pure alcohol and sent for cytological examination.

Clinics offering this service to women are available in most cities in the Western hemisphere. All patients attending gynaecology or antenatal clinics have a cervical smear taken routinely.

High vaginal swab

A swab may be taken from the vagina to test for the presence of micro-organisms so that the correct treatment may be administered.

Figure 10.22
Ayre's spatula

Immunological pregnancy test

This test requires the collection of an early morning specimen of urine. It is used to confirm a diagnosis of suspected pregnancy 2 weeks after a missed period. It may also be used to indicate the level of human chorionic gonadotrophin (HCG) in the urine of a woman who has recently aborted a hydatidiform mole.

Other tests

Blood tests, radiography and skin tests are used to confirm that the patient is not suffering from tuberculosis and are also used in conjunction with 24-hour collections of urine to investigate endocrine abnormalities. The haemoglobin estimation is also very important.

DISORDERS OF THE FEMALE REPRODUCTIVE TRACT

Cervical erosion (ectropion or eversion)

The vaginal portion of the cervix is normally covered with squamous epithelium similar to that lining the vagina. Oestrogen stimulation may cause this lining to be replaced by columnar epithelium similar to that lining the cervical canal, giving rise to the appearance typical of cervical erosion. This condition is more properly named cervical ectropion or eversion.

The erosion appears as a red, circular area covered with mucus surrounding the external os. It is common in women taking the contraceptive pill and during and after pregnancy.

Clinical features

Mucopurulent discharge.
Intermenstrual bleeding.
Postcoital bleeding.
Irritation and discomfort.

Treatment

Cautery of the cervix using diathermy is performed under general anaesthesia. This may be carried out in a day bed area. The patient should be warned that the healing process takes about 3 weeks and that during this time she will have an increased amount of vaginal discharge which may be bloodstained.

Cryosurgery (application of extreme cold) is becoming increasingly popular in the treatment of this condition. It can be performed in an out-patient department since it does not require general anaesthesia.

Pain, similar to that experienced in dysmenorrhoea may occur during the freezing process. The treatment is usually followed by a vaginal discharge, severe enough to require the wearing of sanipads, for 2 to 3 weeks. Postcoital bleeding may occur in a few cases therefore patients are usually advised to avoid intercourse for 2 weeks.

Infections

Infections within the female reproductive tract are very common.

Vulvitis

Lower genital tract infections are usually first seen and treated by the patient's general practitioner. Alternatively, the patient may be referred to an out-patient clinic. Admission to hospital may be required for treatment of a more serious condition to which the infection is secondary.

The vulva is covered with skin and is subject to any skin disorder. It is also the primary site of some sexually transmitted diseases. Discharges from the bladder, vagina and rectum make the vulval area moist and lack of hygiene may allow the vulva to become infected by a variety of organisms. A chronic condition may develop with constant irritation, tenderness and ulceration. This condition may be self-inflicted by the indiscriminate use of deodorants, talcum powders and soaps to which a woman may develop an allergy. The wearing of tights and pantee girdles, particularly if not changed frequently, capture heat and moisture causing sufficient irritation for the skin to break down. These are very difficult conditions to treat and, although not serious, cause considerable discomfort.

Clinical features

In the acute stages of infection the vulva becomes very moist from discharge, inflamed, swollen and tender. The inguinal glands may also become swollen and tender.

Treatment

The aim of treatment is to keep the area clean and dry. Warm baths, vulval toilet and mild, non-irritating antiseptic lotions are useful as well as applications of powders that do not contain deodorants or perfumes. Ointments should never be applied as they make the area more moist and therefore more susceptible to infection.

In some instances vulvitis may be secondary to another condition, such as thrush or diabetes mellitus, and the vulval irritation should improve when the primary condition is treated. If necessary the irritation can be controlled by the administration of mild sedatives.

Bartholinitis

Infection of Bartholin's gland and duct is usually due either to *E. coli*, staphylococcal infection or gonorrhoea. It may however be caused by any pathogen.

Clinical features

A reddened swelling appears on the vulva in the vicinity of Bartholin's gland and the patient complains of acute discomfort.

During the acute stage an abscess may form and once the infection subsides a cyst may develop.

Treatment

In the acute stage treatment is bed rest, analgesia, and a broad spectrum antibiotic.

If an abscess forms, then surgery is necessary to drain the pus. Blockage of Bartholin's duct or gland by an abscess or cyst is an extremely painful condition often requiring emergency admission to hospital. Often the condition is too painful to allow shaving of the area prior to a general anaesthetic being administered for surgery.

Surgery involves suturing the wall of the abscess or cyst to the vaginal wall following incision to drain the pus or fluid. This procedure is called marsupialization and is preferable to incision of the abscess or excision of the cyst.

Postoperatively, vulval toilet is performed every 4 hours during the day. On discharge home the patient is advised to continue regular bathing of the vulva either by use of bidets or baths, and to complete her antibiotic therapy. She may also be advised to avoid any factor which might have contributed to the cause of the condition such as wearing tight trousers or cycling.

Vaginitis

Most female genital tract infections affect the vagina, causing it to become inflamed. The descriptive term used is vaginitis.

These conditions are characterized by pruritus and by the presence of a vaginal discharge possibly causing skin excoriation (Table 10.1).

A low grade non-specific vaginitis will result if the normal bacteria found in the vagina become pathogenic.

Cervicitis

It is difficult to differentiate cervicitis from other lower genital tract infections. However if the cervix is chronically infected then the affected area should be removed by cautery or cryosurgery. The latter would seem to be the more successful method.

Salpingitis

Infection ascends in the genital tract and ultimately organisms may reach the uterine tubes causing salpingitis. Infection may also reach the tubes directly from:

1. The uterus after childbirth or abortion.
2. The bowel.
3. The peritoneal cavity.

Causative organisms

Staphylococcus
Streptococcus
Gonococcus
E. coli
Tubercle bacillus
The resulting infection is usually bilateral and may be either acute or chronic.

Table 10.1
Vaginitis

Type	Organism	Discharge	Special points	Treatment
Monilial vaginitis	Candida albicans	White and creamy	Associated with diabetes mellitus, oral contraceptives, pregnancy.	Nystatin vaginal cream or Nystatin pessaries, one into vagina each night for 14 nights.
Trichomonas vaginitis	Trichomonas Vaginalis	Greenish-yellow, frothy, offensive	Transmitted during coitus	1. Of patient: Metronidazole (flagyl) 200 mg orally t.i.d. for 1 week. Vaginal pessaries such as Locan and Penotrane, one nightly for 2 to 3 weeks. 2. Of sexual partner: Metronidazole 200 mg orally t.i.d. for 1 week. Abstinence from coitus.
Senile vaginitis	Coliform bacilli streptococcus	Brown	Minute ulcers on vaginal walls	Oestrogen Lactic acid: 1. Orally, usually stilboestrol 2. Locally — creams, pessaries such as Dienoestrol cream. Tampovagen pessaries.

Acute salpingitis

The patient suffering from acute salpingitis may be very seriously ill.

Clinical features

Sudden onset.
Pyrexia.
Tachycardia.
Purulent vaginal discharge.
Tenderness and intense pain felt in one or both sides of the lower abdomen.
A mass felt in the same area.
Associated urinary tract infection.

Treatment

A cervical smear may be taken to find the causative organism and appropriate chemotherapy commenced. Complete bed rest is essential to allow the inflammation in the uterine tubes to resolve, if possible, without thickening the walls of these very narrow tubes. Thickening is accompanied by a narrowing or complete blockage of the lumen, a cause of sterility.

Peritonitis may develop, therefore the nurse should observe and report any changes in temperature, pulse and respiration (TPR) or in the site and character of the pain. Surgery is usually contraindicated, because of the risk of infection.

After treatment of a mild infection the inflammatory process affecting the tubes should resolve and the vital structures should revert to normal. In some cases the tubes become blocked. If this occurs at the fimbriated end of the tube the ovary may also become involved.

Chronic salpingitis

Chronic salpingitis may develop after repeated mild infections which have never been completely eradicated.

Clinical features

Pallor due to latent sepsis.
General malaise.
Lower abdominal pain which worsens premenstrually and after exercise.
Backache.
Increased vaginal discharge.
Menstrual irregularities.
Dyspareunia.
The patient is often in and out of hospital having her symptoms investigated.

Treatment

For the young woman rest and chemotherapy are the basis of treatment. Hysterectomy and bilateral salpingo-oöphorectomy may be performed on an older woman once the infection has been controlled by antibiotics and provided she wants no more children.

Abortion

Abortion is the word used to describe termination of pregnancy. It may occur spontaneously or be induced artificially.

Spontaneous abortion

It is estimated that one in four pregnancies abort spontaneously. This commonly occurs about the 12th week of gestation but may occur anytime during pregnancy.

It is thought that more than half the abortions occurring spontaneously are caused by fetal malformation and the remainder are due to some abnormality in the mother, such as progesterone deficiency, uterine fibroids or an incompetent cervix.

It is also possible that a defect in the chromosomes from the spermatozoa may also give rise to defects which may result in abortion.

Threatened abortion

When a woman with a confirmed (or suspected) pregnancy presents with slight vaginal bleeding and, on examination, the cervix is found to be closed she is diagnosed as 'threatening to abort'. If cared for, the pregnancy may be able to continue normally.

Treatment

Complete bed rest in hospital is the only form of treatment. The patient is reassured and given sedation orally or intramuscularly as required. Constipation is avoided by ensuring that the patient takes roughage in her diet and, if necessary, by the regular use of mild aperients or suppositories.

She is discouraged from stretching, bending, vigorous movement and smoking. Visitors are asked not to excite her.

Vaginal examination is not performed for 48 hours, to allow the pregnancy to settle. During this time all sanitary towels and bedpans are saved for inspection in case some placental tissue has been passed. If, on examination, the external os is found to be closed, the patient can be allowed up once the bleeding has stopped.

A positive immunological pregnancy test reassures that all is well and the woman is discharged home. Many authorities advocate rest and all recommend that coitus should be avoided because of the risk of introducing infection.

Inevitable abortion

If the patient presents with lower abdominal pain and vaginal bleeding which is red and contains clots, abortion is usually inevitable.

On examination the external os is usually dilated, which means that the pregnancy cannot continue. If diagnosis needs to be confirmed the Doptone (p. 378) may be used to prove that the fetus is dead, although an immunological pregnancy test should already have produced a negative result.

Complete abortion

In some cases the fetus and placenta are passed complete in the amniotic sac, hence the term 'complete abortion'.

Following a complete abortion rest at home for 1 week is necessary during which time the vaginal discharge is observed. It should be a normal *lochia* lasting from 7 to 10 days.

Complete abortion usually occurs about the 6th or 8th week of gestation.

Incomplete abortion

If the fetus and placenta are not delivered in their entirety the abortion is said to be incomplete.

The vaginal loss may be quite heavy causing the patient to become shocked. The vagina must be evacuated of clots as quickly as possible. The os is inspected using a Cusco's speculum and the products of conception are removed from the cervix and vagina. At this stage ergometrine (0.5 mg i.m.) is given if bleeding is heavy. The patient's haemoglobin should be estimated and blood should be cross-matched in case transfusion is required.

The uterus is evacuated under general anaesthesia as soon as possible and the patient should be able to be discharged home within 2 days.

At the time of the abortion the patient may be considerably upset emotionally and may require sedation as well as reassurance. Both she and her husband should be informed of the facts as they occur and advised to attempt another pregnancy as soon as they wish.

Habitual abortion

The term habitual abortion is used when a woman aborts three or more consecutive conceptions.

Causes

Incompetent cervix.
Uterine abnormalities.
Abnormality in the chromosomes of one or other parent.

For many patients no cause can be found.

Treatment

Correct the cause when possible, for instance an incompetent cervix; it can be treated simply with Shirodkar's suture.

Under general anaesthesia and using the vaginal route, an unabsorbable suture is placed and tied round the cervix at the level of the internal os (Fig. 10.23).

The patient is nursed in bed for 3 to 5 days before being discharged home. She is encouraged to rest as much as possible during the remainder of her pregnancy. The suture is removed 7 to 14 days prior to term and she is permitted to deliver normally.

If abortion becomes inevitable the stitch must be removed.

If the cause is unknown the patient once pregnant should be advised to avoid travel, exertion and coitus, to take a nutritious diet and rest in bed for 2 hours each afternoon.

Figure 10.23
Shirodkar's suture

Ectopic pregnancy

In this condition the fertilized ovum becomes implanted outside (ectopic) the uterine cavity. The commonest site is the uterine tube where it is impossible for a pregnancy to continue much beyond the 10th week of gestation.

Tubal abortion

The fertilized ovum dies. It may be absorbed completely or aborted completely into the peritoneal cavity. It may be absorbed incompletely or it may become surrounded by blood clot thus forming a tubal mole.

Clinical features

The main features of tubal abortion are colicky pain in the lower abdomen followed by a small amount of dark coloured vaginal bleeding. On vaginal examination a small tender lump may be felt to one side of the uterus. Referred pain to the shoulder may be another feature. The patient may be severely shocked. Diagnosis, which may be difficult, can be aided by the patient's history but can only be confirmed by surgery.

Tubal rupture

Ruptured ectopic pregnancy is fortunately rarer than tubal abortion but is easier to diagnose.

Clinical features

The woman experiences sudden severe lower abdominal pain following which she quickly becomes shocked due to haemorrhage into the peritoneal cavity.

Treatment

Sedation and analgesia are required immediately and on admission to hospital blood transfusion is usually necessary prior to surgery.

Both tubal abortion and ruptured ectopic pregnancy are treated with immediate surgery. Either partial or total salpingectomy is performed. The tube is conserved if at all possible, especially if the woman wishes to conceive again.

The postoperative care is that given routinely to a patient following laparotomy. The patient is usually discharged home within 8 to 10 days.

The nurse's most important duty is accurate observation of the patient to assist in diagnosis of this potentially dangerous condition.

Induced abortion

Abortion may be induced criminally by the backstreet abortionist. Most of these abortions are infected and the unfortunate woman is usually eventually admitted to hospital, or at least treated by a doctor, for pelvic inflammation.

Legally in the U.K., the fetus is said to have become viable at the 28th week of gestation. The 1967 Abortion Act allows termination of pregnancy to be performed up to this period of gestation in hospital or licensed nursing homes for therapeutic reasons. It is also required that all terminations of pregnancy are notified on a prescribed form to the Health Department.

In hospital it is preferred that termination of pregnancy be performed before the 12th week of gestation. After this time the placenta is fully developed and the fundus too high in the abdomen to allow the gynaecologist to be certain that he has removed all the products of conception.

Termination techniques: 0 to 14 weeks

The commonest technique used to terminate pregnancies at this period of gestation is **vacuum aspiration** using a special suction machine (Fig. 10.24).

This is a short procedure performed in theatre under general anaesthesia; it is accompanied by minimal blood loss. The patient may be discharged home the day

Figure 10.24
Vacuum suction apparatus

following operation. This technique may be used to treat patients on an out-patient basis during the early weeks of pregnancy. A small amount of bright red blood loss from the vagina for a few days is normal.

If vacuum suction apparatus is not available **dilatation curettage** (D & C) may be performed.

Menstrual regulation which can effectively terminate pregnancy up to the seventh week of gestation is becoming increasingly popular. Three to 10 days following an overdue period a woman who has been at risk of becoming pregnant can have her uterus emptied of endometrium. Thus her menstruation is regulated whether or not she was pregnant.

The uterus is emptied either by aspiration using a 50 ml syringe attached to a narrow catheter, or, by inserting high into the vagina pessaries containing prostaglandins.

Termination techniques: after 14 weeks

Intra-amniotic administration of prostaglandins. This method involves a miniature labour which can be distressing not only to the individual patient but to others in the ward.

Hysterotomy carries a high mortality and is seldom advocated.

Nursing care and observations

Nursing duties include reassurance to all patients distressed by the condition. Observations to be made of the patient undergoing termination are:

Type and site of pain; normally it is in the lower abdominal region and is intermittent.

Type and quantity of vaginal discharge, including inspection of used sanitary towels and bedpans.

When the uterine contents are expelled they should be examined to see if abortion is complete. If incomplete, evacuation of the uterus under general anaesthesia is necessary before the patient can be discharged home.

Complications

Complications which may follow termination of pregnancy are:

Pelvic inflammation.
Salpingitis.
Ruptured uterus.
Secondary infertility.
Psychological disturbance which often manifests itself as a phantom pregnancy.
Death.

The earlier during pregnancy that termination can be carried out the less likelihood there is of any of these complications occurring.

Tumours

New growths other than those originating from endometriosis are commonly found in the female reproductive tract.

Ovarian tumours

A variety of cysts may form on the ovary. Some are small benign cysts which are symptomless. Others may grow very large and disturb ovarian function. The commonest is the pseudomucinous multilocular cyst which has numerous compartments containing a sticky substance. These cysts have a tendency to become malignant.

A bizarre type of tumour is the dermoid cyst which is usually benign. It may contain a variety of structures such as hair, teeth, cartilage, sebaceous glands, brain, bowel or thyroid tissue.

Small benign cysts in young women usually disappear in time without treatment. All other cysts should be excised since, if left, malignant changes may occur.

The operations performed are:

Ovarian cystectomy	Cyst removed and ovary reconstituted
Oöphorectomy	Ovary and tumour removed when it is impossible to save the ovary
Total hysterectomy and bilateral salpingo-oöphorectomy	Removal of uterus, both tubes, vault of vagina, both ovaries and tumour

The last operation is performed in women who have completed their families and who are near the menopause. This extensive operation is undertaken to safeguard against carcinoma of the ovary, which may remain undetected until the late stages of the disease when the signs and symptoms of pelvic cancer appear.

Malignant changes

Ascites is a prominent feature in the later stages and is accompanied by loss of weight and abdominal distension. Severe pain may be experienced when the growth spreads into the peritoneal cavity.

Postoperatively either radiotherapy or cytotoxic drugs may be administered to reduce the rate of growth of the residual tumour. Neither of these methods may be successful and with either, the patient is subjected to a number of unpleasant side-effects to add to her discomfort.

Prognosis is poor. The patient may linger for a comparatively long time. Frequent abdominal paracentesis with consequent loss of protein may be necessary to relieve the ascites. The patient is terminally ill and should be allowed as much activity as she feels capable of and must never be expected to follow a strict timetable. A high protein diet should be encouraged and use made of proprietary foods to tempt the patient. Skin care is essential. The patient becomes emaciated and lethargic and will spend a great deal of time in bed. The abdomen will frequently be distended with ascites, therefore the skin will alternate between being taut and lax. She can be advised to wear maternity clothing which will adapt to her frequent change in girth.

Patient comfort is essential. All questions asked by the patient and her relatives should be answered as honestly as possible to form a basis for psychological support.

Benign uterine tumours

Polypi are small benign tumours which grow on the wall of the uterus and are attached to it by a stem or peduncle. They cause vaginal discharge and menorrhagia and are treated by cautery.

Fibroids

Fibroids are benign new growths of the uterus common in women who have no children; symptoms are commonly produced in the 35 to 45 age group.

They originate within the myometrium as small, encapsulated structures composed of fibrous and muscle tissue. They are classified according to site (Fig. 10.25):

Figure 10.25
Sites of fibroids

Intramural (interstitial): within the muscle wall.
Submucous (extramual): projecting into the uterine cavity.
Subserous (subperitoneal): growing outwards into the peritoneum, sometimes becoming pedunculated.
Cervical (within the cervix): a rare fibroid which ultimately may occlude the cervical canal.

Clinical features

Fibroids may be symptomless for many years. They grow slowly but eventually tend to grow large, causing increased girth and pressure symptoms such as frequency of micturition, stress incontinence, retention of urine, constipation, haemorrhoids and varicose veins. Menorrhagia is common with consequent iron deficiency anaemia, and sometimes the patient complains of metrorrhagia. A submucous fibroid will cause a foul-smelling vaginal discharge. Many women with fibroids are infertile and often their presence is discovered during investigations of infertility.

If symptomless, fibroids should be left alone; otherwise treatment depends on the age of the patient. If she is near the menopause hysterectomy is performed. Myomectomy, cutting the capsule and shelling out the tumour is performed if possible on women who still desire conception.

Carcinoma of the uterus

Body and fundus

Malignant tumours in this area are slow growing and occur most commonly in nulliparous women after the menopause.

They are characterized by postmenopausal bleeding which is always investigated by dilatation and curettage. If the curettings show signs of malignancy, hysterectomy and bilateral salpingo-oöphorectomy are performed. Younger women may present with metrorrhagia. In this instance dilatation and curettage is performed and scrapings are always sent for cytological examination. If malignant cells are present similar radical surgery is performed on the younger woman.

Cervix

Carcinoma of the cervix is the second commonest form of cancer found in women. It can occur at any age but is most commonly found in the 40 to 50 age group and in women who have had a large family early in their lives.

Malignant changes in the cells of the cervix spread locally very quickly. The bladder and rectum are soon involved and metastases to bone and lungs follow rapidly.

Classification

Carcinoma of the cervix is classified as follows:

Stage 0   Nothing abnormal on visual examination of the cervix, but cytological examination shows presence of some malignant cells.

Stage I   Tumour is localized to the cervix. Erosion apparent on naked eye inspection of the cervix.

Stage II   Local spread of the tumour.

Stage III Invasive cancer involving vagina and pelvic wall.

Stage IV   Bladder and rectum involved. Possibly liver metastases.

Clinical features and diagnosis

In stage 0 there are no symptoms. Routine cytological examination has been of great value in detecting this state described as 'carcinoma in situ' or 'the preclinical state'. A positive cervical smear is further investigated by the removal of a cone biopsy from the cervix. In some younger women this often removes the whole area of malignant cells and no further surgery may be necessary. Close follow-up is maintained, cervical smears being taken at frequent intervals.

The most important symptom of invasive carcinoma is vaginal bleeding, which is due to ulceration of the lesion. The examining finger of the gynaecologist may be sufficient to cause bright red bleeding. The bleeding may manifest itself as a brown offensive discharge, as postcoital bleeding, as intermenstrual bleeding or, in the case of the older woman, as postmenopausal bleeding. Diagnosis is confirmed by biopsy. This disease must be diagnosed early to be treated satisfactorily.

Treatment

If the tumour is localized, surgery followed by radiotherapy to destroy residual tumour is the treatment of choice. The extent of the surgery depends on how far the tumour has invaded the tissues. For many patients total hysterectomy and bilateral salpingo-oöphorectomy would be sufficient. In some cases more radical surgery involving removal of the fatty tissue in the pelvis, including the lymph glands, may be necessary. This operation is known as Wertheim's hysterectomy.

Pain is experienced when the nearby organs become involved and may become excruciating when bone metastases develop. Anaemia, loss of weight and emaciation are present as in all carcinomata. Bladder involvement may give rise to symptoms which range from dysuria to leakage of urine from a fistula. Similarly rectal involvement may cause alteration in bowel habit and ultimately may lead to a rectovaginal fistula. In these later stages radiotherapy alone is the treatment of choice.

Prognosis in stages III and IV is poor. In the early stages when it is possible to remove all of the tumour and surrounding tissues prognosis is good.

Carcinoma of the vagina

Carcinoma of the vagina is very rare. It is characterized by post-menopausal bleeding and on examination a firm, hard, ulcerated area is felt in the vagina. It is treated with radiotherapy.

Benign tumours of the vulva

The commonest area of the vulva on which a benign tumour grows is the urethral meatus. It is thought to result from chronic or recurrent infection and is commoner in parous postmenopausal women.

It is very painful, causing dysuria and possibly bleeding. It is treated surgically by excision of the tumour and cauterization of the area from which it grew. Some dysuria must be expected for a few days following this procedure.

Malignant tumours of the vulva

These are relatively uncommon tumours which are usually seen in women over 60 years of age.

Clinical features

The tumour appears as a small, hard, painless ulcer on the labia which, if untreated, will eventually spread to involve the whole of the vulva and will travel, via the lymphatics, to the inguinal and femoral glands.

Such a tumour is preceded by leukoplakia, which is considered to be a premalignant condition. The skin of the vulva becomes white in patches and very itchy, causing the patient to scratch the area. Eventually the skin cracks and malignant change in the cells may follow.

Surgical treatment

Treatment is to excise the diseased area. The operations performed are simple vulvectomy or, more often, radical vulvectomy, which is a very mutilating operation involving removal of the vulva and the inguinal nodes on both sides.

Nursing care

The patient must be prepared for a long stay in hospital and complete bed rest following surgery. She should be encouraged to bring into hospital with her some work or hobby to occupy her during this time.

Routine preparation for major surgery is followed, particular attention being paid to shaving and cleansing the skin of the abdomen, perineum, buttocks and thighs.

Routine postoperative care is required immediately after return to the ward. After 24 hours she is nursed first in the semirecumbent and then in the upright positions. A urinary catheter drains the bladder until the surrounding tissue heals. Bowel movements are controlled by the use of suppositories.

This is not a painful operation but it is a distressing one, particularly as the wound is in an area which can be easily seen by the patient when it is exposed for dressings.

Sterile petroleum jelly impregnated gauze covered by large sterile pads is used to dress the wound. Initially there may be a considerable amount of soakage from the wound necessitating frequent changes of dressing.

As the wound begins to heal the patient is encouraged to move the area to avoid developing skin contractures. In approximately 6 weeks she will be mobile again.

Physiotherapy and general nursing care are vital during the prolonged period of bed rest. Probably most important is the psychological support which can be given by all staff in an effort to make the patient's stay in hospital as pleasant as possible.

Endometriosis

Endometriosis has been mentioned already as a possible cause of infertility. It is described as functioning endometrium outwith the lining of the uterus and has been found in a variety of sites, the commonest of which are the ovary, the myometrium and the pouch of Douglas.

It is subject to the same changes during the menstrual cycle as the endometrium lining the uterus, but the blood flow from this endometrium cannot escape via the vagina. As a result cysts and adhesions form, such as the chocolate cyst on the ovary and the adenomyoma in the muscle layer of the uterus, giving rise to a variety of gynaecological complaints, notably dysmenorrhoea.

The aberrant endometrium ceases to function during pregnancy and the menopause. Endometriosis may therefore be treated by suppressing oestrogen function, so inducing an artificial menopause. In young women it may be possible to remove the areas of endometriosis surgically without damaging healthy tissue. Total hysterectomy and bilateral salpingo-oöphorectomy are performed as the alternative and more radical treatment.

Uterine displacements

The accepted normal anatomical position of the uterus is that it should lie at right angles to the vagina and curve forward over the bladder in a position of anteversion. It is, however, a mobile organ and may adopt a variety of positions within the pelvis.

The commonest abnormal positions in which the uterus may be found are **retroversion**, which is backward displacement, and some degree of **uterovaginal** prolapse, which is downward displacement.

Retroversion (Fig. 10.26)

There are two types of retroversion: mobile and fixed. The former is an uncomplicated condition in which the uterus can be manipulated easily into the position of anteversion; it is usually symptomless.

A fixed retroverted uterus is often complicated by the presence of chronic pelvic inflammation or endometriosis, which causes the uterus to adhere to the pouch of Douglas.

Figure 10.26
Retroversion

Figure 10.27
Hodge pessary

Clinical features

The patient may complain of dyspareunia, backache, dysmenorrhoea and menorrhagia.

To assess whether or not the symptoms are due to retroversion, a pessary test is performed. The uterus is manipulated into the anteverted position, if necessary under general anaesthesia, and a Hodge pessary (Fig. 10.27) is inserted to hold it in this position. The pessary is left in position for 4 to 6 weeks.

If the symptoms are relieved by this measure but recur when the pessary is removed, the uterus falling back into the retroverted position, it can be assumed that the symptoms are caused by retroversion.

Treatment

A ventrosuspension operation is usually performed. This consists of shortening the round ligaments and pulling the uterus forward into the anteverted position.

This operation is performed via the abdominal route and pre- and postoperative care is similar to that required by the patient undergoing abdominal hysterectomy.

Some women with retroverted uteri are infertile and following correction of the retroversion conception may result.

Uterovaginal prolapse

Many older women experience some degree of descent (prolapse) of the uterus through the vagina because of laxity of the vaginal walls and weakening of the muscles and ligaments which support the uterus.

Commonly affected are postmenopausal parous women whose muscles have been stretched during childbirth and in whom lack of oestrogen following the menopause has caused the pelvic organs to shrink and the muscles to lose tone. Prolapse sometimes results when there is a condition present which raises intra-abdominal pressure such as tumours, ascites or obesity.

This condition may present simply as herniation of the walls of the vagina causing swellings in the urethra (urethrocele), bladder (cystocele), rectum (rectocele) and pouch of Douglas (enterocele) (Fig. 10.28).

Figure 10.28
Prolapse of the uterus

The cervix may descend through the vagina until the uterus lies completely outside the vulva. This type of prolapse is called procidentia (Fig. 10.29).

Figure 10.29
Uterovaginal prolapse
(procidentia)

Classification

Three degrees of prolapse are recognized:

1. First degree: cervix still inside the vagina.
2. Second degree: cervix appears outside the vagina.
3. Third degree: uterus lies completely outside the vulva — complete procidentia.

Clinical features

These features may appear in a variety of combinations and are dependent on the site of the prolapse (Table 10.2). Common to all is the sensation of 'something coming down'. In third degree prolapse the displaced uterus can be seen. Other possible features are:

Stress incontinence.
Frequency of micturition.
Retention of urine.
Difficulty in micturition or defaecation.
Vaginal discharge or bleeding due to ulceration of the prolapse.

Table 10.2
Types of prolapse

Name	Area involved	Main symptom	Operation
Urethrocele	Lower anterior vagina	Stress incontinent	Anterior colporrhaphy
Cystocele	Upper anterior vagina	Dysuria Frequency of micturition	Anterior colporrhaphy
Rectocele	Posterior vagina Perineum	Difficulty in defaecation	Colpoperineorrhaphy
Enterocele	Posterior vagina Small intestine	Pelvic discomfort	Colpoperineorrhaphy and removal of the peritoneal sac
Procidentia	Vagina, uterus, pelvic muscles and ligaments	Protrusion of cervix at vulva	Manchester repair and amputation of cervix or vaginal hysterectomy

Figure 10.30
Ring pessary

Treatment

The aim of treatment is to replace the prolapse and keep it in position. Physiotherapy to tighten the muscles of the pelvic floor is sufficient in a few early cases. As a temporary measure, for instance until after a pregnancy or until a patient is fit for surgery, a ring pessary (Fig. 10.30) may be inserted to distend the vaginal walls. The pessary is usually made of polythene and is available in a variety of sizes. The size is chosen according to the length of the vagina, and if it is fitted properly the woman should experience no discomfort and it should not interfere with coitus. Every 4 to 6 months the pessary is removed and the vaginal wall inspected. Any signs of ulceration are treated before the pessary is reinserted.

The most usual form of treatment is surgery to restore the organs to their anatomical positions by removing the excess tissue which forms the herniae and repairing the stretched muscles and ligaments. Surgical treatment of procidentia requires shortening of the cardinal and uterosacral ligaments and possibly amputation of the elongated cervix. In some areas vaginal hysterectomy is performed routinely but in others only if there is some other indication, such as fibroids or postmenopausal bleeding.

NURSING CARE OF PATIENTS UNDERGOING MAJOR PELVIC SURGERY

Via the abdominal route

Female patients undergoing pelvic surgery through the abdominal route require similar nursing care regardless of the precise nature of the operation.

These patients are admitted routinely 2 days prior to surgery. This allows the usual preoperative investigations to be carried out and also gives the patient an opportunity to familiarize herself with her new environment and to see other patients in the different stages through which she will progress. Routine admission procedure is followed during which it is important that the doctor explains the nature of the operation to the patient and, if at all possible, to her husband. This is partly so that the consent form may be signed but primarily to reassure the couple and correct any erroneous ideas about the effects the operation may have on the patient and on their marital relationship.

Preoperative nursing measures

Midstream specimen of urine.
Pubic and perineal shave.
Evacuant enema
Light diet.
Night sedative.

A major complication of pelvic surgery is deep venous thrombosis. To counteract this is an intravenous infusion of *dextran 70* injection (Macrodex) is often administered during and after the operation. Blood transfusion may also be necessary.

Postoperative care

Routine postoperative care is required. The patient may have an intravenous infusion, a urinary catheter, and, in case of a Wertheim hysterectomy, vacuum (Redivac) drainage.

Once the patient has settled in bed, her face, hands and perineum are sponged; then she is helped into her nightdress and her hair is combed. This procedure helps to make her feel more comfortable and boosts her morale considerably.

Pulse and blood pressure are charted every half hour initially. If the pulse rises and the blood pressure falls, the foot of the bed should be elevated immediately and the change in the patient's condition reported. The wound site and the perineum are both inspected in case haemorrhage is responsible for the fall in blood pressure. If there is external haemorrhage, pressure in the form of sterile pads is applied to the area. These measures are usually sufficient; rarely is a patient required to return to theatre.

The morning after the operation the patient is usually able to tolerate fluids and a light diet, so the intravenous infusion is discontinued.

If an in-dwelling urinary catheter has been inserted, it is allowed to drain freely for 48 hours; after this time the patient usually has no difficulty in passing urine normally. If a catheter is not in position the patient should be helped up to the commode from the first morning after the operation. Usually little difficulty is experienced in passing urine.

Strong analgesics are required regularly for the first 48 hours. The administration of these drugs should be timed so that the patient is comfortable but not sleepy at meal times; she will be able to eat, get up to the commode and take a short walk round her bed after eating. To prevent the development of deep venous thrombosis the patient is encouraged to exercise her calf muscles while in bed and to get up for short frequent walks.

By the third or fourth day after the operation, the patient should be allowed up for a bath and a walk round the ward. Deep venous thrombosis is still a danger so she must be discouraged from sitting with her legs dependent for any length of time. A dry dressing on the wound prevents the material of the nightdress from catching on clips and stitches. Clips are usually removed on the fifth day following operation and stitches on the seventh day.

On the second postoperative day the administration of two suppositories helps to disperse the flatus which causes many patients considerable discomfort.

If all goes well the patient should be discharged home 11 or 12 days after operation. She is given an out-patient appointment for 6 to 8 weeks after the operation and she is advised not to do any lifting for at least 3 months, to take plenty of exercise and to resume marital relations as soon as she wishes.

Complications

Chest infection.
Urinary tract infection
Wound infection.
Wound dehiscence (burst abdomen).
Deep venous thrombosis.
Pulmonary embolism.
Death.

Via the vaginal route

Preoperative measures

The usual preoperative measures are required but particular attention must be paid to shaving the vulval and perineal areas.

An ulcerated prolapsed uterus must be treated prior to surgery. In order to do this the patient must be admitted to hospital 1 or 2 weeks prior to the operation. Each day the patient has an immersion bath following which her procidentia is replaced manually. A vaginal pack soaked in magnesium sulphate and glycerine is inserted.

The patient remains in bed with the foot of the bed elevated to allow gravity to aid the process. The following morning the procedure is repeated. Physiotherapy and general nursing care are important since the patient is confined to bed.

Postoperative care

Postoperative care is similar to that required by those undergoing abdominal hysterectomy.

A urinary catheter draining freely will be in position for 48 hours. The patient is encouraged to drink plenty of fluids and her urinary output is carefully measured and recorded. It may be necessary to recatheterize for a further 48 hours if urinary retention develops. Bladder control is usually regained quite quickly.

A vaginal pack may be inserted in the operating theatre to control bleeding. A written order is normally given by the surgeon to remove the pack, usually between

8 and 24 hours after insertion. If left in longer, there is danger of infection developing and the pack will become hard and stick to the vaginal walls, causing trauma when it is eventually removed.

It is essential that vulval toilet be performed 4 hourly for the first 2 days. As soon as her condition permits, the use of bidets, if available, is encouraged. By the third or fourth day the patient should take baths twice daily with salt in the water to promote healing. She should be encouraged to move around as freely as possible and to adopt a normal posture. A cushion or an air ring to sit on greatly aids her comfort.

Stitches inserted in this area are usually of the absorbable type. If not they are removed within 5 days.

Ten to 14 days after the operation vaginal examination is performed to break down adhesions. If satisfactory the patient can be discharged home with an outpatient appointment in 6 to 8 weeks and advice to avoid constipation, heavy lifting and coitus for 3 months.

BREAST

The breast plays an important part in a woman's body image. Some women pay large sums of money for surgical operations that either enlarge their breasts, make them smaller or improve their shape. It follows that removal of a diseased breast will have a profound psychological effect upon a woman.

ANATOMY AND PHYSIOLOGY

The anatomy of the breast is illustrated in Figure 10.31. It is important to note that blood and lymphatic supplies to the breast are liberal; this is of particular significance in relation to some disorders and their treatment.

Blood supply is via the mammary branches of the axillary, internal thoracic and intercostal arteries.

Venous drainage takes place through veins following similar routes to those of the arteries.

Lymphatic drainage is through vessels distributed all over the breast which drain mainly into the axillary lymph nodes.

The breasts develop at puberty under the influence of the ovarian hormones to which they continue to respond throughout reproductive life. Each menstrual cycle therefore brings changes within the breast, premenstrually there is an increase in blood supply and in growth of glandular tissue, which gives rise to the discomfort experienced by many women. The slightly nodular feel of the breasts at this time is also regarded as physiologically normal. The breasts resume a resting phase after menstruation (Fig. 10.31). The cyclic changes continue throughout reproductive life unless pregnancy intervenes, but cease at the menopause with the decline in the production of the ovarian hormones.

Lactation

During pregnancy the secretory cells and duct system develop under the influence of oestrogen and progesterone (Fig. 10.32). About 2 to 3 days after delivery of the baby the blood levels of oestrogen fall. When a certain level is reached the anterior pituitary gland releases prolactin, which is the lactogenic hormone, and the alveoli produce milk.

The milk is propelled along the lactiferous ducts and is stored in the ampullae. When the baby sucks he draws the nipple and areola into his mouth. The action of his jaws empties the ampullae and lower ducts. The sucking stimulus initiates a neurohormonal reflex and the postpituitary gland releases oxytocin, causing the myopethelial cells in the alveoli to contract, and the milk is propelled along the ducts. This process is called the draught reflex and the mother is often aware of the flow of milk towards the nipple.

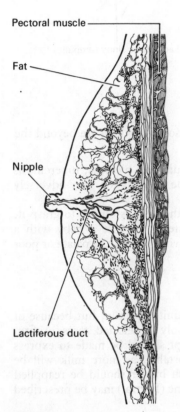

Figure 10.31
Section showing breast in resting phase

Pectoral muscle

Fat

Nipple

Lactiferous duct

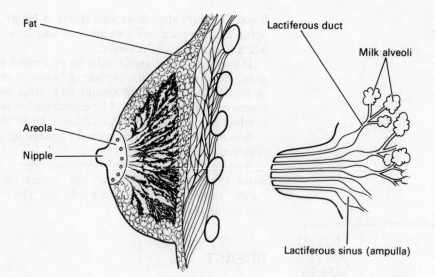

Fat

Areola

Nipple

Lactiferous duct

Milk alveoli

Lactiferous sinus (ampulla)

Figure 10.32
Section showing lactating breast

Suppression of lactation

There are many indications for suppressing lactation, some of which are beyond the scope of this chapter. The commonest reasons are:

1. Medical conditions of the mother, for example diabetes mellitus, tuberculosis or cardiac disease, in which the extra demands made by lactation may adversely affect her health.
2. Malformation of the mother's nipple such that the baby is unable to grasp it.
3. Abnormalities of the baby, for example a preterm baby or a baby with a congenital abnormality that affects sucking and swallowing: cleft lip or palate or poor development of lower jaw.

Method

Oestrogen was widely used to inhibit lactation until quite recently, but because of the risk of thromboembolism it is now prescribed only in selected cases. A firm supporting binder is applied to the breast; no attempt should be made to express milk even if the breasts become hard and uncomfortable, as more milk will be produced. The patient needs reassurance, and a fresh binder should be reapplied frequently. An analgesic such an Panadol or pentazocine (Fortral) may be prescribed by the doctor.

HEALTH EDUCATION AND EARLY DETECTION OF DISORDER

A high proportion of women (sometimes as high as 70%) delay reporting a lump in the breast to their doctor. This may be due to lack of knowledge, but this seems unlikely in view of the proliferation of articles in newspapers, women's magazines and documentary television programmes; it is probable that they are afraid to have their suspicions confirmed.

It is, therefore, imperative that health care professionals encourage all age groups of women to practise self-examination of the breasts at regular intervals. The opportunities afforded for extensive teaching is present in many settings: teaching could be encouraged in well-woman clinics, family planning clinics, doctors' surgeries and ante-natal clinics, and health education in schools could create an awareness of the problem.

Health educators must stress that only one lump in four is likely to be malignant and that early detection, especially in the younger woman, will mean that spread of the disease is less likely and, therefore, the less extensive the treatment that may be necessary. Leaflets illustrating and describing breast self-examination are produced by the Women's National Cancer Control Campaign (U.K.) and the Scottish Health

Education Group; advisory leaflets are available from the Mastectomy Association for women who are about to have or have had a mastectomy.

Breast self examination

Ideally every woman should know what her own breasts feel and look like and be aware that the breasts can naturally feel lumpy because of the glandular and fatty tissues in the breast. Regular self-examination will enable each woman to ascertain what is normal for her and to identify quickly any obvious deviations from normal.

Monthly breast self-examination should be carried out throughout the woman's reproductive life. It should be performed immediately after menstruation when the breasts are softest and in a resting phase.

Any change in shape, asymmetry or puckering of the skin can be noted by performing the examination while standing in front of a mirror (Fig. 10.33A and B).

Palpation is carried out when the woman is lying down on a flat surface with a folded towel under the left shoulder. With the fingers of the right hand held flat (not using fingertips only), the left breast is examined using firm pressure with the fingers and small circular movements. Each quadrant of the breast is systematically examined and then beginning at the nipple and working outwards in small circles, re-examined (Fig. 10.33 C–G). Finally the left arm is brought down to the side and the whole area of the axilla and the area above the breast to the clavicle is palpated.

The right breast should be palpated in the same way using the left hand.

Programmes of screening for breast cancer

Interest was stimulated in screening for breast cancer following the publication of the findings of the Health Insurance Plan trial, New York. Comparison between a control sample of 31 000 women who underwent annual clinical examination and mammography, and a similar size sample who presented for examination following

Figure 10.33
(A and B) Inspection by looking into a mirror (C–G) Systematic self-examination by palpation

self-detection of a lump in the breast demonstrated that much smaller cancers with minimal lymph node involvement could be detected in the screened group. In the 10 year follow-up period a one-third reduction in mortality rates from breast cancer was consistently found in screened women over 50 years of age. Increasing age constitutes the most certain risk factor and consequently the outlook for women in this age group must be hopeful where effective screening methods are available.

In 1975, four centres in Great Britain subsequently instituted screening programmes. In Edinburgh, a screening programme was commenced in conjunction with general practitioners. High initial response rates to an invitation to participate in the programme was obtained (81.8%), and good response rates (84%) in follow-up a year later. On completion of pre-selected screening investigations, 125 women underwent biopsy and of these 18 proved to have cancer.

Screening is a logical progression in preventive medicine, but it is necessary to consider several factors before a programme could be undertaken on a national scale. The cost of screening is high and it would be necessary to find a way of determining which women are at highest risk of developing breast cancer in the population. The acceptability of the techniques used and their effectiveness must be carefully scrutinized before a national programme is introduced.

INVESTIGATIONS

Clinical examination

This is the primary move towards diagnosis. In addition to performing a full physical examination, the doctor will concentrate on:

Observation of the breasts

The woman will be observed while sitting up with her arms at her sides and then with both arms raised above her head. Any skin dimpling, asymmetry or nipple retraction will be noted.

Palpation of the breast

Each breast section will be examined systematically by the doctor. This will help to differentiate between the 'lumpy' benign texture changes that occur in the breast tissue which may be due to pyogenic abcess, fibroadenoma and fibrocystic disease, and the discrete lump which requires immediate investigation. Complete examination is made of the regional lymph nodes. After the suspect breast is examined, the other breast is examined in the same way.

Mammography

This is one of the most widely used and best evaluated X-ray techniques. It has a 90–95% accuracy rate as a screening method. However, in the under 25-year-old age group the breasts are too radiodense and the technique is of no value. After the age of 25 years the radiodensity regresses with age and by the time of the menopause a reasonably good image can be obtained by mammography, and in the elderly (where there is a peak incidence) a very good picture can be obtained.

Thermography and ultrasound are now less favoured techniques.

Aspiration cytology

This procedure (Fig. 10.34) can be carried out on an out-patient basis at the first visit to the clinic. No local anaesthetic is required. An ordinary 10 ml syringe with a 21 gauge needle is used. (This may be held in a metal frame to allow the operator to use one hand only.) Once the needle has been washed through with heparinised saline it can be inserted into the breast cyst and aspirated immediately. The site will be checked in 2 weeks. If the aspirate is blood-stained or if refilling of the cyst occurs, further urgent investigations will be required. The advantage for the woman

Figure 10.34
Procedure for aspiration cytology

is that she may be instantly reassured that she has no cause for concern, or she can receive expert counselling about further investigations.

If the lesion is solid, the same equipment is used with the plunger of the syringe fully withdrawn (maximum negative pressure) and the needle is advanced several times. The needle is then removed and smears are made at once. Interpretation of results can again be made immediately.

Cutting needle biopsy

This is a method used for a solid lump. Local anaesthetic is inserted in the proposed track of the biopsy. The breast is held in a stable position by the assisting doctor and the operator inserts a sterile $4\frac{1}{2}$ inch Travenol Tru-cut needle (Fig. 10.35), thereby obtaining a core of tissue. This specimen is then fixed and stained by utilizing immediate frozen section or placing in paraffin wax.

Figure 10.35
Travenol Tru-cut needle

Open biopsy

This is usually carried out under general anaesthetic because local anaesthetic can reduce definition in the breast. The disadvantages of open biopsy are that haemostasis is sometimes difficult and a small scar is inevitable, but the advantage is that this technique will give the finest determination of diagnosis.

It is important that the nurse is supportive during this stressful period when a definitive diagnosis is being sought. She must remember that in addition to assisting the doctor with the preparation of the patient and the performance of the procedure, she must be aware of the dual threat of cancer and mutilating surgery that the patient anticipates. Patients are vulnerable to emotional distress at the time of diagnosis, before surgery and also postoperatively.

Radiology — chest and axial skeleton

Ordinary X-rays of various parts of the body will show metastases of malignant tumours if present.

Scanning

Skeletal bone scanning and liver scanning are reliable methods of detecting metastases in advanced disease.

DISORDERS OF THE BREAST

The breasts may be affected by a variety of pathological conditions including congenital abnormalities, infections, tumours and diseases that affect the skin. By far the most common and important disorder is cancer, which is, therefore, considered in more detail.

Chronic mastitis

This is a condition in which there is dysfunction of the breast, it is **not** an inflammatory state. The normal cyclic changes that occur during menstruation become out of phase. As a result part or all of the breast becomes fibrous or cystic and the patient experiences pain and discomfort.

Of the various treatments which may be prescribed, reassurance and a well-supporting brassiere are probably the most useful. Should a large cyst form it may require surgical removal. The condition regresses at the menopause.

Acute mastitis

This is an inflammatory condition generally associated with childbirth but rarely occurring before the first 7 to 10 days following delivery. The patient complains of pain and tenderness in the affected breast and on examination there is a clearly defined flushed area. The patient's temperature may be elevated and she feels generally unwell. The infection may be blood-borne or introduced through a fissured nipple.

Early diagnosis and antibiotic therapy have greatly reduced the possibility of abscess formation and in most cases breast feeding may be continued once the local symptoms have cleared up.

Tumours of the breast

These may be either benign or malignant.

Benign tumours (Fig. 10.36)

Fibroadenomata occur as encapsulated lumps, commonly in the breasts of young girls in the 15–25 years age group. They are usually removed although they will not grow very large, because a benign tumour may undergo malignant changes. The usual investigations will be carried out to confirm that it is indeed benign.

Small tumour
- Isolated
- Regular
- Mobile
- Confirmation by histology

Figure 10.36
Benign tumour of the breast

Malignant tumours

Breast cancer is the most common form of cancer affecting women and the leading cause of death among women in the 35–55 year age group. The ratio of women who develop the disease is 1:17, and those who will die from it 1:30. Despite the emphasis on early diagnosis, screening facilities, improvements in surgical expertise and the newer approaches to treatment of breast cancer, the 10-year survival rate has remained relatively constant at 50%. The patterns of breast cancer appear to be changing in that it is now affecting younger women. The search for causal factors in breast cancer is focused at present in four main areas:

1. *Incidence*

It has been shown that there is a much higher incidence in Western Europe and the United States of America than in South-East Asia. Increasing incidence can be demonstrated in South-East Asian women who come to live in the Western developed countries and who adopt Western life-styles. This has led researchers to examine closely the cultural patterns of behaviour regarding diet, age at first pregnancy, subsequent childbearing and lactation practices.

2. *Risk factors*

Women who are at high risk of developing breast cancer usually have an early menarche (before age 13), late menopause (after age 50), and either have their first baby after the age of 35 or are nulliparous (there is a high incidence of breast cancer among nuns).

3. *Exogenous hormones*

There is now evidence that there is some correlation between internal hormone levels and the development of breast cancer. Clinical experimental work is being conducted at present to evaluate the hypothesis that oestrogens, whilst not causing cancer, may provide a receptive environment under particular conditions. Therefore, the effects of the oral contraceptive pill, hormone replacement therapy, the use of hormones in averting abortion, preventing lactation or preventing conception ('morning after' pill) are under investigation to determine whether or not they provide such an environment.

4. *Hereditary factors*

A woman who has a first degree relative who has developed breast cancer has a greater risk of developing breast cancer also. The risks, however, should not be over-exaggerated as it is only in unusual circumstances that this risk factor can double the familial incidence.

Clinical features

1. A small painless lump (Fig. 10.37) or thickening in the breast.
2. Alteration in the shape of the breast.
3. Retraction of the nipple.
4. Dimpling of the skin — *peau d'orange* (orange peel appearance).
5. Ulceration of the skin which will become a fungating mass if left untreated is a late feature.

The cause of these clinical features can be explained in terms of the way in which breast cancer is spread.

Modes of spread

1. Direct infiltration. Malignant tumours may arise within the lobules of the breast or within the ducts. These may be spread from either site to the surrounding

Figure 10.37
Malignant tumour of the breast

tissue. Generally there will be several areas with invasive or pre-invasive changes within the breast. With local spread, the suspensory ligaments (of Cooper) become infiltrated by tumour and the skin is pulled down causing a 'dimple'. Invasion of the lactiferous ducts will cause inversion or retraction of the nipple. Progression of the tumour will cause fixation of the tumour to the skin and to the chest muscle and chest wall. Extensive infiltration causes oedema of the skin and many dimples may be visualised giving the clinically significant and serious *peau d'orange* finding.

2. Via lymphatics and the bloodstream. The lymphatic system and the venous system are closely interrelated and, therefore, single cells or clusters of cells can be shed to involve lymph glands in the axilla or the internal mammary chain and from these sites to a more distant group of lymph nodes. The involvement of the axillary lymph nodes is clinically significant in diagnosis and the spread by the internal mammary chain can result in spread to the chest cavity including the lungs and tissues surround the heart.

Veins draining the breast may be invaded by the tumour and cells may dislodge and be transported to and be found in structures such as the brain, bone, liver and lungs.

Table 10.3
Features of benign and malignant tumours

Benign tumour	Malignant tumour
Well-defined lump	Usually a lump or thickening
Smooth and either firm, cystic or soft	Irregular and hard in consistency
Round or oval	Irregular in shape
Often tender	Painless in early stages
Slow-growing	Rate of growth variable, often rapid
Mobile when examined	Fixed to surrounding tissues; tentacles of tumour grow out in all directions
No spread within body	Metastases spread to various other organs

Staging of tumour

Once the definite diagnosis of breast cancer has been made, the surgeon will require to 'stage' the tumour, that is to specify as nearly as possible the type of cancer present and the extent of any local or general spread of malignancy. Two classifications are used in staging breast cancers — the Manchester staging developed in the 1940s classifies tumours as stages I–IV or tumours may be staged by assessing the status of the tumour (T), lymph nodes (N) and metastatic spread (M).

Stage I T_1 Tumour less than 2 cm.
T_2 Tumour less than 5 cm.
N_0 No palpable axillary nodes.
M_0 No apparent distant metastases.

Stage II T_1 or T_2, N_1 nodes can be felt but are mobile.

M_0 no apparent distant metastases.

Stage III T_3 tumour 5–10 cm

T_4 tumour 10+ cm

$\left.\begin{array}{l} N_2 \\ N_3 \end{array}\right\}$ nodes thought to contain tumour.

Stage IV   Tumour at any stage

N_3 supraclavicular and infraclavicular nodes

M_1 obvious distant metastases

T = tumour status

N = lymph node status

M = distant metastases

Treatment of malignant breast tumours

The most common treatment for breast cancer is excision of the tumour — **mastectomy**. Many alternative methods are currently undergoing clinical trials, for instance, the use of less extensive surgery, adjuvant therapies (radiotherapy and chemotherapy) and the use of anti-oestrogens. Present treatments include breast surgery with or without adjuvant therapy, breast conservation, breast reconstruction and treatment of advanced disease.

Table 10.4 illustrates some of the many options at present under consideration by the breast surgeon. The mode of treatment selected will depend on the type and stage of the tumour, the age of the woman, the reaction of the woman to the options that are acceptable to her at a particular time in consultation with the surgeon.

Breast surgery

The present debate regarding breast surgery is concerned with how extensive the surgery should be but the eventual survival rate varies little whatever the technique used. Staging provides an indication for prognosis but does not give sufficient proof for selecting a particular operative procedure. The surgery currently being practised may be:

a. *Radical mastectomy.* This involves the removal of the breast tissue, pectoralis major and minor muscles and the axillary nodes. It is seldom performed in Great Britain now but is still favoured in the United States of America.

b. *Modified radical mastectomy.* The breast tissue is removed along with the axillary nodes. The pectoral muscles are preserved giving less deformity than the traditional radical mastectomy.

c. *Total (simple) mastectomy.* This is the most common type of operation performed. All breast tissue is removed including the tail of the breast. The pectoral muscles and the axillary and pectoral nodes are left intact. 'Sampling' of the axillary and pectoral nodes at the time of operation and subsequent laboratory reports can be used as indicators for subsequent treatment.

It is recognised that when radiotherapy is not used following mastectomy there is a chance of local recurrence of tumour which can be treated at a later date.

It is not now the practice to proceed from open biopsy to mastectomy in one operation. The woman will, therefore, know definitely prior to surgery what type of operation is to be performed. However, preoperative counselling remains vitally important.

Nursing care

On admission to hospital the patient will be frightened once the diagnosis has been established. Fear of death and its consequences to her family may be uppermost in her mind. Preoperatively she may become aggressive or depressed and tearful. Whatever the manifestations of her anxiety, the thoughtful nurse will afford opportunities for the patient to talk about her fears in privacy and will explain the preoperative routine

Table 10.4
Current alternatives for the management of breast cancer

Investigations
1. Clinical examination
2. Mammography
3. Aspiration cytology or   Out-patient
   cutting needle biopsy
4. Open biopsy — in-patient
↓

**Staging and T.N.M.
classification**

Disease confined to breast	Regional lymph nodes involved	Disease advancing (locally)	Disease advanced (distant metastases)

↓

Additional investigations
1. Biochemical and haematological screening
2. Skeletal bone scan for metastases
3. Liver scan
4. X-rays (chest and pelvis)
↓

Treatment of breast cancer

Breast conservation	*Breast reconstruction*	*Breast surgery*
1. Subcutaneous mastectomy with silastic implant	Mastectomy with wide axillary tail excision plus Latissimus dorsi swing flap graft	(Dependent on axillary node status)
2. Local excision of tumour with radiotherapy		1. Simple mastectomy with delayed radiotherapy
3. Local excision of tumour plus Axillary gland dissection and radiotherapy plus Insertion of iridium wires		2. Simple mastectomy followed by radiotherapy or adjuvant chemotherapy

↓

Advanced breast cancer

Pre-menopausal woman	*Post-menopausal woman*
1. Oöphorectomy	1. anti-oestrogen therapy (Tamoxifen citrate)
2. Adrenal ablation (Aminoglutethamide)	2. Combination chemotherapy (cyclical administration of cytotoxic agents)
3. Hypophysectomy — yttrium 90 implant or cryosurgery	
4. Combination chemotherapy	

in simple terms. She is most likely to give way to her emotions when consent for the operation is obtained, when the skin is being prepared or during the night if sedation has not been effective. The nurse should be alert to these possibilities and ready to deal with such a situation sympathetically and with sensitivity. The hearty 'jolly along' approach is wholly inappropriate. It may help to comfort the preoperative patient if the nurse cites examples of women well known in public life who have had a breast removed and yet continue to look attractive and keep active. During the preoperative period the patient may also be upset by what she hears from other patients in the ward, and, therefore, it is essential that the nursing staff give correct and reassuring information. Each patient should be treated as an individual, and emotional support given relevant to her specific needs at that time.

In general 2 days are sufficient to enable the investigations and routine procedures prior to major surgery to be carried out. Unless visiting is encouraged or the nursing staff make a particular effort to get to know the patient, it can be a time of great loneliness for her.

Steps should also be taken to keep the husband informed and prepared for the change he will find in his wife.

Figure 10.38
Mastectomy showing position of
vacuum (Redivac) drains

At operation the surgeon will have taken great care to seal the severed blood vessels, but because the breast is so vascular some postoperative bleeding is inevitable. Drainage tubes will have been placed in separate stab wounds to prevent blood and serum from collecting under the skin flaps as this would delay healing. It is usual to apply suction to the drains by means of Redivacs (Fig. 10.38) which should be changed at least daily. The drainage must be measured and recorded and the bottles checked at regular intervals in case excessive loss should occur.

The usual postoperative regime for major surgery will be followed. The patient is allowed to sit up gradually and to drink and eat within the limits of nausea.

The dressing should be inspected regularly and is normally left undisturbed for 3 days unless there is evidence of abnormal bleeding or soakage. If the dressing is wet it should be replaced using a strict aseptic dressing technique. Vacuum (Redivac) drains are inspected for patency and the amounts of fluid in the Redivacs measured accurately and recorded on the patient's fluid balance chart.

Care of the arm on the affected side

As soon as the patient has recovered from the effects of the anaesthetic, she should be placed comfortably with sufficient pillows in a semirecumbent position. The arm on the side of the mastectomy incision must be slightly abducted and the forearm supported by a pillow. If the patient is not correctly advised she will tend to hold the affected arm in a rigid position and this may lead to muscle contracture and consequent restriction of arm movement.

Observation of the arms should be made at regular intervals in order that the presence of lymphoedema may be detected. A woman who has had a radical mastectomy will be more likely to develop this distressing complication, but it may also occur following simple mastectomy or in women who have had radiotherapy. If lymphoedema should occur, the use of the Flowtron machine (an inflatable sleeve which utilises intermittent compression) may give some subjective relief initially, although very seldom is there a marked improvement in arm volume for a significant period. Elevation of the swollen arm as often as possible will also provide relief.

Precautions should be taken by the nursing staff not to apply a blood pressure cuff to the affected arm, and no subcutaneous or intramuscular injections should be administered in this arm. Doctors will not use this arm for routine venepuncture or the administration of intravenous drugs or fluids.

When the patient is being lifted in bed or getting out of bed, the nurse should be particularly careful not to compress or grip the axilla especially where there has been lymph node removal during surgery. This will be painful for the patient and may cause dehiscence of part of the incision.

The nursing staff must encourage the patient to maintain good posture once she is mobile. She may develop a tendency to hunch her shoulders, or to hold one shoulder higher than the other. Adequate support in a suitable chair and correct support with pillows when the patient is sitting up, and tactful verbal reminders when the patient is walking will help to eliminate bad posture.

It is advisable for the patient not to wear rings or other jewellery on the affected arm in case lymphoedema develops, and care should be taken when cutting or manicuring fingernails to prevent infection developing in the arm.

Exercises

Providing there are no contraindications to exercise of the affected arm, the surgeon will permit the physiotherapist to commence a regime of gentle exercises on the first postoperative day if the patient is maintaining normal progress. It is beneficial if a nurse is present while the physiotherapist is instructing the patient in her initial exercises so that the nurse may encourage the patient to persevere with the exercises when the physiotherapist is not present.

On the first postoperative day, the physiotherapist will attempt to achieve increasing abduction of the affected arm, gradually obtaining abduction of 90°. The patient is encouraged to use her 'good' arm to help to support the affected arm during these exercises. The physiotherapist and the nurse may also perform the exercises with the patient and, therefore, help the patient to feel that she is not doing all the work, but that a team effort is being made to help her.

When the patient is able to attain abduction of the affected arm, encouragement should be given to move the forearm backwards, and this exercise should be performed bilaterally. This is particularly important if the patient is to receive subsequent salpingo-oöphorectomy

Grasping both hands together in front of the abdomen and gently raising both arms upwards as far as the patient is able is another helpful exercise. These exercises should be given to move the forearm backwards, and this exercise should be performed bilaterally. This is particularly important if the patient is to receive subsequent radiotherapy as this position has to be maintained during treatment (Fig. 10.39).

Once the Redivac drains have been removed, the patient should hold on to the back of a chair with her good arm and practise swinging the affected arm in a pendulum movement. Brushing and combing her hair with the affected arm also assists mobilisation of the affected arm. The provision of a full length mirror in the bathroom will assist the patient to correct any defects in her posture with the help of the physiotherapist. The nurse may help the physiotherapist by unobtrusively watching the patient's posture as she moves about the ward, and report her observations to the physiotherapist.

If the patient is very apprehensive about performing these exercises, other aids may be used. Pulley attachments are available which may be attached to the head of the bed, and the patient instructed to use the pulley in a 'see-saw' motion using the good arm and the affected arm alternately. Education and support of the patient are of paramount importance if good movement is to be obtained following mastectomy.

Radiotherapy

Patients who have carcinoma of the breast with the involvement of lymph nodes will probably be given a course of 20 treatments by irradiation in the course of 1 month. Treatment is usually begun once the mastectomy incision has completely healed.

Figure 10.39
Position of arm during radiotherapy treatment following mastectomy

Healed incision

Consultation between the patient, the surgeon and the radiotherapist is essential during this period. The treatment is usually now carried out on an out-patient basis, the patient being given radiotherapy for 5 days in the week with a period of rest at weekends. Side-effects are few with modern treatment, but occasionally the patient may complain of tiredness and slight blistering of the skin in the irradiated area.

It is important for nurses working in the radiotherapy wards or treatment areas to be aware of aspects of skin care appropriate to patients having treatment to the breast area, and to be able to explain the care necessary both verbally and with the use of appropriate leaflets.

During treatment and for some weeks after treatment, the skin of the area being treated may require special care. Some reaction in the skin as a result of treatment is to be expected in all patients and this will be discussed as treatment progresses. During treatment it is desirable to keep the skin as dry and cool as possible. Sensible light, loose-fitting clothing and the use of a mild starch dusting powder, combined with the avoidance of wetting during washing and bathing are all that are required. Heavily perfumed talcum powder, deodorants, scents or creams are to be avoided.

Any reaction to treatment by the skin is likely to begin towards the end of the course and to continue to develop for some days after treatment stops. It will then begin to regress and should be almost completely settled by the time of the patient's first return appointment.

It is important to instruct the patient that once the skin has apparently returned to normal it remains more sensitive than normal skin to ultra-violet light. Sunbathing to a degree liable to cause sunburn must, therefore, be avoided. The use of medical lamps, such as ultra-violet or infra-red lamps, is not advisable.

Hair washing or hair dressing is permitted provided adequate precautions are taken to avoid wetting the area being treated, so backwards washing is preferable.

There is no contraindication to vaccination or innoculation in the future but the injections should never be given into the arm on the treated side.

Physiotherapy should be continued throughout the period of radiotherapy treatment and classes are held in many departments of physiotherapy once a week to demonstrate suitable exercises.

Prosthesis

Initially a light weight prosthesis will help to improve the patients appearance if it is worn with a well-fitting brassiere and will help her to become less self-conscious about her body image. It will exert no pressure on the area of excision until wound healing is complete. Expert advice may be sought from the appliance specialist in the hospital.

Once healing of the mastectomy site is complete, there is a tendency for the shape of the remaining breast to change and there may be slight contracture of the operated site. It is often wise to delay the fitting of a permanent prosthesis until the size of breast has been established. Many types of permanent prostheses are now available and may be demonstrated by the surgical appliance specialist. An artificial breast made of silicone gel has been found to be most satisfactory by the majority of the patients.

Rehabilitation

It is essential that once the patient returns home she is encouraged to begin to lead as normal a life as possible. It is a period of physical and psychological adjustment. Support should be given by family, relatives and friends. The Mastectomy Association can also help with many problems or services. In many areas local self-help groups are being established which are supportive in nature and concentrate on social rehabilitation, for example fund-raising activities and designing appropriate swimwear and dresses, and exchanging ideas.

Physical rehabilitation is relatively easy for most women. It is important to encourage the continuation of the active exercises that have been taught by the physiotherapist and to perform light household tasks initially such as dusting using a circular motion with the affected arm. Gradually she can resume driving, sewing and domestic tasks. It is important to praise each achievement normally and without overemphasis. Sports, especially swimming, are beneficial. Swimming helps the woman gain confidence in wearing the minimum of clothing and also provides beneficial remedial exercise. Pride in her personal appearance should be encouraged and as she gains in confidence, she should adopt a positive approach to life.

Where lymphoedema persists in the arm, the woman must be particularly careful to avoid burns to that arm. Long oven gloves should be worn and care taken to avoid burns from cigarettes or matches. She should take care not to prick her fingers when sewing or when manicuring her nails and cuticles.

Psychological rehabilitation is a more complex matter. Some time after mastectomy (2–3 months) the woman may experience periods of depression and denial. She may manifest her anxieties by directing her anger at her husband and this may be reflected in her sexual relationships with her partner. The role of the husband is of particular importance at this time. If he is involved in the care of his wife throughout from investigation to surgery, his understanding will be enhanced and his support invaluable. He will be more prepared to cope with the rehabilitation phase of treatment and understand the psychological difficulties which may arise during the period of adjustment, such as his wife's fear of dressing or undressing or her fear of being physically unattractive. Unless these problems are resolved a vicious circle is set up whereby the husband seeks to show his wife affection, she may reject him because she feels he will be repulsed by her surgery and that she is no longer attractive. Subsequently he will then cease to make sexual advances. Both are in fact withdrawing from a situation that should be discussed openly to achieve understanding. The General Practitioner or the Marriage Guidance Council should be consulted where these problems persist. In particular single women with sexual difficulties should seek help which may be resolved by discussion with the Nurse Counsellor at the Breast Clinic. Recurrence of the tumour is a possibility whether in the same or the other breast, and breast self-examination should be continued on the remaining breast. Some women find it difficult to accept that mastectomy does not equate with cure.

Breast conservation

The argument for conservation of the breast for a woman in the early stage of the disease is that there should be no need to subject the woman to mutilating surgery and psychological distress when the long term prognosis will not be altered significantly.

The methods of breast conservation are shown in Table 10.4.

Breast reconstruction

The aim of breast reconstruction is to make good any tissue deficit following mastectomy. This may be achieved in consultation with plastic surgeons when a swing flap graft is used.

Treatment of advanced disease

Treatment at this stage is palliative and aims to give the optimum quality of life to the patient. Disturbing symptoms will present due to metastases in other organs, confusion, breathlessness, bone pain and anaemia.

Different regimes of treatment are used for pre- and post-menopausal women.

Pre-menopausal treatment

1. Endocrine therapy
    Oöphorectomy — this will cause an artificial menopause and a large decrease in the production of oestrogen.
    Adrenal ablation — procured by the use of aminoglutethamide which inhibits adrenal steroid synthesis (Ch. 11)
    Hypophysectomy — the destruction of the pituitary gland by cryosurgery or by implantation of Yttrium 90 in the pituitary fossa (Ch. 11)

2. Chemotherapy
Causes the regression of metastases in most patients who have soft tissue or organ metastases. Multiple drug regimes are used and the cycle of administration is repeated every 28 days.

Post-menopausal treatment

1. Anti-oestrogen therapy
Tamoxifencitrate (Nolvadex) is now proving effective where breast tumours were found to contain high levels of oestrogen receptor protein on 'sampling' at the time of the original surgery. This drug has very few toxic effects.
2. Chemotherapy
As for the pre-menopausal woman, this may consist of a different combination of cytotoxic agents

Terminal care

During this period of palliative care, the nurses' role will be to support the patient and her family. It is at this time when the whole family in consultation with the team of specialists who have been administering treatment may discuss whether the patient may wish to be nursed at home with specialist community support, or whether the remainder of life should be spent in a hospice where personal, pastoral and physical needs can be respected by a team of specialists in the management of terminal care.

The role of the Nurse Counsellor

The role of the Nurse Counsellor is a relatively new idea. It is well recognised that malignant tumours of the breast convey to a woman a threat to her physical appearance which she may consider a serious mutilation and a psychological threat to her femininity. Throughout the period from detection of a lump in the breast, through subsequent treatment and rehabilitation, the Nurse Counsellor should provide emotional support to the woman, gaining trust, acting as a link with the medical team and providing practical support to both the patient and the medical team.

The Nurse Counsellor must be specifically trained in counselling techniques as well as having specialist knowledge in the management of all aspects of the work of the Breast Clinic. This will enable her to assist the patient to come to terms with the disease, to cope during periods of stress and to make the adjustments necessary to enjoy the quality of life that has been achieved. The Nurse Counsellor also has the opportunity to make a valuable contribution to research by defining and investigating problematic areas and producing documentary evidence and scientific conclusions.

SUGGESTED ASSIGNMENTS

1. Find out what facilities exist in your town/city for breast cancer screening. Discuss whether or not you consider the cost of maintaining these facilities can be justified in the long-term.
2. A young married woman with breast cancer is to have a simple mastectomy performed with subsequent radiotherapy. Identify the nursing problems this situation would present and the nursing intervention that would be necessary to assist the patient to achieve optimal health.
3. Infertility is a grave social and psychological problem of many marriages. How can the infertile couple be helped to cope with their difficulties?
4. Isotopes in implants used for treating carcinoma of the cervix have a very long half-life.

a. Discover what provisions are made in your hospital to prevent such materials being lost.

b. What routine steps would be necessary if a radio-active isotope is spilt or lost?

5. The protection of people in radiotherapy units is based on three well-known principles. These are that the dosage of radiation absorbed is dependent on:

a. The duration of exposure.
b. The distance from the source.
c. The use of shielding.

Make a list of those people whom you consider would require protection and ascertain how in your hospital these principles are employed to provide this.

6. Find out how antenatal care is organized in your area. What provisions are made to encourage attendance and what scheme is in use for follow-up of 'defaulters'?

FURTHER READING

Baum M 1981 Breast cancer, the facts. Oxford University Press, Oxford
Faulder C 1982 Breast cancer, a guide to its early detection and treatment, 2nd edn. Virago Press, London
Garland G W, Quixley J M E, Carmeron M D 1971 Obstetrics and gynaecology for nurses, 3rd edn. English Universities Press, London
Garrey M M, Govan A D T, Hodge C H, Callander R 1978 Gynaecology illustrated, 2nd edn. Churchill Livingstone, Edinburgh
Hector W, Bourne G 1979 Modern gynaecology with obstetrics for nurses, 6th edn. Heinemann, London
Jeffcoate Sir Norman 1975 Principles of gynaecology, 4th edn. Butterworth, London
Kleinman R L 1971 Family planning handbook for midwives and nurses. International Planned Parenthood Federation, London
Kleinman R L 1971 Family planning handbook for doctors. International Planned Parenthood Federation, London
Law B 1973 Family planning in nursing. Crosby Lockwood Staples, London
Llewellyn-Jones D 1978 Fundamentals of obstetrics and gynaecology. Gynaecology, vol 2, 2nd edn. Faber, London
Robinson N, Swash I 1977 Mastectomy. A patient's guide to coping with breast surgery. Thorsons, Wellingborough, Northants
Scottish Health Education Unit 1979 The book of the child. SHEU, 21 Lansdowne Crescent, Edinburgh

FOR REFERENCE

Bailey R E, Grayshon J 1983 Obstetric and gynaecological nursing, 3rd edn. Bailliere Tindall, London
Greening W P 1983 Avoiding mastectomy. British Journal of Hospital Medicine 4: 334–336
Report from Edinburgh Breast Screening Clinic 1978 Screening for breast cancer. British Medical Journal 2: 178–180
Stoker T A M 1983 Breast cancer: is screening worthwhile? Modern Medicine 2:10
Walker J, Macgillivray I, Macnaughton M C (eds) 1976 Combined textbook of obstetrics and gynaecology, 9th edn. Churchill Livingstone, Edinburgh.

Chapter Eleven
The endocrine system

The glands comprising this system have in common the fact that they all secrete chemical substances called hormones which are discharged directly into the blood or lymph. The hormones are carried in the circulatory system to a target organ or tissue which responds to the hormonal stimulus. The word hormone means 'to arouse' or 'wake up to' activity.

The endocrine glands which will be considered in this chapter are:

The pituitary.
The thyroid.
The parathyroids.
The pancreas.
The adrenals.

Other glands and tissues produce hormones too, for instance the skin and the kidneys; and one of the glands listed above, the pancreas, secretes pancreatic juice as well as the hormone insulin. Pancreatic juice, however, is discharged via the pancreatic duct into the duodenum (Ch. 5). Insulin is secreted directly into the blood. Hormones can also be produced abnormally, for example ACTH production by oat cell carcinoma of the lung.

After synthesis and secretion by the endocrine glands hormones are inactivated, especially by the liver and to some extent by their target organs, before being excreted. Measurable amounts of some hormones or their metabolites, such as steroids and adrenaline, can be found in urine and this is of help in diagnosis.

There are three main types of hormone:

1. Small proteins composed of amino acids.
2. Amines.
3. Steroids.

Control of endocrine function. The hypothalamus and pituitary together control most of the functions of other endocrine glands, exceptions being parathormone and aldosterone secretion. The pituitary is stimulated by the hypothalamus of the brain, which passes releasing factors and nervous stimuli to the pituitary whose hormones then act on target glands and tissues. The hypothalamus, in turn, is influenced by higher centres of the brain.

Maintenance of normal hormone levels in the body is achieved through negative feedback mechanisms. A good example of such a mechanism in everyday life is a thermostat which controls a central heating system. This device ensures that when the room temperature drops below a predetermined level, the source of heat is switched on, and when the temperature rises above the desired level, the source is switched off.

In the endocrine system, when the level of a hormone rises above or falls below

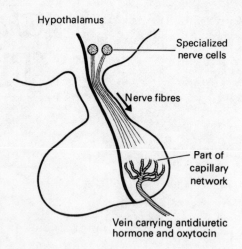

A. Relationship of anterior pituitary to hypothalamus. A portal venous system carries releasing and inhibiting factors from the hypothalamus to the anterior pituitary, stimulating or inhibiting its release of trophic hormones into the bloodstream.

B. Relationship of posterior pituitary to hypothalamus. Oxytocin and antidiuretic hormone are produced by special cells in the hypothalamus, travel along nerve fibres, are stored and released by the posterior pituitary into the bloodstream.

Figure 11.1
The pituitary gland

the normal level, the pituitary gland responds by releasing less or more of the appropriate stimulating hormone.

THE PITUITARY GLAND

This small but vitally important structure is sometimes called the master gland because of its influence on other endocrine glands.

STRUCTURE AND FUNCTION

The pituitary gland (Fig. 11.1) lies in the sella turcica of the sphenoid bone. A stalk connects it to the hypothalamus just behind the optic chiasma, and pituitary enlargement can, therefore, damage vision (Ch. 12). Below are the sphenoidal air sinuses (Fig. 13.1, p. 485). The gland has three lobes, anterior, intermediate and posterior; the intermediate lobe is rudimentary in man.

The anterior lobe

This part of the gland contains two main types of cell which can be differentiated according to the specific hormones secreted and the effect of staining techniques.

Anterior pituitary hormones (Table 11.2)

These secretions (Fig. 11.2) regulate:

1. Growth and activity of the whole body.
2. Other endocrine secretions.

Hypothalamic releasing and inhibiting hormones, which enter the anterior lobe via blood vessels in the pituitary stalk, control the synthesis and secretion of anterior pituitary hormones.

Table 11.1
Types of anterior pituitary cell

	Effects of staining	Functional type	Hormone produced
1. Chromophils	Eosinophil (acidophil)	Somatotroph	Growth
		Mammotroph	Prolactin
	Basophil	Thyrotroph	Thyrotrophic (thyroid stimulating)
		Gonadotroph	Gonadotrophic
		Corticotroph	Adrenocorticotrophic
2. Chromophobes	These are thought to be either potential or resting chromophils. They are normally described as non-secreting but can produce a variety of hormones.		

Table 11.2
Anterior pituitary hormones

Hormone	Regulation of hormone	Action of hormone
1. Growth hormone (GH) (somatotrophin)	Levels are raised by hypoglycaemia, fasting, deep sleep, exercise and emotional stress. Hyperglycaemia suppresses secretion.	Mainly development of bone, muscle and connective tissue. Opposes the action of insulin
2. Thyroid stimulating hormone (TSH)	Regulated by levels of circulating thyroxine	Controls thyroid activity
3. Adrenocorticotrophic hormone (ACTH)	Regulated by corticosteroid concentrations in blood Secretion is controlled by an inhibiting factor from the hypothalamus.	Regulates adrenal cortical activity and release of corticosteroids
4. Prolactin (PRL)	During pregnancy, ovarian hormones inhibit secretion of prolactin	Stimulates milk production postpartum: prolactin released during suckling stimulates milk production for the next feed: the baby 'orders' his next meal.
5. Gonadotrophic hormones a. Follicle stimulating hormone (FSH)	FSH stimulates the ovarian follicle to produce oestrogen: as oestrogen levels rise, FSH is suppressed	Necessary for normal development of male and female reproductive organs: FSH stimulates ripening of the ovarian follicle in the female and spermatogenesis in the male
b. Luteinizing hormone (LH)	The corpus luteum secretes progesterone: as progesterone levels in the circulation rise, LH production is reduced	LH stimulates the development of the corpus luteum in the female and testosterone secretion in the male

Table 11.3
Posterior pituitary hormones

Hormone	Regulation of hormone	Action of hormone
Oxytocin (Greek for sharp birth)	Reflex release is produced by (1) distension of the uterus; (2) stimulation of the nipple by suckling.	Contracts the uterus at term, inducing labour. It is used in obstetrics to stimulate uterine contractions. During lactation oxytocin facilitates milk ejection from breast ducts.
Antidiuretic hormone (ADH) (Vasopressin)	Plasma volume receptors in the great veins of the thorax send impulses to the hypothalamus which responds to (1) increased plasma volume by reducing ADH secretion thus increasing urinary output; (2) dehydration by increasing ADH causing greater reabsorption of water in the kidney. Water balance is maintained, 14 to 18 litres daily being reabsorbed from the kidney, under the influence of ADH.	1. Antidiuretic effect by increasing permeability of walls of distal convoluted tubules and collecting ducts in the nephrons of the kidneys leading to greater reabsorption of water. 2. Contracts smooth muscle of intestine, urinary bladder and blood vessels. Effect on blood pressure is negligible.

The posterior lobe

In this lobe hormones which have been synthesized in the hypothalamus are stored.

Posterior pituitary hormones (Table 11.3)

These secretions (Fig. 11.2) stimulate:

1. The distal convoluted tubules and collecting ducts of the nephrons, causing reabsorption of water (Fig. 11.3).
2. The uterine muscle at the end of pregnancy, causing contraction.

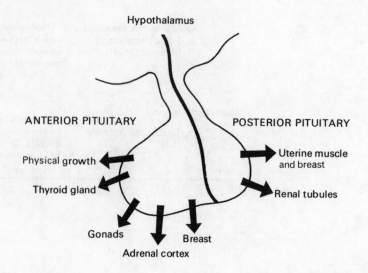

Figure 11.2
Targets of principal groups of pituitary hormones

Increased ADH secretion

Decreased ADH secretion

Increased plasma volume

Decreased plasma volume

Increased water reabsorption in kidney

Decreased water reabsorption in kidney

Urine volume decreased, concentration increased

Urine volume increased, concentration decreased

Figure 11.3
Role of ADH in maintaining water balance

PITUITARY DISORDERS

Disordered function may result in undersecretion (hyposecretion) or oversecretion (hypersecretion) of one or several groups of hormones. If there is undersecretion of all of the anterior pituitary hormones the condition is called panhypopituitarism.

Abnormal secretion of pituitary hormones may be due to disordered function of the gland itself or of the hypothalamus, affecting secretion of inhibitory or releasing hormones.

Causes of disordered pituitary function include:

1. **Tumours.** If the new growth is of secretory tissue, such as a chromophobe adenoma, hypersecretion occurs. Conversely, a craniopharyngioma is of non-secretory tissue and its presence may limit normal function, so causing hyposecretion.
2. **Trauma** such as a fractured base of skull.
3. **Idiopathic deficiency of secretion.**
4. **Therapeutic removal of the gland** by surgery (hypophysectomy) or radiotherapy.

Signs and symptoms vary according to the nature and extent of the endocrine dysfunction and the age of the patient. If the cause of the disorder is a tumour there may also be pressure symptoms, for instance headache and vomiting, and visual disturbance if the optic chiasma is involved (Fig. 12.5, p. 462).

ANTERIOR PITUITARY DISORDERS

These may be summarized as follows:

Hypofunction	Hyperfunction
Bodily growth and activity understimulated	Bodily growth and activity overstimulated
Target glands understimulated	Target glands overstimulated

Hypofunction

Growth hormone (GH)

Insufficient growth hormone during childhood results in failure to grow to normal height. The condition is called dwarfism and the person is normal in all respects except that of stature although puberty may be delayed. The main effect in an adult would be an increased sensitivity to insulin.

Adrenocorticotrophic hormone (ACTH)

Hyposecretion of this hormone produces a secondary adrenocortical failure resulting from lack of stimulation of production of the adrenal cortex hormones, especially the glucocorticoids. Production of aldosterone would not be affected as this is independent of the influence of ACTH. Deficiency could be life threatening. Poor resistance to stress will be present as well as hypoglycaemia and hypotension (p. 455).

Thyrotrophin (TSH) and Gonadotrophin

Hyposecretion of these hormones will present as hypofunction of their respective target organs, the thyroid gland and ovaries or testes.

Prolactin (PRL)

Lack of this hormone will cause failure of lactation for women after childbirth.

Total deficiency (Panhypopituitarism)

This may result from therapeutic removal or destruction of the gland or it may be associated with a pituitary tumour. The signs and symptoms will vary depending on whether the rate of loss of the hormones is sudden or gradual and the order in which they are affected. Since the normal endocrine response to environmental change is absent, coma may follow infection, stress or injury.

Hyperfunction

Growth hormone

Figure 11.4
Acromegaly

Hypersecretion is usually due to an adenoma. If it occurs in childhood, that is before the bony epiphyses have fused, gigantism results. Untreated individuals may reach 2 to 2½ m (7 to 8 feet) in height with proportionately large muscles and organs. Hypertension may be present and diabetes mellitus can develop because of the anti-insulin effect of growth hormone. Giants can also become prone to infection. Pressure from the adenoma may cause headaches, vomiting and blindness. If hypersecretion starts after the epiphyses have fused growth in length cannot take place; instead bone thickening occurs. This is especially noticeable in the jaws, hands and feet, hence the name given to the condition, **acromegaly** (G *akron* extremity, *megas* great) (Fig. 11.4).

Adrenocorticotrophic hormone

Hypersecretion by a pituitary adenoma is one cause of Cushing's syndrome (p. 456).

Prolactin

An excess of prolactin (hyperprolactinaemia) may occur because of pituitary disorder, such as a chromophobe adenoma, or disturbance of hypothalamic control with a reduced level of prolactin inhibitory factor. It may be found in conjunction with acromegaly. The raised level of prolactin suppresses gonadal function and in a female the first indication of this disorder may be amenorrhoea or galactorrhoea (inappropriate lactation).

Investigations

1. Radioimmunological assay of pituitary hormones such as ACTH and TSH.
2. Measurement of target organ response to pituitary hormones. No response

indicates disease of the target organ, not of the pituitary.

3. Insulin hypoglycaemia test. GH, ACTH and PRL are secreted in response to hypoglycaemia. The test can be dangerous when metabolic responses are below normal because of hypopituitarism and it is not done if heart disease or epilepsy are present. The patient is fasted overnight except for water and has an indwelling intravenous cannula inserted at least 30 minutes before the test is started. He is also told that he will feel drowsy and may sweat during the test. Blood is collected for basal measurement of hormone levels then soluble insulin is given intravenously, the dose being calculated in relation to the patient's body weight. Blood specimens are taken at regular intervals over the next $1\frac{1}{2}$ to 2 hours. A carbohydrate-containing meal is given at the end of the test. The patient must not be left unattended during the test and 50% glucose for intravenous injection must be available at the bedside to correct severe hypoglycaemia, should it occur.

4. Oral glucose tolerance test (OGTT). Normally GH levels will fall during this test but in acromegaly little or no suppression of the GH levels will be seen after the glucose load is given (p. 443).

5. X-rays. These may show enlargement of the sella turcica due to an expanding tumour and the bony abnormalities characteristic of acromegaly.

6. Computerised axial tomography (CAT scan). This will show up any extension of the tumour above the sella turcica (p. 86).

7. Visual field examination. A tumour in or near the pituitary gland may produce pressure on the optic nerve (pp. 461–462).

Methods of treatment

Radiotherapy

A tumour may be destroyed or removed by radiotherapy emanating either from: *yttrium 90 implants* inserted via the nose and sphenoidal sinus, or *conventional radiotherapy*, usually after surgery.

Hypophysectomy

This may be done by excision of the tumour or by destruction of tissue using a probe with a freezing tip. Microsurgery techniques make this possible using the transsphenoidal approach. A small piece of tissue may be taken from the thigh area to seal the opening made in the dura mater. The transfrontal approach is sometimes used where there are signs of pressure on adjacent structures such as the optic nerve — otherwise access is via the sphenoidal sinus (Fig. 11.5).

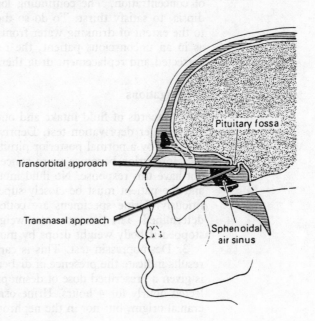

Pituitary fossa

Transorbital approach

Transnasal approach

Sphenoidal air sinus

Figure 11.5
Hypophysectomy

Drugs

Bromocriptine will reduce levels of PRL and GH. Where infertility is present in hyperprolactinaemia, this is also likely to be corrected and the patient may need to be given advice on contraception. For treatment of acromegaly, bromocriptine is normally used as an adjunct to surgery or radiotherapy. The drug should be taken with food to minimize side-effects which can include nausea and vomiting.

Replacement therapy

The replacement may be of one hormone only or of several. When hyposecretion of TSH or ACTH is affecting thyroid and adrenalcortical function, the secondary hormones — thyroxine, hydrocortisone and oestrogen or testosterone — are usually administered instead of giving pituitary trophic hormones.

POSTERIOR PITUITARY DISORDERS

Diabetes insipidus

This may occur alone or in combination with other pituitary deficiencies.

The cause is usually hyposecretion of ADH (or, rarely, failure of renal tubules to respond to the stimulus of the hormone — nephrogenic diabetes insipidus).

Causes of hyposecretion

1. Pituitary tumour.
2. Infection such as meningitis.
3. Fractured base of skull.
4. Surgery on or near the pituitary gland.
5. Idiopathic malfunction.

Either sex and any age may be affected. The condition may be transient following hypophysectomy or head injury.

Clinical features

These stem from the fact that water is not reabsorbed by the distal convoluted tubules and collecting ducts of the kidneys (Fig. 11.3). In consequence, abnormally large amounts of urine enter the bladder and the urinary output may exceed 5–10 litres in 24 hours. The urine is pale and clear with a very low osmolality due to lack of concentration. The continuing loss of fluid results in frequent drinking (polydipsia) to satisfy thirst. To do so the patient will go to considerable lengths, even to the extent of drinking water from flower vases. Where thirst cannot be satisfied, as in an unconscious patient, the result is life-threatening unless the fluid loss is corrected and replacement drug therapy begun.

Investigations

1. Records of fluid intake and output.
2. Water deprivation test. Deprivation of fluid intake will stimulate production of ADH by a normal posterior pituitary gland leading to a rise in urine osmolality, therefore urine becomes more concentrated. A person with diabetes insipidus will not have this response. No fluid intake is allowed at all for the duration of the test and the patient must be closely supervised to ensure that no fluid is taken surreptitiously. Urine specimens are collected at specified intervals and the osmolality determined. The patient is also weighed before and during the test which must be stopped if body weight drops by more than 3%.
3. Desmopressin test. This is carried out after the water deprivation test when results indicate the presence of diabetes insipidus. Following rehydration the patient is given a prescribed dose of desmopression (*DDAVP*) and urine specimens are collected hourly for 4 hours. Urine osmolality will rise if the diabetes insipidus is of cranial origin, but not in the nephrogenic form.

Treatment

1. Replacement therapy is by desmopressin, a long-acting ADH analogue, which is taken intranasally 2–3 times daily. This can also be given by intramuscular or intravenous injection where the patient is unconscious or in the early stages after trans-sphenoidal hypophysectomy.

2. Chlorpropamide and carbamazepine. These substances enhance the action on the kidney of any endogenous antidiuretic hormone.

Syndrome of inappropriate antidiuretic hormone secretion (SIADH)

Abnormal amounts of ADH are secreted causing a reduced level of sodium in the blood (hyponatraemia) due to dilution of body fluids by retained water and increased excretion of sodium. Urine is relatively concentrated. The condition can arise from a bronchial carcinoma which produces ectopic ADH. Where the tumour cannot be removed, demeclocycline or lithium carbonate can be given to produce a nephrogenic diabetes insipidus. Fluid restriction to 0.5 litre in 24 hours is occasionally effective but is very unpleasant for the patient.

NURSING CARE IN PITUITARY DISORDERS

Disturbances in function are shown in many ways and prolonged or continuing treatment may be needed. Abnormalities of stature and appearance may result in much distress. In dwarfism, for instance, the small person may be handicapped socially, psychologically and physically. The developing mind is imprisoned in a child's body. Anxiety about slow growth is often greatest in boys: a youthful appearance with delayed pubertal development may add to embarrassment and lead to much unhappiness. It is important to accord the small person the same respect one gives other individuals.

In dwarfism, the child and his parents should be told about the expected pattern of growth and advised that adult stature may be greater than expected. Learning and social and athletic activities at which they may excel should be suggested. The person should be encouraged to dress and behave in accordance with his age.

Sensitivity, too, should be displayed to the patient with acromegaly who has become unhappily aware of his altered appearance and speech.

Special aspects of preoperative management

The gland is often approached via the nose, and nasal swabs can be taken to ascertain if antibiotic therapy should be started. Antiseptic nasal creams may also be prescribed to control organisms, and the nose may be packed with cocaine and adrenaline 1:1000 to prevent bleeding. Caring for the patient in a single room will help to keep him free from infection.

Special aspects of postoperative management

Any activity leading to an increase in intracranial pressure should be avoided. The patient is nursed flat initially and then gradually allowed to sit up. Coughing, nose blowing and bending down are discouraged. Measures are taken to prevent constipation. There should be very little pain as such but a headache may be present or discomfort from nasal packing.

In all procedures for pituitary destruction hydrocortisone is prescribed to prevent symptoms of adrenal cortex deficiency from developing.

Nursing observations and records

Complications which are of particular importance after this type of operation are intracerebral compression and bleeding, leakage of cerebrospinal fluid, infection, and abnormal endocrine function.

Particular attention is paid to observations relating to:

1. Intracranial pressure (p. 92).
2. The nose, for CSF leakage — look for repeated swallowing.
3. Temperature, pulse and respiration, for signs of infection.
4. Urinary output and osmolality for signs of diabetes insipidus.

Continuing supervision

Following an operation for pituitary destruction the patient is readmitted, after an interval of 3 months, and hydrocortisone therapy is stopped to see whether it is necessary to continue the drug. Pituitary destruction or hypofunction, from any cause, may demand the replacement of one or several hormones.

Hydrocortisone may have to be taken for life. The patient will be advised to increase the dose in times of infection or stress and always to carry a card bearing the diagnosis and details of current drug therapy in the event of an emergency.

Thyroxine is given if hypothyroidism is detected.

Sex hormones. Oestrogens for women, testosterone — by implants in the abdominal wall — for men, and gonadotrophins to restore fertility, may be needed.

Desmopressin is prescribed to treat diabetes insipidus. Should the patient be a diabetic his insulin requirements will probably become less.

THE THYROID GLAND
STRUCTURE AND FUNCTION

This gland lies in the neck, in front of the trachea (Fig. 11.6). It has a very rich blood supply. Embedded in its **posterior surface** are four parathyroid glands. Passing very close to the thyroid is the recurrent laryngeal nerve, supplying the muscles of the larynx. These anatomical relationships are important in surgery of the gland, because of the danger of accidental damage.

Microscopically the gland is composed of spherical vesicles made up of thyroid cells. Thyroid hormone secreted by these cells is stored in the form of colloid in the vesicles and is released into the bloodstream when required. Iodine is necessary for the formation of the hormone and must be supplied in the diet. The two major thyroid hormones are tri-iodothyronine (T3) and tetraiodothyronine (thyroxine or T4). The gland is stimulated to release these by thyroid stimulating hormone (TSH), which is in turn produced by the anterior pituitary in response to thyroid releasing factor from the hypothalamus. Regulation of production of thyroid hormones is brought about by a feed-back system, such as is described on page 425. In this case circulating levels of thyroid hormone influence the output of thyroid releasing factor by the hypothalamus. On release into the bloodstream, most of the hormones are carried bound to plasma proteins. A small quantity circulates in the free form.

Figure 11.6
Thyroid gland showing position of parathyroids

Thyroid cartilage
Parathyroid glands
Parathyroid glands
Trachea

The main functions of thyroid hormone are summarized below:

1. It controls the basal metabolic rate.
2. It is essential for normal mental and physical development of children.
3. It influences the functioning of the nervous system, deficiency of the hormone causing slowing down and sluggishness, excess causing overactivity and excitability.
4. It potentiates the effects of adrenaline and sympathetic nervous activity. An excess is seen as features of overactivity.
5. It is necessary for the formation of vitamin A from carotene.
6. It lowers levels of blood cholesterol.
7. It increases the absorption of glucose from the intestines.

Tests of thyroid function

These are carried out to determine whether the gland is over- or underactive. Since most of the tests presently in use are of a sophisticated biochemical type and do not involve the nurse to any great extent, only a brief description is provided.

1. ^{131}Iodine (I) uptake test. A measured dose of ^{131}I is given, and the proportion taken up by the thyroid gland is measured by a counter. Provided patients are not suffering from iodine lack, an increased uptake indicates hyperthyroidism, a decreased uptake, hypothyroidism. In the latter a greater than normal amount of ^{131}I is found in the urine, which must be collected for specified periods after the initial dose.

2. Direct measurement of circulating thyroid hormone can be carried out. This test has largely replaced the protein-bound iodine (PBI) test, which was easily disturbed by a number of factors.

3. Tests of the function of hypothalamus-pituitary-thyroid interrelationship. Normally the administration of thyroid releasing hormone (TRH) stimulates the pituitary to produce thyroid stimulating hormone (TSH). If hyperthyroidism is present the feed-back mechanism activated by high levels of thyroid hormone prevents this response. The test involves measuring blood levels of TSH after administration of TRH.

4. Basal metabolic rate. This test is not often used, as it is an inexact indicator of thyroid function. It is based on the patient's utilization of oxygen under controlled circumstances, from which his energy consumption can be calculated. The result is compared with normal people of the same age, size and sex.

DISORDERS OF THE THYROID GLAND

Goitre

The term goitre refers to enlargement of the thyroid gland. A simple goitre is not associated with excess secretion of thyroid hormone. Normally these patients are euthyroid or have degrees of hypothyroidism.

Aetiology

1. Iodine deficiency. This limits the amount of thyroid hormone made and causes, enlargement. Endemic goitre is found in areas remote from the sea, where diet is deficient in iodine. Some 'fad' diets also lack iodine, while in pregnancy there can be a relative iodine deficiency because of increased urinary excretion and the demands of the fetus.

2. Goitrogens. Certain substances inhibit the uptake of iodine by the gland, bringing into play the mechanism described above and leading to goitre. Among these substances are the thiouracils, carbimazole, potassium perchlorate (all used in the treatment of hyperthyroidism), sodium aminosalicylate (para-aminosalicylate — PAS), lithium compounds and phenylbutazone.

Clinical features

As a rule, there is only a painless swelling in the neck. Gross enlargement may press on the trachea causing cough and dyspnoea, and on the oesophagus leading to dysphagia.

Treatment

The administration of iodine in the form of potassium iodide to children suffering from deficiency prevents further enlargement. It does not reduce the size of the gland. Adults are given thyroxine 0.1 to 0.25 mg daily, which has a similar effect and may reduce the size of the thyroid. Goitrogens are, of course, avoided. Surgery (subtotal thyroidectomy) is carried out when the gland becomes unsightly or causes difficulty in breathing or swallowing (see below for further details). Following surgery, thyroxine may be given to prevent symptoms of hypothyroidism.

Hyperthyroidism

Sometimes referred to as thyrotoxicosis, or exophthalmic goitre, the main features of this condition (except exophthalmos, see below) are caused by increased secretion of thyroid hormone. Although the cause is uncertain, it is thought that a form of antibody, a long-acting thyroid stimulating substance (LATS) found in the blood, may be responsible.

Clinical features

Increased heat production, sweating and excitability are typical. Patients suffer weight loss, although they usually have a good appetite. Heart rate is increased even while sleeping. In a long-standing condition, disturbance of heart rhythm and heart enlargement may result. Exophthalmos (protrusion of the eyeballs) is often the most obvious sign. The cause of this is still uncertain. Mood disturbance can resemble acute anxiety states, with restlessness, agitation and tremor. Varying degrees of elation may also be seen.

Treatment

The results of treatment are extremely satisfactory though the distressing exophthalmos is not usually eliminated. Three well-established methods are used. Each is more suitable than the others in certain circumstances.

Antithyroid drugs. These interfere with the production of thyroid hormone in various ways. One of the most widely used drugs is carbimazole. Its side-effects are not common but, if they occur, propylthiouracil can be used instead. Higher doses are given for up to 4 months to reduce hormone production to normal, then lower maintenance doses are given. After a year or two it is possible to see if remission has occurred by gradually withdrawing the drug. Another drug which may be used occasionally is potassium perchlorate if allergy to other drugs occurs. In severe hyperthyroidism, disturbances of cardiac rhythm may be controlled by propranolol. Drug therapy is most suitable for young children, for adults with smaller goitres and for pregnant women.

Radioactive iodine therapy. This method is most suitable for people of older age groups on recurrence of symptoms after partial thyroidectomy, or in cases of pre-existing debilitating disease such as rheumatic heart disease. It is never used in pregnancy and is undesirable for persons of reproductive age. The treatment consists of administering orally a radioactive isotope of iodine (^{131}I). This is taken up by the thyroid gland, where the emitted radiation is concentrated on thyroid cells, destroying some of them. The risk of producing hypothyroidism is a significant complication. The use of such radioactive materials requires special handling facilities and staff trained in the necessary precautions.

Surgery. Partial thyroidectomy is used mainly in adults and particularly where drug therapy has not controlled the condition. About seven-eigths of the gland is removed. Prior to operation, drugs are used to reduce thyroid function to normal. Potassium iodide is given for 14 days to reduce the vascularity of the gland. This makes operation easier and safer since excessive bleeding does not occur and large amounts of hormone are not released into the bloodstream.

Nursing care

A point which must be uppermost in the nurse's mind is that her attitude towards her patient must not be coloured by those features of the disease, such as mood elevation, anxiety and restlessness, which can be demanding and difficult to deal with.

Rest. The maximum provision for rest is essential. This includes a quiet, non-stimulating environment and a quiet, calm approach by staff. A limited amount of activity is useful to minimize boredom and frustration. Restriction on the number of visitors may also help by reducing stimulation. Extreme restlessness may require the use of sedatives. Other patients in the ward, who may be disturbed by a restless, overactive patient, must not be forgotten.

Diet. There are a number of reasons why diet is important. The overactive patient with increased metabolic rate requires increased amounts of carbohydrate to meet his energy requirements. Weight loss may indicate a need for increased protein. Sweating results in greater than normal fluid loss, which must be replaced by increased intake. A few patients will not have good appetites and will require special consideration. Stimulating drinks such as coffee and even tea may need to be avoided.

Observation. This should include:

1. Pulse rate (radial and apex) including rate when asleep.
2. Temperature and respiratory rate. An increased temperature may indicate infection, particularly if drug therapy has caused leucopenia.
3. Weighing, which should be carried out at least weekly.
4. Rashes due to drugs, which should be noted and reported at once.
5. Mood and behaviour.

Comfort. To a great extent, the patient's comfort depends on allowing for his extra sensitivity to heat. Adequate ventilation is helpful, and very light bedclothes should be used. Frequent changes of clothing and linen and frequent baths help to cope with excess sweating. Protection of the eyes is essential if the patient has exophthalmos.

Nursing in surgery of the thyroid

A period of medical treatment is always given to ensure that no signs of hyperthyroidism are present when the operation is carried out. Electrocardiography is also carried out to detect any cardiac abnormality. Laryngoscopy may be performed preoperatively to detect possible vocal cord paralysis, especially if there has been previous thyroid surgery. Preparation for surgery is essential, as for other forms of operation. It must be remembered that reassurance about the cosmetic result is of importance, especially to younger women. Preoperative education of the patient should include information and explanation of what he may expect after operation. This should be provided in a way which will not cause alarm. Reassurance will be derived from knowing that all discomforts will be dealt with promptly. He will need to know that he will have an intravenous infusion, that his throat will be uncomfortable and that he may have some difficulty in swallowing. Practice before surgery in supporting his head and neck is valuable. Preoperative administration of potassium iodide or Lugol's iodine for 2 weeks prior to operation renders the gland firmer and less vascular, thus minimizing the risk of postoperative complications. Propranolol may be given to block the effects of high hormone levels on the heart. This may be continued for up to a week after operation.

Except in cases of malignancy, about five-sixths of the gland is removed. Sufficient gland tissue is thus left to provide an adequate supply of hormone. The incision is made along a natural skin fold in the neck and is closed with stainless steel clips. There are often small wound drains — these are usually removed after 24 hours, and all the clips in about 3 days.

There is a normal tendency for patients to be frightened to move their heads after this operation. They should be reassured by careful support of the head, protecting the wound from strain, whenever position is changed. During the first day, patients will not feel like eating, but frequent small drinks should be encouraged. These will help the sore throat, which is a normal feature. From the second day on, increasing mobility is allowed and the diet progresses from soft to normal.

Postoperative observations

Observation after operation is for the purpose of detecting complications: these are, fortunately, uncommon.

1. *Haemorrhage*. In the early postoperative period pulse and blood pressure readings should be taken every 15 minutes. Dressings should be examined for signs of bleeding and, since blood may run round behind the neck and shoulders, these areas should also be examined. Blood may not escape from the wound but may collect in the tissues. Nurses should therefore be alert to breathing or swallowing difficulties caused by pressure of blood on the trachea and oesophagus. In cases of serious respiratory difficulty, the wound should be reopened with clip removers, which should be kept at the bedside. The patient should be put into a lateral position. Blood vessels will have to be religatured in theatre, and if the degree of respiratory difficulty warrants it, a tracheostomy may be performed.

2. *Damage to nerves*. Because of the proximity of the recurrent laryngeal nerve, temporary signs of interference may appear. Permanent damage is rare. Hoarseness and sore throat are to be expected after operation, but if they increase in severity or if respiratory difficulty occurs, nerve injury may be indicated. *Dysphonia* (difficulty in speaking) can also occur, as a result of vocal cord paralysis. If both cords are paralysed, breathing difficulties may require tracheostomy.

3. *Tetany*. Accidental removal of parathyroid glands leads to depression of blood calcium levels. The features of this rare but serious complication may take up to a week to appear. Severe cases are manifest within 24 hours. Paraesthesia of extremities develops, with painful muscle contractions. Painful flexion of wrists and ankles also occurs (p. 441). The condition is quickly relieved by intravenous calcium gluconate.

4. *Thyroid crisis*. This is now extremely rare because of improved preoperative preparation. It is heralded by a rapid increase of pulse and temperature occurring within 24 hours of operation accompanied by restlessness and delirium.

5. *Hypothyroidism*. This long-term complication occurs in a few cases. Treatment is by administration of thyroxine.

Hypothyroidism

This term implies underactivity of the thyroid gland. Causes include ^{131}I therapy and surgery. Primary hypothyroidism associated with a goitre (Hashimoto's thyroiditis) is of autoimmune origin.

Cretinism

Hypothyroidism in children is known as cretinism. Maternal hormones supply a baby's needs for up to 3 months after birth. Then, if the baby is hypothyroid, features due to deficiency begin to appear. These are a general stunting of mental and physical growth. If left untreated the child becomes a mentally retarded dwarf with coarse facial features. Early detection and administration of the deficient hormone leads to great improvement in physical growth and, in some cases, mental development. In others, mental retardation persists.

Myxoedema

This term refers to the clinical state resulting from prolonged severe hypothyroidism. As would be expected, many of the features are the converse of those of hyperthyroidism. These include lack of energy, apathy, sensitivity to cold, reduced sweating and a slowed pulse rate. Accumulation of mucin in tissues gives the appearance of oedema, especially around the eyes. Mental slowness is obvious. Hair becomes dry and brittle and may be thin. Amenorrhoea may develop and anaemia may also be present. Treatment by the administration of thyroxine must be given for life. Careful adjustment of dosage is necessary to avoid symptoms of hyperthyroidism.

Nursing care

To a large extent this depends on the symptoms. The patient's slowness of thought and action requires much patience and understanding. Sensitivity to cold indicates the need for a warm environment and adequate clothing and blankets. Dry skin is helped by using bath oil and suitable lotions. Constipation, which is common, suggests the need for more roughage in the diet and, if necessary, suitable aperients. In general, what makes the patient comfortable is a good guide. If thyroxine is being administered, watch should be kept for signs of hyperthyroidism. Diet should have adequate protein and iron content, but excessive carbohydrate should be avoided.

THE PARATHYROID GLANDS
STRUCTURE AND FUNCTION

The four parathyroids lie behind the thyroid gland (Fig. 11.6); branches of the thyroid arteries provide their blood supply. In the embryo, the parathyroids occasionally migrate elsewhere, for example to the mediastinum. Their number can also vary. They secrete **parathormone**, which maintains plasma calcium levels within a narrow range despite the large daily exchanges of calcium between intestines, bloodstream, kidneys and bones.

Parathormone secretion is not regulated by the anterior pituitary but varies inversely with plasma concentration. Plasma phosphate concentration is inversely related to that of calcium.

The main functions of parathormone are:

1. To mobilize calcium and phosphate from bones into blood (Ch. 4).
2. To reduce renal excretion of calcium.
3. To promote intestinal absorption of calcium aided by vitamin D. (These actions raise the plasma calcium.)
4. To reduce phosphorus reabsorption by the kidneys, thus promoting its excretion and lowering plasma phosphate. This is necessary, since calcium and phosphate together tend to precipitate out of solution and could thus damage tissues and especially arterial walls.

PARATHYROID DISORDERS

Hyperparathyroidism

This term denotes excessive parathyroid activity; the condition is uncommon, the highest incidence being among females and between the ages of 30 and 50 years. The disease may be familial.

Primary hyperparathyroidism. The cause is usually a benign adenoma or adenomas (90% of cases), occasionally hyperplasia and more rarely cancer. There is oversecretion of parathormone, regardless of plasma calcium concentration. Calcium and phosphorus are mobilized from bone, renal absorption of calcium is increased, plasma calcium levels rise and urinary phosphate excretion is increased.

Secondary hyperparathyroidism. In some diseases where there is depression of the plasma calcium, there is compensatory enlargement of the parathyroids. The underlying disease may be intestinal, causing malabsorption of vitamin D and calcium, or renal, where there is excess calcium excretion.

Clinical features of primary hyperparathyroidism

Raised plasma calcium causes lethargy and anorexia. It weakens and eventually paralyses muscles. The paralysing effects of excess calcium on the gut wall may cause abdominal pain and constipation. Polyuria occurs, since the kidneys are filtering and excreting excess mineral salts. The nauseated patient may be reluctant to drink, but he should be encouraged to do so to prevent dehydration and formation of renal stones. Renal disorders are common, with formation of calcium-containing kidney stones due to high urinary calcium. Calcium-depleted bones become brittle. Osteitis fibrosa (replacement of bone by fibrous tissue) causes vague pains, which may be mistaken for rheumatism and can lead to bone deformities. Cyst formation in bones adds swelling to deformity. Calcium 'ring' deposits can occur in the cornea, and effects on nervous tissue may cause agitation, confusion or depression.

Nurses should ensure that patients whose bones are so fragile are protected from accidents.

Investigations

1. Measurement of plasma calcium with the patient at rest and fasting. (Calcium absorption following meals would affect the readings.) Plasma calcium is raised and plasma phosphorus reduced in primary hyperparathyroidism.
2. Measurement of parathormone levels by radioimmunoassay when possible.
3. Bone X-rays. These may reveal cysts and low bone density.
4. Bone biopsy. This may show reabsorption of trabeculae by osteoclasts and replacement by fibrous tissue (oesteitis fibrosa).
5. Intravenous urogram. This may demonstrate calcium deposits in the renal tract.
6. Urinary calcium, measured on a normal diet, is increased because the increase in the amount filtered overwhelms the effect of renal reabsorption under the influence of parathormone.

Treatment

Secondary hyperparathyroidism. Oral vitamin D will raise plasma calcium levels by enhancing absorption and so remove the stimulus to parathyroid hyperplasia. Operative treatment is seldom indicated.

Primary hyperparathyroidism is treated by surgical removal of abnormal parathyroid tissue. If hyperplasia of all four glands exists, three and a half are removed.

Preparation for operation

Preoperatively, the patient may be infused with methylene blue to facilitate recognition of parathyroid tissue. This procedure causes skin and mucous membrane to develop a greenish tinge. The patient should be warned about this beforehand and assured that the colour will disappear quickly. Ward staff without experience of this operation should also be prepared for this change in appearance.

Postoperative observations

Hypoparathyroidism occurs if much parathyroid tissue is removed and because calcium-depleted bones take up free calcium. Plasma calcium levels are monitored by:

1. Taking blood samples.
2. Frequent observation of the patient for signs of latent tetany, using Chvostek's and Trousseau's signs (p. 441) and noting any tingling sensations in the limbs.

Should signs of hypocalcaemia develop, an intravenous injection of 10% calcium gluconate is given. Dihydrotachysterol (DHT), an analogue of vitamin D, is sometimes given in large doses postoperatively (8 mg daily for 2 days). As they act more slowly than DHT, vitamin D preparations are less satisfactory for immediate postoperative management. Aluminium hydroxide may be given orally with meals to reduce phosphorus absorption. (Since blood calcium levels are now reduced phosphorus levels rise). Later, a high calcium diet is given, the calcium usually consisting of calcium salts, because these patients often have renal disorders and milk is inadvisable because of its high protein and phosphorus content.

Postoperative complications

These are similar to those which may follow thyroidectomy (p. 438), for example a slipped blood vessel ligature resulting in a haematoma which compresses the trachea. Clip removers should be available for such an eventuality, so that pressure on the trachea may be relieved. If the surgeon has explored the mediastinum chest complications may arise.

Rehabilitation

Maintenance therapy with DHT is continued, with out-patient supervision of dosage, until bone healing occurs. If hypocalcaemia persists, the patient may require life-long calcium supplements and vitamin D_2. Existing stones do not dissolve so renal function may be impaired permanently.

Hypoparathyroidism

Hypoparathyroidism may either arise spontaneously or follow disease or injury, but more often it results from accidental removal of the parathyroids during thyroidectomy.

Clinical features

1. **Tetany** develops when plasma calcium falls significantly below the normal 2.12–2.62 mmol/l. There is increased excitability of nerves and muscles. Motor and sensory nerve impulses fire off spontaneously. Abnormal sensory impulses cause tingling sensations (paraesthesiae), while the motor impulses cause involuntary muscle twitches. These twitches are most obvious in the muscles of the inner forearm and hand supplied by the ulnar nerve. There is flexion of wrist and knuckles with extension of the fingers (carpal spasm, Fig. 11.7). As a result of defective muscular control, the patient is more liable to fall and requires careful observation. Two signs of latent tetany are:

Chvostek's sign. Tapping the facila nerve at the jaw angle produces twitching of facial muscles.

Trousseau's sign. Applying a blood pressure cuff to the arm causes muscular spasm of forearm and hand.

2. **Laryngospasm** may be severe enough to obstruct the airway.

3. **Epileptic convulsions**, due to increased excitability of nerve cells in the brain, may be the first symptom.

4. **Psychological disturbances** may range from minor disorders to major psychoses.

Figure 11.7
Carpal spasm

Investigations

These are carried out when the patient's condition permits. They include the following:

1. Fasting plasma calcium.
2. Serum inorganic phosphate.
3. Renal phosphate clearance.
4. 24-hour urine collection to measure urinary calcium excretion. Nurses must explain to the patient the importance of an accurate 24-hour urine collection and of fasting before certain blood specimens are taken. It may also be necessary to collect faeces. Some investigations may make it imperative that the calcium intake is known and, if this is so, a special diet will be supplied.
5. Electrocardiograph may demonstrate variations in cardiac muscle function.

Treatment

Emergency treatment

Calcium salts such as 10 ml of 10% calcium gluconate are given intravenously to raise the plasma calcium level when symptoms are severe and require urgent relief. If epileptic convulsions occur, the patient must be protected from injury.

Replacement therapy

Parathormone injections are ineffective since the patient soon produces antibodies neutralizing their action. Vitamin D_2 (calciferol) can be given daily to increase calcium absorption or, alternatively, DHT 0.5 mg–1 mg daily.

The inverse relationship between calcium and phosphorus means that phosphorus levels fall as calcium levels rise. A low phosphorus diet may be given initially, to reduce the work of the kidneys in excreting excess phosphorus. As these two minerals are found in the same foods, calcium-rich foods are restricted at first.

Aftercare

Out-patient supervision will be needed to carry out the following:

1. Periodic serum calcium estimations to monitor drug dosage.
2. Periodic observation of renal function. Overdosage of vitamin D can cause hypercalcaemia with consequent risk of renal calculi.

Serious intellectual impairment cannot be restored by treatment, hence the need for early diagnosis to prevent such complications.

THE PANCREAS
STRUCTURE AND FUNCTION

The endocrine secretions of the pancreas are produced by groups of cells called the islets of Langerhans. They contain two cell types:

1. Alpha (α) cells secreting **glucagon**. This promotes glycogen breakdown, thereby raising the blood glucose.
2. Beta (β) cells (75% of the islets) secreting **insulin**. This lowers the blood glucose by:
   a. Promoting glycogen synthesis particularly in liver and muscles.
   b. Increasing cellular utilization of glucose in many tissues.
   c. Inhibiting gluconeogenesis from protein.

Both hormones are secreted in response to changes in blood glucose levels. Insulin is produced when levels are rising and glucagon when levels are falling.

PANCREATIC DISORDERS

The only condition which will be discussed results from the failure of the pancreas to secrete sufficient insulin to meet the body's requirements. This failure may be either partial or total. The disorder is called diabetes mellitus.

Diabetes mellitus

Diabetes mellitus is the commonest endocrine disorder. Prevalence in urban societies is 2 to 6%, many people being unaware of their condition. The disease is commoner in prosperous societies and among certain races.

Aetiology

1. Genetic endowment is important in those contracting diabetes. In all age groups environmental factors may determine which of the genetically predisposed develop clinical diabetes.
2. Age: 80% of cases occur in those over 50 years.
3. Obesity and diabetes are associated but uncertainty exists as to whether obesity causes or results from diabetes.
4. Physical stress may induce diabetes in susceptible people, mainly by increasing corticosteroid production. Corticosteroids are antagonistic to insulin.

A few cases result from:

1. Pathological processes such as carcinoma of pancreas.
2. Certain treatments, for example with corticosteroids.

3. Increase of hormonal insulin antagonists. This may occur during pregnancy or because of overproduction of pituitary growth hormone (an insulin antagonist).

Clinical features

Diabetes affects the metabolism of proteins, fats, carbohydrates, water and electrolytes. Without the secretion of a sufficient amount of insulin, glucose cannot pass into tissue cells and instead accumulates in the circulation, with the following results:

1. The blood glucose level rises (**hyperglycaemia**).
2. The kidneys are unable to reabsorb all the glucose passing through them and glucose appears in the urine (**glycosuria**).
3. The high concentration of glucose in the filtrate exerts an increased osmotic pressure which hampers the reabsorption of water by the renal tubules, so that a much larger volume of urine than normal is formed (**polyuria**).
4. Polyuria leads to dehydration and thirst. The patient drinks large quantities (**polydipsia**).
5. Fat is utilized for energy production instead of carbohydrate, but is incompletely metabolized since for its total combustion, carbohydrate must be metabolized simultaneously. Toxic acid products of incomplete fat metabolism (**ketones**) accumulate in blood and urine and are also excreted in breath, giving it a characteristic smell.
6. Ketoacidosis causes vomiting and drowsiness and may lead to coma and death.
7. Increased gluconeogenesis occurs, causing weakness and wasting of muscles.
8. Extreme tiredness from inability of body to produce energy normally.

Investigations

Urine tests. Glycosuria suggests diabetes.

Blood glucose tests. High blood glucose levels (over 8.3 mmol/l) indicate diabetes in anyone displaying other classical symptoms of the disease. Most people need no other tests.

Glucose tolerance tests (OGTT). Glucose 75 g is given orally to the fasting patient and blood samples are taken half hourly for 2 hours. A fasting venous blood glucose level of 7 mmol/l or more and a 2 hour level of more than 10 mmol/l are diagnostic of diabetes mellitus. Nurses must ensure that the glucose is properly dissolved and diluted to the same strength since the concentration affects the absorption rate. The mixture is more palatable when flavoured with pure lemon juice and chilled. The patient must drink all of the mixture and he should not reduce his carbohydrate intake in the days prior to OGTT since the test should reflect insulin response under normal dietary conditions. He should also refrain from smoking and remain at rest throughout the test as smoking and exercise will influence blood glucose levels. Urine may be tested hourly during OGTT but little extra information is gained.

In Figure 11.8, the OGTT shows a comparison of blood glucose and insulin levels in normal people, mild diabetics needing only diet therapy, moderately severe diabetics needing diet and oral hypoglycaemic drugs (OHD) and severe diabetics needing diet and insulin therapy.

Methods of treatment

For treatment purposes, diabetics form two groups:

1. Insulin dependent diabetics (IDDM).
2. Insulin independent diabetics (NIDDM).

Insulin dependent diabetics are often young, underweight people who will rapidly develop fatal ketoacidosis if not given insulin. Some older people are also insulin dependent. Onset of diabetes is acute.

Insulin independent diabetics are more often middle-aged or elderly and obese. Most of these patients produce some insulin and are less prone to developing ketosis. However, complications associated with long-standing diabetes can occur in both types: many mature onset diabetics have histories of mild symptoms which have

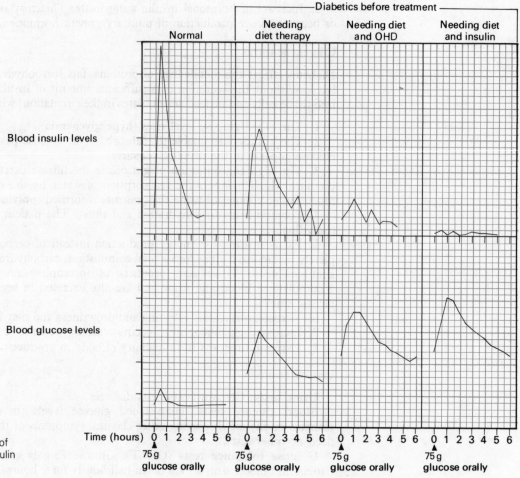

Figure 11.8
OGTT showing comparison of blood glucose and blood insulin levels

been overlooked, thus delaying treatment. The aim of treatment is to re-establish normal metabolism. There are three methods:

1. Diet alone.
2. Diet and an oral hypoglycaemic drug.
3. Diet and insulin.

Diet alone

Dietary control alone is suitable for most mature onset diabetics. Weight reduction is important and a diet ranging from 3400 kJ to 5000 kJ daily is prescribed according to individual needs. The carbohydrate allowance is about 50% of the total with the emphasis on foods with a high fibre content (p. 448). Research shows that small snacks spread over the day are more effective for weight reduction than three large meals, since there is adequate insulin response to smaller meals. Often the patient must learn new eating habits, especially if he has a 'sweet tooth'. With elderly people, changes need to be easy to follow and acceptable. The diet is reviewed regularly.

Oral drugs and diet

Oral hypoglycaemic drugs are prescribed for the few insulin independent diabetics who cannot be controlled by diet alone. Hypoglycaemic attacks are less likely on oral therapy than on insulin therapy, but are still possible. In times of illness, these drugs may be inadequate to control diabetes, insulin being required until diabetes is stabilized. The principal groups of drugs are:

The sulphonylureas (Table 11.4) (sulphonamide derivatives) reduce the release of glucose from the liver: the duration of action varies. Serious side-effects are rare. Chlorpropamide can cause jaundice. All can cause hypoglycaemia and in the case of chlorpropamide the hypoglycaemia, if severe, can be difficult to treat or even fatal.

Table 11.4
The sulphonylureas

Action	Pharmaceutical name	Proprietary name	Daily dose
Short	tolbutamide	Rastinon	0.5–3 g
Intermediate	acetohexamide	Dimelor	500–1500 mg
	glibenclamide	Daonil	5–15 mg
	glymidine	Gondafon	0.5–1 g
	tolazamide	Tolanase	100–500 mg
Long	chlorpropamide	Diabinese	100–500 mg

The biguanides (Table 11.5) lower the blood glucose level possibly by increasing glucose uptake in the tissues. Side-effects are nausea, vomiting and diarrhoea.

Table 11.5
The biguanides

Pharmaceutical name	Proprietary name	Daily dose
metformin	Glucophage	0.5–3 g

If a patient becomes resistant to sulphonylureas alone, a biguanide may be added. Diabetics on sulphonylureas tend to gain weight, although their diabetes is well controlled. Obesity is a health risk. Another danger is that individuals may come to depend on drugs rather than diet to control diabetes.

Insulin and diet

Insulin dependent diabetics require insulin injections and diet prescribed to match their physical activities and to maintain their weight. Blood glucose and urine tests indicate whether a balance between carbohydrate intake and insulin dosage is being achieved. Weight loss, hyperglycaemia and high glycosuria indicate the need for more insulin, while hypoglycaemia demonstrates that too much insulin is being injected for the carbohydrate ingested. (A scale balance is the symbol of the British Diabetic Association; their motto is 'Balance is life'.)

Stabilizing diabetes

Injected insulin cannot eliminate the glycosuria which occurs after meals in severe diabetes. Insulin dosage is adjusted to keep blood glucose levels as near normal as possible.

1. Urine testing for glycosuria in insulin dependent diabetics is performed immediately before meals since glucose levels should be nearly normal if insulin therapy is adequate.

2. In the case of patients on oral therapy or diet, blood glucose is lowest after overnight fasting and rises during the day, peaking after meals. A urine test performed 2 hours after the largest meal reflects the highest blood glucose level of the day. Satisfactory control exists when tests are persistently negative or show only occasional glycosuria. When the patient is receiving low doses of tablets or none at

all, testing urine thrice weekly suffices, provided that the diabetes remains stable.

3. Testing for ketones is important during illnesses and when over 2% glycosuria exists.

Urine testing: the nurse's role

The test specimen must be urine which has been recently formed. The patient should empty his bladder, and half an hour later the test specimen should be obtained. If this is not done test results will relate to urine that has been in the bladder for some time (Table 11.6). Results may be less reliable in elderly people due to poor bladder emptying and a rising renal threshold for glucose.

Blood glucose monitoring

The introduction of this technique for use by nurses and patients can lead to a much better degree of control. However, it is important that instructions are followed precisely and that test strips are stored correctly.

The side of the finger tip is pricked and squeezed to allow a good-sized drop of blood to fall on to the test strip. After a set period of time, the blood is washed or wiped off and after a further set time the colour change is read visually, against a colour code on the test strip bottle, or with the aid of a meter (Fig. 11.9). Some types of strip are easier to read visually than others and meters are expensive to buy so a careful choice of equipment and an accurate technique are essential to produce reliable blood glucose readings. The meter must also be suitable for the test strips being used.

Table 11.6
Urine testing results shown in relation to insulin dosage in a person having Actrapid (short duration) and Monotard (medium-long duration) twice daily.

	Time of urine testing			
	before breakfast	before lunch	before tea	before bedtime snack
Insulin dose effective at this time	evening Monotard from previous day	morning Actrapid	morning Monotard	evening Actrapid

Figure 11.9
Blood glucose meter

Figure 11.10
The need to adjust insulin
dosage

Strenuous exercise | Stress | Infections

Reduce insulin
dose beforehand
as instructed

Increase insulin
dose as instructed

Coping at home

Stabilization of diabetes is best achieved on an out-patient basis; otherwise, when
the patient returns to a more energetic routine than in hospital, increased energy
output will cause insulin requirements to fall. The patient may learn to adjust his
insulin dosage when necessary (Fig. 11.10). Generally, he should reduce his insulin
when hypoglycaemia occurs (p. 451) and increase his insulin when glycosuria occurs
over a similar period, but if in doubt medical advice should be sought.

The daily dose of insulin must **never** be missed even if food intake is reduced.

Types of insulin

Many types of insulin are available (Table 11.7); there are three main differences
between them.

1. Origin. Animal species, beef or pork, and the much newer semi-synthetic
human insulin, are all available. The human insulin is not showing any real advantage so far over highly purified porcine insulin. It appears to be absorbed and used
faster.

Table 11.7
Some examples of U 100 insulin

Soluble insulins (short-acting)		Modified insulins (medium or long-acting)	
Hypurin neutral	(beef)	Hypurin lente	(beef)
Neusulin	(beef)		
Actrapid MC	(pork)	Insulatard	(pork)
Velosulin	(pork)	Semitard MC	(pork)
		Monotard MC	(pork)
Human actrapid	(semi-synthetic)	Human	(semi-synthetic)
		monotard	

Figure 11.11
Injection sites for insulin

Figure 11.12
Automatic injector

2. Level of purity. Older types of insulin contain tiny amounts of other substances which, over a period of time, can lead to antibody formation resulting in a need for larger insulin doses. Highly purified or 'mono-component' (MC) insulins such as Actrapid, Semitard and Monotard should overcome problems of insulin resistance and skin allergies. The patient should in any case know the animal source of his insulin since hypoglycaemia may occur if this is changed.

3. Duration of action. This is described as short, medium and long-acting. These times will vary from one individual to another and to some extent the most suitable dose for any given person can only be found by a combination of experience and 'trial and error'.

Soluble insulin is quick-acting but short-lasting. At least two injections daily are needed when used alone. Soluble insulin alone is often prescribed until acute illness has subsided and diabetes has been stabilized. Some people remain healthier using soluble insulin, particularly if they have suffered any complications of diabetes.

Modified insulins (Table 11.7) are combined with other substances to prolong their action.

Injections

As insulin is a polypeptide hormone, and would be inactivated if taken orally, it must always be given by injection.

The patient learns to inject himself on the outer parts of the thighs, the upper arms and the lower abdomen (Fig. 11.11). Automatic injectors (Fig. 11.12) can be used with one hand, thereby increasing the number of potential injection sites. Repeated use of the same site may lead to fat atrophy and interfere with insulin absorption.

In 1983 insulin became available in U100/ml strength (Table 11.7), that is, 1 ml contains 100 units. The older strengths of 20, 40 and 80 U/ml are being phased out. New syringes are also available in 2 sizes, marked directly in units. The 0.5 ml model has 50 marks measuring 1 unit for each mark while the 1 ml model will measure 100 units with 2 units for each mark (Fig. 11.13). Both glass and metal (reusable) and plastic disposable syringes are available made to BS1619/2. Glass and metal syringes should be stored in industrial methylated spirit. The piston is moved up and down in the barrel several times to remove any trace of spirit before drawing up insulin. Disposable syringes can be safely reused for several days if put back into their original covers and stored in a refrigerator.

Glass syringes, non-disposable needles and urine testing kits are available on prescription. Syringes, preset to inject a certain insulin dose, are available for blind diabetics. The setting should be checked frequently by a sighted person. Equipment, especially syringes and needles, should be kept out of reach of children to avoid accidents. The insulin vial in current use can be stored at room temperature but kept away from very warm areas such as a radiator or heated airing cupboard. Spare vials should be kept in a refrigerator and a new vial taken out a few hours before it is required.

Cleanliness of equipment is essential to avoid infection.

Diets and nutrition

Foods labelled 'diabetic' cannot be taken freely and are not essential. They are also expensive to buy. Their kilojoule value and carbohydrate content must be considered.

Diets should meet bodily needs for energy, repair and growth. A manual worker will require a larger diet and more insulin than a sedentary worker. For all diabetics a high fibre diet is recommended giving about 50% of the kilojoule allowance as carbohydrate. The high fibre content leads to slower absorption of the available carbohydrate and a less pronounced rise in blood glucose level following a meal. Suitable foods include wholemeal bread, pulses, fruit and vegetables. These foods also have the advantage of being more satisfying to eat although anyone just starting on this type of diet may be troubled with flatulence for the first few days.

Refined carbohydrate, such as sweets or Lucozade, should be reserved for use in

Figure 11.13
U 100 syringe, 1 ml size

hypoglycaemia. Dietary fat should be taken in moderation. Protein may be unrestricted but the amount may be specified to ensure that a suitable amount is taken in relation to the person's total energy intake (kilojoules).

A diabetic who is already established on some other form of diet should seek professional advice before changing to a high fibre diet so that control of blood glucose levels is not noticeably upset.

Dietary carbohydrate must be measured accurately to balance the dose of insulin taken.

Nurses, and diabetic patients, should be able to adjust diets to avoid monotony and provide maximum freedom; this adjustment requires a knowledge of carbohydrate exchanges.

Foods with a carbohydrate content which cannot be estimated should be avoided, for instance thickened soups and sauces. Where no choice of menu is likely to be available, say, in a friend's home, prior consultation is advisable.

Other energy sources include:

1. **Alcohol**. Dry wines and spirits have a high kilojoule count because of their alcohol content and are restricted for those on reducing diets.

2. **Sorbitol**. This is commercially prepared from glucose. It is absorbed very slowly in the body and does not seem to raise the blood glucose level in diabetes mellitus. However, intake of sorbitol must be limited as it has a kilojoule content similar to that of sucrose and it also causes diarrhoea when taken in large amounts due to its slow rate of absorption and the effects of osmosis.

Diabetes and pregnancy

There is no reason why a diabetic should avoid pregnancy if she receives adequate medical care. Genetic counselling is advisable. Pregnancy carries certain risks — in particular there is a greater risk of stillbirth or neonatal death. Induction of labour or caesarian section is usually necessary. The chances that a diabetic mother will have a diabetic child are increased.

Elective surgery

The patient is admitted about 3 days preoperatively to assess his diabetes. Intravenous glucose may be given if fasting blood glucose levels indicate it is needed. Postoperatively, insulin is given according to the degree of glycosuria and blood glucose concentration. Insulin independent diabetics may need to be given insulin temporarily.

Diabetic ketoacidosis

Other terms used include diabetic coma and severe hyperglycaemia.

When there is insufficient insulin for glucose metabolism, the sequence of events shown in Table 11.8 occurs.

The severity of the crisis is proportional to the acidosis, not to the blood glucose level.

Possible causes

1. Neglect of treatment through ignorance or carelessness.
2. Illness or stress which increases insulin requirements.

Table 11.8
Ketoacidosis

Biochemical changes	Symptoms and signs
1. Glucose accumulates in the blood in large quantities (hyperglycaemia)	Thirst
2. Hyperglycaemia causes osmotic diuresis with excess loss of water and electrolytes in urine	Polyuria Low BP Raised pulse Dehydration Dry tongue Inelastic skin
3. Body cells use fat as an alternative fuel. Fat is incompletely metabolized and ketones appear in blood and urine (ketosis). Ketones affect the brain — causing drowsiness and eventual coma — and the respiratory centre — stimulating rapid, deep breathing	Anorexia Vomiting Drowsiness Loss of consciousness Deep respirations Acetone smell on breath

Treatment

Analysis of blood samples enables blood glucose, electrolytes and carbon dioxide combining power (an indication of the degree of metabolic acidosis) to be measured.

1. Precipitating causes are treated when known (for example antibiotics are given for infections).

2. Dehydration is corrected by intravenous infusion (for example, normal saline followed by 5% dextrose to prevent further breakdown of fat and protein).

3. Carbohydrate metabolism is re-established by giving soluble insulin intravenously or intramuscularly. The subcutaneous route is ineffective due to circulatory collapse. Insulin doses are calculated 3 to 4 hourly according to blood glucose level. Insulin can also be given by continuous intravenous infusion when much smaller doses are required, for example, six units per hour.

4. Intravenous sodium bicarbonate or lactate is occasionally given to correct acidosis.

5. After insulin therapy and correction of acidosis, potassium begins to enter the cells, depleting blood potassium levels. This may cause cardiac arrhythmias, therefore potassium is given intravenously.

Nursing care involves all the techniques employed in care of the unconscious patient (Ch. 3). A nasogastric tube may be inserted to minimize risk of inhaling vomitus. When conscious, the patient is allowed oral fluids containing carbohydrate. Later, he progresses to a solid diet. These patients are particularly liable to develop pressure sores so preventive measures must be started early.

Aids to nursing observations

1. An oscilloscope to detect cardiac arrhythmias.
2. A self-retaining catheter to facilitate urinalysis for the unconscious patient.

Records

It is an important nursing responsibility to maintain accurate records. Special charts (Fig. 11.14) on which all information is correlated should be provided; entries should always be made promptly and clearly.

Figure 11.14
Diabetic ketosis chart

Hypoglycaemia

A diabetic learns to recognize symptoms of hypoglycaemia. Onset is rapid when the blood glucose level falls below about 2.7 mmol/l.

Possible causes include:

1. Meal missed or delayed.
2. Full amount of carbohydrate not taken.
3. Unexpected exercise.
4. Incorrect insulin dose.

Clinical features

Clinical features result from abnormal brain function due to shortage of its vital 'fuel' — glucose. Unlike other body tissues, the brain can use only glucose as its energy source. Symptoms vary and include rapid heart rate, sweating, hunger, unsteadiness of gait, truculent behaviour and alterations in consciousness. During sleep signs may include nightmares, sleepwalking or damp bedclothes. If hypoglycaemia develops more slowly there is usually lethargy, reduction of spontaneous activity, conversation and movement, and behaviour similar to that produced by alcohol intoxication. This type of hypoglycaemia occurs more commonly in patients treated with 'long-acting' insulins or oral hypoglycaemic agents.

Treatment

Treatment must be prompt. Blood glucose levels fall below those necessary to maintain metabolism of brain cells and prolonged attacks may produce irreversible cerebral changes. The underlying cause of hypoglycaemia can be determined later. The hypoglycaemic diabetic should have carbohydrate, such as glucose sweets or a glass of milk and a biscuit. The patient may need to be fed if he refuses to take the food and should not be left alone until he returns to normal. If he loses consciousness, intravenous glucose or intramuscular glucagon is injected. (Glucagon raises the blood glucose level by increasing glucose release from the liver. By giving a child glucagon, parents are often able to restore consciousness sufficiently to give glucose orally.)

The diabetic should always carry a card (Fig. 11.15) or other form of identification indicating his condition and insulin regime to anyone who may find him in a distressed condition. An unconscious diabetic should be treated as if he were hypoglycaemic unless proved otherwise. Incorrect treatment of hypoglycaemia with insulin can be fatal, whereas permanent damage is unlikely to result from giving glucose to a patient in a hyperglycaemic coma. When a diabetic is about to undertake unusually strenuous exercise, he should reduce his insulin dose beforehand or take extra carbohydrate to prevent hypoglycaemia.

I am a diabetic

If I am found ill or fainting please
read the instructions overleaf . . . .

I am a diabetic

If I am found ill or fainting please give me two tablespoonfuls of sugar in water. If this does not revive me please call a doctor or an ambulance immediately.

Name

Address

Telephone No.

Name of Doctor or Hospital

Address

Telephone No.

My usual dose of insulin is   units of
                                                    (type of insulin)
brand

given at
          (time(s) of day)

Figure 11.15
Diabetic card

Continuing care

Diabetes mellitus may be controlled, but not cured. People living with this disorder may be confronted with difficulties and complications.

Emotional problems

It is difficult to accept cheerfully the need for daily insulin injection and to struggle with a rigid diet. Knowledge will help the diabetic achieve greater flexibility and confidence in his diet and other features of his life-style, hence the importance of education about all aspects of his condition. This means team work, involving doctors, nurses, dietitians, the patient and his family. The British Diabetic Association (BDA) provides information on self-help and includes advice about diets, the life of a diabetic, holidays and car insurance. The organization finances research into diabetes and helps to dispel prejudice against diabetics, for instance among employers.

Most occupations are open to diabetics. Those where there may be injury to themselves or others if hypoglycaemia occurs, such as driving public vehicles or working on scaffolding, are unsuitable.

Adolescents may resent the 'discipline' of diabetes and fluctuating control may result. The adolescent may not always be at fault since nervousness, fear and infection can cause hyperglycaemia.

A child's emotions and activities fluctuate more than an adult's. This may cause instability. Children should not constantly be made to feel different from their peers. Provided they are taught the necessity of dietary control, they should be allowed to choose from the full range of foods for which a reliable carbohydrate value is available.

Control problems

These need to be investigated as they arise but some likely causes include:

1. Faulty injection technique.
2. Using a different make of syringe from normal. The dead space in the syringe will be different and this alters the amount of insulin given although the correct number of units of insulin have been drawn up in to the syringe.
3. Use of an unsuitable site, for example where tissue has become thickened. This inhibits absorption of the insulin.
4. Out of date insulin.
5. Poor dietary compliance.
6. Lack of understanding.

Early complications

Blurred vision may result from instability of blood glucose levels. This condition is transient but may take several weeks to clear after treatment is begun.

Infections may occur since hyperglycaemia and glycosuria provide an ideal growth medium for bacteria. Common infections are vulvovaginitis, urinary infections, pyelonephritis, infections in skin creases of the obese person and conjunctivitis.

Long-term complications

These occur more often but not exclusively in poorly controlled diabetics and the incidence of complications is directly related to the degree of control.

Visual defects

Three visual defects resulting from diabetes are cataract, retinal disease and vitreous haemorrhage (Ch. 12). Regular eye checks will help in the early detection of retinal disease so that treatment can be carried out before permanent damage and possibly blindness develop.

Neuropathy

1. Autonomic neuropathy (p. 84) can affect any system of the body and produce wide ranging problems such as postural hypotension, impotence, diarrhoea and loss of awareness of hypoglycaemia.

2. Peripheral neuropathy mainly affects the lower limbs and leads to gradual loss of both ankle and knee reflexes and of sensation. Involvement of motor fibres may lead to muscle wasting and difficulty in walking. Lack of sensation makes the limbs very vulnerable to injury resulting in trophic ulcers.

Atherosclerosis

The risk of coronary artery, cerebral vascular and peripheral vascular disease is increased in diabetics.

A combination of peripheral vascular disease and neuropathy, especially in older people, means that injury or infection to devitalised limbs can quickly lead to gangrene. Diabetics should take special care of their feet which need to be washed, dried and inspected daily, including the soles, for any sign of damage. Toe nails should be cut straight across and level with the end of the toe for protection. When poor circulation, difficult toe nails, corns or similar foot problems are present, the person should attend a qualified chiropodist.

Shoes and stockings should allow for easy toe movement. New shoes need to be broken in gradually. The diabetic person should feel inside shoes for any rough areas before putting them on. Where peripheral neuropathy is present, the person's hands will still be able to feel rough areas. The diabetic should be discouraged from walking barefoot, especially on wooden floors or other potentially rough surfaces. Bed socks should be worn instead of using a hot water bottle.

Renal changes

Nephropathy may occur in diabetics of long standing and can result in death from chronic renal failure (p. 337).

THE ADRENAL GLANDS

These two glands are located on top of the kidneys.

STRUCTURE AND FUNCTION

Each consists of two separate functional parts, the cortex and the medulla (Fig. 11.16).

The adrenal cortex. Three groups of hormones are secreted:

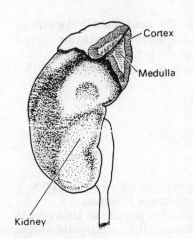

Figure 11.16
Section of adrenal gland

1. *Glucocorticoids*. Of these, the most important is cortisol (hydro-cortisone). This is secreted in response to the adrenocorticotrophic hormone (ACTH) from the anterior pituitary. In turn, ACTH secretion is brought about by a releasing factor secreted by the hypothalamus and controlled by a feed-back mechanism based on blood levels of cortisol. Cortisol stimulates gluconeogenesis (the formation of glucose) from protein. It antagonizes the action of insulin. It is important for the excretion of water by the kidneys, for the manufacture of red blood cells, to help maintain blood pressure and for the body's ability to respond to stress. Excess cortisol inhibits the inflammatory reaction, interferes with protein synthesis causing muscle and bone weakness and leads to hyperglycaemia.

2. *Mineralocorticoids*. Aldosterone, the most important of these, is concerned with maintaining normal levels of sodium in the body. A fall in body sodium leads to increased secretion of aldosterone. The effect of this is to increase the kidney's reabsorption of sodium from the urine, thus conserving it.

3. *Androgens*. These are sex hormones produced in both sexes which are concerned with muscular development and the growth of pubic and axillary hair.

The adrenal medulla. Functionally separate from the cortex, medullary activity has much in common with sympathetic nervous activity. The hormones secreted are noradrenaline and adrenaline which have the effect of preparing the body for physical exertion. Thus, when the need arises, heart rate increases, blood pressure rises, blood is diverted to essential organs (heart and muscle), energy is made available by converting liver and muscle glycogen to glucose, the bronchial smooth muscle is relaxed to allow greater air entry and the metabolic rate is increased.

DISORDERS OF THE ADRENAL GLANDS

These may result from abnormalities of either the cortex or the medulla.

Underactivity of the adrenal cortex

Addison's disease is a chronic condition of underactivity. It may be the result of tuberculous destruction of the gland or of atrophy.

Clinical features

These derive from the failure to secrete the necessary hormones. Serious loss of sodium occurs in the urine. Low blood pressure is characteristic, and patients may faint on standing up. There is also a tendency to develop hypoglycaemia and a raised blood urea. Skin pigmentation will develop. Tiredness, anorexia and nausea are common. Weight loss and menstrual disturbances may occur. Response to stress is impaired and patients may succumb to infections, injury or exposure to cold.

Treatment and nursing care

Management of Addison's disease is mainly the replacement of the missing hormone. Initially cortisol 20 mg is given twice daily. It may also be necessary to give fludrocortisone to maintain fluid and electrolyte balance. Monthly follow-up sessions are necessary to monitor and adjust the dosage if necessary. Patients must be instructed on what to do if a minor illness occurs, for example a heavy cold or influenza. In such circumstances, the daily dose of cortisol should be doubled by the patient. Each patient should have a supply of intramuscular hydrocortisone to be given by his doctor in an emergency. A card should be carried at all times, indicating that the bearer is taking corticosteroid therapy.

Acute adrenal failure

This crisis calls for urgent and intensive treatment. A severe degree of shock develops with a dramatic fall in blood pressure. Oliguria or anuria may result. Vomiting may occur with weakness, apathy and confusion. Unless treated quickly and adequately, coma and death will follow. Measures to combat the fall in blood pressure should be taken. The patient is nursed flat, with the foot of the bed elevated. Intravenous fluids are given to maintain water and sodium balance; up to a litre of normal saline may be given quickly. It may also be necessary to give intravenous glucose. Cortisol is administered intravenously for up to 48 hours. In most cases remarkable improvement will occur within 24 hours, and once the patient's progress is certain and gastrointestinal disturbance has settled, cortisol may be given orally.

During the initial period the patient remains very ill and much depends on the accurate observation and recording of vital signs. Particularly important are blood pressure readings, observations of level of consciousness and measurement of fluid intake, urinary output and amount of vomitus. There is an increased risk of infection for these patients and precautions should be observed which will protect them. In addition, the patient's comfort depends on thoughtful nursing care. Such episodes are very frightening for patients, so a quiet, reassuring and confident approach by the nurse is essential. Nursing should be carried out in a quiet atmosphere with the minimum of stimulation. Patients will benefit from the reduction of emotional and physical disturbance. Once the crisis is over, management continues as described for Addison's disease.

Overactivity of the adrenal cortex

A variety of syndromes may result from overproduction of the various hormones of the cortex. Among these is Cushing's syndrome, the result of excess quantities of circulating cortisol.

Cushing's syndrome

This complex disorder is usually the result of bilateral adrenal hyperplasia, which may be caused by a tumour of the adrenals or by a tumour of the pituitary secreting excess ACTH (p. 430). The syndrome is uncommon but merits some discussion because its symptoms may easily be produced by the therapeutic use of corticosteroids, a not uncommon means of treating a variety of disorders.

Figure 11.17
Cushing's syndrome

Clinical features

Clinical features of Cushing's syndrome include muscle wasting and symptoms of diabetes mellitus (glycosuria, polyuria and thirst). Obesity of the trunk is marked, the contrast with the thin legs and arms giving a characteristic appearance (Fig. 11.17). Obesity is contributed to by sodium and water retention, which also leads to hypertension. Patients develop a moon-shaped face, women grow facial hair and may cease menstruating. In men, impotence may develop. The skin bruises easily and shows striae (purple markings). Osteoporosis leads to fractures and the collapse of vertebrae.

Investigations

Investigations, including plasma cortisol and ACTH levels are normally carried out to confirm the diagnosis. A skull X-ray may show abnormality of the pituitary fossa in the event of the cause being of pituitary origin. Further investigations include blood glucose levels and urinary steroid measurement, the latter requiring 24-hour urine collections. The dexamethasone suppression test involves giving in the evening an oral dose of dexamethasone, equivalent to a normal day's cortisol production. This in normal patients suppresses ACTH and therefore cortisol secretion. If the level of cortisol in blood taken the next day has not fallen below a specific point, Cushing's syndrome is indicated.

Methods of treatment

The approach clearly depends on the cause. If the syndrome was induced by corticosteroid therapy, the dosage is adjusted. Pituitary tumours may be removed or irradiated (p. 431). Adrenal hyperplasia may be treated by unilateral or bilateral adrenalectomy (the latter rendering life-long replacement therapy a necessity). Total adrenalectomy can be a serious operation, since it removes the patient's ability to respond to stress. This effect is minimized by administering cortisol intramuscularly for a day or two before operation, and continuing for a period after surgery.

Preparation for surgery

Correction of hyperglycaemia by diet and insulin therapy may be necessary. Surgery can be made safer by preoperative administration of metyrapone, a drug which blocks the synthesis of cortisol. Replacement therapy with dexamethasone is required. Preparation in this way may take some weeks before the patient is ready for surgery. When one adrenal gland is diseased, the high levels of cortisol it produces will suppress ACTH production. Thus the normal gland is without stimulation to produce cortisol. When unilateral adrenalectomy is carried out, replacement therapy, intravenously during surgery, and orally afterwards is therefore essential. This is continued until the remaining gland recovers its function.

Postoperative therapy

Following operation, an intravenous infusion is necessary to prevent electrolyte imbalance. Sodium and potassium levels in the plasma will be monitored in order to decide on the appropriate intravenous regime. Once the condition has stabilized, cortisol may be administered orally, together with fludrocortisone to regulate sodium and water balance.

Postoperative nursing care

The patient is nursed lying flat for a period to prevent hypotension and circulatory failure. Blood pressure recordings are necessary at least every 15 minutes, until it is certain that his condition is stable. Observation of other vital signs, skin colour and urinary output are essential, as well as of the wound and any drainage. Coughing and deep breathing are painful because of the wound, so a great deal of encouragement, together with chest physiotherapy, is necessary. Note should be taken of any chest pain or dyspnoea. When the patient is ready for mobilization, a frequent check of his blood pressure must be made once he gets up. If hypotension occurs he should be returned to bed and the doctor notified. The nurse must also note any signs of hypoglycaemia (p. 451), which may necessitate intravenous glucose. **Adrenal crisis**, the most serious complication of this form of surgery, is most likely to occur between 9 and 12 hours after operation. Symptoms of this complication are nausea, weakness, abdominal pains and signs of shock. The administration of a vasoconstrictor drug such as metaraminol will be necessary, and patients should be managed as described for acute adrenal failure (p. 455).

Overactivity of the adrenal medulla

This is usually caused by the presence of phaeochromocytoma, a rare tumour of the medulla which secretes large quantities of the medullary hormones.

Clinical features

Effects are hypertension, which may be sustained or intermittent, features of increased metabolism or hyperglycaemia and glycosuria. Serious consequences such as heart failure and cerebrovascular accident may result from the hypertension.

Treatment

As most tumours are benign, removal usually results in cure. Surgery carries with it a serious risk of severe hypotension once the tumour has been removed.

Surgical management

Before surgery, drugs which counteract the effect of adrenaline are given. Included in these is propranolol which blocks the effect of adrenaline on the heart. During surgery, bouts of hypertension are controlled by intravenous phentolamine, while after removal of the tumour, hypotension is controlled by metaraminol. This is continued into the postoperative period. Careful observation of blood pressure is crucial after surgery.

SUMMARY AND IMPORTANT NURSING CONSIDERATIONS IN ENDOCRINOLOGY

Treatment of any endocrine disorder consists of the following:

1. Decreasing hormonal ouput of hyperactive glands by, for example, surgery or radiotherapy. If the pituitary is stimulating the secretion of an overactive gland it may be destroyed surgically or by other means.

2. Supplementing hormones of underactive glands or stimulating the gland to produce the hormone by, for example, giving pituitary trophic hormones.

If any endocrine glands are completely removed or destroyed, essential hormones must be supplied for life.

It must be remembered that all patients are different, and contributing to these differences are the endocrine glands. Malfunction of these glands produces changes in behaviour or appearance, the basis of which the nurse should understand. Features of the disease are often very obvious and may be a source of embarrassment to the individual, one example being exophthalmos in thyrotoxicosis. Endocrine disorders can profoundly affect a person's life and the lives of those around him, as in the early senescence induced by hypopituitarism.

Education of the patient and of others involved is a vital part of treatment of endocrine disorders. The greater the understanding of the situation by all concerned, the more assured the patient will be of his ability to cope with his disorder and the more flexible can be his way of life. The patient must know that his treatment does not usually provide for excessive hormonal demands resulting from physical and emotional stress. He should try to avoid such situations and should know how to cope if they arise inadvertently.

Probably the most significant part of the nurse's role is her observation of the patient for complications resulting from his disease, his surgery or hormone replacement therapy. Of special importance are appearance, sweating, pulse rate, blood pressure, respirations, urinary output and symptoms such as headache, vomiting and pain. Prompt recognition of any abnormality can be life-saving. It should be remembered that not only are individual readings of pulse rate and blood pressure important, but also the upward or downward trend observed over a period.

The continuing scientific advances in endocrinology and the plethora of tests and equipment that results should never be allowed to lessen the nurse's sensitivity to her patient. Through all the drama of caring for such seriously ill patients, it must never be forgotten that the patient's basic needs must be attended to — his skin, diet and comfort. He needs reassurance and information about his condition, as do his relatives.

SUGGESTED ASSIGNMENTS

1. Patients having long-term hormonal replacement therapy may, from time to time, experience problems. Explain how in the case of (a) thyroid hormone replacement and (b) cortisone replacement these problems can be detected early.

How should patients be helped to recognize the early symptoms?

2. A diabetic must be knowledgeable about his condition if he is to lead a normal and active life. Investigate the education of diabetics in your hospital, in particular:
   a. Which personnel are involved?
   b. What is taught to diabetics?
   c. How are allowances made for patients of differing abilities to understand what is being taught?

3. What associations for diabetics are there in your locality? As an exercise, find out how such an organization endeavours to meet the special needs of diabetics.

4. Explain how thyrotoxicosis might come to be confused with a particular psychiatric illness.

When a patient is being treated for thyrotoxicosis in a medical ward, some of the clinical features of the illness are liable to affect fellow patients and staff. What do you think the effects might be, and how as a nurse can you seek to minimize them?

FURTHER READING

Barnes S 1983 Primary hypothyroidism. Nursing Mirror (May 4th): 46–48

Bloom A 1983 The diagnosis and management of late-onset diabetes. Geriatric Medicine (March): 187–194

British Diabetic Association 1972 The diabetics handbook. British Diabetic Association, London

Farquhar J W 1982 Diabetes in your teens. Churchill Livingstone, Edinburgh

Gotch P M 1981 Teaching patients about adrenal corticosteroids. American Journal of Nursing (January): 78–81

Lewis J G 1983 The endocrine system, 2nd edn. Penguin Library of Nursing Series. Churchill Livingstone, Edinburgh

Mann J, Oxford Dietetic Group 1982 The diabetics' diet book. Martin Dunitz, London

Nursing 2nd series The add-on journal of clinical nursing 1983 Hormones part 1. (May)

Toft A D, Campbell I W, Seth J 1981 Diagnosis and management of endocrine diseases. Blackwell Scientific, Oxford

Watkins P J 1983 ABC of diabetes. British Medical Journal

Marris, P. (1974) Loss and Change. London: Routledge & Kegan Paul.
Maslow, A.H. (1954) The Farther Reaches of Human Nature. Geriatric Medicine
  March, 457-459.
British Diabetic Association, 1978 The diabetes handbook. British Diabetic Association, London
Parsons, T.K. (1987) Diabetic care. Nursing Times Occasional Paper. Edinburgh
Weller, B.F. (1981) Tackling nurse education. Nursing Mirror, Midwifery Supplement
  January, 22-23.
Wilson-Barnett, J. & Kalideen. (1981) The new factor book and Rogers Nursing, Singapore Churchill
  Livingstone, Edinburgh.
Mead, J., Diford, J. Smith Group. 1981 The essentials handbook. Macmillan Education. London
Patients and relatives The education of a handicapped family. 1981 Home nurse part 1. Army
Tait, A. Campbell, G. & Soe, 1981 Diagnosis and management of palliative disease. Blackwell
  Scientific, Oxford.
Wright, S.W.J. 1985 ABC of diabetes. British Medical Journal

Chapter Twelve
The eye

The study of the eye and its disorders is called ophthalmology, a fascinating and intricate specialty. This chapter is not, however, written for those intending to specialize in ophthalmic nursing but for students who, as part of their basic training, may spend a month or two working in an eye hospital or ophthalmic clinic of an out-patient department. It may help the student with a patient admitted to general or mental hospital who, by chance, happens also to have an eye condition.

The aim is, therefore, to provide an introduction to some common eye disorders and to the principles which underlie their treatment and nursing care.

ANATOMY AND PHYSIOLOGY

Figures 12.1 to 12.3 show the structure of the eyeball and the associated parts of the eye.

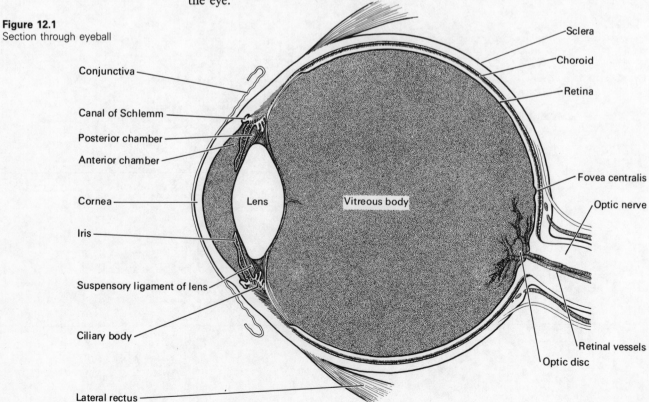

Figure 12.1
Section through eyeball

Conjunctiva

Canal of Schlemm

Posterior chamber

Anterior chamber

Cornea

Iris

Suspensory ligament of lens

Ciliary body

Lateral rectus

Lens

Vitreous body

Sclera

Choroid

Retina

Fovea centralis

Optic nerve

Retinal vessels

Optic disc

Figure 12.2
Eyelids and conjunctiva

Figure 12.3
Lacrimal apparatus

The eyeball

The eyeball is an almost spherical structure which has three layers:

1. The outermost coat consisting of the transparent **cornea** and the tough, strong, opaque **sclera**. It protects the delicate structures within the eye.

2. The middle layer consisting of the vascular, pigmented **choroid** which is continued forwards as the **ciliary body** and the **iris**. Together these structures form the uveal tract.

3. The innermost, nervous layer, the **retina**, containing the light-sensitive cells, the rods and cones. In the centre of the retina is the **macula lutea** (yellow spot), within which lies the **fovea centralis**, an area of acute vision where cones are very numerous.

The entry point of the optic nerve and retinal vessels, the **optic disc** (Fig. 12.4), lies to the side of the macula lutea. The retina is the only place in the body where blood vessels can readily be seen. It can display abnormal changes in generalized diseases such as hypertension, some disorders of the nervous system and, of course, in diseases of the eye itself. In each **optic nerve** two sets of fibres supply the visual fields on opposite sides of the body; for example, the left temporal and right nasal fibres combine to form the right half of the right visual field (Fig. 12.5). The diagram also shows how pressure on the **chiasma**, for example from a tumour of the pituitary gland, can cause loss of half the field of vision from each eye (bitemporal hemianopia).

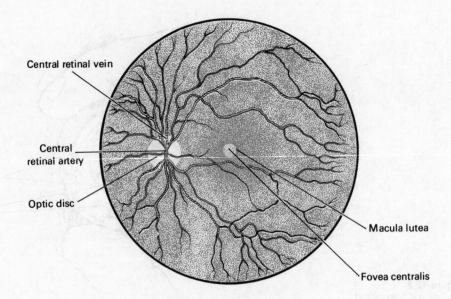

Figure 12.4
Ophthalmoscope view of optic disc, macula and retinal vessels (fundus)

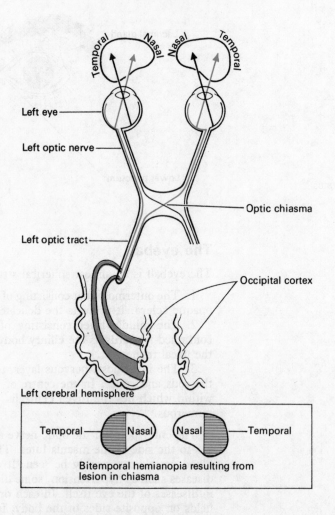

Figure 12.5
Visual pathways and visual fields

Within the eyeball the lens divides the **anterior chamber** containing aqueous fluid from the **vitreous body** which lies behind.

Aqueous humour is secreted by the ciliary body; it circulates around the anterior chamber and is drained away via the **Canal of Schlemm**.

Associated structures

The accessory parts of the eye are the **eyelids, lacrimal apparatus** for production and drainage of tears and the **conjunctiva**, a fine mucous membrane which lines the lids and continues over the eye as the corneal epithelium. All of these structures function to protect the eye and to facilitate vision.

Each eye is rotated within the orbit by means of the six extrinsic muscles which are inserted into the sclera.

Normal vision

The design of the eyeball allows light reflected from objects within the range of vision to fall on to the retina. Light travels in straight lines so that, in order to fall exactly on to the retina, these rays of light must be refracted (bent). Refraction occurs as light rays pass from one medium to another, for example from air to water or vice versa. Light entering the eye is refracted in the same way, starting with the anterior surface of the cornea.

The parts of the eye through which light must pass before reaching the retina are called the **refractive media**. They are: the cornea, the aqueous, the lens and the vitreous body.

The cornea plays the greatest part in refraction; the lens, however, has an important role because by accommodation, that is, alteration in its shape, the degree of the refraction can be varied.

Figure 12.6
(A) Normal eye focusing a distant object (over 20 feet away)
(B) Normal eye focusing a near object (note alteration in shape of lens)

In a normal eye both near and distant objects can be focused (Fig. 12.6A and B). This normal refractive power is termed **emmetropia**. To be able to see detail of an object clearly, an inverted image must be brought into exact focus on to the macula lutea. The cones in and around this area are sensitive to daylight and enable us to see colour and detail of objects (central vision). The rods situated nearer the periphery of the retina enable us to be aware of our surroundings (peripheral vision) in the daytime and to permit some night time vision.

The formation of a nerve impulse for transmission to the brain is the result of a biochemical process in the retina. Once formed the impulse is conveyed via the optic pathways (Fig. 12.5) to the visual area of the occipital cortex for interpretation as sight.

Vision with errors of refraction

Myopia (short sight)

The length of the eyeball is greater than normal, therefore light rays are brought to a focus at a point which falls short of the retina. The person can see by holding objects close to the eyes, but objects at a distance appear blurred. Correction is achieved with a concave lens which focuses the image on to the retina (Fig. 12.7).

Figure 12.7
Myopia

Figure 12.8
Hypermetropia

Hypermetropia (long sight)

The length of the eyeball is shorter than normal, therefore light rays are brought to a focus at a point behind the retina. Objects are seen clearly at a distance but appear blurred close to the eye. Correction is by a convex lens which brings the image forward on to the retina (Fig. 12.8).

Astigmatism

In this condition the eye is optically oval, so that horizontal and vertical planes of light are brought to a focus at different points. Correction is with a cylindrical lens.

Presbyopia (old sight)

This occurs in normal aging and should not be confused with failing vision. From approximately 45 years of age onwards the lens gradually loses its elasticity so that its ability to alter its shape to accommodate for near and distant objects gradually diminishes. The person sees more clearly at a distance where only passive accommodation is required; so objects are held further away from the eye in order to see detail. A common example is an older person who needs to have a newspaper at arm's length in order to be able to read the small print (Fig. 12.9). Correction is achieved by means of a convex lens.

Figure 12.9
Presbyopia

Drugs used on the eye

There are a number of drugs which, apart from their general effects, also cause changes in the eye, notably those which stimulate the parasympathetic nervous system. Patients heavily sedated with opiates have constricted pupils; conversely, persons intoxicated with alcohol will have pupils which are widely dilated. Some antidepressants and powerful analgesics such as pethidine produce unwanted side-effects on the eye which can be a nuisance to the patient.

There are two very important groups of drugs used in the treatment of eye conditions:

Mydriatics

These drugs dilate the pupil (Fig. 12.10A). They work by paralysing the muscle which constricts the pupil thus leaving the dilator muscle unopposed. Some mydriatics also paralyse the ciliary muscle which controls the shape of the lens so that the individual cannot focus for near vision.

Examples of mydriatics are:

1. **Atropine sulphate** ½–2%. It takes about 30 minutes to dilate the pupil fully and its effects, which cannot be counteracted, last for 10 days. It is used to limit the formation of adhesions between the iris and the structures which lie behind in, for example, inflammatory conditions involving the iris or following intraocular operations such as cataract extraction. Occasionally people are hypersensitive to atropine. The eye becomes red and irritable and an allergic-type rash develops on the lids and conjunctiva.

2. **Mydrilate** (cyclopentolate hydrochloride) 1% is a recent preparation and is used in many departments for examination purposes. This drug has maximum effect in 30–60 minutes, and recovery occurs in 24 hours.

3. **Phenylephrine hydrochloride** 10%. This drug takes about 20 minutes to dilate the pupil and lasts for several hours. Mydrilate and Phenylephrine may be used in combination to dilate the pupils for examination purposes. Their action can be counteracted by Pilocarpine 1 or 2%.

Miotics

These constrict the pupil. They have a stimulating effect on the constrictor and ciliary muscles so that in addition to constriction of the pupil the lens accommodates for near vision (Fig. 12.10B). Miotics increase the drainage of aqueous humour by

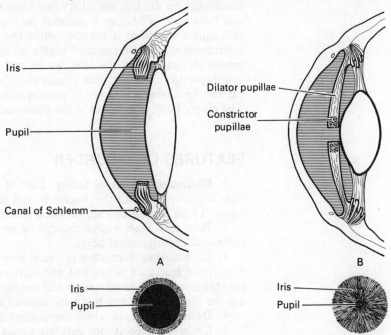

Figure 12.10
(A) Effect of mydriatics
(B) Effect of miotics

some unknown mechanism and because of this they are of particular use in the treatment of glaucoma (p. 472). An example of a miotic drug is pilocarpine 1–4%.

Other drugs used may be specially prepared for local (topical) application or they may be given systemically. These include:

Antibiotics

Topical preparations of many antibiotics are available but the most commonly used are chloramphenicol 0.5% and Framycetin (soframycin) 0.5%.

Carboanhydrase inhibitors

Acetozolamide (Diamox) given systemically to inhibit the production of aqueous is the most widely used drug in this group.

Beta blockers

These well known drugs are used in the treatment of hypertension. As topical preparations such as Timolol 0.25% or 0.5% they are useful in reducing intraocular pressure. It should be remembered that the patient can exhibit the same side-effects, for example, bradycardia and hypotension as if he was taking the drugs systemically.

Steroids

Eye drops containing a steroid are often prescribed to lessen inflammatory reactions following intraocular operations. They may also be ordered in the treatment of some non-infected inflammatory conditions such as iritis. Betamethazone (Betnesol) 1% is an example.

AETIOLOGY OF DISORDER

As most of the tissues within the orbit are similar to those found elsewhere in the body — skin, hair, vessels, nerves, muscles and mucous membrane — it follows that the eye and its associated structures can be affected by many of the same disorders that affect other organs.

The highly specialized tissues of the eye, the cornea, the lens and the complex that makes up the iris, the ciliary body and the choroid are unique in their structure and behaviour. The cornea contains no blood vessels and is dependent upon tears and aqueous to keep it healthy, while the lens depends solely on aqueous for its nourishment. The presence of toxins in aqueous can give rise to haziness of the cornea or opacities in the lens, which will in turn affect vision. Trauma will also cause opacities. The iris, ciliary body and choroid are contiguous vascular structures, the former having no power of regeneration if partially removed, as in iridectomy. The ciliary body is involved in the phenomenon of *sympathetic ophthalmitis* (p. 471).

FEATURES OF DISORDER

1. **Diminution of visual acuity**. Loss of sight can be so gradual that the patient does not notice it until the disease is well advanced; this is typical of chronic glaucoma. There can, of course, be sudden and complete loss of vision.

2. **Pain** may arise within the eye or be associated with pain of the face as in disease of the trigeminal nerve.

3. **Lacrimation** (formation of tears) may be excessive and cause watering of the eye. If the tear duct is blocked and lacrimal secretion is unable to pass down and into the nose in the usual way, it will overflow down the cheek. Alternatively if there are too few tears the eye becomes dry and the cornea is endangered.

4. **Double vision**, in which the patient does literally see 'two of everything'.

5. **Cosmetic defects**, for example ptosis (drooping) of the lid.

EXAMINATION AND INVESTIGATIONS

Enquiry is made into the patient's general health and detailed examination of other parts of the body is carried out as required. The ophthalmologist will make a systematic examination of the eye from the eyelashes to the optic disc. Investigations may include the following:

Tests of visual acuity

The ability of the eye to perceive the shape of objects is assessed for both near and distance vision.

Near vision

Ordinary printer's types are used in testing near vision.

Distance vision

Special test-types are used, with the patient placed at a standard distance for testing distance vision. A nurse may be asked to carry out this test.

In the Snellen test-type letters are arranged in rows of diminishing size (Fig. 12.11A). The normal eye would see the top letter at 60 metres and subsequent lines at decreasing distances. For convenience the patient stands 6 metres away from the vision board and he is asked to read down the chart until he can go no further. His visual acuity is measured according to the number of lines of letters he can read accurately. This is then expressed as a fraction, the upper 6 being the test distance in metres. Thus $\frac{6}{6}$ is normal vision, but if it is $\frac{6}{36}$ then he can only see at 6 metres what he should be able to see at 36 metres. Ability to see to top letters only is $\frac{6}{60}$. If the patient is unable to see the top letters even when moved closer to the board, his ability to count the examiner's fingers or see hand movements is tested and, failing this, his perception of light. The person is regarded as totally blind if he is unable to perceive light.

Figure 12.11
(A) Test type — Snellen (B) Test type — 'E' test (C) Test type — recognition of objects

The vision of each eye is tested separately with and without glasses, if worn. The eye which is not being tested is occluded.

For children or non-English speaking adults the 'E' Test (Fig. 12.11B) can be used. The person is given a wooden E which he moves to correspond with the position of the E on the test-type. For the very young child a test involving recognition of simple objects on the test-type (Fig. 12.11C) is more suitable.

Ophthalmoscopy

An ophthalmoscope (Fig. 12.12) is an instrument which permits a view of the interior of the eye. This view is referred to as the fundus. The examination can be carried out on any patient without prior preparation, but it is preferable for the pupils to be dilated and a darkened room is ideal. The nurse should always screen the patient from direct sunlight which makes examination impossible.

The very specialized technique of indirect ophthalmoscopy is particularly useful in retinal detachment surgery.

Slit lamp examination

The aim is to allow examination of the structure of the eye magnified by means of a narrow beam of light. The patient is seated with the head fixed in a suitable rest with a forehead bar and adjustable chin rest (Fig. 12.13). The examiner is seated opposite the patient, looking through a binocular microscope. Light from the slit lamp is condensed into a narrow sharp band which will show up the parts of the eye to be examined, for example the cornea, anterior chamber, lens, iris detail and anterior vitreous.

Measurement of intraocular pressure

In health the pressure within the eye is maintained by the flow of aqueous into and out of the anterior chamber at approximately 15 to 20 millimetres of mercury. A rough estimation can be made by palpation. Accurate measurement is achieved by a tonometer attached to the slit lamp and is important in the diagnosis of glaucoma.

Figure 12.12
A direct ophthalmoscope
(A) Back view (held to examiner's eye) (B) Side view

Figure 12.13
A slit lamp

Estimation of the visual fields

This is done either by using a special apparatus called a perimeter or more simply by comparing the patient's fields with that of the examiner, one eye at a time. With one eye closed or covered and the open eye fixing on the examiner's eye the patient's ability to see hand movements is compared with that of the examiner.

Perimetry is essential for determining the loss of vision in certain eye conditions, notably chronic glaucoma, and also for localizing an intracranial lesion which involves the visual pathway.

Staining the eye

A dye such as fluorescein sodium dispensed in liquid or strip form (Fig. 12.33, p. 479) will stain the cornea a bright, luminous green where there is loss of corneal epithelium as in corneal abrasion from an ulcer or foreign body. If a Fluoret strip is used it should first be moistened with sterile normal saline and then applied to the inside of the lower lid. Fluorescein drops are instilled in the usual way but should be followed by one or two drops of normal saline. Multidose bottles of fluorescein are highly dangerous because the dye harbours and promotes the growth of pyocyanaeus.

Bacteriological investigation of lacrimal secretion

A sample is taken from the lower conjunctival sac and sent to the laboratory for culture. This is carried out routinely before many operations and is used to find the causative micro-organisms and their sensitivity where there is infection of the eye, for example in conjunctivitis. The lower lid should be well everted so that the specimen is taken only from the conjunctival sac. Care must be taken to label the specimen indicating right or left eye.

COMMON DISORDERS OF THE EYE

Conjunctivitis

Inflammation of the conjunctiva has many causes including bacterial infection by the *Staphylococcus aureus*, the pneumococcus, occasionally the gonococcus and allergic reactions to eye make-up, drugs, dyes, and so on. It may also occur in association with general illness such as measles, asthma and some skin conditions.

Clinical features

The patient will complain of gritty pain but usually **no visual loss**. The whole of the conjunctiva is red and sore and possibly oedematous. In severe cases there is a purulent discharge which causes the lids to stick together especially after sleep. The cornea is always clear and the pupil normal.

Treatment

The cause is removed where possible. Local antibiotics are prescribed in cases of infection and a culture may be taken of the discharge. The eye is left uncovered.

Keratitis

Inflammation of the cornea is fairly common at all ages and can be serious. It can be a recurring condition thus causing the patient a good deal of misery as well as visual loss. There are many causes of keratitis including infection, response to allergy and injury.

The most usual sequence of events leading to keratitis in one eye is an abrasion caused by a foreign body or superficial injury which has become infected causing corneal ulceration. A virus infection due to the herpes simplex ('cold sore') virus

Figure 12.14
Dendritic ulcer

Figure 12.15
Circumcorneal injection

characteristically gives rise to a dendritic ulcer (Fig. 12.14) which is not easily seen unless stained with fluorescein. Occasionally keratitis is due to some endogenous illness such as syphilis in which case the condition is non-ulcerative and both eyes are affected.

Clinical features

There is pain in the eye, excessive watering, loss of vision and spasm of the lids. The redness is classically circumcorneal (ciliary injection) due to engorgement of the deep blood vessels (Fig. 12.15). An accompanying iritis is common and the patient may feel generally unwell. Severe keratitis of any type can cause extensive destruction of the cornea; if perforation follows then aqueous humor will leak out and the infection spreading inwards will cause further damage to internal ocular structures.

Treatment

This depends on the cause and on the severity of the condition. The patient may require hospital admission.

The sensitivity of any organism present should be determined by culture. The doctor may prescribe antibiotics to be given locally either by drops or, if there is severe infection, by subconjunctival injection and systemically. A mydriatic such as atropine 1% will be ordered (see iritis, p. 471).

Local heat usually by hot spoon bathing or by electric eye pad affords some relief of pain. Between treatments the eye is kept closed and covered with a pad for the patient's comfort and to protect the vulnerable cornea. If the infecting agent is the herpes virus, an antiviral agent prepared in drop or ointment form is used intensively. Sometimes cauterization is indicated. This may be done by a qualified ophthalmic nurse on medical instruction, by application of pure carbolic on the tip of a sharpened orange stick. If the cornea has lost its sensation a tarsorrhaphy may be carried out. In this operation the lids are joined together centrally over the cornea to give it protection (Fig. 12.16). Extensive corneal damage may require corneal grafting (keratoplasty), the donor material having been taken from a cadaver eye. Exposure keratitis (Ch. 3) is preventable and, if it occurs in hospital, it should be regarded as a lapse in nursing care.

Figure 12.16
Tarsorrhaphy

Lid margin removed and left raw ∴ when suture removed lids will remain in contact

Rubber tubing to prevent tension suture cutting through delicate skin

Suture tightened. Raw lid edges touching. Suture removed 10–14 days

Iritis

Iritis, inflammation of the iris, is usually associated with inflammation of the ciliary body (**cyclitis**) and therefore often referred to as **iridocyclytis**.

As the layer of the eye involved in this process is called the uveal tract the inflammation may also be called **uveitis**.

Anterior uveitis is inflammation of the iris and ciliary body.

Posterior uveitis or choroiditis is inflammation of the choroid.

A combination of anterior and posterior uveitis is known as **pan-uveitis**.

The causes include trauma, local infection and systemic conditions like rheumatoid arthritis, gonorrhoea, ankylosing spondylitis or sarcoidosis, but in most cases no underlying cause is found. The course of the inflammation parallels the behaviour of inflammation elsewhere; it may be acute, clearing away as quickly as it came, or it can wear on with fibrotic replacement of specialized tissues and adhesions between the iris and the lens (posterior synechiae). This latter course can obviously disturb vision and, less obviously, block the flow of aqueous causing a secondary glaucoma.

Clinical features

The redness resembles that of keratitis and indeed iritis can well be secondary to keratitis. The cornea is clear and the pupil may be small (due to inflammatory spasm or distortion by inflammatory adhesions). There is blurring of vision, pain and photophobia.

In severe iritis the exudate from the inflamed iris, consisting of cells and protein, may sink to the bottom of the anterior chamber to form a layer of pus, known as **hypopyon**. Secondary glaucoma may arise due to interference with the aqueous flow.

Treatment

Guttae (G) atropine 1% is prescribed twice daily because the pupil must be dilated to lessen the risk of anterior synechiae (adhesions between the iris and cornea). Dilating the pupil also lessens the pain by preventing sphincter spasm.

Provided the cornea has no abrasion and infection does not contraindicate their use, steroids such as G. betnesol 0.5% are given locally to suppress inflammation. The appropriate antibiotics are given for any obvious infection.

Secondary glaucoma is treated with systemic acetazolamide (Diamox) 250 mg: this reduces the flow of aqueous.

If the condition persists or does not respond to treatment subconjunctival injection of steroids and mydricaine may be necessary. Oral steroid therapy is indicated in choroiditis and the usual precautions with these drugs must be adhered to.

Sympathetic ophthalmitis

This is inflammation of the uveal tract of one eye following a perforating injury involving the uveal tract of the other eye causing similar inflammation. The injured eye is called the 'exciting eye' and the subsequently affected eye is called the 'sympathizing eye'.

This condition does not usually arise until 10–14 days after the injury has occurred but it can occur after several years have elapsed. In some circumstances the removal of the exciting eye may be necessary especially if the eye is not likely to regain useful vision. Local and systemic steroids are used in treating the sympathizing eye and prognosis has been improved by the use of these drugs.

Panophthalmitis

This is an intense, purulent inflammation of the uveal tract usually following a penetrating injury. Pus accumulates within the eyeball with eventual destruction of its contents. The only treatment is early and adequate systemic antibiotics, but once vision is lost removal of the contents of the eyeball (evisceration) is indicated. This procedure avoids severing the optic nerve which would increase the risk of infection travelling to the brain.

Glaucoma

This term means a raised intra-ocular pressure causing hardness of the eye. Untreated it will reduce the blood supply to the optic nerve with resulting progressive loss of visual field. Any circumstance which blocks the flow of aqueous through the pupil or out of the eye will cause glaucoma. All types of glaucoma have serious consequences for the patient.

Acute glaucoma (closed angle or congestive glaucoma)

Characteristically acute glaucoma affects middle-aged, edgy women with long sight. As long-sighted eyes are small the anterior chamber is shallower than usual and the filtration angle consequently narrower. With increasing age the lens increases in size thus giving less room for the filtration of aqueous into the canal of Schlemm.

Some precipitating factor, either local or general, which causes the pupil to dilate is all that is required for such persons to develop acute glaucoma. Since the pupil normally dilates in the dark or in response to stimulation of the sympathetic nervous system, watching a horror film could provoke an attack in susceptible individuals.

As shown in Figure 12.17 contact between the iris and cornea results in complete blockage of the filtration angle.

Figure 12.17
Blockage of filtration angle in acute glaucoma

Clinical features

There is a sudden onset of severe pain which radiates out from the eye. The patient becomes generally ill with nausea and vomiting, the latter feature very occasionally being responsible for misdiagnosis. The eye is deeply engorged. Vision is markedly decreased. **The cornea is steamy and the pupil fixed and dilated**. A considerable increase in intra-ocular pressure will be found on examination.

Treatment

The tension is reduced as a matter of urgency; if it is left for as long as 4 hours the patient may well become blind.

Medical

Conservative treatment is started on admission using:

1. Acetozolamide to decrease the production of aqueous by the ciliary process. It is usual to give a loading dose intravenously or intramuscularly followed by oral administration. The patient will be prescribed a potassium supplement to counteract the loss of potassium in the urine (see diuretics, Ch. 7).

2. Miotic drugs such as G. pilocarpine 1–4% are instilled intensively until the pupil is a pinpoint. As a result the iris is drawn away from the cornea and the angle which was closed is opened, allowing some drainage of the aqueous. G. pilocarpine is usually prescribed 6 hourly for the unaffected eye as a prophylactic measure. Systemic administration of drugs which alter the osmotic balance between the plasma and aqueous, for example intravenous infusion of mannitol or oral glycerol, may be used.

Surgical

Afterwards surgery is carried out on both eyes. First a drainage operation is performed on the affected eye to allow aqueous to flow through a permanent fistula to the subconjunctival space. Later a peripheral iridectomy (Fig. 12.18A and B) is performed on the second eye to allow aqueous to reach the drainage angle despite a dilated pupil.

Figure 12.18
(A and B) Peripheral iridectomy

A   B

Chronic glaucoma (simple or open angle glaucoma)

A gradual rise in pressure in the eye causes symptomless but progressive loss of visual fields. This is one of the most common blinding diseases in the Western world.

Clinical features

The patient is usually over 50 years. As the retina is destroyed slowly and progressively from the periphery the patient can still read until the condition is well advanced. For this reason the disease tends not to be noticed in the early stages. It is usually picked up on casual examination.

Treatment

The patient is usually treated medically as an out-patient.

The response to treatment is noted by checking the intra-ocular tension, the visual fields and the optic disc. Failure to respond to medical treatment is an indication for a surgical drainage operation similar to that performed for acute glaucoma.

Secondary glaucoma

This is a rise in pressure due to disease or injury to the eye, for example in iritis where cells and exudates are thrown off into the aqueous, slowing or stopping drainage at the angle of the eye. Treatment is to deal with the cause.

Congenital glaucoma (buphthalmos or 'ox eye')

This is glaucoma occurring in a baby due to a developmental defect of the aqueous drainage system. The tissues in a young child are so elastic that the whole eye enlarges as the result of pressure within the eye.

There is considerable risk of reduced vision if the condition is neglected. The treatment is both surgical to correct the malformation and medical to reduce the intra-ocular pressure using drugs similar to those for chronic glaucoma. The risk of visual loss remains high even with treatment.

Cataract

A cataract is any opacity of the lens; some types may give rise to gradual loss of vision.

Types of cataract

Cataracts are classified according to their various causes.

Senile cataract

Degenerative changes occur in the lens with advancing age, starting from about 55 years. It may take several years for the lens to become completely opaque.

Diabetic cataract

Patients with diabetes mellitus (p. 453) have an increased tendency to cataract. The changes are similar to those of senile cataract but tend to start earlier (45 to 50 years).

Young diabetics are prone to develop cataracts, particularly if their diabetes is not well controlled.

Congenital cataract

If a mother contracts rubella during the 9th to 12th week of pregnancy the baby may be born with congenital cataracts. Rubella vaccine (Ch. 1) has reduced the incidence.

Traumatic cataract

A penetrating injury or blunt injury which causes rupture of the lens capsule will allow aqueous to seep in, thus causing opacity of the lens.

Treatment

Treatment is surgical extraction of the lens and replacement of the lost focusing power by a suitable spectacle, contact lens (Fig. 12.19) or intra-ocular lens. In an adult the lens is generally removed in its capsule using forceps or a *cryotherapy* probe. (Details of care before and after the operation are given on p. 480).

In younger patients (under 35) the lens and its capsule are broken up and aspirated piecemeal.

Figure 12.19
Corneal contact lens

Detachment of the retina

Detachment occurs when the innermost layer of the retina containing the rods and cones becomes separated from the pigment epithelium layer below (Fig. 12.20). A breach in the retina allows fluid to accumulate beneath it so causing further separation.

Detachment occurs most commonly in myopic eyes because the myopic retina becomes especially thin and is liable to develop breaks; it is also common after cataract extraction. It may be secondary to trauma, inflammation or, less commonly, presence of a malignant growth in the choroid. Retinal detachment may occur at any age.

Figure 12.20
Detached retina

Clinical features

The patient complains of seeing flashing lights as the retina tears, and then a feeling of a curtain across the vision. There is no pain but serious loss of vision if the retina is not returned to and secured in its normal position.

Treatment

Some kind of surgery is usually indicated because the hole needs to be sealed off and the sub-retinal fluid removed. Occasionally a patient may be admitted for a period of complete bed rest, with the head positioned to allow the retina to fall back into place and the subretinal fluid to be absorbed. Various methods of surgical repair may be employed, depending on the surgeon and on the type of detachment, for example if there is just a hole or a tear with no sub-retinal fluid present then light coagulation, laser or cryotherapy may be used to seal the edges of the hole. The tear is sealed with cryotherapy, then a ridge is formed opposite the hole by a band of silicone sewn over the sclera altering the shape of the eye and bringing the sclera

Figure 12.21
Example of operation for retinal detachment

and choroid into contact with the hole (Fig. 12.21). The sub-retinal fluid can be drained or left to absorb. More recent developments include the use of intravitreal air and silicone oil.

Trauma

Foreign bodies

Particles may enter the conjunctival sac and give rise to irritation. Usually they are easily removed but occasionally one may become impacted in the conjunctiva of the upper lid. If so, eversion of the upper lid (Fig. 12.22) is necessary in order to remove it. The competent first aider can generally dislodge the particle using a corner of the patient's handkerchief. Irrigation using a household eye bath is usually effective if the foreign body is loose.

Foreign bodies which embed in the cornea are much more serious and require prompt specialist attention. After removal of the particle, the eye must be stained to ascertain the extent of corneal abrasion. An antibiotic is then instilled and if necessary a mydriatic. The eye is covered with an eye pad and the patient is asked to return for a check-up, usually the following day. Should a particle of metal be left in the cornea for more than 4 hours, rust will appear which is difficult to remove.

Perforating injuries

Any sharp instrument may perforate the cornea or sclera and damage the structures within the eye. Young children may stick knives, darts or arrows into the eye. Fireworks are a hazard and road traffic accidents where there is shattering of the windscreen may cause a perforating injury.

The first aid treatment is to put a sterile dressing over the injured eye and transport the patient to hospital as quickly as possible, keeping him flat and his head still.

A history is taken in the accident and emergency department, and the patient is admitted and sent to the operating theatre for examination under general anaesthetic as soon as is practicable. Consent for an anaesthetic and also consent for removal of the eye, if necessary, is required.

In theatre the eye is examined carefully and assessed, then cleaned and sutured.

If the eye is too badly injured to have any useful vision and if it is likely to act as a source of inflammation to the other eye (sympathetic ophthalmitis) then the eye is enucleated (removed).

Figure 12.22
Eversion of the upper lid to disclose subtarsal foreign body

Figure 12.23
Hyphaema

Non-perforating injuries

Direct violence

A severe blow from a fist close to the eye or to the eye itself may not perforate the eyeball but will probably cause damage to the delicate structures within. The same is true of objects such as a flying squash ball or shuttle-cock which are common causes of eye injury. If the small blood vessels of the iris are torn, blood will collect in the anterior chamber giving rise to the condition of hyphaema (Fig. 12.23). Treatment is to admit the patient to hospital for a period of complete bed rest to allow the blood to be absorbed. It the blood is not absorbed it may interfere with the drainage of the aqueous, thus causing pain in the eye and a rise in intra-ocular pressure (secondary glaucoma).

A cataract can result from this type of injury — so too can retinal detachment and vitreous haemorrhage. A 'black eye' or periorbital haematoma may look dramatic but provided the eye itself is not damaged the condition is not serious. Bruising will normally subside in about a fortnight without treatment. The patient should however be encouraged to have his eye examined by a doctor and always to see an ophthalmologist if there is any disturbance of vision.

Burns

Burns may be thermal or chemical (Ch. 14).

Thermal burns often involve other parts of the patient's body, but a firework may cause damage mainly to the eye and lids.

Chemical burns are more common and arise because an acid or alkali has entered the eye. Of these, lime burns, occurring frequently at building sites, are among the most serious. The pain is so severe that the patient is often quite unable to co-operate with any first aid measures designed to remove the lime.

The most important duty of the first aider is to get the patient to hospital with the minimum delay. Copious lavage using water or normal saline from whatever utensil is at hand, for example, a jug or teapot, will help if this treatment is possible. In the accident and emergency department the eye will be irrigated immediately with saline (anaesthetic drops having first been instilled to relieve pain and reduce spasm of the lids). Particular care is taken to see that no particle is retained within the upper or lower conjunctival sac where it would continue to cause tissue necrosis.

Following medical treatment the patient is likely to require surgery to deal with the scarring which results.

Burns caused by caustic soda should be irrigated with normal saline.

Strabismus (squint)

In normal vision the two eyes are used together; two images are formed, one on each retina, and they are fused by the brain so that one image is seen in three dimensions. This is called binocular vision.

If during development of vision in the young child there is failure to fuse the two images because of weakness of one of the extra-ocular muscles, then one eye deviates or squints. To prevent double vision the brain suppresses the image formed by the wandering eye, which begins to lose its acuity. Eventually the squinting eye will lose its central vision altogether, and for this reason it is important that treatment is carried out before the child is 5 years of age. The commonest type of squint is a convergent squint where the eyeball turns inwards giving the patient a 'cross-eyed' appearance (Fig. 12.24).

Treatment

A combination of both medical and surgical treatment may be necessary.

Figure 12.24
Convergent squint

Figure 12.25
Congenital ptosis

Figure 12.26
External stye

Figure 12.27
Meibomian cyst

Figure 12.28
Eversion of lid with meibomian cyst prior to evacuation of cyst

Medical

Conservative treatment involves correction of refractive errors, occlusion of the 'good eye' to make the 'lazy eye' work and exercises supervised by the orthoptist. If the child's eye is covered, co-operation of the mother is essential as the child will need almost constant supervision in order to prevent him from removing the patch.

Surgical

This involves either weakening or strengthening one or more of the eye muscles, for example a muscle may be severed and reinserted into the sclera behind its original point of attachment, thus in effect lengthening the muscle.

As the operation is extra-ocular, little preparation is necessary. Since it is not always carried out on the squinting eye and several operations may be necessary, the parents should be forewarned and reassured.

Recovery is usually speedy and uneventful. A baby or very small child may rub his eye but this does not usually cause any damage. In older patients with long-standing squints the operation is carried out mostly for cosmetic reasons.

DISORDERS OF THE EYELIDS

Eyelids are delicate structures which all too readily become permanently disfigured if damaged in some way. Even quite minor conditions are uncomfortable for the patient and obvious to the onlooker.

Ptosis

This is a congenital condition in which the upper eyelid droops (Fig. 12.25). Ptosis is often bilateral and if severe enough to cover the pupils will interfere with vision. This results in the child tipping his head backwards in order to see.

Surgical measures are required to correct the condition.

Damage to the lid or its nerve supply in, for example, myasthenia gravis (p. 125) may also cause ptosis later in life.

Inflammatory disorders
A 'stye' (hordeolum)

Staphylococcal infection of one of the glands at the base of a lash causes a small boil to develop (Fig. 12.26). The lid becomes red, swollen and painful particularly when its owner blinks. After a few days a bead of pus is discharged spontaneously. No treatment is necessary but local heat is soothing and helps speed the discharge of pus.

Antibiotic cream applied to the lid margin may help to prevent spread of infection to other lash folicles when the condition is recurrent.

Meibomian cyst (chalazion)

This is a type of retention cyst (Fig. 12.27). A meibomian gland becomes distended with secretion due to blockage of its duct, the initial cause being infection. The condition is sometimes referred to as an 'internal stye'. The fibrous wall of the cyst prevents spontaneous discharge of its contents so that surgical evacuation is required (Fig. 12.28).

Removal of the cyst is performed quite simply in the out-patient department using a local anaesthetic.

Blepharitis

A generalized inflammation of the lid margin causing redness, formation of scales and irritation is called blepharitis. In its simplest form blepharitis is associated with dandruff of the scalp. Superimposed staphylococal infection makes the condition more serious and may cause ulcer formation with subsequent scarring. Blepharitis tends to run a chronic course and is difficult to cure. Treatment includes control of dandruff and for the more serious forms, local application of hydrocortisone and antibiotics.

CARING FOR OPHTHALMIC PATIENTS

It is not within the scope of this book to describe nursing procedures which, in any case, require to be demonstrated and practised in the clinical situation. There are, however, some principles of care which will be considered.

General care

Ophthalmic nursing is in many ways very different from general nursing. Eye patients often do not feel ill but nevertheless may be required to lie still for some time. For example, a patient with a retinal detachment may have to be nursed post-operatively in a particular position where he is unable to amuse himself or watch television. The hours will pass very slowly. Since some patients have well-founded fears of loss of sight the period spent in hospital is likely to seem long, tedious and anxious. The nurse can help such patients by talking to them, keeping them informed of what is going on in the ward and in the world outside and encouraging them to talk about their worries. The ward should be kept quiet and patients should be protected from sudden noises, but the atmosphere should be cheerful and optimistic. Newly admitted patients are likely to be nervous, as are many of those the nurse meets in out-patient or accident and emergency departments. A quiet, calm, confident nurse will help them to feel more at ease and to co-operate.

Before local procedures are carried out the patient must have his head well supported. If the patient is not in bed then he is best placed on a couch with his head slightly raised for any but the most minor undertakings. The nurse can then work from behind with the aid of a good light (Fig. 12.29). Since the patient should be discouraged from contracting his facial muscles, flinching or making unexpected movements while care is being given, it is sensible to start with him in as comfortable a position as possible and to spend a little time in helping him relax.

Figure 12.29
Positioning patient and light prior to giving eye care

Local care

When carrying out treatment to the eye the nurse must:

1. Use flawless, aseptic techniques at all times.
2. Be gentle and precise in her movements.

Figure 12.30
Instillation of drops into lower fornix

3. In all cases of infection or inflammation, care for the unaffected eye first. In this way she will avoid contamination from the infected eye and the patient will know what to expect before his painful eye is touched.

4. Remember that the cornea is the most sensitive part of the eye. She will therefore avoid touching it in any way. If, for example, drops are to be instilled she will ask the patient to look up and allow the drops to fall gently into the lower conjunctival sac (Fig. 12.30). If she is going to remove a foreign body from under the upper lid she will ask the patient to look down to his toes before attempting to evert the lid and so avoid pressure on the cornea.

5. Check carefully any preparation to be instilled in or applied to the eye (correct patient, correct drug, **correct eye**, correct time).

6. Ascertain whether ointment is to be placed in the conjunctival sac or applied to the lid margins.

7. Ask the patient to close his eye before placing an eye pad in position. This is particularly important if the eye has been anaesthetized as the pad could rub the cornea without the patient's knowledge.

Local preparations

These include:

1. **Drops** (guttae) which may be dispensed in either aqueous or oily solutions. The patient should have his individual bottle if individual doses (Fig. 12.31) are not dispensed.

2. **Ointments** (occulenta). These may be dispensed in single dose containers (Aplicaps) (Fig. 12.32). If the ointment is contained in a multidose tube the risk of contamination is considerably increased.

3. **Fluoret strips** (Fig. 12.33). See the section on staining the eye, (p. 469).

Figure 12.31
Individual preparations — minim drops

Figure 12.32
Individual preparations — Aplicaps

Figure 12.33
Individual preparations — Fluoret strip

Care of the surgical patient

Until recent years most intra-ocular operations were performed using a local anaesthetic. This was because a general anaesthetic carried the risk of postoperative vomiting and the subsequent danger of hyphaema (p. 476) and iris prolapse.

Preoperative care of a patient having an intra-ocular operation

For the elective operation requiring an incision into the eyeball, such as cataract extraction, a patient is admitted 2 nights before the operation. This allows time for orientation, examination and investigations.

Orientation

This includes measures taken for any surgical patient, but an elderly patient, especially if in hospital for the first time, needs extra care and fuller explanation. If he is not familiar with the use of a bedpan, urinal or feeding cup before the operation, then he is likely to become agitated and confused when confronted with such things for the first time immediately after it and his recuperating eye will be endangered. Time should be taken to show him how to lift himself up the bed gently and also how the nursing staff will lift him.

Explanations of the postoperative programme and its restrictions may need to be repeated several times.

Examination and investigations

A general physical examination is carried out by the doctor. Should the patient have a cough the operation may have to be postponed not only because of possible respiratory complications but because of the risk to the eye wound. Haemorrhage within the eye is more likely if the patient's blood pressure is high, so measures may have to be taken to reduce it. As part of the campaign to prevent infection the patient must be generally clean. If the hair has been neglected it should be washed during this period. The nurse can explain that it would be inadvisable for the hair to be washed for a week after the operation. Urine will be tested as a matter of routine; the presence of sugar or albumin is of particular significance and should be reported without delay.

At the time of obtaining consent for the operation, reassurance can be given that it will be the operated eye only which will be covered after the operation. The relatives should be seen and their co-operation sought in such matters as approaching the patient very quietly from the patient's sighted side.

Smears are taken from the conjunctival sacs for culture. Afterwards antibiotic drops are usually prescribed for instillation as a prophylactic measure. The lashes of the eye for operation may be trimmed short using sharp-bladed but blunt ended scissors. A calm, relaxed manner, a steady hand and some petroleum jelly on the blades of the scissors (so that the lashes adhere to them) are prerequisites for success. Some surgeons like the lacrimal sacs to be syringed preoperatively to ensure patency.

On the morning of the operation the routine is similar to that for any patient about to have a general anaesthetic.

Postoperative care

While the patient is in the theatre, the bed area is cleared, the oxygen and suction points are checked and the bedside locker is placed on the side of the unoperated eye. Once he comes round from the anaesthetic, the patient is nursed in the dorsal position with one pillow for approximately 6 hours. At the end of this time, provided the patient's condition is satisfactory, he will be sat up gradually with more pillows and supported with a back-rest.

It is necessary to make sure the patient has a bell to call a nurse for anything which is needed as it is important that the head is kept fairly still following an intra-ocular operation. Hands and face will be washed gently postoperatively, but he will be left in his operation gown until the following morning to avoid unnecessary movement, unless of course the gown is soiled.

The patient will need reassurance that the operation went according to plan and that, provided he keeps reasonably still and avoids touching his eye, there is every chance it will be successful. He may need to be reminded that he should not try to reach anything from his locker. Careful observation is needed during the night because he is more likely to become confused if he wakes.

On the first postoperative morning the first dressing is carried out usually with the surgeon present. Stitch cutters may be required to remove the lid suture so that the eye can be examined. The eye is gently swabbed with sterile normal saline solution and compared with the unoperated eye. The lids, wound, conjunctiva and the anterior parts of the eye are all inspected and any abnormalities are noted in the nursing records. The doctor will usually prescribe a local antibiotic and a steroid to counter postoperative inflammation and mydriatic drops to prevent this inflammation from causing adhesions with a constricted pupil.

If the first dressing is satisfactory, the patient is given a bed-bath and allowed to sit out of bed. He may be helped to the toilet if he is sufficiently recovered from the anaesthetic. Provided the meal is cut up and placed well within reach so that he has no need to bend his head down, he is usually allowed to feed himself.

Dressings are carried out and treatment is given as prescribed. On the second postoperative day the patient can be given a general bath with help and he can walk to the toilet unaided. A male patient may shave from the second day taking a little extra care around the operated eye. He needs to be warned not to bend down to pick things up, such as slippers out of his locker, not to rub his eye or make sudden jerky movements of his head. From the first postoperative day dressings may be removed and dark glasses worn particularly if vision is poor in the unoperated eye. A pad or Cartella shield (Fig. 12.34) is applied over the eye at night to avoid damaging it while asleep. Providing there are no complications he is ready for discharge on the fifth to seventh postoperative day.

On discharge, drops are still generally required and it is important that the person who will instill the drops at home is instructed as necessary. If he is worried about rubbing his eye the patient can be given a supply of eye pads to wear at night only. If the patient already has his own glasses the lens for the operated eye is occluded so that he can use his spectacles to see with his non-operated eye.

An out-patient appointment is made for some 2 weeks after discharge. If he is discharged to his own home arrangements may have to be made to provide a home help, 'meals on wheels' and possibly visits from a district nurse. If it is impossible to provide such help and if there is no one with whom the patient can stay, a period of convalescence may be required. Advice includes reminders not to bend, stoop or lift heavy weights. Normally about 2 months following lens extraction the eye will be sufficiently quiet to permit refraction for the necessary spectacles.

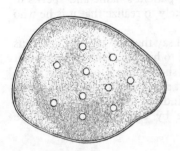

Figure 12.34
Cartella shield

CARING FOR THE VISUALLY HANDICAPPED

A patient may be completely blind, that is to say he cannot distinguish light from dark, or he may be partially sighted but have such limited vision that it is of little use to him. Whether or not he qualifies for registration as a blind person is a decision for an ophthalmic specialist to make.

Blindness may arise in a variety of ways from either injury or disease. In old age it is most often due to disease of the blood vessels within the eye or to disease of the retina. Initially loss of sight causes the patient to become profoundly depressed and in some instances he may develop suicidal tendencies.

If blindness develops quickly and unexpectedly in an elderly person he may become literally too terrified to move and be found wretched and immobile in a chair. Young people, given time, skilled supervision and encouragement, usually come to terms with their blindness and it is well known that some develop increased acuity of their other senses such as hearing and touch. While some remain bitter and resentful there are many more who acquire such serenity and optimism that they are sources of inspiration to their sighted friends and relatives.

Blind persons often manage to move around unaided in their own homes or in familiar surroundings, but when admitted to hospital they become bewildered and afraid to venture about the ward. The nurse must therefore take time to explain the geographical layout and the location of the things the patient needs to use. He must be warned of any hazards, for example equipment in the ward over which he could trip or hurt himself. This is of particular importance if blindness is incidental to some other condition for which the patient has been admitted and he is therefore being nursed in a general ward not specially geared to his needs. Doors which are left half open, and this includes locker doors, are dangers to the blind; so too is anything left out of its accustomed place. Orderliness is important.

Provided that he is well enough and safety precautions have been taken, the blind patient should be encouraged to walk about. When guiding him it is best if, having first offered him a bent arm to hold, the nurse then walks slightly ahead.

At meal times he should first be told what is in the meal; then the clock face can be used to describe the whereabouts of the various portions of food — for example potatoes at 12 o'clock, peas at 8 and meat at 5 o'clock.

A sighted person who is dozing should be approached by quietly saying his name and then by a gentle touch on his head or arm; it is the same with a blind person. Failure to give adequate warning may startle the patient who may 'jump'. The imaginative nurse will realize that unless she uses the patient's name and speaks to him directly when in the company of others he is unlikely to realize that it is he who is being addressed.

Similarly, when about to leave the room, she should say that she is going and thus avoid the embarrassment of leaving the patient talking to himself. Unless the patient is known to be deaf it is not only unneccessary but shows a lack of sensitivity to shout. She must always remember to tell him first what she is about to do. Sympathy and understanding are essential when caring for the blind but to offer pity is unkind. The nurse will do the patient the greatest service by encouraging him to be independent.

Services for the visually handicapped

The services available to blind and partially sighted persons vary from country to country. In Great Britain some are provided by welfare services and others through a number of voluntary organizations. It is only upon registration that the full range of facilities become available in Britain so that, although it is not obligatory for the visually handicapped to register, it is to their advantage to do so.

The register for blind and partially sighted persons is maintained in Britain by the local authorities. If a person wishes to become registered he must first obtain a certificate from an ophthalmic specialist, who will examine him free of charge. Responsibility for the visually handicapped is shared between the health, education and social work departments. The services provided by them and the voluntary organizations collectively include:

Special primary and secondary education in either day or residential schools.
Various training facilities, for example in Braille, typewriting or handcrafts.
Industrial rehabilitation and sheltered workshops.
Personal services such as home visits and individual advice.
Financial benefits and special concessions, for example reduced rates on public transport, income tax and radio licence relief.
Free loan tape recorders, radios and books in Braille and Moon type.
Social clubs.
Holiday homes.
Guide dogs and training facilities.
Special equipment including white walking sticks, Braille clocks, watches and controls for stoves.

SUGGESTED ASSIGNMENTS

1. Ask a friend to co-operate in the following exercise.

Blindfold yourself (no cheating!) for a whole evening and carry out as many of your normal activities as you can without help (ask your friend to intervene only if you are in real danger of harming yourself). Try to imagine that your inability to see is permanent and then consider how this would affect your life.

If possible visit a special school for the blind to find out how they teach people recently blinded to live with their handicap.

2. What are the commonest causes of accidental injury to the eye in your area? Are there any industries or sports played which put the eyes at special risk? Without being too restrictive, suggest practical safety measures to reduce the incidence of injury in either of the above.

Make a simple list of precautions suitable for young boys using an adventure playground.

3. Plan a programme for a week to help to relieve the monotony and boredom for partially sighted elderly patients in a hospital ward.

4. How would you advise someone who wishes to donate his eyes for medical use after death? For what purposes can cadaver eyes be used?

FURTHER READING

Chawla H B 1981 Essential ophthalmology. Churchill Livingstone, Edinburgh
Darling V H, Thorpe M R 1981 Ophthalmic nursing, 2nd edn. Bailliere Tindall, London
Dobree J H, Boulter E 1982 Blindness and visual handicap. Oxford University Press, Oxford
Gardiner P A 1979 ABC of ophthalmology. British Medical Association, London
Parr J 1982 Introduction to ophthalmology, 2nd edn. Oxford University Press, Oxford
Paven-Langston D (ed) 1980 Manual of ocular disease and therapy. Little Brown, Boston
Thomas P 1978 Pharmacology of the eye. Lloyd-Luke, London
Trevor Roper P D 1981 Ophthalmology. Grant McIntyre, London

Chapter Thirteen
The ear, nose and throat

Ear, nose and throat (ENT) surgery and nursing, in common with other fields, have benefited from advances in science and technology.

The introduction of antibiotics and other chemotherapeutic agents has revolutionized the treatment of many formerly troublesome ENT affections, with a subsequent reduction in morbidity. Also, radiotherapy and cytotoxic drugs are being used increasingly in the treatment of malignant conditions as an adjunct to surgery. The use of the operating microscope has opened up new frontiers for ear, nose and throat surgeons and, of course, for their patients. To improve or re-establish a person's hearing is indeed a rewarding exercise. The scope of ENT surgery is very wide, ranging from microscopic reconstruction of the middle ear, to emergency life-saving tracheostomy. These two procedures have implications for nurses in terms of both basic nursing care and more technical nursing skills, as do most other procedures undertaken by the ear, nose and throat surgeon.

Patients admitted to hospital for the treatment of ear, nose and throat conditions are seldom detained long in hospital. Even though this is the case it is still important for the nurse to get to know her patients as well as is possible. A good nursing history and assessment is essential for planning the nursing care and ensuring their stay in hospital is safe and that the treatment is successful. Patients requiring ear, nose and throat surgery require the same preparation as any patient having surgery. Special pre- and postoperative requirements are discussed in relation to each specific disorder.

Obviously in a book of this nature not all of the pre- and postoperative nursing care is discussed in detail, so suggestions for further reading are given at the end of the chapter.

Some of you may be puzzled as to why ear, nose and throat surgery should be a comprehensive speciality; a discussion of the anatomical relationships between these three areas will perhaps convince you of the rationality of the specialism.

The ear, nose and throat make up a large, irregular cavity in the skull (Fig. 13.1) which has openings into the middle ear via the auditory tube, into the larynx and hence into the lungs. The pharynx is continuous with the oesophagus and so there is an opening into the stomach. Openings are also found leading from the sinuses, to allow drainage of mucus, and from the orbits, so that tears can drain into the nose.

This complicated cavity (or cavities) is lined with epithelial tissue. Most of the epithelial lining is of ciliated columnar epithelium, while in the pharynx and leading into the oesophagus it is of the stratified variety.

THE NOSE AND PHARYNX

The nose and the upper part of the pharynx form the upper section of the respiratory tract; the lower part of the pharynx is common to both the respiratory and alimentary tracts.

Figure 13.1
Saggital section through nose,
nasopharynx and larynx

Figure 13.2
Ciliated epithelium showing
goblet cells which produce
mucus

Anatomy and physiology

The anterior part of the nose is called the vestibule (Fig. 13.1). It is lined with squamous epithelium. Coarse hairs, vibrissae, are found in this part (Fig. 13.1). These prevent large dust particles and insects from entering the nose. The remainder of the nasal lining is of ciliated columnar epithelium (Fig. 13.2) which is interspersed with 'goblet' cells which secrete mucus. The mucus traps bacteria and other foreign particles that impinge on the mucous membrane; the action of the cilia is to sweep this unwanted material to the natural orifices. The mucous membrane has another role besides preventing the entry of foreign bodies into the respiratory system: to warm and moisten the incoming air. The structure of the nose, with its various bones projecting into it, presents a large surface area with a rich blood supply, enabling this function to be performed adequately. The sensory nerve endings of smell (olfactory nerves) protrude into the attic of the nose (Fig. 13.1).

The sinuses, which are lined with ciliated epithelium, are normally filled with air. They give resonance to the voice and lighten the weight of the skull. Because of the very small and sometimes awkwardly placed openings from them (Fig. 13.3) and because the mucous membrane can easily become swollen and congested, acute and chronic sinusitis are fairly common disorders.

DISEASES

Epistaxis

Bleeding from the nose is a very common form of haemorrhage, especially in children and the elderly. It is not a disease in itself but may be a sign of disease. The bleeding may be spontaneous from any area but especially from Little's area. The

Figure 13.3
Ostia draining paranasal sinuses

Figure 13.4
Blood supply to the nose
showing common bleeding sites

nose has a very rich, blood supply (Fig. 13.4). Any blow on the nose may obviously result in bleeding as may fractures of the nasal bones, facial bones or base of skull. Also new growths in the nasal cavity such as polyps, benign haemangiomata and carcinomata may bleed. Various inflammatory disorders, for example, acute and chronic rhinitis and sinusitis and perhaps more rarely syphilis and tuberculosis, may be responsible for the bleeding. Of the more general disorders cardiovascular diseases, such as hypertension and telangiectasis, are likely causes, the former being a common reason in the more elderly person. Blood diseases such as leukaemia, thrombocytopenia and agranulocytosis should also be excluded if the epistaxis is recurrent. Patients on anticoagulant therapy may experience very refractory nose bleeds.

Clinical features

The onset of bleeding is sudden in most cases and may be from one small area or from several. As was mentioned, Little's area is very often the bleeding site. If bleeding is profuse and prolonged the patient will exhibit signs of shock. The patient may also vomit quite large quantities of blood if the bleeding point is at the back of the nose and the blood is swallowed.

Treatment and nursing care

The patient should sit down with the head slightly forward over a basin and the clothing well protected. The nostrils should be cleared by blowing one at a time;

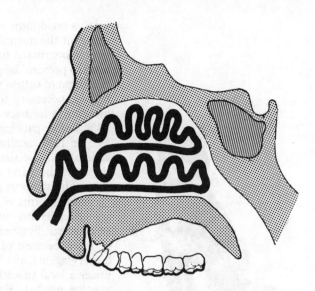

Figure 13.5
Nose pinched during bleeding

Figure 13.6
Nasal pack in position

Figure 13.7
Postnasal pack

using a good light the nasal passages should be inspected. If the bleeding area is at the front the nostrils should be pinched for 10 minutes exactly (Fig. 13.5). The patient is instructed to breathe through the mouth. A cork may be placed between the teeth to prevent the patient from swallowing any blood which enters the nasopharynx. A pledget of cotton wool may be placed in the nostril before applying the pressure. It may be necessary to pack the nose if pressure does not stop the bleeding or if the bleeding is far back in the nose. The arrangement of the packing is shown in Figure 13.6. Before packing, the nasal passages are first sprayed with a local anaesthetic such as 5 or 10% cocaine or, more often, 4% lignocaine in an equal amount of 1: 1000 adrenaline. The success of packing depends to a large extent upon adequate anaesthesia of the nasal mucosa. 25 mm ribbon gauze which has been soaked in BIPP (bismuth iodoform paraffin paste) or Calgitex is inserted under direct vision.

Various forms of packs and epistaxis balloons such as Simpson's and Brighton's are available although some ENT surgeons favour the use of Foley catheters to stop an epistaxis. Systemic antibiotics must be given if packs are to remain in for 24 hours or more because of the danger of infection. The surgeon may also use chemical cautery agents, for instance silver nitrate stick or trichloroacetic acid, administered under a local anaesthetic; for more persistent and recurrent bleeding, electrocautery may be needed. Following cautery there may be a degree of local infection and crusting. A child may then pick off this crust causing a recurrence of the bleeding. The application of petroleum jelly for a few weeks will help to prevent crusts forming so preventing further trauma allowing the epithelium to thicken and heal and protect the blood vessels. In the majority of patients bleeding will be controlled by the measures outlined. Other techniques will be required where bleeding is persistent; one of these is the insertion of a post-nasal pack (Fig. 13.7). This is a very uncomfortable procedure and the patient needs an anaesthetic. Very special attention to the airway is required whilst such a pack is in situ. A few patients will require clipping of the blood vessels supplying the nose, for example, the anterior ethmoidal artery as it emerges from the orbit.

If no local cause for the bleeding is found the patient will usually be referred to a physician for further investigation.

Hay fever — allergic rhinitis

This is a very common condition: an estimated 3 million people in Britain are afflicted to a greater or lesser extent. Each year around half a million patients require medical attention. Many also suffer from some degree of asthma. The condition is often due to an allergic response to a foreign protein in pollen (Fig. 13.8). In this case it will be seasonal being worst in spring and especially during the summer. It may also be a reaction to various animal proteins when it is usually more dramatic in its course.

Clinical features

There are bouts of sneezing, eyes water and are itchy and nasal linings are red and swollen causing blockage of the nose.

The condition is a fairly typical antigen-antibody reaction. The pollen acts as an allergen stimulating the susceptible individual to produce specific antibodies. These antibodies become fixed on to the tissues of the eyes, nose and lower respiratory tract. When this happens the patient is said to be sensitized; when he is next exposed to pollen he develops the signs and symptoms described above.

Prevention and treatment

Various centres perform pollen counts to give potential sufferers an early warning of when they will be most at risk. Individuals who are known to be allergic should take precautions to prevent overexposure to the pollens. Wearing spectacles or sunglasses keeps pollen out of the eyes and reduces the discomfort of photophobia. Doors and windows should be kept shut. The doctor may prescribe a simple antihistamine, which may be effective in relieving the symptoms. Patients should be discouraged

A Domestic cat

B House dust mite

C Timothy grass

D Bread mould

Figure 13.8
Some common allergen sources

from using decongestants continuously and should use them only in urgent situations to relieve severe congestion. Once the acute episode has been resolved the condition can sometimes be prevented from recurring by using a drug called sodium cromoglycate. This substance which is in fine powder form is thought to stabilize the 'mast' cell membrane preventing its degranulation and hence the release of histamine and other substances which disturb the function of the blood vessels. The release of histamine and other substances from the mast cells cause the mucosa to become oedematous and to produce large amounts of serous and/or mucoid secretions in the nasal cavity, a prominent feature of allergic rhinitis.

Nurses are often involved in investigating the cause of the hay fever and other causes of chronic rhinitis, of which there are many. Investigations include skin tests to find possible allergens. If the causative allergen is isolated a course of desensitizing injections is given over a period of several weeks. In the case of pollen sensitivity the course is best given in the weeks before the pollen season begins.

The outlook for patients whose lives are made miserable by allergic rhinitis has improved considerably over the last few years and is likely to improve even more.

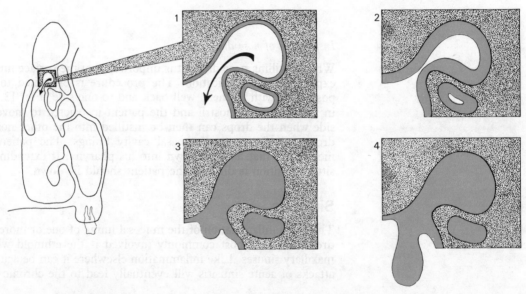

Figure 13.9
Formation of polyps

Polyposis

Figure 13.10
Polyps protruding in nasal cavity

One outcome of chronic congestion of the mucous membranes is the formation of polyps. Figure 13.9 shows schematically how polyps are thought to develop. There is nearly always an allergy related vasomotor disorder. The polyps consist of grossly oedematous mucous membrane with internal spaces filled with fluid. The polyps (Fig. 13.10) are covered by a layer of epithelial tissue which may be of squamous or ciliated columnar epithelium. There is a marked infiltration of plasma cells, lymphocytes and eosinophils which is typical of chronic allergic conditions. The blood supply to the polyp is often very scanty.

Clinical features

The main complaint is of nasal obstruction. There is always a discharge which ranges from mucoid to frank yellow pus. There is a deep seated sinus infection and complaints of headaches. The polyps may be clearly seen (Fig. 13.10) as a large pale grey mass. They may be multiple and are often bilateral.

Treatment and nursing care

Treatment is by surgical removal. Decongestant drops are given for 1 week and steam inhalations will also help to reduce congestion and give symptomatic relief of discomfort.

Figure 13.11
Instillation of nasal drops

Instillation of nose drops

When instilling nose drops it is important that the surface mucosa of the nose is well exposed to the medication. The procedure is explained to the patient and he is positioned with his head well back and to one side (Fig. 13.11). A drop is instilled in the uppermost nostril and the patient instructed to move his head to the other side when the drops can then be instilled into the other nostril. By doing this the drops will flow over the nasal cavity linings. The patient should spit out any medication that has run down into his pharynx. If extending the head back in the sitting position is difficult the patient should lie down.

Sinusitis

This is an inflammation of the mucosal lining of one or more of the sinuses. In children the sinus most commonly involved is the ethmoid whilst in adults it is the maxillary sinuses. Like inflammation elsewhere it can be acute or chronic. Repeated attacks of acute sinusitis will eventually lead to the chronic condition (Fig. 13.12).

Figure 13.12
Normal and congested mucous membrane in nasal cavity

Clinical features

The majority of cases are secondary to acute rhinitis or the common cold or, more rarely, to measles and influenza. A child will often get an attack of acute sinusitis following swimming if he has been jumping into the water without holding his nose; this is especially so if the child has an infection. Infection may also spread from an infected tooth socket or be a sequel to fractures of the facial bones. The signs and symptoms, dependent to some extent on the sinuses involved and usually appearing a few days after the primary infection has apparently cleared, are:

Increasing nasal obstruction.

Purulent nasal discharge if the sinuses are draining, which causes irritation in the throat and halitosis.

A sense of fullness in the cheek if a maxillary sinus is infected.

The patient feels toxic and has a headache, especially in the morning, which may clear as the day goes on.

The temperature may be raised.

The nasal mucosa is congested and the anterior nostrils are excoriated. In children with ethmoidal involvement a degree of orbital cellulitis may be present.

The diagnosis can be confirmed by *transillumination of the sinuses* in a darkened room; by X-ray pictures or proof puncture (see p. 492).

Treatment and nursing care

During the toxic and febrile stage the patient should have all the nursing care of the febrile patient (Ch. 1). If possible, nasal swabs should be obtained for culture and sensitivity tests. Strict attention should be paid to nose blowing and, if necessary, instructing the patient on the proper method, which is to blow one nostril at a time. Paper handkerchiefs should be provided and a disposal bag conveniently placed for collecting them. The room temperature and humidity should be kept fairly constant as changes in either affect nasal mucosa. Moist inhalations are helpful for adult patients but should not be given to children because of the danger of scalding. Specific medical treatment includes the administration of nasal decongestants. Antibiotics will also be prescribed according to the results of bacteriological investigations. Analgesics such as soluble aspirin and paracetamol will give symptomatic relief. Some patients may require antral puncture and lavage. This procedure is described below.

In the majority of cases the inflammatory changes clear up completely with adequate treatment and the ciliated columnar epithelium recovers its functions. Sometimes the condition becomes more chronic, especially when the maxillary (antral) sinuses are infected, because of their poor drainage (Fig. 13.3).

Antral puncture and lavage

This is the introduction of a special trocar and cannula (Lichtwitz) into the antral sinus (Fig. 13.13). It is a common procedure in ENT departments and is used in both diagnosis (proof puncture) and the treatment of sinusitis. The procedure, which is carried out by the doctor, is usually done under local analgesia, the anaesthetics of choice being either lignocaine 4% with adrenaline 1 in 1000 (coloured pink) or cocaine 5 to 10% with adrenaline. Cotton-tipped probes are soaked in the anaesthetic and inserted under the inferior turbinate bone for 10 to 15 minutes. Some doctors prefer 2% lignocaine by injection because it gives a more profound anaesthesia. In children a general anaesthetic may be required. Specimens of the sinus contents are usually sent for bacteriological examination or, if cancer is suspected, for cytological studies.

For some patients the doctor may leave a fine polythene tube in position in the antral sinus which greatly facilitates repeated lavage. Repeated lavage may be necessary in chronic sinusitis to clear sinuses of debris, giving the mucosa a chance to recover. This procedure is often carried out by an experienced ENT nurse. The complications of antrum puncture are fainting — it is not a pleasant experience

— other more rare complications include perforation of the orbit, cellulitis, surgical emphysema and osteomyelitis. Following antral lavage, conservative treatments are continued.

In some unfortunate patients the condition does not respond to repeated lavage and chemotherapy. These patients require more radical surgery in the form of an intranasal antrostomy or Caldwell-Luc operation (Fig. 13.14). In this procedure the antral lining is removed. For more details of this procedure a more specialized text should be consulted.

Complications of sinusitis

Various complications can arise from acute and chronic sinusitis. These include spread of infection to the orbits and osteomyelitis of the frontal and maxillary bones. Infection can also spread by various routes to the cranium, causing a variety of intracranial complications. For discussion of these complications a more specialized text should be consulted.

Fracture of the nose

This usually follows a blow on the nose. The nasal bones (Fig. 13.15), which are not very robust, break easily. Depending on the force of the blow the sinuses and facial bones may also be involved.

Bruising and swelling are seen on examination, and bleeding from the nose may be profuse.

No active first aid treatment should be given other than cold compresses to relieve pain and swelling and to stop bleeding.

The extent of bony injury is confirmed by X-ray. If the bones are out of alignment the fractures are reduced by manipulation. This is best done as soon as possible. The nasal area, being vascular, is prone to haematoma formation, which separates the fragments of broken bone. If this is allowed to develop fully it is more difficult to stabilize fragments in position after manipulation. Fractures of nasal bones heal fairly quickly, which is an important consideration for the surgeon in deciding when to reduce the fracture. A plaster of Paris splint may be required for a few days to keep the bones in position (Fig. 13.16). If bone and cartilages heal in an abnormal position, the free flow of air may be obstructed and this may give rise to difficulties.

Figure 13.16
Plaster of Paris nose splint

Most patients will be admitted to hospital if reduction is necessary. The patient is nursed in the upright position supported by pillows. If there is a history of loss of consciousness the patient should be observed for changes in conscious level (Ch. 3). The nurses should also observe for cerebrospinal fluid rhinorrhoea. If this is suspected the discharge should be tested for sugar with a Clinistix.

Analgesics will be required for relief of pain. Antitetanus prophylaxis and antibiotics are also prescribed.

If there are no complications only a short stay in hospital is necessary. In the case of more extensive damage to the facial bones referral to a plastic surgeon may be necessary. The patient may also require correction of any deformity at a later date, for example, to relieve nasal obstruction or for cosmetic reasons.

Deviations of the nasal septum

Deviations of the nasal septum are quite common. The fault may lie in the cartilaginous septum, turbinate or palate bones. It is often congenital; there is unequal growth of the bones giving rise to asymmetry of the nasal cavities or it may be a sequal to trauma.

Clinical features

These include complaints of nasal obstruction, frontal headaches and recurrent attacks of sinusitis. The obstruction is generally worse in one side than the other but is not usually so bad as to affect the sense of smell.

Treatment and nursing care

The treatment is surgical and the two operations most commonly performed are:

1. submucous resection (Fig. 13.17A)
2. septoplasty (Fig. 13.17B)

Figure 13.17
(A) Submucous resection
(B) Septoplasty

Preoperative care

The general care is the same as for any operation. X-rays are taken of facial bones. Any active infection is treated before operation. In the period immediately before the operation the surgeon may wish the nasal cavities to be anaesthetized. One method of achieving this is by Muffeting. This consists of instilling 5 ml equal parts of adrenaline 1: 1000 and lignocaine 4% in each nostril. The patient has to hold this solution in the nasal cavity for 20 minutes. Alternatively if the patient is not able to co-operate the nasal cavities can be packed with 25 mm ribbon gauze (Fig. 13.6) which has been soaked in equal parts of adrenaline 1: 1000 and lignocaine 4%. The aim of these procedures is to reduce the amount of bleeding at the operation.

The patient is warned that there will be packs in the nose after the operation.

Postoperative care

Special attention is paid to the airway as packs will be in situ; these are left in for 2 days and then removed. Packs are of two types either, 'finger cot' packs with a 'bullring' nose pack or nose pad. Alternatively 25 mm ribbon gauze which may be impregnated with petroleum jelly. Observation for bleeding either post nasally or anteriorly is essential. Following removal of the packs, decongestants and steam inhalations may be helpful in giving relief from symptoms. The nose is often extremely tender following the operation and analgesia may also be required. Before discharge the doctor will inspect the nasal passages for haematoma formation and adhesions between the nasal septum and turbinate bones. The patient should be instructed to return if there is any bleeding, not to pick his nose and to blow it gently. One other important point, because of oedema there may not be much obvious improvement in the first week or two following the operation and the patient should be warned about this. He should avoid smoking, extremes of temperature and crowded, enclosed spaces.

Acute tonsillitis

Acute inflammation of the tonsils and adenoids is a common disease. The condition is seen more often in children than adults, as the tonsils atrophy with age. Chronic tonsillitis and infectious diseases such as measles and scarlet fever predispose to acute tonsillitis. The causative organisms vary, but the haemolytic streptococcus is the most common.

Figure 13.18
Normal structure of the mouth

Clinical features

The severity of the condition may range from a mild catarrhal inflammation (Fig. 13.19) to a severe septic infection. A feeling of fullness in the throat, leading to soreness and pain on swallowing, is the usual sequence. Earache, with enlargement and tenderness of the lymph nodes, is also common. The patient has all the signs of a febrile illness, and in severe cases he feels very ill.

Treatment and nursing care

The patient is usually under the care of a physician rather than an ENT surgeon. As the condition is infectious he should be isolated. He will require all the nursing care of the febrile patient (Ch. 1). Gargles are given to keep the mouth and throat clean. Analgesics provide symptomatic relief. In severe cases an antibiotic is prescribed after ascertaining sensitivity of the causative organism. The condition usually clears away completely, but in some cases a peritonsillar abscess (quinsy) develops (Fig. 13.20) and more active antibiotic treatment is required after incision of the abscess to allow drainage of the pus. This relieves the pain almost immediately the recovery is speeded up. Strict attention to oral hygiene is necessary.

Chronic tonsillitis

This condition may follow acute tonsillitis and can cause considerable general ill-health due to the absorption of toxic substances from the tonsils The tonsils are persistently reddened as are the pillars of the fauces. A caseous substance accumulates in the crypts, which are ulcerated, and liquid pus can be expressed from them with a spatula. There is often a bad taste in the mouth and the patient has foul breath. Some patients experience persistent soreness of the throat with acute exacerbations. There is swelling of the lymph nodes and the patient feels vaguely unwell. The toxic substances absorbed from the infected tonsils are thought to be a factor in causing many diseases such as rheumatic diseases, nephritis, chest infections, fibrositis, neuritis and iritis.

Hypertrophied nasopharyngeal tonsils or adenoids

The adenoids, which, like the tonsils, are composed of lymphoid tissue, lie on the posterior wall of the nasopharynx (Fig. 13.21). The adenoids often become inflamed, and because of their position various signs and symptoms arise. These include mouth breathing and snoring and frequent prolonged head colds. Complications can and do frequently follow, the most serious being sinusitis and blockage of the auditory tubes leading to secretory otitis media (glue ear). The same general ill-health found in chronic tonsillitis occurs. Depending on the frequency and severity of the attacks conservative treatment is tried first. If the child develops complications and fails to thrive, removal of the adenoids is indicated.

Figure 13.19
Acute tonsillitis

Figure 13.20
Peritonsilar abscess

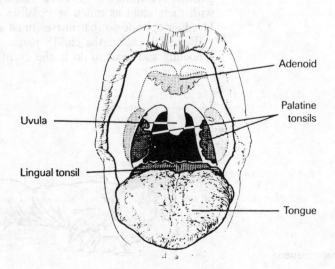

Figure 13.21
Waldeyer's ring
(tonsils and adenoids)

Adenoid

Palatine
tonsils

Uvula

Lingual tonsil

Tongue

Treatment and nursing care

In children both tonsils and adenoids are usually removed at the same time (adeno-tonsillectomy). In adults, only the tonsils are removed, the adenoids having atrophied. The patient is admitted the day before the operation. If there is any evidence of upper respiratory tract infection or history of acute tonsillitis in the previous 3 weeks the operation will have to be postponed. If there is active infection this would put the patient at risk of respiratory complications during the anaesthetic and also increase the likelihood of postoperative bleeding. Any history of a bleeding tendency should be noted and in the case of children the teeth should be inspected to see that none is loose as they may be dislodged during the operation and inhaled.

The general preoperative care is the same as for any other operation under a general anaesthetic. For details of the operations performed — dissection and, now much more rarely, guillotine — a textbook on ear, nose and throat surgery should be consulted.

Postoperative care

Patients are nursed in the post-tonsillectomy (semi-prone) position (Fig. 13.22) so that any blood from the tonsil bed can drain freely from the mouth. If bleeding is suspected, evidence being swallowing and an increase in pulse rate, a careful inspection of the tonsil area is made using a good light; unless bleeding is profuse, cold compresses are applied to the cheek in the hope that the clot will stabilize. If the bleeding is profuse the nurse must maintain a clear airway, clear blood by gentle suction and inform the surgeon. Maintenance of a clear airway is vital and it is important to pull the tongue forward if this falls back. There is no use in giving oxygen if the airway is obstructed. The patient's colour will show signs of improvement as soon as the airway is properly cleared. Half hourly pulse and blood pressure readings are recorded. The normal postoperative care and attention are given. Some surgeons prescribe paracetamol to relieve pain. Salicylates are not normally used as they interfere with blood clotting and may predispose the patient to haemorrhage from the tonsil bed. Pain is often felt in the ear following tonsillectomy; this is referred pain and not due to otitis media. Adults may require two or three injections of pethidine or other strong analgesia. The routine of different units varies considerably, but most units encourage patients to take a normal diet as soon as possible following operation. 3 to 4 hours after the operation the patient should be changed into his own night clothes after washing the hands and face and given a refreshing mouth wash. The patient is then given a drink and ice cream or jelly. The cool ice cream is soothing and the swallowing prevents the muscles becoming tense. Gentle but firm insistence is often required to persuade the patient to take anything by mouth but if he persists he will soon find it easier and within 24 hours the worst of the discomfort will be over. The length of stay in hospital also varies. As most tonsillectomy patients are children, extended visiting periods are allowed to enable parents to be with their child as much as possible. A very small number of patients do have a bleeding episode so that nurses must be alert at all times for this possibility.

Before discharge the child's parents should be given instructions regarding diet, schooling and what to do in the event of bleeding from the tonsil bed.

Figure 13.22
Post-tonsillectomy position

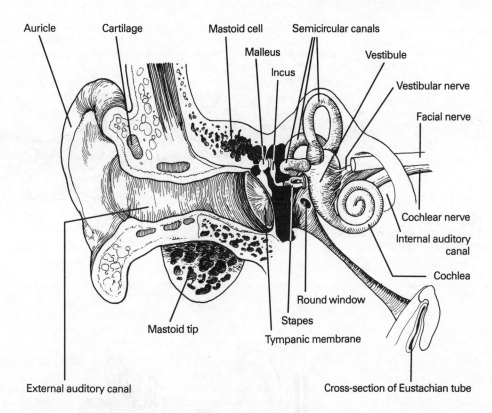

Figure 13.23
External, middle and internal ear

THE EAR

The ear is concerned with hearing and balance.

Anatomy and physiology

As can be seen from Figure 13.23, the ear can be conveniently divided for descriptive purposes into three areas, the external, middle and internal ear. The **auricle** of the ear directs sound waves along the **external auditory canal**, where the waves cause the **tympanic membrane** to vibrate. This vibrating membrane in turn causes the three auditory **ossicles** to oscillate. The footplate of the **stapes** is fitted into the **oval window** of the vestibule (Fig. 13.24) and the vibrations transmitted by the ossicles pass into the fluid in the **cochlea**.

The effect of conducting sound waves through this elaborate structure of canals, membranes and ossicles is to amplify the sound waves bombarding the pinna (Fig. 13.25). This is necessary in order to stimulate the sensory nerves. Any congenital or acquired disruption of these structures causes conductive deafness (Table 13.1).

Figure 13.24
Transmission of sound. Sound waves cause the tympanic membrane and ossicles to vibrate enabling the sound to pass into the endolymph of the cochlea. The sound waves are magnified about 20 fold by this mechanism

Figure 13.25
Translation of sound waves into
meaningful sensations

Figure 13.26
Method of distinguishing
between sensorineural and
conductive deafness

Table 13.1
Main causes of deafness

Conductive deafness		Perceptive deafness	
External ear	Middle ear	Inner ear	Intracranial
Congenital atresia	Congenital deformities	Hereditary cochlear defects	Tumours in cerebellopontine angle
Acquired atresia	Otosclerosis	Presbycusis	Multiple sclerosis
Accumulation of cerumen	Perforated eardrum	Intrauterine causes	Encephalitis
Foreign bodies	Dislocation of ossicular chain	Labyrinthitis	Meningitis
Inflammation — otitis externa	Acute otitis media	Ménière's disease	Cerebral tumours
Furuncle	Chronic suppurative otitis media	Meningitis	Psychogenic
New growths	Secretory otitis media	Viral infections	
	Cholesteatoma	Trauma	
	New growths	Noise-induced	
		Allergy	

Sensory nerves arising from a structure within the cochlea — the **organ of Corti** — are thus stimulated and sensations of sound are transmitted along the cochlear division of the auditory nerve to the temporal lobe in the brain, where sounds are interpreted.

Congenital and acquired abnormalities of the auditory nerves give rise to a type of deafness known as sensorineural or perceptive deafness (Table 13.1) (Fig. 13.26).

Closely approximate to the cochlea is another very complex arrangement of canals and caverns, the **utricle, saccule** and **semicircular canals**, which make up the **labyrinth**. The semicircular canals are arranged in three planes. The whole complex arrangement is filled with fluid, and specialized nerve endings project into this fluid. Some of the nerve endings have **otoliths** attached to them which move with any currents set up in the fluid.

The sensations caused by stimulating these nerve endings are conveyed along the vestibular division of the auditory nerve to the cerebellum and other parts of the brain. The sensations arise when movements of the head cause the fluid to flow and so provide the brain with information about the position and movements of the head and body.

Deafness

As can be seen from Table 13.1 deafness has many causes. Deafness is a serious social handicap and possibly because it is not as conspicuous as blindness, the deaf do not always get the sympathy and understanding they deserve. What is perhaps not obvious from the table is that deafness can be congenital or acquired. Generally speaking, few of the congenital causes of deafness, respond to medical and/or surgical intervention. Of the acquired forms of deafness many are very amenable to treatment and some of the procedures for improving hearing are described below.

The deaf person will find it easier to understand what is being said if he can see the face of whoever is addressing him. Some people with hearing difficulty rely mainly on lip reading, so lip movements are important and obviously conversations should be carried on in a good light. In all instances — whether deafness is partial or where a hearing aid is worn — speech should be slow and distinct; shouting is not helpful and, in cases of sensorineural deafness, may be counterproductive. If hearing is better in one ear then another the patient and his bed or chair should be placed so that anyone speaking to him directs the voice to the better ear.

Hearing aids

Hearing aids are designed to amplify sounds so that the deaf person can hear them more clearly. They do not of course reproduce the sounds as well as the normal ear would; even the very best hearing aids distort the sound to a certain extent

Figure 13.27
A deaf person, who relies on lip-reading, needs to see the lips clearly

Howling noise

Unwanted feedback

Wanted sound

Leak

Figure 13.28
A common cause of interference when using a hearing aid is a poorly fitting mould

Auriscope

Jobson Horne probe

Tilley aural forceps

Dressed orange sticks

Ear syringe

Figure 13.29
Instruments for removing wax

(Fig. 13.28). Many types of hearing aid are available and nurses should familiarize themselves with them. They should learn how to test and adjust them to enable each person to get optimum use from his aid. Many of the modern aids whilst being very discreet and barely noticeable have very small controls so that people who have poor vision, or who are disabled or elderly may experience difficulty in adjusting them. Instruction should also be given on how to clean the ear piece which can become blocked with wax and or debris.

DISEASES

Foreign bodies in the ear

All general practitioners and casualty departments are accustomed to dealing with foreign bodies in the external canal of the ear. Often there are few symptoms except perhaps slight deafness.

Treatment

The canal is inspected using an auriscope (Fig. 13.29). Provided the foreign body is not impacted and is not organic in nature, syringing will usually remove it.

Wax

Wax or cerumen is a normal secretion from wax glands in the cartilaginous part of the external auditory canal (see Fig. 13.23). In some patients wax accumulates and causes such symptoms as deafness, earache, discharge, tinnitus and vertigo. If the wax is soft it is easily removed using a Jobson Horne probe tipped with cotton wool. Hard wax must first be softened, for which various preparations such as olive oil or proprietary cerumenolytic agents may be used. These should be warmed to body temperature (37°C) before instilling so as not to cause dizziness. These agents are used prior to syringing the ear. In some patients where the wax has become very hard and covered by a layer of keratin it may be necessary to give a general anaesthetic in order to remove it.

Figure 13.30
Ear syringing

Syringing the ear

This is generally a safe and simple method of removing wax and other foreign bodies from the external auditory canal (Fig. 13.30). It is well within the competence of the nurse but should not be done without prior instructions from the doctor. The procedure should not be carried out if the patient is known to have a dry perforation of the tympanic membrane or where there is an acute inflammation of the external or middle ear. The main solutions used are normal saline for irrigation, 1% sodium bicarbonate solution or, most frequently, plain tap water. The doctor will advise on the lotion to be used.

The lotion should be at 37°C when it is in the external canal; otherwise convection currents will be set up in the labyrinth and the patient will become dizzy. The nurse should not undertake this procedure before:

1. Having observed an experienced person perform it.
2. Having performed it herself under supervision.

Complications are giddiness, perforations of the tympanic membrane, trauma from the syringe nozzle and otitis externa.

Otitis externa

This may be either localized or diffuse.

Localized external otitis

This is usually due to infection of a hair follicle (furunculosis) in the cartilaginous part of the external canal (see Fig. 13.23).

Clinical features

There is severe earache, a red and swollen orifice and an increase in pain especially over the tragus when the ear is touched.

Treatment

Various forms of packing are used, such as wicks of glycerin and magnesium sulphate BP paste. Symptomatic relief is obtained from analgesics. An antibiotic may be prescribed for some patients.

Diffuse external otitis

This condition can occur in one or both ears. It is often associated with the scalp condition seborrhoeic dermatitis or dandruff. The inflammation results in intense irritation; the patient tries to relieve the irritation by poking in his ears, which only exacerbates the condition.

Treatment

If dandruff is thought to be a predisposing factor, the patient should use a medicated shampoo. Various drugs are used locally, including antibiotics and steroid preparations. The condition is very difficult to cure and the patient should be discouraged from poking in his ears. (Similarly, mothers should be warned of the risks of unnecessary use of cotton wool buds when caring for their infants.)

Acute otitis media

Acute inflammation of the middle ear is a very common complaint; to avoid serious sequelae it must be promptly and adequately treated.

Predisposing factors

These include blocked auditory tubes, enlarged adenoids, stomatitis, rhinitis of any origin, sinusitis, faulty nose blowing, tumours of the nasopharynx, diving into infected water and perforations of the tympanic membrane.

Clinical features

It follows from what has just been said that infection of the middle ear is nearly always via the auditory tube. The auditory tube becomes blocked and the air normally in the middle ear and mastoid cells is absorbed; mucus collects and later becomes purulent. On examination of the ear the tympanic membrane is seen to be inflamed and bulging. The patient has earache, is deaf and, if a child, becomes febrile. There may be a discharge of blood and pus from the ear with immediate relief of pain if the tympanic membrane ruptures.

Treatment

If the inflammation does not respond to antibiotics or if perforation of the membrane seems likely, the surgeon may perform a myringotomy (an incision of the tympanic membrane) to allow drainage of pus. This avoids the laceration of the membrane which occurs should it rupture spontaneously. This procedure, which necessitates a general anaesthetic, is not often required because of the effectiveness of antibiotics in resolving the infection. Nasal decongestants are prescribed to relieve congestion and to allow drainage via the auditory tube. This also allows air to pass up the tube and so equalizes the pressure on either side of the tympanic membrane.

Complications of acute otitis media

These are always serious, the most dangerous being chronic suppurative otitis media with mastoiditis, destruction of the ossicles and perforation of the tympanic membrane.

Secretory otitis media

This condition arises because of blockage of the Eustachian tubes, often by enlarged adenoids. It is mainly a disease of childhood. The middle ear cavity becomes filled with a thick mucinous material hence the alternative name of 'glue ear'. The child becomes deaf, a fact which may not always be readily appreciated by parents and teachers.

Treatment and nursing care

The surgeon makes a small incision in the tympanic membrane (myringotomy) and sucks out the mucinous material using a **Zollner** sucker. This is often quite difficult to accomplish as the material is very tenacious. Once cleared a grommet (Fig. 13.31) is fitted into the incision and this ensures adequate ventilation of the middle ear cavity.

Figure 13.31
Grommet inserted into tympanic membrane following myringotomy and clearance of secretions

Myringotomy incision

Grommet in situ

(Actual size)

Figure 13.32
Site of perforation in (A) Simple
CSOM (B) dangerous CSOM

The pre- and postoperative care is essentially the same as for other ear operations (see below) only in this instance there are usually no packs or external dressings. Only a short stay in hospital is needed. On discharge the child's parents are advised to avoid getting the external auditory canal wet, hence no swimming until it is healed. Flying is also prohibited. The grommet gets pushed out by the healing tympanic membrane, by which time normal ventilation and drainage via the Eustachian tube should be re-established. Regular follow-up is arranged as the disorder may recur.

Chronic suppurative otitis media

This is a chronic inflammatory disorder in which pus is produced. There are two types, namely simple and dangerous chronic suppurative otitis media (CSOM) (Fig. 13.32).

Most patients come to surgery with a long history of chronic middle ear disease relating a sad story of progressive deafness and a foul smelling aural discharge. The discharge is often intermittent and the patient will report periods when the ear has been dry especially following treatment.

In the more dangerous form there is cholesteatoma formation (Fig. 13.33) with destruction of the ossicular chain. As with any chronic inflammatory process there is always the danger of extension to neighbouring tissues and structures. Chronic mastoiditis, lateral sinus thrombosis, cerebral abscess, meningitis and facial paralysis are all possible serious complications of this disorder.

Treatment and nursing care

Better primary health care and the advent of antibiotics have reduced the incidence of chronic ear disease. Nevertheless the busy otorhinolaryngology department still sees many patients with chronic ear disease. The introduction of the binocular operating microscope has enabled the ENT surgeon to perform more reconstructive surgery instead of the radical surgery of the past.

The main operations performed are cortical mastoidectomy, modified radical mastoidectomy and radical mastoidectomy. These are all operations to clear out necrotic and infected tissue. One of the main reconstructive operations is myringoplasty — repair of the tympanic membrane: for this operation a small piece of fascia is often used (Fig. 13.34). The other operations are tympanoplasty and ossiculoplasty in which the ossicular chain is restructured using a variety of techniques and prostheses (Fig. 13.34). The nursing care is much the same for all procedures differing only in a few details. The surgeon will make his wishes known.

Preoperative care

The patient will be admitted a few days before the operation so that a full range of audio-metric tests can be performed. Sometimes these tests are done on an outpatient basis. Either way they are essential for pre- and postoperative comparison.

Cholesteatoma

Break in ossicular chain

Blocked auditory tube

Ruptured tympanic membrane

Otosclerosis

Acute suppurative otitis media

Figure 13.33
Common causes of middle ear
deafness

A Myringoplasty

B Stapedectomy—Teflon strut
and vein graft repair

C Ossiculoplasty using
a bone strut

D Stapedectomy—wire strut
and fat used for reconstruction

Figure 13.34
Four examples of microscopic
surgery of the middle ear
Bottom row — A selection of
prostheses developed for
reconstructing the ossicular
chain

——— Correct
.... Incorrect

Hair kept in
position by
hair fixative

Myringoplasty

Mastoidectomy

Stapedectomy

Figure 13.35
Skin preparation before ear
surgery

The patient requires all the normal preoperation care given before major surgery. In addition hair is shampooed using a medicated shampoo and the head is shaved on the affected side (Fig. 13.35). The scalp and postauricular sulcus must be cleaned with an antiseptic solution. Care must be taken to keep any of the solution from running into the ear. The hair is kept in place using hair fixative and the area covered using a head bandage. (Fig. 13.35).

Postoperative care

In the immediate postoperative period the patient is usually nursed flat. Despite this he may experience nausea and vomiting due to disturbance of the labyrinth.

Nursing observations are of particular importance:

The patient's temperature, pulse, respirations and blood pressure are recorded half hourly.

Signs of increasing intracranial pressure (see Ch. 3) must be reported immediately.

The patient must be observed for signs of facial palsy, denoted by asymmetry of the face. This is because the muscles on the affected side are unable to counteract effectively the pull of muscles on the unaffected side.

The patient should be asked to 'show his teeth' and any paresis (weakness) of the facial muscles is usually obvious. Should this complication develop the bandage is loosened and the surgeon and operating theatre staff are informed. To counteract the vertigo and the dizziness which many patients experience the patient is sat up gradually using one additional pillow at a time. If the dizziness persists a pillow is removed for a time. Occasionally a labyrinthine sedative may be required. If dizziness and or vomiting are very severe the doctor should be informed. The first dressing is commonly done by the surgeon and usually requires a general anaesthetic. The dressing may be left in position for up to 5 days following some types of mastoidectomy. The patient's temperature and pulse should be recorded 4 hourly throughout this period. Any complaints of pain or evidence of inflammation should be reported to the doctor. Not all operations will be instantly successful; some may not be successful at all and patients should be warned that it may be some time before the anticipated improvement materializes.

Ménière's disease

Ménière's disease is a very distressing condition caused by a disturbance in the labyrinth. Excess fluid accumulates in the membranous labyrinth causing distension. This results in malfunction of the nerves of balance and hearing. There are three main symptoms of which the patient complains:

1. Increasing deafness.
2. Tinnitus.
3. Repeated attacks of vertigo.

The diagnosis is made on the basis of the history, audiometry, caloric tests and X-rays of the petrous bone. More specialized X-rays, for instance computerized axial tomography (p. 86), may be required if tumours of, or in the region of, the acoustic nerve are suspected.

Treatment and nursing care

Medical treatment is tried first, consisting of dietary modification such as reduced salt intake and labyrinthine sedatives. The dreadfully distressing symptom of tinnitus — sometimes called the roaring deafness — may be helped by special 'masking' hearing aids. If medical treatment fails a small number of patients may benefit from surgery. Several different surgical procedures have been devised. One of the more popular at the present time is decompression of the endolympahatic sac. Vestibular neurectomy and stellate ganglionectomy are also performed. Selective destruction of the vestibular labyrinth is another procedure which is possible using ultrasound, the aim being to preserve the hearing. The disease often becomes bilateral so that procedures which destroy hearing on one side cannot be undertaken lightly. Remission does occur in some patients making the longer term prognosis very difficult. The pre- and postoperative care is essentially the same as for other major ear surgery.

Vertigo and Tinnitus

Vertigo can also occur as a symptom of other ear diseases and because of tumours of the 8th cranial nerve and cerebellar lesions such as tumour or an abscess. Tinnitus which is a subjective sensation of sound in the ear is a very common and distressing disorder. It is a sign of irritation of the cochlear mechanism. The symptom is described as hissing, buzzing or hammering in the ear and can be so unpleasant as to cause severe depression and even suicide. It is worth remembering that some drugs are ototoxic, for example, salicylates and streptomycin so that complaints of tinnitus from a patient receiving these drugs should be reported immediately.

THE THROAT

The lowest part of the pharynx and larynx comprises the throat.

Anatomy and physiology

The larynx is composed of several cartilages (Fig. 13.36) which give it a rigid structure to prevent it from collapsing easily. The opening into the larynx is closed during swallowing by a flap of elastic cartilage tissue called the epiglottis. Stretched across the inside of the larynx are the vocal cords. The vocal cords are attached to the movable arytenoid cartilages of the larynx. A complex arrangement of muscles is attached to the arytenoids and cartilages and these muscles 'open' and 'close' the vocal cords. As air passing from the lungs is forced over the tensed vocal cords, sound is produced. The different pitches of sound depend on the degree to which the cords are stretched and the flattening or thickening of the cord edge. Speech, which is a learned activity, is controlled by an area in the left frontal lobe called Broca's area. The nerve supply to the larynx and vocal cords is via the recurrent laryngeal nerves which arise from the vagus nerves in the thorax, and branches of the superior laryngeal nerve.

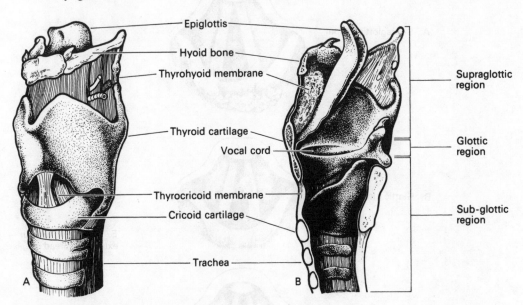

Epiglottis
Hyoid bone
Thyrohyoid membrane
Thyroid cartilage
Vocal cord
Thyrocricoid membrane
Cricoid cartilage
Trachea

Supraglottic region

Glottic region

Sub-glottic region

A   B

Figure 13.36
The larynx (A) Front view
(B) Saggital section

Tumours of the throat

Benign tumours of the throat such as papillomata and fibromata are uncommon but can be troublesome when they do occur. In a child they may easily obstruct the free passage of air and on occasion may necessitate a tracheostomy. There is always a danger of damage to the vocal cords when such tumours are removed.

Various polyps (Fig. 13.37) nodules and cysts also arise mainly on the vocal cords and may require surgical intervention.

The nursing care is the same as that given to any patient requiring surgery. Great care must be taken postoperatively on recovery from anaesthesia to ensure that the patient can swallow properly. The surgeon will advise the nursing staff on this and may well forbid food and fluid for several hours following the operation. Histopathology of the tissue removed is necessary so that the patient can be reassured that the growth was benign.

Carcinoma of the larynx

Carcinoma of the larynx makes up about 2% of reported cases of malignant disease. The condition is more common in males than females. It has been suggested that the undesirable habit of smoking is a predisposing factor. There are also racial differences in the incidence of laryngeal carcinoma. The prognosis of the condition varies according to the site of the primary tumour. This is because of the anatomical arrangement of the larynx, its blood supply and in particular its lymphatic drainage. Spread is by local invasion of the growth and via the lymphatics to the neck and mediastinum; blood-borne metastases are uncommon.

Clinical features

These depend on the site of the tumour (Fig. 13.37). If the cords are not involved a vague discomfort in the throat, thickness of the voice, irritable cough, swollen lymph nodes in the neck and occasionally difficulty in breathing are the most common presenting features. If the cords are involved hoarseness is the main feature initially. Even in the very early stages, there is some alteration in the voice no matter how small the lesion. Hoarseness persisting for more than 14 days should always be investigated.

A. Supraglottic tumour

B. Glottic tumour

C. Polyp on cord

D. Paralysis

E. Subglottic tumour — extensive spread

Figure 13.37
Lesions of the larynx

Diagnosis

This is not always easy, as several conditions can present with similar clinical pictures. These conditions include chronic laryngitis, syphilis and tuberculosis. The diagnosis is made on the basis of a careful history, direct laryngoscopy and tissue biopsy for histological examination. X-ray examination of the chest and neck are also carried out, the former to exclude bronchial carcinoma which may be causing pressure on the recurrent laryngeal nerves.

Treatment and nursing care

Once the diagnosis is established there are two main forms of treatment — surgery and irradiation.

For tumours in supra-and subglottic regions of the larynx the usual treatment consists of a combination of irradiation and surgery. Many patients do not seek treatment early enough because of the vagueness of the symptoms. Patients with supra- and subglottic tumours undergo a course of irradiation followed by surgical removal of the tumour. Localized glottic tumours respond very well to radiation exposure, with a high cure rate. The voice returns more or less to normal.

Preoperative care

The surgery required is extensive; for this reason the patient must be as fit as possible before the operation. As with all major surgery the management of the patient is very much a team effort involving surgeons, radiologists, physiotherapists, speech therapists and nurses as well as the resources of many other departments within the hospital. The patient is admitted a few days before the operation. This enables the team to get to know him and to prepare him to manage without a larynx, with all that this entails. The speech therapist instructs the patient in oesophageal speech; even quite elderly patients show a remarkable ability to master this form of communication. The physiotherapist instructs the patient in breathing exercises as the patient will have a permanent tracheostomy following removal of his larynx (Fig.13.38) and chest infections must be avoided.

The doctors and nursing staff are responsible for carrying out all the normal preoperative care. A positive, optimistic approach by all members of the team will do much to instil confidence in the patient and his relatives. An opportunity to meet a former patient who has had a successful laryngectomy will do much to instil confidence. Most patients accept the situation philosophically, having already undergone irradiation therapy, an exhausting experience in itself. The anaesthetist will also visit the patient as the nature of the surgery presents him with several problems in providing adequate ventilation of the lungs during operation.

Figure 13.38
Extent of surgery in laryngectomy

The general preoperative care is the same as for all major surgery. Some surgeons may request that a nasogastric tube be passed before the patient goes to theatre; other surgeons pass the tube during some stage of the operation.

Postoperative care

On return from theatre the patient should be under constant surveillance; for this reason and to protect him against infection he will be nursed in an intensive care area or in a side room in the ward. Once back in the ward the patient will be nursed in the upright position well supported by pillows, as soon as it is safe to do so. He will have a tracheostomy tube in position; usually this will be a plain plastic or rubber tube (Fig. 13.39). Some surgeons prefer to use cuffed tubes to prevent blood and other secretions from flowing down the trachea into the lungs (Ch. 6). Pressure from the cuff on the walls of the trachea quickly causes a troublesome necrosis (a pressure sore), which can erode through to the oesophagus causing a tracheo-oesophageal fistula. For this reason a regime for regular release of the cuff must be established. The other alternative is a two-cuffed tracheostomy tube, only one cuff needing to be inflated at a time. Most surgeons will fit the patient with a silver tube later in the postoperative period (Fig. 13.40).

The tracheostomy tube will require very frequent cleaning using suction every 15 or 30 minutes. (Ch. 6). Strict asepsis must be observed. As the normal humidification of incoming air by the nasal passages is absent, some form of humidification will be required. There are various means of achieving this. If the secretions become very thick and tenacious 5 ml of normal saline may be instilled into the trachea before suction. This will help to loosen the secretions and make them easier to suck out. A tray with sterile spare tubes and all necessary equipment should be available so that should the tube become dislodged or blocked it can be replaced immediately. As the ostomy is to be permanent it is fashioned in such a way that it will not close or collapse as might an ordinary tracheostomy. Special attachments for giving oxygen via a tracheostomy tube are available.

The wound should be inspected for any sign of haemorrhage and the dressing changed using a strictly aseptic technique. There are usually two vacuum drains in situ. These are required to drain away blood and haemoserous fluid from beneath the very extensive skin flaps necessary for removal of the larynx and repair of the pharynx. Haematoma formation under the skin flaps may cause respiratory distress, difficulty in swallowing and predispose to infection and fistula formation. If a vacuum drain is in place, it must be maintained to prevent the accumulation of blood and serum within the wound area, which could give rise to pressure resulting in respiratory distress.

Figure 13.39
Tracheostomy tubes (A) Single cuffed tracheostomy tube — balloon (cuff-inflated) (B) Medasil silicone stoma button (C) Plain plastic tracheostomy tube

Figure 13.40
Silver tracheostomy tubes
(A) Obturator
(B) Inner tube
(C) Outer tube

The patient's intravenous infusion will be maintained as prescribed. The stomach contents are aspirated hourly via the nasogastric tube to prevent regurgitation during the initial period. Frequent and careful oral toilet is essential to prevent infection from developing in the mouth. Prescribed analgesics are given as required to control pain. The usual postoperative observations and blood pressure should be recorded half hourly.

Depending on how well the patient progresses — and every patient behaves differently — the intravenous fluids may be discontinued on the first or second postoperative day. The patient's fluid and nutritional needs are given via a nasogastric tube. This method of feeding is maintained up to the tenth post operation day. This allows the wounds to heal properly and lessens the risk of infection.

Before oral feeding is recommenced it must be ascertained that there are no fistulae communicating with the respiratory system. This is common in patients who have undergone radiotherapy treatment, and it tends to delay healing. The existence of fistulae can be established by, for example, running a few drops of an aqueous solution of gentian violet on to the patient's tongue and asking him to swalllow. The tracheostomy and wound are then observed to see if any gentian solution appears. If no solution appears, normal feeding is gradually introduced. The patient may be allowed up to sit in a chair by the second or third post operation day and may even manage a short walk. Early ambulation is desirable. The physiotherapist and speech therapist will attend to fulfil their respective roles and the patient should be ready for discharge by the end of the second week or even earlier.

Unfortunately, not all patients respond to treatment either because they have been slow to seek medical aid or because of the position and nature of their tumour. In a few instances the tumour erodes through the skin, becomes infected and causes an offensive odour. Many patients remain in this unpleasant state for quite a long time causing great distress to their families. Necrosis of the skin and fistulae are common features in patients who have undergone irradiation. There are often difficulties in swallowing and breathing and palliative surgery may be necessary. Pain is not a common feature. Many of these patients die of uncontrollable haemorrhage. During this terminal illness drugs to relieve any pain and allay anxiety will be necessary.

The many successful treatments make the management of these patients a rewarding exercise especially when one sees the patient months and then years later, having mastered oesophageal speech and leading an almost normal life. Even swimming may be possible as several different types of attachment are available to enable this. Patients should be encouraged to lead as full a life as possible within their physical and mental capacities.

SUGGESTED ASSIGNMENTS

Projects

1. What services and facilities are available for the deaf and hard of hearing in the community in which you live and nationally?

2. From your knowledge of speech production and from listening to people communicating orally, list the qualities of speech. From this list predict which qualities you think will be absent in the patient who has had a laryngectomy and has learned oesophageal speech.

If possible interview a patient who has had a laryngectomy or listen to a tape recording of a patient using oesophageal speech and see if your predictions are valid.

Discussion topics

1. Should the government pass laws compelling people to wear ear defenders to prevent deafness or is this an individual responsibility?

2. Loss of hearing is a worse handicap than loss of vision

FURTHER READING

Birrell J F 1982 Diseases of the nose, throat and ear, 9th edn. Wright, Bristol

Hall Simson I, Colman B H 1981 Diseases of the ear, nose and throat, 12th edn. Churchill Livingstone, Edinburgh

Ledman H 1981 ABC of ear, nose and throat. British Medical Association, London

Miles Foxen E H 1980 Lecture notes on diseases of the ear, nose and throat, 5th edn. Blackwell Scientific, Oxford

Pracy R, Siegler J, Stell P M, Rogers J 1981 Ear, nose and throat surgery and nursing. Hodder and Stoughton, London

Saunders W H, Havener W H, Keith C F, Havener G 1979 Nursing care in eye, ear, nose and throat disorders, 4th edn. Mosby, St Louis

Chapter Fourteen
The skin

This chapter deals with some ways in which skin damage occurs. It also gives an introduction to the principles of nursing care and treatment of some common skin disorders. The reader seeking more specialized knowledge will find an increasing number of excellent textbooks becoming available.

STRUCTURE AND FUNCTION OF THE SKIN

Figure 14.1 shows clearly the component parts of the skin and its appendages. The outer layer, the **epidermis,** has a **basal cell layer.** These cells are constantly dividing and moving towards the surface. Here they become *keratinized* and are constantly being removed by friction and washing. Other cells, called **melanocytes,** are in the basal cell layer. These produce a pigment, **melanin,** which gives the skin its colouring; it is increased by the action of sunlight.

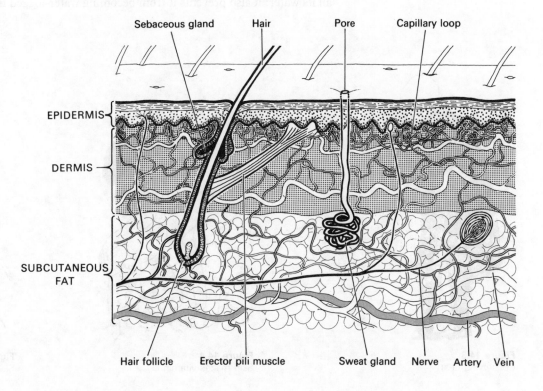

Figure 14.1
The skin

Hair follicles are invaginations of epidermis into the second layer of skin, the **dermis**. Growth of hair occurs in a cycle, with three phases. The growing phase (anagen) is followed in turn by an inactive phase (catagen) when no development of the bulb occurs. In the third phase (telogen) the hair is shed. Regrowth follows and since follicles behave independently there are always some in each phase. Normal scalp hair grows at a rate of 1 to 3 millimetres per week; elsewhere growth is slower. In certain circumstances, for example during treatment with some cytotoxic agents, or in the course of radiotherapy treatment when the head is involved, hair will fall out temporarily. Patients so affected can be assured that regrowth, though it may be slow, will occur. **Sebaceous glands** open into hair follicles secreting **sebum**, a fatty substance which keeps hair and skin soft and pliable.

Sweat glands are found in the dermis. These are coiled tubes the ducts of which open on to the skin surface. Two types are found, smaller **eccrine** glands all over the skin, and larger apocrine glands concentrated in the skin of the axillae, pubic region and the areolae of the breasts. **Apocrine** glands are inactive until puberty. Water is lost to the body by means of sweat produced by these glands. This in turn, while evaporating provides a method of cooling the body. Thus, when heat needs to be lost, more sweat is produced and evaporated. When conservation of heat is required there is less sweat (Figs 14.2 and 14.3).

The dermis has a network of collagen fibres providing support for blood vessels, lymphatics and special sensory nerve endings. Undulations at the junction of the dermis with the epidermis are called **papillae** and prevent separation of the two layers. They also allow for nourishment of the basal cell layer of the epidermis by dermal blood capillaries. The rich blood supply to the skin enables rapid healing to occur, while the ability to increase and decrease the blood flow in skin vessels is a valuable factor in the regulation of body temperature.

Skin manufactures **vitamin D** as the result of the action of sunlight upon it (Fig. 14.4). At one time, when low living standards and inadequate, low-vitamin diets were common, children living in smoky towns often had rickets as a result of being deprived of sunlight.

Another important function of skin is **protection**, not only against microorganisms but also against other harmful agents such as acids and alkalis (Fig. 14.5). Occasionally, however, a hair follicle becomes infected producing a boil.

Skin is also **waterproof** (Fig. 14.6). Not only does it prevent the body from losing all its water; it also prevents it from becoming water-logged in the rain or in the bath.

Figure 14.2
Losing heat

Figure 14.3
Conserving heat

Figure 14.4
Skin makes vitamin D

Figure 14.5
Skin protects

Figure 14.6
Skin is waterproof

Some water is lost in a controlled way by sweating, but uncontrolled loss, as might occur in severe burns, is very serious and can lead to death.

Special nerve endings in the skin also keep the brain informed about the environment. Different sensations, such as heat, cold, touch, pressure and pain, are caused by the nerve endings being stimulated, stimuli then being transmitted to the brain.

The changing skin

Everyone admires the soft, smooth skin of babies, yet softness means tenderness, so special care must be taken of the skin of infants. It should be remembered that the surface area of a baby's skin, in relation to its weight, is much greater than that of an adult so proportionately more heat is lost. As the heat-regulating mechanism in infants takes time to develop, heat loss can be dangerous. Environmental temperatures for babies must therefore be adequate and constant, and exposure avoided (Ch. 17).

As years go by, changes occur in the skin. Often the first remarkable change is during the period of adolescence when acne may be a problem (Fig. 14.7). Not only is it unsightly but it occurs at a time when young people are at their most sensitive. Acne usually clears up by the mid-twenties, but in the meantime, sympathetic treatment is essential. The cause of acne is believed to be related to the increase in androgens which occurs at this time of life and leads to an abnormal response within the sebaceous glands. There is no firm evidence to indicate that diet has any long term influence on acne but normal washing of the skin with soap and water should be encouraged, and patients should be warned against picking the spots as this habit may result in scarring. Any treatment prescribed must be used on a long term basis. An oral antibiotic, commonly tetracycline, is prescribed daily for moderate or severe acne and maximum absorption occurs if the medication is taken with water before meals. Topical treatments such as benzoyl peroxide or retinoic acid tend to be effective in reducing the number of lesions. Initially the skin may become reddened with some scaling but perseverance with the treatment usually leads to an improvement.

During the menopause further skin changes may occur. This, too, is a period of endocrine change often accompanied by emotional upsets. Thinning of the hair may be noticed, as well as the appearance of facial hair. Weight gain increases the possibility of intertrigo (inflammation occurring in folds of skin). *Pruritus*, especially around the external female genital organs, may also begin to be troublesome.

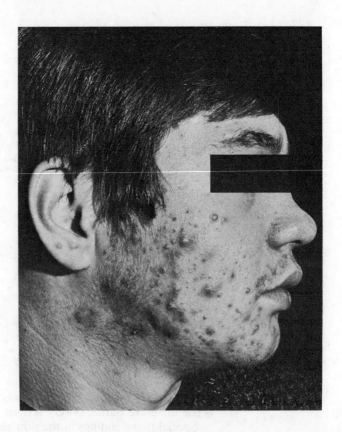

Figure 14.7
Acne vulgaris (Courtesy of Mr
McIntyre, Department of
Medical Photography, Victoria
Hospital, Kirkcaldy)

The effects of ageing on the skin are probably in part due to changes in the dermis, the supporting part of the skin. Contrasted with that of a baby, aged skin is wrinkled and loose. Often it is very thin and almost transparent. Patches of brown pigmentation occur. Dietary deficiencies leading to symptoms of pellagra or scurvy may be the result of poverty or apathy (Ch. 4). In old age, there may be nail thickening and distortion as well as skin changes. This problem is best dealt with by a chiropodist.

KEEPING SKIN HEALTHY

Washing

Skin becomes covered with sweat, sebum, dust and dead epithelial cells. Decomposition of sweat by bacteria gives rise to unpleasant odours, particularly in the axillae and groins. Daily washing with soap and water is required and many people find deodorants helpful. (By and large, expensive brands of deodorant tend to be no better than cheaper ones.) Special attention must be paid to folds of skin — between toes, and in the groin, scrotum and anal regions. This is particularly true of the helpless patient being nursed in bed for whom the old maxim 'as far down as possible and as far up as possible' is not good enough. 'Possible' must also be washed thoroughly. Occasionally a person's skin may react to certain soaps and deodorants, and these must then be avoided.

Nutrition

No special diet is required to keep skin healthy, only one containing the necessary nutrients. Protein deficiency, seen in underdeveloped countries, causes kwashiorkor, one feature of which is skin ulcers. Vitamin C deficiency causes scurvy, while pellagra, the result of nicotinic acid deficiency, has among its features skin disorder. Of these three, the only one likely to be seen in developed countries is scurvy, which may occur among the elderly (Ch. 20).

Clothing

Although warmth is important, clothing should be comfortably loose. Undue tightness causes chafing and damages the skin. Nylon and other synthetic materials are not very absorbent and are therefore not suitable for wearing next to the skin. They also tend to keep the body too hot in summer and too cool in winter. Tight-fitting shoes and elevated heels can cause untold damage to feet, the least of which will be corns. Socks should be changed daily, more frequently if the feet sweat profusely. Metal hooks and fasteners, especially if nickel-plated, cause skin reactions in some people.

Cosmetics

Although cosmetics are useful for covering blemishes and often enhance the appearance, it is nonetheless true that most women have no idea what they are putting on their skins. Many ingredients go into cosmetics, and occasionally some people will find that their skin reacts to certain varieties. These they must avoid.

BREACHES IN THE SKIN

Skin normally remains intact unless damaged in some way. A common form of injury is burning. An inadequate blood supply due to impaired arterial circulation will also lead to skin death; so too will inadequate venous drainage such as occurs with varicose veins. A common result of skin damage is an ulcer. This is defined as a circumscribed lesion in which loss of skin and possibly subcutaneous tissue has occurred.

Pressure sores

Patients who are confined to bed for long periods and who have a limited degree of movement are liable to suffer damage to skin and possibly also to underlying tissue. Pressure sores, or decubitus ulcers, are mainly the result of prolonged pressure being exerted on the skin at various points. This localized pressure diminishes the blood supply to the skin, which becomes devitalized and susceptible to damage by even the most trivial injury. Often a reddening of the skin appears first, then a break in its integrity. Unless vigorous measures are taken, an ulcer, which is often infected, develops. A distinction is sometimes made between this and the death of deeper tissue, which can extend to bone; but in both cases pressure is the principal cause.

Figure 14.8 shows the parts of the body most likely to be affected by prolonged pressure. These are parts where tissue is compressed between bone and the surface on which the person is lying. The surface can vary in hardness. Operating tables

Figure 14.8
Pressure areas

tend to be fairly hard in spite of cushioning; so too do stretchers in ambulances. A long period spent on such surfaces can begin the process that results in the development of sores. Softer surfaces that change to fit the body contours will achieve a more even and wider distribution of body weight and are consequently less likely to be damaging.

Causes

Although pressure is the main cause of pressure sores, there are several other contributory factors. These can be divided into two groups; those relating to the condition of the patient himself, and those relating to his environment, for example his bed.

Factors relating to the patient

Malnutrition, especially protein and vitamin C deficiency.

Other diseases — diabetes mellitus, anaemia, malignant disease, obesity, oedema of any origin.

Changes particular to old age — hypertension, lowered resistance to infection, impaired sensation, impaired consciousness.

Slipping down the bed because of lack of support.

Factors relating to the environment

Wrinkled or patched sheets.

Rubber mackintoshes on beds.

Draw sheets of rough texture.

Bread crumbs or other particles in the bed.

Soiled or wet sheets.

Friction caused by incorrect lifting.

Excessive skin massage.

Excessive use of soap on skin.

Bedpans.

Prevention

Prevention of pressure sores is a nursing priority. Provided preventive measures are begun before damage occurs, sores need not develop. The most important part of prevention is to recognize those patients who are prone to develop sores so that preventive measures of the appropriate intensity can be taken at the earliest possible moment. Research has provided an extremely useful method of measuring the degree to which any patient is at risk. The method, shown in Table 14.1, consists of assessing the patient on a scale from 1 to 4 on five different aspects of his condition. Those patients who score a total of 14 or less on these scales are considered to be at risk and require intensive measures to prevent pressure sores developing.

Traditional preventive methods of treating pressure areas include massage using soap and water, barrier creams and sometimes the application of surgical spirit to the skin. With the exception of gentle washing for hygiene and the use of barrier creams for incontinence, there is probably little or no value in any other of these measures. Indeed, excessive massage and the overuse of soap and water can be harmful.

Useful preventive measures include:

Regular changing of position (2 or 4 hourly).

Inspection of pressure areas at each change.

Keeping the skin clean and dry.

Avoiding friction and abrasion.

Changing linen when wet or soiled.

Using barrier creams for the incontinent.

Avoiding patched sheets.

Improving the patient's nutritional state.

Table 14.1
Assessment of a patient's risk of forming pressure sores (*From* Exton-Smith, A. N., Norton, D. & McLaren, R. (1962) *An Investigation of Geriatric Nursing Problems in Hospital*. Originally published by the National Corporation for the Care of Old People. Reprinted in 1975 by Churchill Livingstone, Edinburgh.)

Physical condition		Mental condition		Activity		Mobility		Incontinence	
Good	4	Alert	4	Ambulant	4	Full	4	Not incontinent	4
Fair	3	Apathetic	3	Walks with help	3	Slightly limited	3	Occasionally incontinent	3
Poor	2	Confused	2	Chair-bound	2	Very limited	2	Usually — urine	2
Bad	1	Stuporous	1	Bed-fast	1	Immobile	1	Doubly incontinent	1

Preventing sliding down the bed by use of a foot board, or slightly elevating the bed foot.

Lifting patients properly (Ch. 2).

Providing local protection for heels and elbows.

Where the patient's illness limits his ability to move or be moved, other aids may be necessary, for example:

Air rings.
Latex foam pads.
Sheepskins.
Pillow packs.
Ripple mattresses or water beds.

There is also a range of more sophisticated equipment, such as the Stryker frame, which is used in nursing spinal injuries (Ch. 3). Other devices include variations on the theme of the fluid-filled mattress. Whichever method is used, there is no substitute for the basic principles of prevention already mentioned, especially the early detection of 'at risk' patients.

Pressure sores should therefore never be regarded as inevitable. Though some will occur, early detection of skin damage and relief of pressure will prevent a superficial lesion becoming deep. Once established, every possible step must be taken to make sores heal as quickly as possible. Obviously further pressure must be avoided entirely. A diet rich in protein with sufficient carbohydrates and supplementary vitamins will aid tissue repair. Anaemia must be corrected, with blood transfusions if necessary.

Attention to the ulcer involves aseptic dressing technique, as would be practised for any wound. Infection is frequently a problem, so cleansing is necessary as well as the removal of dead tissue (sloughs). Swabs for bacterial examination must be taken to detect infection. A wide range of methods have been used in the treatment of pressure sores, in order to remove necrotic tissue and debris, to clear up infection and to promote healing. As cleansing agents, cetrimide, hydrogen peroxide and numerous others have been shown to be effective. Debrisan, composed of tiny porous beads, can be used in a paste form. Dressing materials used include melolin, silastic foam and Op-site. Other methods tried include sugar paste, karaya gum, ultra-violet radiation, massage with ultra-sound and hyperbaric oxygen. Again all are claimed to hasten healing. All in all, there is a bewildering range of substances and methods which have been tried, though little evidence available as to the most effective. A series of photographs or measurements taken during particular methods of treatment will help in evaluating their effectiveness.

Pressure sores heal more quickly if patients can be mobilized. This minimizes the effects of pressure and improves blood flow. Sores which are difficult to heal may eventually require plastic surgery.

Leg ulcers

Chronic leg ulcers are caused mostly by defective venous drainage from a limb. Adequate drainage depends on the pumping action of surrounding skeletal muscle and the presence of valves in the veins. It is significant that the only mammal to suffer from such ulcers is man, who is also the only one to have adopted the upright posture completely. Impairment of drainage often results from thrombophlebitis of deep leg veins (Ch. 7). Eventually valves become defective and blood becomes stagnant in the veins. Varicosities of superficial leg veins and chronic oedema of the lower part of the leg occur. Skin becomes undernourished and devitalized and may become eczematous. Sooner or later an ulcer forms, frequently precipitated by a trivial injury.

Other factors, such as pregnancy, obesity or intra-abdominal tumours, may also hinder venous drainage and lead to ulceration. Ulcers may also result from insufficiency of arterial blood supply. Arteriosclerosis of large arteries in the lower limb cuts down blood flow and, if severe enough, leads to gangrene. Small areas of skin gangrene will develop into ulcers on the legs and feet. Infection of ulcers frequently complicates the situation and hinders healing.

Figure 14.9
Leg ulcer in early stages of healing

Management

The management of varicose ulcers is aimed mainly at relieving the local oedema and improving venous drainage. If drainage is improved, oedema will subside and healing will begin (Fig. 14.9).

Reduction of weight

Since obesity is often a causative factor of ulcers, weight may have to be lost and the loss maintained.

Diet

A balanced diet containing protein and vitamins will also aid healing.

Exercise

Treatment of varicose ulcers in bed is rarely necessary. Walking should be encouraged and, when standing, calf muscles should be kept contracting and relaxing. When resting, keeping the legs above the level of the trunk promotes venous drainage.

Local treatment

Most methods of treating venous ulcers involve the use of compression bandages and may include local massage. First the ulcer crater is cleaned thoroughly with a solution such as normal saline or potassium permanganate. The skin around the edges may then be massaged, gradually working away from the ulcer. Strips of an impregnated bandage such as Uraband, Quinaband or Ichthaband are used to pack the crater. The same bandage is used to bandage the leg up to the knee. An adhesive bandage such as Lestreflex, with lengthways stretch only, is used as a compression bandage applied from the base of the toes up to the knee. Other substances used to promote healing after cleaning include karaya gum and zinc ointment. Charcoal preparations are sometimes used to reduce odour from an infected ulcer.

A week is allowed to elapse before the next treatment. After healing, support is still needed. *Tubigrip* is an alternative to elasticated stockings, which may be difficult for patients to put on properly. Recurrence of the ulcers means that varicose veins must be treated.

If the ulcers are due to impaired arterial supply, treatment is often doomed to failure and amputation may be necessary. Some ulcers will heal, but only with difficulty. It is important to screen such patients for diabetes mellitus (Ch. 11).

Patients with impaired arterial circulation must be educated in the care of the *ischaemic* limb in order to avoid injury. Cleanliness is essential, with daily washing in warm water and careful drying. The skin between the toes should receive particular attention. Woollen socks are less harmful than nylon but should be free from darns. Well-fitting footwear is necessary, and in cold weather fur-lined boots, though expensive, are valuable. Extra care is needed with corns and toe-nails; these should be left to the skills of a chiropodist.

BURNS

A burn is an injury to tissues which results from the application of heat (moist or dry), electricity, chemicals (acids or alkalis), radiation or friction. When a burn is superficial only the epidermis has been destroyed leaving some of the basal layer. Healing occurs without scarring within a few days. A deep dermal burn destroys the epidermis but leaves epithelial structures such as hair follicles and sweat glands in the dermis and spontaneous healing is still possible within a few weeks if infection does not occur. A full thickness burn involves complete skin destruction and possibly destruction of deeper tissues as well. This burn will only heal quickly and effectively with the aid of skin grafts.

Once skin has been destroyed two of its most important functions are lost — the prevention of loss of fluid from the body and protection against infection. Obviously, the more skin that is destroyed the greater will be the effects of losing these two functions. Thus in estimating the seriousness of a burn, the area of skin lost is a very useful guide. It is also useful initially as an indication of how much fluid has been lost and which must, therefore, be replaced quickly. Calculation of the area burned is easily and quickly carried out using the percentages given in Wallace's 'rule of nine' (see also Fig. 14.10). The size of the patient's hand is approximately 1% of the body surface. This method of measurement is useful when estimating small areas.

Estimation of the depth of a burn to establish the need for skin grafting is less straightforward. Guides to diagnosis include the temperature of the substance causing the burn, the time of contact, the site of the burn and whether or not the patient can feel a sharp prick with a sterile needle over many points of the burned area. When only epidermis is destroyed, regeneration will occur from epidermal cells left in sweat glands and sebaceous glands, as well as any remaining basal cell layer. However, if the dermis is also destroyed, regeneration cannot take place. A small amount of epithelium will grow inwards from the margin of the burns, but most healing will be by granulation followed by scar formation. The only way of minimizing this is by skin grafting.

Head 9%

Neck 1%

Arm 9%

Trunk: front 18%
back 18%

Leg 18%

Figure 14.10
Wallace's 'rule of nine'

Table 14.2
Percentage of body area of various parts

Area of body	% of body area
Surface of head	9
Surface of each upper limb	9
Surface of front of trunk	18
Surface of back of trunk	18
Surface of each lower limb	18
Surface of neck	1

Prevention of burns

There are many cases of burning each year and a great number are preventable. Most occur in the home and could be prevented by the exercise of a little common sense. The vulnerable groups are children between the ages of 1 and 15 years and the elderly. The following are among the most obvious preventive measures:

Young children should never be left alone in the house.
All fires should have approved guards.
Flexes of electrical appliances should be out of the reach of children.
Matches or lighters should never be left out.
Saucepan handles should be turned away from the front of cookers (which should preferably be fitted with guard rails).
Gas cookers are safer if placed away from draughts.
All electrical equipment and flexes should be properly maintained.
Inadequate lighting should be corrected.
When not in use, electrical appliances should be switched off and unplugged, especially at night and on leaving the house.
Care must be taken not to overload power points with too many appliances.
Containers of hot water should not be left unattended nor put on table-cloths, which may be pulled on by a child.
Flame-resistant clothing and nightwear is advisable for children.
Hot water bottles should be protected with a suitable cover.

First aid for burns

The first step is to remove the cause of the burns or extinguish the flames. This can be accomplished by wrapping the part or person in a rug or blanket to exclude air (providing the rug is not made of synthetic material). The first step in dealing with electrical burns is to switch off the current and, if necessary, stop any machinery. Burning clothing must be removed, though not if charred and adherent to the body.

Burned patients are severely shocked. Initially this is neurogenic shock due to pain, but it quickly becomes *oligaemic* as a result of fluid loss and reduction in the volume of circulating blood. Casualties should therefore rest, preferably lying down. Superficial burns should be immersed in cold water or held under cold running water. This cools the part and reduces pain. Also important in minimizing shock is reassurance. Oral fluids may be given, though only small quantities at a time are advisable in case of vomiting.

Scalds will necessitate the removal of soaked clothing. All that is necessary is for the burned area to be covered with clean, dry material, such as part of a clean sheet or a pillow-case. No other substance should be applied.

With chemical burns, as much of the chemical as possible should be washed off with cold running water. A bath or shower may be necessary if large areas are affected.

Finally, there must be no delay in getting the victim to hospital. It must be borne in mind that even a burn of a small area can cause considerable shock, so the patient should be seen in a hospital casualty department.

Hospital care

Shock

In hospital, the primary objective of treatment is to lessen shock, which may be life-threatening. Burns of 10% or more in children and 15% or more in adults can produce shock severe enough to kill. Before treatment begins, a quick assessment of the patient is necessary, though it should not delay treatment. Records of temperature, pulse, respiration rates and blood pressure are essential and should be taken at 15-minute intervals. A blood sample is taken in order to carry out a haemoglobin estimation and *haematocrit*. Fluid replacement begins with an intravenous infusion. A self-retaining catheter is inserted into the bladder and measurement of urinary output is carried out hourly, as well as a record of all fluid intake. The extent of the surface area burned is also considered when deciding on the amount of fluid which should be replaced. Most fluid is lost in the first few hours, so replacement is greatest at that time. Less fluid can be given after the first 24 hours. Nasal, throat and rectal swabs are taken from the patient because of the risk of autoinfection. Pain is severe, particularly in superficially burned areas where nerve endings have not been destroyed, therefore analgesia is given. Regular observation of the patient's vital signs and fluid balance are continued until his condition improves. If the patient was burned in a house fire it is particularly important to note any difficulty in breathing which might arise following inhalation of fumes from burning upholstery.

Fluids

As was noted before, replacement of fluids is a matter of urgency. Since plasma has been lost, plasma is the most suitable replacement. This will maintain osmotic pressure within capillaries and prevent leakage of water into the tissues, a process which would decrease the circulating blood volume and increase shock. *Dextran* solution (high molecular weight), sometimes referred to as a 'plasma expander', has a similar effect. The oral intake of fluids should be encouraged unless vomiting occurs. In the early stages, restriction to 30 or 60 ml of fluid per hour by mouth will help prevent vomiting.

Infection

Prevention of infection is second only in importance to controlling shock and initially the burned areas are covered with sterile sheets. When the patient's condition permits, the burn is cleaned carefully under general anaesthesia. All dead tissue and foreign material are removed. Blisters are snipped with sterile scissors. As well as the risk of septicaemia, infection delays healing and may cause unsatisfactory results. Important among preventive principles are:

Routine nasal swabs from all staff.
Exclusion and treatment of nasal carriers of pathogens.
Exclusion of all staff with respiratory infections and septic skin lesions.
The use of barrier nursing techniques.
The use of sterile bed linen if the exposure method of treating the burn is used.

It should also go without saying that a high standard of environmental hygiene is imperative.

Local treatment

After the initial treatment of a burn, two principal methods of management are available.

Exposure

This allows cooling and drying of the burned surface. Bacterial growth is inhibited by drying and a protective *eschar* forms. In time this will separate and infection beneath it is likely. Surgical excision of the eschar is carried out before this can happen, followed by skin grafting. The advantage of the exposure method is that the risk of infection is minimized and a clean wound suitable for skin grafting is provided. Patients are also generally more comfortable. Total barrier nursing is essential, in a room where the air is filtered and a temperature of 25° or 26°C can be maintained because considerable heat loss occurs. Sterile bed linen is also necessary.

Occlusion

This method, using occlusive dressings, has many disadvantages. The most serious being that dressings quickly become saturated with exudate from the burn and are an admirable medium for bacterial growth. The dressing agent must be non-irritant and non-toxic such as silver sulphadiazine cream and gauze to prevent sticking. It must be covered with layers of sterile absorbent material in a thick pad. The dressing must extend 8 or 10 cm beyond the edges of the burn and be held in place with a crepe bandage. Infection is difficult to prevent, and the patient is uncomfortable. The frequency of redressing depends on the type of medication used and whether there are signs of infection.

Hand burns. To allow the maximum movement of hands the following method of dressing is valuable. Silver sulphadiazine cream (Flamazine) is applied to the burn and the hand covered with a polythene bag. The bag is secured loosely at the wrist by a bandage applied over a layer of cotton wool. At least once each day the hand is cleansed with for instance Betadine followed by reapplication of the cream and a new bag. In this way movement is unhindered, the risk of contractures reduced, and the patient afforded some independence. Elevation of the hands when not in use will minimize swelling.

Skin grafting. Destruction of the skin means that its regeneration is impossible. Unless a skin covering is provided, infection is inevitable and scar tissue will form. A covering for the raw area is provided by split-skin grafts taken from elsewhere on the body and placed on the surface in sheets. The donor area will regenerate its own epithelium from that left in hair follicles and sweat glands; the process takes 2 to 3 weeks. It may be difficult to find sufficient skin to cover a large area, so to provide immediate covering in very extensive burns where the situation is urgent, a *homograft* may be used. This will be rejected in time but can be life-saving.

Skin grafting is usually carried out from 5 to 10 days after the injury. During this time, dead tissue will have been removed, infection controlled and the patient's nutritional state improved. The main concern in caring for the grafted area is to prevent displacement of the graft. Unless infection occurs it may be left covered for about a week then dressed under general anaesthetic, when sutures are removed.

It has been found that deep dermal burns will heal more quickly if grafts can be applied directly on to living dermis, having first removed the surface of the burn by successive slices of damaged tissue. This is known as tangential incision and is carried out, one area at a time, starting within the first few days of injury. Short parallel cuts in the skin graft applied allow it to expand to form a mesh. This enables a larger area to be covered and the epidermis spreads to cover the mesh spaces. Initially following application of the graft blood and serum need to be evacuated frequently but this method reduces infection risks and accelerates healing.

When healing has occurred, usually 3 to 4 weeks, elasticated pressure garments or crepe bandages are worn during the day for several months. These help to minimize swelling and prevent breakdown of the grafted area. Gentle massage of the graft with hand cream such as Atrixo or Nivea helps to keep the skin soft. The donor area is protected by a dressing of Sofra-tulle and left undisturbed for about 2 weeks. When healing is complete the dressing automatically separates from the skin.

Nutrition

Burned patients require a diet rich in protein and high in kilojoules. Daily protein intake should be as high as 150 g, and 16 000 or more kJ should be supplied, depending on the patient's weight. Extra vitamins, especially vitamin C, are also necessary. Correction of anaemia may necessitate the administration of oral iron.

In the early stages, the situation is likely to be complicated by the fact that the patient is severely ill and unlikely to be able to take a normal diet. Nasogastric feeding may then become necessary. Extensive burns may lead to some red cell destruction and the need for blood transfusion, requiring the appropriate care (Ch. 8).

Nursing the burned patient

All the above points require considerable expertise and technical skill. It must also be remembered that basic care, such as washing and treatment of pressure areas, is necessary and will demand considerable patience. Even apparently simple matters such as making the patient comfortable in bed require imagination and ingenuity. Inconceivable difficulties can arise for the patient even when using the bedpan or feeding himself.

The aspect of nursing burned patients most likely to tax the nurse's skill to the utmost is that of maintaining the morale of the patient. It is stating the obvious to say that kindness, sympathy and patience are essential qualities; however, firmness and the ability to encourage self-help rather than dependence are also necessary. Above all, the nurse must remember that the eventual objective is to rehabilitate the patient, returning him to as near normal a life as possible.

NURSING CARE OF PATIENTS WITH SKIN DISORDERS

Rashes, spots and blisters on the skin can be so readily seen that patients are extremely conscious of them, and also very sensitive to the reactions of others to their appearance.

Patients with severe skin disorders will therefore benefit from being nursed in a dermatology unit. Here they will see other patients with similar conditions making progress, and be cared for by nursing and medical staff with expert knowledge. In these units the emotional needs of patients are taken into account, and, as they are not usually incapacitated, they can mix together on a social basis.

Many patients with diseases of the skin do not need to be admitted to hospital, but can be treated as out-patients and care for their skins at home with the help of the family. Regular attendance at clinics provides the psychological support and practical advice necessary. Admission to hospital only occurs as the result of an acute exacerbation of the disease.

Although it can be very demanding, nursing patients with skin disease can be greatly rewarding and enjoyable. It is one of the branches of nursing where the nurse is frequently involved in the long term support of a patient and often his family as well. By taking a problem solving approach to care it is possible to meet the individual needs of the patient more readily. Several skin disorders present with itching and, or the presence of a rash or bullae and the aims of care are to reduce the itching to a minimum and promote good healing, with the minimum of emotional trauma. The following principles of care will help the nurse to achieve these aims and to understand the problems encountered by patients and their families. She can help them both at home and whilst in hospital, and she can evaluate the effectiveness of her care by noting the patient's progress.

Alleviation of itching

Itching can be exhausting and frustrating for the patient. It is first of all essential to observe when itching occurs and to attempt to discover the reason for it. The problem may be more severe at night for example, or be aggravated by a particular food or drug. Rest is as important for an inflamed skin as for any other inflamed organ of the body. While it may seem unnecessary to the patient, he should rest in bed initially for a short period to reduce any external stimuli. Mild sedation is sometimes prescribed to help achieve this rest.

The environment should not be too hot, with adequate ventilation, light bed clothes and loose cotton nightwear rather than nylon or wool. Foods that may

Figure 14.11
Avoid overheating

Figure 14.12
Avoid foods causing flushing

Figure 14.13
Adequate fluid intake

Figure 14.14
Avoid 'self-medication'

produce flushing of the skin such as hot, strong tea or coffee, spices or alcohol should be avoided.

The danger of causing secondary infection by scratching must be explained to the patient. Sometimes it is necessary, with a very young child, to apply splints or cotton gloves to prevent the skin being damaged in this way.

If lotions or creams are to be used they should be applied directly after the patient has had a warm bath (33.5–35.5°C) and his skin has been gently dried.

An over anxious patient will be more prone to scratching and if the nurse can help him to identify and deal with his problems he will become more relaxed, and in turn the intensity of itching will be reduced.

Maintenance of body fluid

When a large amount of fluid is lost due to formation of *bullae* or in the form of exudate then there must be adequate replacement of fluid by mouth. The patient will also require a diet high in protein to replenish losses.

Emotional adjustment

The nurse can be an active agent in promoting and helping her patient to achieve a state of mind and an attitude towards his skin condition which not only will hasten recovery, but may minimize recurrences of it. She can develop a relationship with her patient which is characterized by his confidence in her, and in which he becomes an equal partner in his care. She must know the effects of skin disease, both conscious and unconscious, on her patient's emotional state. She must also be able to relate these to the severity of the disorder and to the patient's behaviour. Only in this way can the nurse maintain an approach to her patient which is supportive, positive and objective yet sympathetic. The nurse's own behaviour is of paramount importance. She must overcome the natural revulsion that occurs on seeing some forms of skin disease for the first few times, and on no account allow any expression or implication of revulsion or distaste to occur.

Positive steps can be taken to establish communication by taking the patient's hand to examine his fingers or nails. Some of the simple creams can be applied directly by hand if they do not contain steroid preparations. The nurse can also encourage relatives to take part in applying treatment and therefore getting used to touching the patient's skin.

Taking time to sit and talk to her patient also implies that the nurse is not reluctant to spend time in his company.

Apart from the disorders mentioned on page 534 few conditions are infectious or contagious. Patients and relatives need to be aware of this and patients should be encouraged to mix freely together to chat or watch television once they are no longer confined to bed.

Avoidance of further skin damage

When the patient is bathed it is important to remove moisture from the skin gently by patting dry with a soft towel rather than rubbing a towel briskly on a tender skin. Simple Soap or Emulsifying Ointment B.P. are both suitable cleansers for use in the bath.

No form of 'self medication' should be used by the patient, for example proprietary antiseptics, which if added to the bath water may cause further damage to the inflamed skin. Aperients containing phenolphthalein should also be avoided because it may cause a drug eruption.

Topical treatment should be applied to lesions only, not the surrounding healthy skin.

Efficient application of medication

The nurse must follow the instructions of prescriptions carefully when applying topical medication. If a patient is to apply medication at home it is usual to give him written instructions which he can read and refer to at leisure. It is important to

Figure 14.15
Patch test — positive. (Courtesy
of Department of Medical
Illustration, North Staffordshire
Hospital Centre)

ensure that he fully understands these and this is a further opportunity to involve
relatives and help them to understand how best they can assist the patient.

Rehabilitation

When an acute exacerbation of a skin disorder has settled, the patient should return
to work whenever possible. Occasionally it may be necessary for him to consider a
different occupation if it is established that work conditions or some form of irritant
or allergen related to his work caused the exacerbation. In cases of this sort,
substances known to irritate the skin must be avoided. Sometimes identification of
the irritating agent can be confirmed by the use of *patch tests* (Fig. 14.15).

Where the skin of the hands is involved, then it is advisable that they are
protected when carrying out wet work by wearing rubber gloves lined with cotton
ones.

Special cover creams are available which will help to disguise scars or marks on
the skin. This is particularly important if the skin of the face is involved. Young
adolescents with acne for example need a great deal of help and encouragement to
maintain a normal life-style.

Topical skin treatments

These are varied as no one treatment is beneficial to all patients or beneficial for the
same patient when a skin disorder is at different stages.

Baths, paints, lotions, creams, ointments or pastes may be prescribed singly or
sometimes for use in conjunction with each other. It is important to use the treatment in the prescribed form.

Baths

A bath for the patient before application of dressings will help to remove any exudate
or crusts that have formed on the skin. Dilute potassium permanganate solution may

Figure 14.16
Wet dressings
1. Soak strips of linen in solution
2. Apply strips to overlap each other
3. Cover with tubular gauze bandage

Figure 14.17
Ointment spread dressings
1. Prepare the spread
2. Apply the strips of linen, each piece overlapping the previous strip by two-thirds
3. Secure with tubular gauze or elasticated net

be prescribed for addition to the bath to reduce the risk of secondary infection developing, and other medicated baths may also be prescribed.

Paints

These may be applied directly to the area required using cotton wool or a small soft brush.

Lotions

Lotions are cooling to the skin and will frequently help to relieve itching. Simple lotions e.g., Calamine Lotion B.P. may be dabbed on the skin as frequently as the patient desires. Some lotions may be applied in the form of wet dressings (Fig. 14.16) of cotton or linen soaked in the solution. If this method is used then the dressings must be constantly kept in a wet state by adding further lotion or renewing them daily or twice daily. The patient's bed may need to be protected by use of a polythene sheet during treatment.

Creams

These also have a cooling effect on the skin as the water content evaporates but they may need to be reapplied liberally three to four times daily. If dressings are used they should be of cotton or linen as gauze allows the cream to seep through the mesh and is therefore ineffective.

Ointments

Ointments are greasier and may be rubbed in gently and covered with tubular gauze. An ointment may also be spread thinly on to a piece of linen, torn into strips and applied to the area, each strip overlapping the previous one (Fig. 14.17). These are renewed daily and if large areas are to be covered then ideally the patient will wear a pair of old cotton pyjamas in place of the linen strips.

Pastes

Pastes are much thicker and may be applied either using a wooden spatula or a gloved hand. The area is then covered with the tubular gauze.

Paste impregnated bandages are also available which may be left in place for 1 to 3 weeks. Pastes will not wash off the skin but can be removed gently using swabs soaked in olive or arachis oil.

Steroid preparations

When these are prescribed they must be used sparingly and with care and on the relevant lesions only, the nurse being sure she does not get them on her own skin. Steroids are also prescribed in a diluted form.

Occasionally, polythene occlusive dressings are prescribed to enhance the effect of these preparations. The area to be treated is smeared with the prescribed cream and covered with a piece of polythene. The air is excluded from beneath and the edges sealed with adhesive tape. This dressing is left in place for several hours. This method of treatment tends to be reserved for particularly stubborn lesions because of the possible complications, which include increased absorption of steroids, development of infection in the area covered, atrophy of the skin, and development of striae in the area treated.

SOME COMMON SKIN DISORDERS

It has been said, and often quoted that the skin can be affected by anything under the sun, including the sun. Practically any substance which comes into contact with the skin may cause a reaction in some individual. Particularly potent in this respect are chemicals, more of which are being manufactured daily, and used with increasing frequency both in the home and in industry.

Eczema

Eczema and dermatitis are interchangeable terms describing a process taking place in the skin. The epidermis develops small areas of oedema called primary vesicles. Serous fluid escapes when these vesicles are damaged. As the condition becomes more chronic the epidermis becomes thickened, especially if the patient rubs or scratches the area continually. Painful cracks may also appear.

Classification of eczema is difficult because there are so many types, with characteristics of more than one type sometimes appearing in the same patient. The eczema may follow repeated contact with substances such as chemicals or plants causing an allergic or hypersensitive reaction. This is known as contact eczema (Fig. 14.18). Some nurses develop it following handling of penicillin solutions or wearing rubber gloves. Although contact may be at one point of the body only, the entire skin may become sensitized. Therefore a patient might be in a very distressed state because areas of his skin are weeping and itching, not associating this reaction with a single point of contact.

Figure 14.18
Contact eczema from rubber in bra (Courtesy of Department of Medical Illustration, North Staffordshire Hospital Centre)

When the reaction has settled down then *patch tests* help in identifying the substance, which can then be avoided. Some substances, known as primary irritants, will produce an eczematous reaction on any person's skin if left in contact for a sufficient length of time. These may be caustic substances such as strong chemical solvents or weaker ones such as detergents.

Table 14.3
Substances commonly leading to sensitisation

Cosmetics	perfume or lanolin
Clothes	rubber, dyes
Plants	primula obconica
Chemicals	antibiotics, topical antihistamines
Metal	nickel studs on jeans, ear-rings
Cement	
Resins	

Table 14.4
Some types of endogenous eczema

Type	Age group	Area of body involved
Atopic	Usually appears at approximately three months	Face, scalp, arms, legs
	Toddlers, young children May persist into adult life	Flexures
Seborrhoeic	Infants	Scalp, forehead, napkin area
	Adults	Face
Nummular or discoid	Young and middle aged	Limbs
Pompholyx	Young adults	Palms and soles
Varicose/stasis	Elderly, poor circulation	Lower leg

In endogenous or constitutional eczema the classification tends to be related to the pattern and distribution of the lesions on the body surface (see Table 14.4). One of the commonest types is atopic eczema (Fig. 14.19) which appears in babies a few weeks after birth. As the child grows the flexures become involved and itching may be intense. There is frequently an associated hay fever or asthma in the patient and a family history of similar disorders.

Figure 14.19
Atopic eczema (Courtesy of Department of Medical Illustration, North Staffordshire Hospital Centre)

Treatment

Treatment of eczema is elimination of any aggravating factor if possible, rest and sedation if the eczema is widespread and application of prescribed medication according to the state of the skin. Wet dressings or paints are applied when the skin is very inflamed, and creams, ointments or pastes when the skin is dry and scaly.

Psoriasis

In normal skin the cells of the epidermis move upwards from the basal layer and are shed in approximately 25 to 28 days. In psoriasis this process is speeded up and

Figure 14.20
Chronic psoriasis, elbow
(Courtesy of Department of
Medical Illustration, North
Staffordshire Hospital Centre)

areas of the skin have an increased proliferation of epidermal cells presenting as raised red plaques covered by silvery scales. The extent of the lesions may vary from one or two small patches, which present little problem, to widespread chronic plaques causing major disability. Fingernails, toenails and the scalp may also be involved. Pustular psoriasis of the palms and soles may occur with or without involvement elsewhere and tends to be very resistant to treatment. The scalp is particularly difficult to treat because of the hair.

Treatment

This is aimed at remission of the disorder as there is no permanent cure. Individual patients may benefit from different treatments. Topical and systemic steroids are only occasionally used because quite often there is a rebound occurrence of the lesions when treatment is stopped. Dithranol may be prescribed topically in soft yellow paraffin or Lassar's paste. This is suitable for patients who have to be admitted to hospital because their psoriasis is particularly disabling. At the present time photochemotherapy (PUVA) is being used in some areas of Britain with success. Its effect is to reduce cell *DNA* synthesis and therefore slow down cell proliferation. The treatment involves patients taking a psoralen preparation followed after approximately 2 hours by exposure to long wave ultra-violet light (UVA) for a short time. Initially three treatments weekly are given, reduced to one at intervals of 1 to 3 weeks as maintenance. An artificial source of UVA is used with a bank of lamps arranged either over a couch or in a booth in which the patient stands (Fig. 14.21). It is very important that the patient's eyes are protected by polaroid goggles during treatment. Eyes and skin must be protected against direct sunlight for approximately 12 hours following treatment as the psoralen preparation increases skin photosensitivity. The long term effects of PUVA treatment are still being evaluated with reference to premature ageing of the skin, skin cancer and cataracts.

Systemic treatments that may be used for exceptionally severe psoriasis are anti-mitotic drugs such as methotrexate or Razoxane. These are generally effective but may have adverse effects on the bone marrow and, in the case of methotrexate, on the liver. Therefore any patient receiving this treatment must be closely supervised medically. Etretinate is also undergoing clinical assessment for treatment of psoriasis

Figure 14.21
PUVA treatment

but this, as antimitotic drugs, is only used for selected patients under close supervision and never in pregnancy. Many patients with psoriasis continue to persevere at home with tar preparations or other topical treatments. They can gain much psychological and practical support from the Psoriasis Association, 7 Milton Street, Northampton NN2 7JG.

Basal cell carcinoma

This is a malignant local tumour which arises from the basal cell layer of the epidermis but rarely metastasizes. It is often known as a rodent ulcer which in its commonest form begins as a small *papule* spreading outwards leaving a central ulcer that fails to heal. The edges are raised and pearly. Basal cell carcinoma usually occurs on the face and is a condition mainly of the middle-aged or elderly. It affects, particularly, fair skinned people who have spent a great deal of time in sunshine. It is a very common condition in Australia: in Britain it tends to occur in people who have spent most of their working lives out of doors or who have had some form of arsenic therapy many years before.

Treatment

Following biopsy to confirm diagnosis, radiotherapy or surgical excision are the main treatments of choice and patients will normally be treated on an out-patient basis.

Squamous cell carcinoma

Squamous cell carcinoma also arises in the epidermis but is more likely to metastasize. The tumour begins as a small *nodule* which grows to become oval or circular. It may develop into an ulcer with rolled edges. This cancer may arise on the face, lips or back of the hand. These are areas exposed to sunlight but they could have been exposed to chronic trauma or carcinogens such as oil or tar.

Treatment

Following diagnosis by biopsy, treatment is either surgical excision or radiotherapy or both and if treatment is carried out early then prognosis is good.

Figure 14.22
Basal cell carcinoma, nose
(Courtesy of Department of
Medical Illustration, North
Staffordshire Hospital Centre)

Figure 14.23
Squamous cell carcinoma, ear
(Courtesy of Department of
Medical Illustration, North
Staffordshire Hospital Centre)

Drug reactions

Almost any drug given systemically is capable of causing a skin reaction. Some people taking penicillin may develop *urticaria* or a widespread *erythema*, whereas sulphonamides may produce a bullous eruption. Not all drug reactions are allergic. Individuals may have an intolerance to some drugs due to impaired function of the liver or kidney. In this instance the drug cannot be excreted. It builds up to a toxic level and a skin reaction may occur. The drug may have been taken for some time before the reaction occurs. It is important to remember that patients may not even class medications as drugs if they are very familiar with them, for example aspirin.

Treatment

Once the suspected drug has been discontinued, treatment is largely symptomatic. This is a condition in which the nurse who adheres to the previously mentioned principles of skin care can really feel rewarded at seeing the speedy recovery of her patient.

The patient must be made aware of the name of the suspected drug so that he can avoid taking it in the future. Information on drug reactions should always be recorded clearly in the patient's case notes.

INFECTIONS OF THE SKIN

Impetigo

The common causative micro-organism is the staphylococcus, although frequently the streptococcus is also present. Impetigo is usually the result of autoinfection, staphylococci carried in the nose being transferred to the skin by the hands and inoculated by scratching. The scratching may be caused by itching rashes, scabies or lice. Children are especially liable to damage the skin in this way. In men, impetigo may be spread over the face by shaving. Vesicles form, followed by crusting; removal of crusts may actually impede the healing going on beneath. The

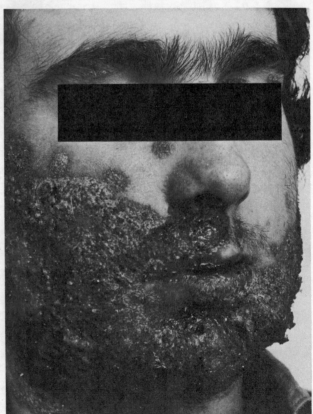

Figure 14.24
Impetigo (Courtesy of Mr McIntyre, Department of Medical Photography, Victoria Hospital, Kirkcaldy)

condition is more unsightly than dangerous (Fig. 14.24) except in babies, in whom it can be fatal. Usually an antibiotic ointment such as Aureomycin clears the condition quickly; widespread lesions may respond to antiseptic baths or may require systemic antibiotic therapy.

Spread of infection to others must be prevented by keeping face flannels and towels separate. Bed linen must not be used by anyone else, and hair-brushes and combs should be used only by the infected person.

Boils

These common infections of hair follicles occur singly or in groups and may recur. As susceptibility to infection is a complication of diabetes mellitus, people who have outbreaks of boils should be screened for this disease by having their urine tested. Eventually a boil will come to a point, rupture and discharge its contents. This will be followed by healing. Interference with boils should be kept to a minimum. Boils on the face are potentially serious, as septic material may find its way into the bloodstream if they are squeezed and this infection may spread to the brain. The only local treatment necessary is cleansing with antiseptic and application of a protective dressing. Locally applied antibiotic creams may help. Nasal swabs may be taken to identify micro-organisms carried in the patient's anterior nares and to enable specific treatment to be applied.

Spread of infection is especially likely when the boil is discharging. Therefore, frequent change of dry, sterile dressings is important. Carbuncles are similar to boils except that a large area of *necrosis* occurs; they point at a number of places and discharge through multiple *sinuses*. Patients are usually ill, have a pyrexia and should rest in bed. Systemic antibiotic therapy is usually needed.

Erysipelas

The same micro-organism which causes scarlet fever, the haemolytic streptococcus, also causes erysipelas. It usually enters through a break in the skin. At the onset, patients are usually quite ill and pyrexial. The skin around the point of entry becomes inflamed and swollen and there is direct spread of infection to adjacent skin. The face is the commonest site of infection with the organism entering through a small crack in the nostril. The condition responds well to penicillin, administered orally or intramuscularly.

Warts

These are very common virus infections of the skin. They occur often among school children, probably because of the opportunity to spread via towels, swimming pools and gymnasium floors. Most children lose their warts within a few years. Warts on the soles of the feet are known as verrucae or plantar warts. They are painful because of the pressure on them. Warts may be treated in a variety of ways, including the application of carbon dioxide snow, silver nitrate or podophyllin combined with salicylic acid in jelly form. Diathermy can also be used. Verrucae are usually treated with carbon dioxide snow or removed surgically.

Herpes simplex

A cold sore in the lip is a common example of herpes simplex. It is believed that, once acquired, the virus lies dormant, erupting only from time to time and often in association with the common cold, influenza or pneumonia. The lesion clears up in about 10 days. There is no specific treatment although antiviral agents might be prescribed and an antibiotic cream will prevent secondary bacterial infection.

Herpes zoster

Commonly known as shingles, this painful rash is caused by the virus of chickenpox. The patient is usually adult and not uncommonly elderly when both the rash and the pain, which may persist long after the skin lesion has cleared, cause considerable distress. The virus attacks a posterior root ganglion of the spinal cord and travels along a sensory nerve fibre to reach the nerve endings. A vesicular rash outlines the path of the affected nerve. Treatment consists of analgesics for the very severe pain which occurs. Isolation from as many people as possible prevents spread, especially to children. If, as occasionally happens, the trigeminal nerve is involved, vesicles occur on the face and may cause corneal ulceration on the affected side (Ch. 12).

Fungus infections

The commonest fungus infections of the skin are ringworm and athlete's foot (tinea pedis). Ringworm usually affects the scalp but may affect other parts of the body as well. Recently there has been a decline in scalp ringworm, which is mainly caused by a variety of fungus acquired from cattle. Griseofulvin, an antifungal antibiotic, is effective in treating ringworm but involves a long process of treatment.

Athlete's foot is almost impossible to eradicate completely. Griseofulvin will allay the symptoms but the infection invariably reappears. It may be impossible to decide if it is a relapse or a reinfection, for instance, by other members of the household. Various local applications, each containing a fungicide in a cream base, are available. Castellani's paint helps, as does *Whitfield's ointment*, but neither is used much now.

SKIN INFESTATIONS

Scabies and lice are two of the most common infestations of the skin.

Scabies

Figure 14.25
Acarus scabiei

Scabies is caused by a mite, the acarus scabiei (Fig. 14.25), and is acquired by direct contact with another person. Several weeks elapse before the main characteristic — itching — commences. Meanwhile the female mite burrows her way into the skin and lays her eggs. These hatch into mites. The burrows can be seen as dark lines about 1½ cm long, usually between fingers, on wrists and in flexures. Scratching causes excoriation and may lead to secondary bacterial infection. Spread to others can occur as a result of prolonged, intimate contact, and nurses and doctors are at risk from infested patients.

Treatment is effective if carried out properly and if it includes all members of the family. First a bath is taken and the whole body thoroughly washed. The whole body surface is painted, from the neck down to the toes, with Quellada. When this has dried, the patient may dress in clean clothing. Each time the patient's hands are washed the paint must be reapplied to them. After 24 hours, a bath may be taken again. Usually one treatment is adequate, though a second may be given if necessary.

Table 14.5
Examples of common drugs prescribed topically in skin disorders

Drug	Brand name	Preparation	Condition
Betamethasone valerate	Betnovate	Lotion, cream, ointment	Eczema
Crude coal tar		In Lassar's paste	Psoriasis
Dithranol	Dithrocream	Cream	Chronic psoriasis
Gamma benzene hexachloride	Quellada	Paint	Scabies, lice
Hydrocortisone acetate	Hydrocortone	Cream, ointment	Eczema
Zinc paste and ichthammol	Ichthopaste	Impregnated bandage	Eczema
Potassium permanganate solution		Wet dressings, baths	Eczema

Figure 14.26
Pediculus capitis

Lice

Three types of lice infest the human body, **head lice** (pediculus capitis) (Fig. 14.26), **body lice** (pediculus corporis) and **pubic lice** (pediculus pubis). Head lice are the most common and, in spite of generally good standards of hygiene, are still prevalent among many children. Spread occurs easily in schools, so that lice may be found on children whose standard of hygiene at home is high. Head lice live on human blood and lay eggs (nits) which adhere to the hair with a cement-like substance. DDT preparations, never effective for nits, have become less harmful to lice also. However, malathion, in the form of Prioderm lotion, kills both lice and nits.

Body lice lay their eggs in the seams of clothing, and an effective way of dealing with them is by dusting with DDT powder. A bath, followed by dressing in clean clothing should result in freedom from infestation.

SUGGESTED ASSIGNMENTS

1. Draw and label a diagram of the skin and the underlying structures. Show the position of the needle when an intramuscular injection has been given correctly.

2. How would you respond in the following situations?

   a. A friend has a 75-year-old grandmother being nursed at home following a 'stroke' and is worried about pressure sores developing.

   b. You are asked to talk to a group of teenagers at their school and to discuss the effect on the health of the skin of cosmetics and some types of occupation.

3. The skin, being on the outside of the body, is exposed to many harmful agents. It may also reflect internal disturbances, both physiological and psychological. Discuss the value of observing the skin of patients to the diagnosis and treatment of their illnesses.

4. A 17-year-old girl in your ward is recovering from extensive burns to her right arm and neck. Give an account of the emotional problems you might expect her to experience and of how you would help her to cope with these.

FURTHER READING

Cason J 1981 Treatment of burns. Chapman and Hall, London

Fry L, Wojnarowska T, Shahrad P 1981 Illustrated encyclopaedia of dermatology. Update Publications London

Huckbody E 1977 Nursing procedures for skin diseases. Churchill Livingstone, Edinburgh

Mackie R 1983 Eczema and dermatitis. Martin Dunitz, London

Marks R 1983 Psoriasis. Martin Dunitz, London

Pegum J S, Baker H 1979 Dermatology, 3rd edn. Bailliere Tindall, London

Torrance C 1983 Pressure sores, aetiology, treatment and prevention. Croom Helm, London

Wilkinson D S 1977 The nursing management of skin diseases, 4th edn. Faber, London

Chapter Fifteen
Mental handicap

This chapter is merely an outline of mental handicap. It is intended as an introduction for nurses who will be gaining experience in this field during training.

A student nurse's first experience in a unit for mentally handicapped people may be somewhat of a surprise, for a number of reasons. These units are run as homes, since most of the residents will spend the greater part of their lives in them. Mentally handicapped people are not to be expected to adapt to an existing ward routine; indeed they may be quite unable to do so. A primary objective of care is to meet their psychological needs, and their environment is arranged with this in mind.

It may also seem strange, to discover that the staff are far less concerned with diagnosis than with each person's abilities and potential for development. The arrangement of material in this chapter takes account of this difference in emphasis. The general approach to the management and care of mentally handicapped people appears first. A brief description of the causes, methods of diagnosis and the general features of individuals with mental deficits is given towards the end of the chapter.

CARE OF THE MENTALLY HANDICAPPED

At one time care consisted of providing a secure environment. It is realized now that many of these people have capacities for development; consequently opportunities and stimulation should be provided to enable and encourage them to attain their highest potential.

Philosophy

The mentally handicapped person is a human being with not only the right to life but the right to a quality of life in keeping with human dignity. Services for the mentally handicapped ideally should have the attainment of this right as their main objective. This presupposes the development of potential no matter how limited the final achievement may be.

The multidisciplinary approach to assessment

Assessment is carried out on a multidisciplinary basis. The mentally handicapped person's needs are assessed and individual programmes are tailored to meet these needs. Reassessment is an essential part of any programme to evaluate progress and for further planning.

Medical assessment is carried out by paediatricians, psychiatrists and orthopaedic and ENT surgeons. Clinical and educational psychologists have much to contribute in assessment, programme planning and remedial advice. Speech therapists, physiotherapists, occupational therapists, remedial gymnasts musical therapists, and teachers all have expertise which is invaluable in assessment. The social worker takes a full social history, which is necessary in identifying family problems. The nurse specially trained in mental handicap nursing is in a unique position in the assessment team. Nurses collectively are with the person 24 hours a day and are therefore able to observe behaviour patterns, frequency and types of epilepsy, communication problems, abilities in the activities of daily living and reactions to medication.

In recording behaviour, one of the most popular and useful charts available is the Gunzburg Progress Assessment Chart of Social Development. There are several types. Each type contains a useful chart of abilities related to self-help, communication, socialization and occupation and, properly used, these records show at a glance the areas in which the person has developed skills and where progress has yet to be made.

The multidisciplinary approach to management

Mental handicap is a 'life-sized' problem because in most cases there is no cure; therefore, the mentally handicapped person needs programmed management that extends from birth throughout his life. Mental handicap is a multifaceted problem: it occurs in childhood, but mentally handicapped children grow up; therefore services must provide for all age groups and for varying levels of intelligence.

Efficient management can only be achieved through a multidisciplinary approach where each 'specialist' uses his skills to develop the individual's potential to the fullest. Services should be the responsibility of a multidisciplinary team serving an area. The family with a mentally handicapped child is a family with stress: for the parents there is the strain of knowing that the problem will remain throughout their child's life, and for the other children a handicapped brother or sister can cause various problems. The family needs to be in touch from the very beginning with some person or group who can not only give support but also offer concrete, practical advice about programmed management all along the line. Ideally, services should provide early identification of the handicap, assessment of the potential development, a planned schedule from childhood through to adulthood and genetic counselling. The pivot of such services would be residential accommodation on either a long- or a short-term basis.

The physical environment

The ward, home unit or group home should be imaginative and as home-like as possible, with colours, textures and ornamentation used skilfully to provide sensory stimulation; but there should also be a more subdued, restful area where patients can relax and be quiet on occasion. This is important for all age groups. Where rooms are set aside for specific learning activities, however, it is more practical to have the minimum of distracting stimuli so that the person with the patient does

Figure 15.1
Restful area where patients can relax

not have to compete for his attention. Necessary materials can be brought in for the session. In this way the environment can be manipulated to promote learning.

Adequate ventilation, heating and lighting are also very important. In some instances extractor fans may be necessary to allow the air in a room to be changed quickly. Lighting can be used effectively in adding to the overall home-like effect. Surfaces should be easily cleaned. Facilities for bathing and toilet training should be adequate both functionally and in providing privacy. In children's units play equipment of a suitable type should be provided as well as the space to store it.

Experiments have shown that ideally patients should be cared for in small groups in a family-like situation with good staff ratios. The environment must also be safe as the mentally handicapped are very accident prone due to physical clumsiness and their inability to judge distances. They are also unable to recognize a potentially harmful situation.

Nursing care

Nursing care means doing for patients what they are unable to do for themselves. However, nursing the mentally handicapped also includes teaching patients to do these things for themselves. It involves providing for the physical, psychological and social well-being of the patient. There are two main areas of nursing activity. One is to ensure that the person's basic needs are met; the other is to see that the patient uses and develops, as fully as possible, whatever abilities he possesses. Considerable importance is attached to the surroundings in which these activities take place and much thought is expended to make the milieu as normal as possible.

The concept of normalization, which was first developed in the Scandinavian countries, is that the mentally handicapped individual should be allowed to develop in as natural a setting as possible and be given access to facilities, pleasures and comforts enjoyed by ordinary people.

The aim of a nursing care programme for the mentally handicapped is to develop potential in such a way that the person is capable of returning to the community or, if this is not possible, of living a useful and contributory life in a sheltered environment. In very high dependency patients where the above aims are unrealistic, the objective is to improve the quality of life in any way possible; for example a patient who is mobile, if only in a wheel-chair, has more opportunities than a patient confined to bed.

Nursing care of a high quality is the first step in socialization. Good basic cleanliness does much to dispel the all too familiar image of hospitals for the mentally handicapped. Careful attention to grooming can camouflage defects, and the individual consequently becomes more socially acceptable. Attention must be paid to skin care. Daily bathing is essential and the use of a cream to keep the skin soft and supple is recommended, particularly in patients with Down's syndrome; older patients can be taught to attend to their own skin care. Oral and dental care is of

Figure 15.2
A small group of patients
enjoying a game of bingo

particular importance for all patients; it becomes of even greater moment when certain anticonvulsants are being given. Phenytoin, for instance, causes gingivitis.

Care should be taken of the eyelids with emphasis on the prevention of blepharitis. The nose should be kept clean and, where possible, children should be trained to do this for themselves. A persistent discharge from the nose or ear should be investigated since it could mean the patient has pushed a foreign body into one of these orifices (Ch. 13), which might not be obvious on initial examination. Nails should be kept short and clean. Clothing is very important and should be attractive, well-fitting, individual and durable, with colours and materials properly matched.

A well-balanced diet is important and foods likely to cause diarrhoea, particularly in the high dependency patient, should be avoided. On the other hand, the inclusion of roughage can help prevent constipation. Adequate fluid intake must be maintained because patients are often unable to indicate thirst. Special diets are necessary in certain conditions such as phenylketonuria (Ch. 4). In the management of bladder and bowel the objective is, if possible, to train the patient to control these functions. Where this is impossible, nursing ingenuity is taxed in caring for the incontinent patient and, at the same time, maintaining a fresh, well-ventilated environment.

Special nursing care is necessary in the management of many conditions such as Sturge-Weber syndrome (p. 552), hydrocephalus (p. 552) and the biochemical disorders. It is also necessary in conditions which complicate mental handicap.

Complications of mental handicap requiring special care

Epilepsy

Epilepsy is a symptom of an underlying cerebral disorder. There are various types of epilepsy but the same principles of nursing management apply for all. It is important to ensure that blood levels of anticonvulsants are maintained and to observe the effects and side-effects of these drugs. Special care is necessary when anticonvulsants are being changed.

Cerebral palsy

This term refers to muscular disabilities resulting from either damage to or impaired development of the brain. The most important single cause is brain damage during birth. The special management of cerebral palsy includes the prevention of deformity, the management of appliances and the nursing care following orthopaedic surgery.

Hyperkinesis

The hyperkinetic syndrome describes a state of hyperactivity or violent motor unrest. It occurs in children, is associated with cerebral damage and is a condition requiring skilled management. The fostering of the nurse-patient relationship is all important in reducing the level of anxiety in the child. These children need periods of calm during the day when they can sit quietly with a nurse. Soothing background music is helpful. Constant observation is necessary to prevent accidents.

Treatment includes drug therapy, diet and, in severe cases, brain surgery.

Disturbed sleep patterns

Disturbed sleep patterns call for ingenious nursing management. Patients are often unable to say if or why they are uncomfortable or that they are in pain. It is the nurse's responsibility to recognize and interpret the patient's behaviour, for instance screaming and head scratching may denote toothache. The development of observational skills is very important in caring for mentally handicapped people because of their difficulty in communicating normally.

Aggression

Aggressive behaviour can be very disruptive in a therapeutic environment. The nurse must first deal with the immediate situation and then find out the cause of the outburst. Management may need to be modified as a preventive measure.

Mental illness

Neuroses and psychoses (Ch. 16) may be superimposed on mental handicap and these conditions need special management.

Physical illness

Congenital heart defects, diseases of the respiratory system and skin conditions are fairly common among the mentally handicapped and require special nursing management. In some instances patients are returned to their parent hospital 48 hours after an operation and will need appropriate nursing care.

Promoting the development of abilities

Physical

Due to delay in maturation the mentally handicapped person's physical rate of growth is slowed down. Control of head movements, sitting and walking are delayed; muscle co-ordination is poor and patients with Down's syndrome have hypotonic (flabby) muscles. When cerebral palsy is present there is an added problem of muscle spasm interfering not only with limb movement but also with swallowing and speech.

In some instances the development of muscle control and co-ordination is a preliminary to acquiring elementary self-help skills. The nurse, working in conjunction with the physiotherapist and remedial gymnast, can do much to aid physical development. Passive and active exercises and positioning to prevent or correct deformities can be programmed to meet individual needs. Muscle relaxation exercises using water play — if possible in a swimming pool — are beneficial. Movement to music can make exercises more fun. Allowing children scope and opportunity to walk, climb, balance, skip and sometimes ride ponies can also help and give confidence. For children who have not learned to walk the use of standing and walking frames allows the experience of weight-bearing and balance and the development of *proprioception*.

Figure 15.3
Opportunity for climbing and balancing in an adventure playground

Figure 15.4
Using a floor level mirror to
teach posture and body image

Psychological

Psychological development can be considered in two areas — *emotional* and *cognitive*.

Emotional

An important aspect of nursing care is to provide an emotional climate which is warmly accepting, where the person is first of all an individual and only secondly a mentally handicapped individual. In this way a sense of security, which is necessary before any learning can take place, is developed. A positive approach where praise rather than blame is used can be strongly motivating.

Consistency in approach is important because inconsistency causes confusion in the mentally handicapped person who has difficulty in adapting to change. When environmental changes have to be made, the patient should be well prepared for them by simple explanations. Such measures can do much to prevent the emotional outbursts that are caused by frustration when the patient is unable to cope with differing demands.

Expectations of achievement should be realistic: patients can feel hopeless and give up trying if they sense staff disappointment, and low dependency patients can be surprisingly perceptive. Nurses and other team members should be able to establish rapport with the patients as this is essential in meeting and assessing emotional and other needs. Parents or parent substitutes should if possible be kept in close contact with children. The nurse's role is that of a therapist and not a parent substitute. However, when a child has no parents the nurse should ensure that he does not suffer emotional deprivation while in the nurse's care.

Cognitive

A knowledge of cognitive development is necessary in understanding the mentally handicapped person's difficulty in learning. The mentally handicapped person receives information through the senses, but he has difficulty in interpreting and giving a meaning to these sensations. The nurse in constant contact with mentally handicapped children should ensure that all the various aspects of a situation are clearly seen, felt and heard so that *perception* is made easier. Meaningful perception also depends on past experiences; therefore, the nurse should give the children as wide a variety of experiences as possible so that the introduction of new stimuli can be more easily assimilated.

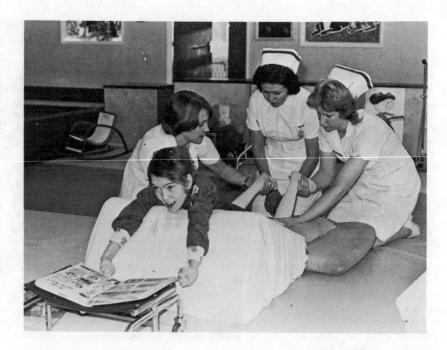

Figure 15.5
Positioning to correct deformity

As a child's language ability helps him to correlate his memory of past experiences and his understanding of new ones, it is important to extend his vocabulary. He should be encouraged to use words in ordinary conversation. Signs or other forms of communication should not be accepted if a patient is capable of verbalizing, but when there is no verbal ability it is important that the nurse talks to these patients and develops a communication link on non-verbal levels. Since these children have a short *attention* span, simple sentences should be used in giving instructions; the child's name should be called first to attract his attention; and where possible the nurse should sit or kneel in front of the child on his physical level. If such methods are not used, verbal instructions may be lost in the background noises surrounding the child. The nurse, speech therapist, psychologist and teacher work closely together in developing language ability.

Figure 15.6
Water, a necessary therapeutic tool

Social

It is generally accepted that almost all human behaviour is learned including basic skills such as walking, eating, washing, dressing and control of elimination. These skills are generally recognized as the activities of daily living. In normal children this learning takes place informally at home. In mentally handicapped children, however, these skills will not be acquired automatically but will need to be taught, that is informal learning is unlikely. Nursing care, therefore, must include the assessment of stages of readiness for training, provide base line data and record and report accurately observations on behaviour, both orally and in writing. Nurses must be able to programme and facilitate the learning of these basic skills.

THERAPEUTIC TECHNIQUES

An outline of skill training

Some basic principles can be applied in teaching either simple or (later) more complicated tasks:

1. The target behaviour should be defined and an assessment made of the individual's readiness for the particular type of response.
2. The task should be analysed, that is the skill to be taught should be closely examined and broken down into simple steps.
3. Each step should be taught using the same sequential pattern at each performance.
4. As each step is being taught, simple verbal instructions should be given together with a demonstration, making sure the child can see clearly and follow what is being done. It may be necessary to sit or stand beside the child to avoid confusion between right and left.
5. Corrections should be made where necessary, but at first slow, clumsy attempts should be accepted until the child becomes more adept. Encouragement should be given when the child shows even the slightest approximation of the desired result.
6. The child should be allowed to practise the skill until it is overlearned, that is until it becomes habitual.
7. Later, observation will be necessary to ensure that the skill is maintained.
8. Mirrors can be used in teaching skills such as hair care and dressing.
9. Distractions should be removed while trying to gain the child's attention.

Behaviour modification

Behaviour modification is the application of learning theory to the changing of human behaviour. It is based on the stimulus-response (S–R) theory. The principle involved is that if a behaviour is reinforced or rewarded it will be repeated.

Reinforcements

Reinforcements can be positive (pleasant) or negative (unpleasant); it is usually better to use positive reinforcements. Before deciding on reinforcements an assessment must be made as to what will be rewarding to the person. For children incentives such as sweets, social praise or social approval can be used. In some instances tokens are given which can be exchanged later for money or other suitable rewards.

The reinforcer should be given as soon as the desired behaviour has occurred. Care must be taken not to reinforce undesirable behaviour that may occur at the same time. It is also very important to be invariably consistent in the use of reinforcements. Initially one cannot expect a perfect response, but when the child's response approximates desired behaviour he is rewarded; this is called shaping. In this way the behaviour required is gradually 'shaped' or built up. A negative reinforcement is used when correcting undesirable behaviour and could take the form of suitable punishment such as ignoring attention seeking when it occurs.

Behaviour modification is becoming more widely used in the care of the mentally handicapped. Nurses are involved in these programmes and need to understand the

Figure 15.7
Most children enjoy playing in a
tree house

underlying psychological principles. In conjunction with psychologists they help to devise and supervise these programmes.

Play therapy

Children learn through play; therefore nurses with the help of psychologists should devise and carry out play programmes suitable for individual children to help develop imagination, language, body image and sensory and motor abilities. It must be understood that play will not occur spontaneously in mentally handicapped children but must be developed by adults who guide but do not intrude. A box of clothes for dressing up, a full-length mirror, a play house, dolls that can be dressed and undressed are among useful, easily obtained equipment.

An adventure playground planned with imagination and insight into children's developmental needs can be an asset. Most children love a tree house where they can really let their imagination run riot. Safety precautions must, however, be implemented.

The use of 'self' as a therapeutic tool

'Imitation is the sincerest form of flattery'

Mentally handicapped persons also learn by identification and imitation; the nurse, therefore, can use her own personality as a therapeutic tool in teaching sociothera-

Figure 15.8
Fun and games in a safe
environment

peutic skills either to individuals or to groups. In this way the nurse can help the patient to establish meaningful relationships, behave in a socially acceptable way in a group situation and communicate his needs and opinions to others. Depending on the strength of the nurse-patient relationship the nurse is in a position to use social approval as a reinforcer and to counsel and guide patients. For teenagers and older mentally handicapped persons group therapy can provide a useful learning situation.

Socialization

For both children and adults more sophisticated social training should take place as far as possible outside the hospital, using community resources. When the hospital has a holiday home at its disposal there is a tremendous opportunity for social orientation. Resourceful staff can allow patients to shop, plan menus and organize leisure activities in much the same way as do normal people. However, much teaching must go on at hospital level before this kind of adaptation can occur. For adult patients training in self-help and self-care form the basis for socialization. Ideally children should be so trained that when they reach adulthood they will have achieved at least marginal independence, provided they have the initial potential.

Education and training

Since the mentally handicapped are late developers it is only reasonable that education should be nearly continuous. Further education in areas such as cookery, housewifery, dressmaking, beauty culture, as well as academic subjects is invaluable for women. Various areas in the hospital can be used for occupational training. The laundry, kitchen and wards provide training opportunities which, if planned, supervised and evaluated, can provide patients with practice in various household and occupational skills.

Figure 15.9
Riding

Occupational and industrial therapy departments can provide both training for rehabilitation and work for long-stay patients. The ability to work and to receive financial remuneration for it satisfies an individual's ego. Acquiring self-confidence and social poise can be helped by recreational activities such as dancing, ice skating, clubs and other suitable forms of entertainment. Music appreciation, hand work and games can also be taught so that leisure time can be used constructively.

Sex education is important and for young adults individual and group counselling sessions are useful.

Music therapy with the mentally handicapped

Mentally handicapped people are isolated people: their capacity for communication and for self-expression can be severely restricted by their handicap. The frustration arising from this restriction frequently becomes expressed in 'socially unacceptable' behaviour. This adds a secondary handicap to that already present, so that the mentally handicapped person becomes even more isolated from other people and from society at large.

Music has qualities of communication which make it uniquely suited as a medium for therapy: it is a non-verbal language which is socially acceptable; it is present in all cultures and in all ages since the beginning of human development; it is a universal phenomenon and people, everywhere, respond to it in some way. Music is also an emotional language capable of matching human emotions in all their varied subtleties and sudden changes.

In music therapy the therapist uses improvised music to meet the mood of the patient and to awaken a musical response on the tambourine, cymbal, drum or vocally. Once the patient begins to participate the therapist can support and develop these responses so that the music therapy situation becomes a mutual shared and creative experience.

The clinical goals in music therapy develop as the patient reveals more and more of himself through his music-making, and this gives the therapist clues as to what kind of music an individual needs and which direction the therapy will take.

In a hospital setting the music therapist should balance the work between individual and group sessions, and participate in case-conferences and multi-disciplinary team meetings. The music therapist's observations often complement that of other professionals and can be invaluable in contributing towards a more complete understanding of the mentally handicapped person.

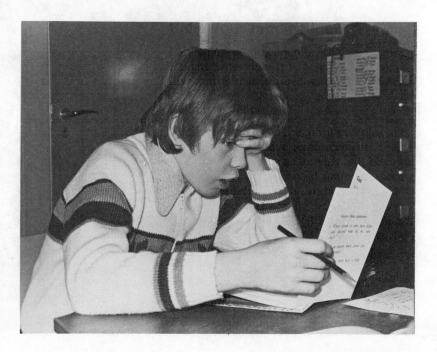

Figure 15.10
An individualized educational programme meets the child's needs

Figure 15.11
Interesting work will gain
children's attention

SUPPORT FOR THE FAMILY

The nurse trained in the field of mental handicap needs to be able to counsel, support and advise parents and others in aspects of caring and training. She should be able to identify stress in the family. Parents often have a guilt complex about their handicapped child especially if they are unable or unwilling to care for the child at home. Empathy alone is not enough, and the nurse must be able to support, guide and give practical help. It is possible for a ward sister to help to support a mother whose child has been discharged home, either by visiting or simply by being available at the other end of a telephone. In this way skills, knowledge and attitudes can effectively be imparted to parents and others.

The services available in Great Britain to patients living at home are noted in Chapter 18. Help may be offered by voluntary organizations too: the National Society for Mentally Handicapped Children gives help and advice whenever possible.

The emergence of the community nurse trained in mental handicap has been an added support for the family of a handicapped child living in the community. Her role is to assess the needs of the child in the home, devise programmes for the child's development and advise the parents about specific problems such as behavioural problems or physical problems. (Nurses can also use opportunities to educate the public in the understanding of mental handicap. Involvement in voluntary organizations gives an opportunity for education and support.)

CO-ORDINATION OF CARE

The nurse is in a position to co-ordinate the efforts of the other members of the therapeutic team. A patient's programme must be co-ordinated to gain the maximum effect from all the various specialist therapists. In some instances stimuli received from other therapists will need to be interpreted for the child. He will also need help and encouragement, as well as the opportunity, to practise new-found skills, and will need a considerable amount of time, support and understanding when struggling with new learning experiences.

SOME CAUSES OF MENTAL HANDICAP

Genetic anomalies

This is a general term for a large group of conditions. There are two main subdivisions:

1. Conditions associated with abnormalities of *chromosomes*, either the *autosomes* or the sex chromosomes.

2. Disorders of metabolism. This range of maladies results from an inability to make normal use of a normal constituent of the diet.

Disturbances of development

Fetal development may be adversely affected during gestation (prenatally). *Perinatal* (around and during birth) and *neonatal* (within the first month of life) misfortunes may also result in mental handicap.

DIAGNOSIS

A history of the pregnancy and of the perinatal and postnatal periods is essential. Details of other pregnancies and of the mother's general health are taken. A physical examination including a full neurological examination is performed. Various diagnostic tests such as chromosome counts, haematological investigations, chromatography, X-rays and EEGs may be carried out. In the case of children a full developmental history should be taken.

GENERAL FEATURES OF MENTAL HANDICAP

A mentally handicapped person seems 'odd' because of appearance and behaviour.

Physical appearance

Many abnormal physical features can be present especially when mental handicap is as a result of genetic factors. (For an example, see p. 551 Down's syndrome.)

Psychological features

Psychologically the mentally handicapped person cannot think or formulate ideas adequately; these defects together with a short attention span make learning difficult. Normal people appear to have a filtering mechanism whereby they can concentrate on one of several presenting stimuli. The mentally handicapped person is often unable to select the appropriate stimulus and therefore tries to pay attention to several at one time; he is consequently easily distracted.

Behavioural disorders

A mentally handicapped person may also suffer from behavioural disorders such as distractedness, hyperactivity, hyper-reactivity, perseveration, awkwardness, destructiveness and aggression. Motor performance habits such as head banging, rocking and other stereotyped mannerisms may be present.

Social immaturity

As learning is slow in all areas, social maturity is delayed or non-existent. For the normal person much social learning is acquired informally in the family situation and later among peer groups. The mother, once she begins to say 'no' to her child, is interpreting society's standards for him and he consequently learns what is acceptable and unacceptable in the society. For the mentally handicapped child this kind of learning is a very slow process. He lives very much in the 'here and now' and is unable to carry over learning from past experiences and to foresee the results of his actions, thereby impairing the acquisition of social maturity.

Associated conditions

Associated conditions such as epilepsy, cerebral palsy, congenital heart defects, susceptibility to chest infections and visual and hearing defects may also be present.

Emotional disturbances resulting from socially inadequate or culturally defective homes or from disturbances in the mother-child relationship may also occur.

THREE EXAMPLES OF COMMON CLINICAL PROBLEMS

The following disorders are among the commonest conditions associated with mental handicap.

Down's syndrome

People with Down's syndrome have many obvious physical characteristics in common. The thick, everted lips, large, fissured tongue, eyelids with an *epicanthic fold* and flattened bridge of nose give the typical 'mongoloid' features. The short stature, clumsy gait due to poor muscle co-ordination, awkwardness of hand movements and undersized stature complete the picture. Hands and feet show *dermatoglyphic* peculiarities. These characteristics are so noticeable that a preliminary diagnosis will probably be made soon after birth.

Nursing care

Many physical defects are associated with the syndrome, notably heart malformations (Ch. 7), susceptibility to mouth and gum infections and, most marked of all, predeliction to respiratory disease. About half the children born with Down's syndrome die of bronchopneumonia (Ch. 6) in the early years of life. The physical manifestations of disease require the same care and treatment as that accorded to any other child.

The degree of mental retardation varies considerably. Some children are severely handicapped, others may become self-supporting, especially if employment can be offered in a sheltered workshop.

It is generally accepted that children with Down's syndrome need intensive mental and physical stimulation during the first year of life. Marked improvement in development has been claimed when this form of therapy has been used.

The happy and affectionate dispositions of these children evoke correspondingly warm and tender responses from their families and from other people who become responsible for their care.

Figure 15.12
Down's syndrome

Figure 15.13
Sturge–Weber syndrome

Sturge-Weber syndrome

Sturge-Weber syndrome is a condition of obscure aetiology associated with mental handicap. The essential pathology is angiomatosis of the skin and the leptomeninges. The facial haemangioma is usually confined to half the face in a pattern similar to that of the branches of the trigeminal nerve. It may, however, be bilateral and present on other parts of the body. The areas of meningeal thickening with venous angiomatosis are usually found over the occipital lobe and on the same side as the facial naevus. Most patients have focal motor seizures. They may also have spastic hemiplegia.

Nursing care

Special nursing care involves care of the eyes and the mouth. Following epileptic seizures observations are very important as intracranial bleeding may occur. The same precautions are necessary if the child should fall and have even a slight head injury.

Hydrocephalus

In hydrocephalus there is an increased accumulation of cerebrospinal fluid within the ventricles of the brain (Ch. 3). There are many possible underlying causes, some of which may be treated surgically. The resulting pressure causes the bones of the skull to separate, the skull circumference to increase, the ventricles to become distended and the brain substance to be compressed.

Nursing care

If the head is grossly enlarged these children are unable to move from their cots. Therefore, imagination is necessary to improve the quality of life they can enjoy; in particular, they like to be able to see people and their surroundings and their posture in bed should permit this. The weight of the head causes great pressure on the scalp and pressure sores can occur; careful positioning with the use of soft pillows can prevent them.

When lifting the child from the cot the head must be supported before moving the child's body. It must be remembered that a hydrocephalic child has the same need for love and cuddling as a normal child and this need not be neglected provided the nurse acquires skill in handling the child.

GROWTH POINTS

There is need for much more research in the field of mental handicap particularly in the area of behavioural management. Community care needs to be extended far beyond that available at present. There should be more support for the mentally handicapped and their families, more training centres for children and adults in the community and more sheltered workshops. Emphasis must be placed on the rights of the handicapped person who is entitled to normal patterns of life in society and has a right to be respected for his human dignity. Finally it is important to realize that mental handicap is a multifaceted problem for which no one discipline has all the answers. There is need for efficient co-operation and participation on the nurse's part as a member of a therapeutic team.

SUGGESTED ASSIGNMENTS

Project

1. Think about a patient with Down's syndrome you are helping or have helped to nurse in hospital. Could she have been looked after in her own home? What help would the family have needed? Was it available? What would the advantages and disadvantages have been for your patient and her family?

2. Select one or two patients who for some reason have been prevented from carrying out their usual occupation for a period of time. Study carefully the effect this has had upon the behaviour of each individual and the reactions of his family and other patients.

Discussion topics

1. How has the experience you gained during your time in a unit for the mentally handicapped helped you to improve nursing care in other clinical areas?

2. Mental handicap is commonly regarded as causing a range of disadvantages. Consider ways in which mentally handicapped persons make a positive contribution to our society.

FURTHER READING

Crome L, Stern J 1972 Pathology of mental retardation, 2nd edn. Churchill Livingstone, Edinburgh
Finnie N R 1968 Handling the young cerebral palsied child at home, 2nd edn. Heinemann, London
Gunzburg H C 1973 Social competence and mental handicap, 2nd edn. Bailliere Tindall, London
Kirman B, Bicknell J 1975 Mental handicap. Churchill Livingstone, Edinburgh
Marais E, Marais M 1976 Lives worth living. Souvenier Press Educational and Academic, London

Chapter Sixteen
Mental disorder

To be sick in body evokes sympathy; to be sick in mind incurs laughter, disgust and ridicule, bringing shame to the individual and his family. In the early nineteenth century such sentiments resulted in the building of huge, self-contained asylums, places of refuge for the mentally disturbed. The asylums were built on the outskirts of towns, surrounded by high walls and camouflaged by trees. Their inaccessibility discouraged frequent visits and, once committed there, the inmates soon became the forgotten people.

Remnants of the stigma attached to mental illness linger on, but fortunately more people are recognizing that treatment in the early stages of mental disease can make life more worthwhile for the patient and his family. Instead of hiding the sick relative from prying eyes, they are bringing him forward for treatment. The development of the community psychiatric nursing service has helped considerably in this change of attitude. The community psychiatric nurses (CPNs) are proving to be effective therapists both in recognizing symptoms of an acute onset of neurotic or psychotic illnesses and in the treatment process.

This change in attitude is reflected in the change in psychiatric hospitals from places of custodial care to places providing a therapeutic environment around which the whole range of psychiatric services can revolve.

Much active treatment is done in out-patient departments and Health Centres, particularly for people suffering from the 'stress' diseases of modern living. With the help of new treatment methods, including drug therapy, more and more people are managing to cope with their illnesses at home, perhaps requiring only short periods in hospital.

Long-term psychiatric hospital patients are mainly psychotics who have lived most of their adult lives in hospital and now have nowhere to go. Many of these have been rehabilitated — or could be if sufficient places were available — to live in half-

Figure 16.1
Changing face of psychiatric treatment Left: Asylum 1950s Right: Psychiatric department 1980s

way houses, which provide a form of community living away from the hospital environment but not completely out of its control. This move towards community psychiatry has been aided considerably by organizations which, among other services, provide essential transport for patients to out-patient clinics, day hospitals and recreational activities. They give care and support where it is desperately required.

Mental disease can be just as debilitating as physical disease and can cause even more disruption to the life of the patient and his family. The psychiatric services try to improve and maintain not only the patient's mental health but also that of the family unit.

The WHO has prepared a classification of mental disorders (Table 16.1), and the nursing care of patients with the commonest of these conditions is outlined in this chapter. The nurse should realize, however, that it is very difficult to categorize psychiatric illnesses because a patient's symptoms do not always fit neatly into pigeon-holes.

The **neuroses** are a group of mental disorders, without any demonstrable organic basis, in which the patient may have considerable insight and unimpaired reality testing; that is, he usually does not confuse his morbid, subjective experiences and fantasies with external reality. Behaviour may be greatly affected, although usually remaining within socially acceptable limits; personality is, however, not disorganized. The principal manifestations include excessive anxiety, hysterical symptoms, phobias, obsessional and compulsive symptoms and depression.

Table 16.1
Mental disorders (Based on WHO international classification)

Neuroses	Psychoses	Dementia
Reactive depression	Endogenous depression	Presenile
Anxiety states	Involutional depression	Senile
Obsessive compulsive states	Manic depressive psychoses	Arteriosclerotic
Phobias	Organic psychoses	
Hysteria	Schizophrenias	
Anorexia nervosa	Paranoid states	
	Alcoholism	
	Drug addiction	
	Personality disorders	

The term **psychoses** encompasses those conditions in which impairment of mental functions has developed to a degree that interferes grossly with insight and the ability to meet some of the ordinary demands of life or to make adequate contact with reality.

Mental disorder can also be described in relation to normal behaviour. Normal behaviour can be defined as socially acceptable behaviour in a given culture. Any exaggeration of or deviation from this concept of mental health can be described as mental illness.

Many people are unable to cope with the stresses of everyday living and express their difficulties through an extravagant response that is termed a neurotic illness. Neurosis is based on learnt behaviour and does not involve the whole of the personality; it is a reaction to stressful circumstances in a personality predisposed to such a reaction by previous learning.

Most neurotic patients are able to distinguish between reality and the symptoms of their individual illness, for instance the compulsive hand-washer can admit that what he is doing is absurd but cannot stop doing it. Insight is generally present in neurotic illness, but it can be absent, notably in hysteria, where the patient has no insight at all into his illness.

Psychotics are generally regarded in lay terms as being mad. For them reality becomes so distorted as to be out of the range of normal experience. Their behaviour is bizarre, and in the more severe cases they are unable to distinguish between reality and the disorders of perception which are a feature of the illness. This lack of insight is sometimes considered diagnostic of psychosis, but this is not completely accurate, since many schizophrenics and depressives in the early stages of their illness are aware that they are ill.

Aetiology

Mental illness results from stress within the social environment aggravated by personality traits and heredity factors. It is commonly thought that the inherited factors consist not only of a genetic element but also of a pattern of behaviour learnt from example.

Other factors related to the causation of mental illness are:

Local damage to the brain, such as tumours, head injuries, viral infections and deterioration accompanying arteriosclerosis.

Certain physical illnesses, in particular pernicious anaemia and myxoedema which cause depression, and thyrotoxicosis which causes an anxiety state.

Chemical factors, in particular alcohol, drugs and poisons. A great deal of research is being done in the field of biochemistry in an attempt to isolate causative factors of mental illness.

Clinical features

The clinical features of mental illness are manifestations of disordered function of mood, behaviour, perception, thought and memory. The most commonly seen features are the following:

Anxiety

Anxiety expresses a distressed mind. It is the commonest of the unpleasant human emotions and is fear of an unknown situation. It arises from a basic insecurity and is accompanied by lack of concentration, insomnia and physiological disturbances such as sweaty palms, dryness of the mouth, indigestion, frequency of micturition, diarrhoea, palpitations and headaches.

Agitation

Agitation is associated with anxiety. The distress is expressed in constant motion which may take a variety of forms, often drumming of the fingers, movements of the lips and groaning sounds. The individual gives the impression of being constantly 'on edge', twittering, anxiously moving about, never able to rest.

Depression

Depression is a state of deep sadness, dejection and despondency. It is accompanied by lethargy and the slowing down of body functions, resulting in dry skin and hair, anorexia, constipation, tiredness, insomnia, lack of energy and loss of libido. Emotions are flattened and the individual, who appears dull and uninteresting, is usually unable to explain or justify such apparent misery. Suicide attempts are always a possibility.

Elation

Elation is an elevation of mood which may be inappropriate to the individual's present circumstances.

Obsession

An obsession is a fixed thought or idea which persists in the patient's mind although he is aware that it is often illogical and out of keeping with his beliefs.

Compulsion

A compulsion is an act which the patient feels compelled to carry out regardless of how painful or illogical it seems. A common example is washing hands after touching anything other than the patient's own body.

Phobia

A phobia is an abnormal fear of a particular object or situation. It may be based on early learning — for instance a fear of dogs or a fear of crowds — or it may result from an early, forgotten, unhappy experience.

Insomnia

Insomnia or sleeplessness is a very common complaint of the mentally ill. Irregularities may include:

> Difficulty in getting to sleep.
> Waking early.
> Sleeping during the daytime but being unable to sleep at night.
> Nightmares.

Anorexia

Poor appetite is a feature of depression, chronic alcoholism and drug addiction. Delusions and hallucinations may cause a patient to refuse food.

Delusions

A delusion is a false belief which has no rational basis and which is out of keeping with the individual's educational and cultural background.

Illusions

An illusion is a misinterpretation of an external stimulus, for instance a bush in the dark interpreted as being someone skulking.

Hallucinations

An hallucination is a false perception dependent upon one of the senses: hearing, smell, taste, touch, sight. In this instance there is no external stimulus present: the patient may smell the scent of flowers when neither flowers nor perfume is present.

Thought disturbance

Thought disturbance takes a variety of forms and is observed in the patient's talk:

> Neologisms: coining new words.
> Thought blocking: sudden gaps in the thought process.
> Flight of ideas: a constant stream of different ideas with little connection between them.

The patient may also be seen to exhibit a strong emotional reaction to particular topics.

Memory disturbance

A patient showing signs of memory disturbance may simply appear to be easily distracted and lacking in concentration. His memory may be good for events long past but poor for recent events. There may be gaps in his memory to which he admits, or he may confabulate, that is fill in the gaps with imagined events. There may be clouding of consciousness, confusion and disorientation shown by the patient being unsure of his identity and unable to estimate rationally time and place. He may also have complete loss of memory (amnesia).

Normal psychology

It is essential for the nurse to have some understanding of the normal psychology of the human maturation process so that she can appreciate where the patient deviates from the normal. This knowledge will also help the nurse to understand her own behaviour and to appreciate the effect she may be having on the behaviour of others, particularly colleagues, patients and their relatives.

Psychological defence mechanisms

It is also useful for the nurse to be aware of the recognized psychological defence mechanisms.

Rationalization is a means of self-deception by which facts are distorted to produce satisfactory and socially acceptable reasons for bad conduct.

Sublimation is the direction of socially unacceptable or forbidden tendencies into more acceptable channels. For example, sport can be an outlet for unconventional sexual and aggressive desires.

Projection is the attribution of one's own unacceptable feelings and attitudes to someone else or to the environment.

Repression is an unconscious symbolic expression of an unconscious impulse which is incompatible with one's ideals.

Regression means reversion to earlier stages of individual and social development, reacting and behaving accordingly.

The nurse may also find it useful to know some of the terminology associated with the various schools of analytical psychology led by figures such as Sigmund Freud, Carl Jung, Alfred Adler and Melanie Klein.

Investigations

The investigations required to diagnose psychiatric illness are carried out concurrently with initial treatment, which may be in an out-patient clinic or may follow admission to hospital, whichever is more suited to the needs of the patient and his family. An attempt is made to assess the patient's personality and environment, which may provide indications as to how the symptoms have occurred.

This detective work usually involves a number of professional staff. The doctor compiles a history of the patient's physical and mental illness. He wants to know if there is a family tendency towards a particular disease or a common behavioural pattern passed on from one generation to the next. Assessment of the patient's present physical and mental state is necessary. Psychologists' reports on the patient's intelligence, abilities, aptitudes and personality traits are submitted. The psychiatric social worker is asked to compile a report on the patient's home background and work situation. It may be possible for the psychiatric social worker or community nurse to meet the patient in his own environment and to observe the family's interaction. The general practitioner's help is sought to confirm the social and medical history of the patient and his family. The psychiatrist interviews relatives. These discussions often give a totally different perspective to statements made by the patient.

If the patient is admitted to hospital during this period, the nurse's role may be most crucial. Nursing staff are with the patient 24 hours a day observing all his daily activities. In many centres the nurse may also participate with the patient in occupational and recreational therapy. As a result nursing staff have continuous exposure to the patient during all his activities and, provided their method of reporting is efficient, all relevant observations can be communicated to the whole team, particularly those observations which might indicate a change in the patient's behaviour pattern.

Any significant encounter between the patient and a staff member, a relative, a friend, a workmate or another patient should be reported to the therapeutic team for consideration.

A physical illness may cause psychological disturbances, and the possibility of such a disorder will be taken into account when considering the differential diagnosis. For this reason a thorough physical examination is performed on all psychiatric patients and any indications of somatic disorder are followed up, for example pernicious anaemia mimicking depression or thyrotoxicosis resembling an anxiety state.

Assessment

Once the patient's case history is compiled a possible diagnosis can be reached and the treatment deemed suitable for the individual decided on. This decision is arrived at in ways which vary, depending on the administration and philosophy of the hospital or unit.

Hierarchical structures

The decision-making process depends on the structure of the particular unit or hospital. In a hierarchical structure a junior doctor examines the patient and compiles his history. He then confers with his senior colleagues regarding the diagnosis and possible treatment, which he then prescribes. Treatment is administered by the appropriate member of staff.

Therapeutic community

Most psychiatric units pay at least lip service to the concept of the therapeutic community, which is described as a multidisciplinary approach to patient care. In this community all members of staff, from the consultant to the ward maid, have a role to play in creating an environment conducive to treatment and all must have an opportunity to present their views.

Case presentation

About 1 week after admission the junior doctor presents his case history of the patient to the psychiatric team, which includes doctors, nurses, psychologists, social workers, occupational, industrial and recreational therapists and learners from all these professional groups. Most of the team know the patient by this time and are able to contribute to the discussion concerning his treatment, which should be based on an agreed, consistent approach known and understood by all staff.

Review session

A similar group meeting is held at regular intervals to review each patient's progress and to assess the effect of treatment. Also, consideration is given to new developments and decisions are made concerning, for instance, a patient's fitness to go home for weekends prior to discharge.

Treatment methods

Group psychotherapy

Within a therapeutic community treatment invariably includes participation in group psychotherapy. When treating neuroses these sessions should be analytical in character, making the patient dissect his problems and recognize the part his own behaviour plays in their occurrence. Psychotic patients benefit from supportive psychotherapy, which provides reassurance, encourages and supports 'good' and positive behaviour and gently points out 'bad' or negative behaviour. (This is in contrast to analytical psychotherapy, in which patients themselves are pressurized to interpret their own behaviour.) Supportive psychotherapy should be honest and realistic so that the patient is helped to live as full a life as possible.

In addition to staff, other patients act as therapeutic agents in group psychotherapy. Indeed, patients are often more persistent in pressurizing one of their members than are staff.

Figure 16.2
Verbal and non-verbal
communication during group
psychotherapy

Such a group should be directed by a staff member recognized as a leader, who encourages group members to comment and analyse throughout the meeting. The leader or another staff member who participated in the group is encouraged either to write a summary of the meeting or to give an oral report to the rest of the team.

A staff meeting usually follows each group meeting to pick out relevant points relating to the progress of individual patients and to provide material for discussion of the interaction and feeling in the unit at that particular time. These sessions can be used as teaching sessions for the learners.

The nurse observer may write in the nursing notes of the patient's record a summary of the part individual patients played in the group meeting.

Didactic or individual psychotherapy

This is psychotherapy on a one-to-one basis. Many psychiatrists consider this the only true psychotherapy. It is a very time-consuming method and only a few patients can be treated in a given period, whereas in the same amount of time a psychiatrist can treat many patients using the group method.

Family or marital therapy

The marriage partner or other family members may be included in the talking session between the patient and the therapist, particularly if it is considered that these people have been involved in causing or aggravating the patient's illness or can help in any way to resolve it. It can be very difficult to get some patient's relatives to accept responsibility for their contribution to the patient's conditions.

In some units, such as the Cassel Hospital in England, entire families are admitted to hospital for treatment.

Figure 16.3
Individual psychotherapy

Figure 16.4
Family therapy

Behaviour therapy

Behaviour therapy is based on learning theories and is a deconditioning or desensitization process by which the patient is retrained to cope with a situation which has previously illogically distressed him. This may take the form, for instance, of a fear of leaving home that causes the patient to become a prisoner within his own house. In behaviour therapy a therapist must work for a period of time almost exclusively with one patient, exposing the patient to ever increasing doses of the fear-provoking situation. For example, in the case of the patient who will not leave home, at first the therapist accompanies him on short excursions from the home. Then, once he can cope with going out with an individual he trusts, the next step is for the patient to out alone but with the therapist not far away. Ultimately the patient will be able to leave home knowing that the therapist is not in the vicinity.

Nurses have been found to be very good at this type of work, possibly because they are used to spending long periods of time with the patients as part of everyday living in hospitals. Some nurses, after special training in these methods of treatment, are able to practise as an alternative to the psychiatrist. There is a potential for the development and application of this approach to treatment of the behaviour problems presented by patients with a variety of mental illnesses.

Abreaction

Abreaction can be used in the treatment of hysteria and in other conditions where it is thought that the patient may be sublimating. This can be a long drawn-out procedure and requires careful explanation to the patient.

An intravenous injection of sodium thiopentone or sodium amylobarbitone induces the patient to relax sufficiently to speak without inhibition. It is hoped he will reveal long-forgotten incidents from his childhood that may be relevant to his present condition.

This is usually in a one-to-one situation between the patient and the psychiatrist. The nurse may only be required to assist with the administration of the drug. She may be excluded completely from the proceedings or allowed to remain as an observer or chaperone. During a long session the nurse may be expected to relieve the therapist, particularly during the early stages when the patient is allowed to talk freely about whatever comes into his mind. In such a case the nurse must be given guidance by the therapist as to what tactics to employ if the patient requires direction.

Figure 16.5
Behaviour therapy successfully used in the treatment of agoraphobia

Aversion therapy

Aversion therapy is rarely used nowadays, although some therapists find it useful in treating alcoholism and sexual deviations. The object is to guide the patient's stimulus in a healthier direction by giving him an aversion to what was formerly a pleasurable activity. This is achieved either by drug-induced distressful vomiting or

Figure 16.6
Encounter group

by subjecting the patient to electric shocks when practising the asocial behaviour. Psychological support is required if this treatment is to be effective.

During this procedure the nurse may have to monitor the patient's physical condition regularly in case the side-effects of the treatments are too harsh.

Encounter groups

Many patients suffering from neurotic illnesses are extremely inhibited. Some psychiatrists and psychologists, particularly in the United States, advocate the use of encounter groups to encourage people to express their feelings through physical contact with each other. Encounter groups have not been used to any great extent in the U.K. where most psychiatry is provided by the National Health Service, possibly because the sexual overtones inherent in this treatment method could be at variance with what is commonly regarded as professional etiquette.

Cultural differences are noticeable when people meet in a group. For instance British people tend to stand farther away from those they are talking to than do people from Eastern countries. At a party it can be amusing to watch an Englishman backing away from a persistently advancing Arab. Each is trying to maintain what he considers to be the correct social distance from the other. So, in spite of valiant efforts by both to observe the proprieties the unfortunate consequence of the encounter is embarrassment and disharmony. We in Britain also tend to reserve touching for our intimates whereas touching is part of conversation in some parts of the world. In areas where there are multi-racial societies such as in many large hospitals an encounter group can be a valuable teaching tool in promoting understanding and awareness of cultural differences.

Electroconvulsive therapy (electroplexy)

This procedure, known simply as ECT, is effective in the treatment of endogenous depression and early schizophrenia.

The patient is prepared as for a general anaesthetic. Electrodes are applied to the temples and an epileptic-type fit is induced, controlled by a short-acting anaesthetic, sodium thiopentone, and a muscle relaxant such as suxamethonium chloride.

The initial care is the same as for an unconscious patient. Once he has regained consciousness following the anaesthetic the patient is allowed to sleep for a few hours and then is encouraged to get up, dress and participate in the usual ward activities. If the procedure has been performed on an out-patient basis he will then be allowed home, accompanied by a friend or relative.

Temporary confusion and memory loss often follow this procedure, which is otherwise painless. A course of ECT usually provides for eight treatments, but the number may vary. Sometimes one electrode only is applied to one temple, but more often one is applied to each temple. Controversy has always raged over the ethics of using this form of therapy.

Drug therapy

Drug therapy does not cure mental disorders, but most psychiatric symptoms can be relieved by the judicious use of drugs.

The main groups of drugs used in the treatment of the anxiety states and depression are the antidepressants (Table 16.2) and the mild tranquillizers (Table 16.3). The major tranquillizers (Table 16.4) are used in the treatment of confusional and delusional states and hallucinations.

The tricyclics are effective antidepressants which take 10 to 14 days to act. The monoamine oxidase inhibitors (MAOI) are not generally effective antidepressants, but some patients respond well to them. If taken in conjunction with tyramine-containing foods such as cheese, yoghurt, alcohol, broad beans, meat extracts (Bovril) and yeast extracts (Marmite), a severe hypertensive reaction can result. A similar reaction is caused if the MAOI group of drugs are taken at the same time or within 2 weeks of completing a course of tricyclics.

Table 16.2
Antidepressant drugs

Tricyclics	Monoamine oxidase inhibitors (MAOI)
imipramine (Tofranil)	phenelzine (Nardil)
trimipramine (Surmontil)	tranylcypromine (Parnate)
amitriptyline (Trypizol)	

Table 16.3
Mild tranquillizing drugs

Benzodiazepines	Barbiturates
chlordiazepoxide (Librium)	phenobarbitone
diazepam (Valium)	amylobarbitone

Table 16.4
Major tranquillizing drugs

Phenothiazines	Butyrophenomes
chlorpromazine (Largactil)	haloperidol (Serenace)
thioridazine (Melleril)	trifluperidol (Triperidol)
trifluoperazine (Stelazine)	
promazine (Sparine)	
fluphenzine enanthate (Moditen enanthate)	
fluophenazine decanoate (Modecate)	

The benzodiazepines are very effective in the treatment of anxiety states, particularly if the patient is agitated. They are much safer to use than the barbiturates, small doses of which are effective in relieving anxiety. The barbiturates produce drug dependence and tend to make elderly patients confused.

The phenothiazines first came into use in 1951. They are effective particularly in schizophrenia, but are palliative only and the symptoms reappear if the drug is discontinued. Moditen and Modecate are long-acting drugs administered intramuscularly at intervals of 2 to 4 weeks; therefore they are particularly useful to the chronically ill patient living in the community. There are many side-effects to the drugs, notably pseudoparkinsonism, which is treated with antiparkinsonism drugs, for instance orphenadrine (Disipal). Jaundice, skin rashes and photosensitivity are other side-effects.

The butyrophenomes are newer drugs which are effective in treating schizophrenia and particularly in controlling mania. If prescribed in a low dosage, anxiety can be alleviated. The important side-effects of these drugs are also extrapyramidal symptoms, which include rigidity, shuffling gait, lack of facial expression, coarse tremor of the hands and head at rest, excessive salivation, rocking of the body backwards and forwards and posturing.

Most patients suffering from mental disorders are victims of insomnia and hypnotic drugs are usually prescribed to induce sleep.

THE LAW AND MENTAL DISORDER

The law related to mental disorder is designed to protect the patient, his property, his family, the people looking after him and the public.

The Mental Health Act 1959 (1960 Scotland) revolutionized people's attitudes to mental illness by making admission and discharge to a mental hospital as informal as admission and discharge to a general hospital.

Within the Act, provision has been made to detain compulsorily patients who require treatment but do not recognize they are a danger to themselves or others. Amendments were passed to strengthen the Act to enable potentially dangerous patients to be detained in institutions. These Acts have now been consolidated in the Mental Health Act 1983 (1984 Scotland).

Application for detention can be made by the person's nearest relative or by an approved social worker (a Mental Health Officer in Scotland) and must be supported by medical evidence. Whenever possible this advice is obtained from two doctors, the patient's general practitioner and one appointed by the local authority for the purpose.

At any time, if his condition warrants it, the patient can be discharged or can be accorded informal status. Under these sections of the Act the patient can be discharged by a doctor, or on written application from his nearest relative, or by the Mental Health Tribunal.

Under the Act, the police have the power to take a person to a place of safety, which may be a mental hospital if they consider it most appropriate, for a period of up to 72 hours until appropriate arrangements can be made to take care of the person.

Various health agencies issue leaflets setting out the rights of patients detained in hospital, which should be given to the patient and his relatives. The doctor should explain to the patient the conditions of detention and how he may appeal against detention.

In some cases the criminal courts seek medical advice regarding the mental state of a person accused of an offence. If the court concurs that the person concerned would benefit more from psychiatric treatment than from a prison sentence, a hospital order is issued.

A patient committed under a hospital order is treated as if he had been admitted on the date of the order in pursuance of an application for admission except that the power to order the discharge of the patient shall not be exercisable by the nearest relative. The patient can be discharged by a doctor or the Mental Health Tribunal.

If the person is detained under a hospital order for the safety of the public, then he should be placed under a restriction order. By this order decisions about the patient's movements and freedom are delegated to the Secretary of State. A restricted patient may apply directly to a Mental Health Review Tribunal after 6 months. Every case should be reviewed by the Mental Health Review Tribunal once in 3 years. The Secretary of State alone has the power to discharge this patient.

If a detained patient absconds from hospital, the police, social worker and the patient's nearest relative are informed. Under the Act psychiatric nurses may detain a patient in these circumstances until the arrival of the doctor.

The Mental Health Act is a comprehensive coverage of all aspects of the law that could possibly affect the patient. One aspect which may concern nurses in hospital is the section dealing with the correspondence of detained patients.

The doctor can censor letters and stop letters from being posted if they are obscene or if the individual, to whom they are being sent, requests that they should not be posted. The doctor has no authority to open a letter or prevent its being posted if it is addressed to any person representing a government or legal body including the following:

The Department of Health and Social Security.
A Member of Parliament.
The Mental Health Review Tribunal.
The Court of Protection.
The patient's solicitor.
The Managers of the hospital in which the patient is detained.
The European Commission of Human Rights or
The European Court of Human Rights.

State mental hospitals are provided for the care of the criminally insane. The Secretary of State is responsible for admission and discharge, and provision is made for transfer both to and from the area hospitals. There is one in Scotland at Carstairs and three in England and Wales: Broadmoor in Berkshire, Rampton in Nottinghamshire, Moss Side in Liverpool.

MENTAL DISORDERS

Depression

Depression is one of the most common conditions encountered in psychiatric hospitals. In lay terms it is a mood, but in psychiatric terms it is a syndrome with a number of variations:

Reactive (exogenous) depression.
Manic-depressive psychosis.
Endogenous depression.
Obsessional depression.
Involutional depression.
Puerperal depression.

Reactive depression is regarded as a neurotic condition. The other variations have psychotic features.

Reactive depression. This is described as exogenous because there are precipitating stressful factors outside the individual's personality that provide an understandable psychological cause for the behavioural response. Examples of precipitating factors are circumstances such as bereavement and loss of status. The reaction is, however, exaggerated.

Such a reaction usually occurs in individuals who are hypersensitive, anxious and resentful and who have difficulty coping with stressful situations. It could be said that reactive depression occurs in people with a predisposed personality who are subjected to adversities.

Most people have experienced the mood of depression and can therefore understand the patient's feelings, but they will have difficulty in appreciating the distorted response of the syndrome.

Reactive depression can be distinguished from other types by its accepted clinical picture: there is a recognized cause for the deep unhappiness experienced by the individual, who is usually anxious and resentful, blaming others for his illness; he will have great difficulty in getting to sleep, but if diurnal variation is present he will feel better in the morning, becoming more depressed as the day wears on.

Endogenous depression, manic-depressive psychosis. In contrast, endogenous depression usually occurs in the absence of any apparent environmental stress. There is usually a heredity factor and there may be a history of recurrent attacks of mania. The condition is known as manic-depressive psychosis.

It is a severe depression marked by strong delusions of guilt, unworthiness,

Figure 16.7
Depression

hypochondriasis and persecution. Sometimes hallucinations are present. The patient usually gets to sleep easily enough but experiences early morning waking. The risk of suicide is considerable.

Spontaneous recovery will eventually occur.

Obsessional depression. This is a mild depression commonly occurring for the first time in middle-aged obsessional personalities with no family history of the disease. In women, it is often associated with the menopause.

Involutional depression. Rarer, but seen in the same type of people, is a severe depression labelled involutional depression. The features of this condition are intense agitation and delusions of guilt, persecution and hypochondriasis (usually concerning the bowels). Sometimes nihilistic delusions are present, when the patient insists that everyone including himself is dead. No attempt should be made to reason with the patient regarding his delusions.

Puerperal depression. During the first few days of the puerperium (Ch. 10), because of the rapid changes taking place in the woman's endocrine balance, many women are slightly depressed and emotionally labile. This should not be confused with the severe depression called puerperal psychosis, which may occur early in the puerperium.

The main features of this illness are suicidal tendencies and a strong compulsion to kill the child. Admission to hospital is essential to prevent harm to the baby and to avoid suicide attempts. The other children in the family are usually safe.

Whenever possible, the baby is admitted with the mother, so that she can continue to look after it with the help of the nursing staff.

Complete recovery usually occurs within a month but relapse is common.

General features of depressive illness

All depressed patients suffer from a sad, despairing mood characterized by a feeling of hopelessness which lasts for weeks, months or even 2 or more years. Misery and dejection are apparent in the facial expression, stance and the way the clothes are worn. The patient looks weary, tired and lethargic and is unable to react with a normal show of emotion to events around him. He finds life dull, unexciting and worthless. He is unable to concentrate and experiences memory impairment and loss of libido.

This flattening effect on the spirit also affects his physical health. He complains of anorexia, loss of weight and constipation.

Some individuals become so retarded that they sit silent and immobile, while others become so tense and anxious that they become agitated.

In spite of their underlying depression some patients are able to put on a smiling, chatty, but usually brittle, front to conceal their inner despair. These patients are suicide risks because they have the inclination and the initiative to be able to commit suicide successfully.

Treatment and nursing care

Many patients can be treated effectively by the general practitioner with antidepressant drugs. In addition to drug therapy some patients may require sessions with the psychiatrist on an out-patient or day-patient basis, during which they can discuss their feelings and relationships.

Hospital admission is desirable for the severely depressed individual who cannot be safely managed at home, possibly because of the high degree of agitation he displays or because he constitutes a potential suicide risk.

Antidepressant drugs form the basis of treatment. Hypnotics are invariably prescribed to counteract insomnia, and agitated patients require mild tranquillizers to control their restlessness and distress. Endogenous depression responds well to electroconvulsive therapy but it is rarely used in the treatment of reactive depression unless agitation is a feature of the illness, in which case it can be useful.

Didactic and group psychotherapy can be usefully employed in assisting depressed patients to analyse their distress and pinpoint problem areas. Social problems can often be identified and, if possible, corrected, with the patient being helped to reach a new freedom of discussion with family members.

Occupational and recreational therapy provides some mental stimulation for the patient, giving him the opportunity to mix with other people.

Depressed patients are apathetic and will deteriorate if allowed to sit alone in a dingy, unstimulating environment. Their mood may be lightened slightly if the ward is light, sunny and furnished attractively and comfortably. Homely touches such as fresh flowers and carefully tended houseplants help to provide a pleasant, caring atmosphere. The aim is to create an environment in which it is possible for patients to meet with understanding and to be assured that the staff are interested in them as individuals.

Apathetic patients have difficulty in making simple decisions. To help them the nurse must develop a positive approach, insisting gently but firmly that basic principles of hygiene and nutrition are observed and that the various therapies are attended. These patients should be encouraged to participate in ward activities but should never be forced to do so. They will take the line of least resistance and can be guided into a passive response provided someone takes the initiative for them. The nurse should encourage conversation, talk to them even when they do not respond, reinforce their accomplishments and try to boost their self-confidence.

Those who are filled with resentment, blaming anyone other than themselves for their illness, need to regain their trust in people. The nurse can best help these patients by being consistent and matter of fact in her approach. These patients are sometimes subject to panic attacks (see anxiety states, p. 573).

Every depressed patient can be regarded as a potential suicide risk and should therefore be observed carefully but unobtrusively day and night. The nurse must observe any change in the patient's appearance or behaviour and report any suicidal tendencies.

All personnel in the ward, including patients, should be made aware if a particular person has contemplated suicide and their co-operation should be sought in preventing future incidents. Discussion of the subject should be free but not laboured, especially in group situations. Nursing responsibilities are:

To ensure that the patient is not left alone.
To know if he has in his possession items with which he could injure himself.
To be prepared to challenge him about his intentions.
To ensure he swallows medication and does not secrete tablets until he has a sufficient number for an overdose.

Constant observation of this type of person is an extremely arduous duty, but negligence is dangerous. Most of these patients observe the staff more rigorously than the staff observe them particularly as their apathy lifts. At this time a patient may appear to be improving, but hopelessness and despair may remain and the patient is now able to plan coolly and calculatingly the strategy which will lead to his death.

Such constant observation may increase the patient's depression, therefore he must gradually be trusted to be on his own. This should be a deliberate policy agreed on by all staff.

A suicide attempt is often a cry for help.

Manic states

In manic-depressive psychosis attacks of depression may alternate with the opposite mood state of mania. The first attack of mania is often precipitated by a crisis, and further attacks may occur at regular intervals or may accompany stressful situations.

Hypomania is a state of less severe excitement and overactivity than mania. All the symptoms of mania are present but they are less severe and the condition lasts longer than mania.

Clinical features of mania

Mania usually occurs in people who have a warm and friendly personality. With the illness these traits become exaggerated and the person becomes extremely elated and full of self-confidence, voicing complicated and ambitious plans which it would be impossible to fulfil.

They leap from one place to another with large, graceful movements, constantly moving and talking and dispersing largesse. They are unable to be still and cannot concentrate on any one task or topic of conversation. Their speech is sometimes difficult to understand because they talk rapidly and loudly using puns and rhymes and displaying 'flight of ideas'. They become hypersensitive to noise and space, feeling hemmed in, particularly indoors. They often feel that their skin is easily irritated even by clothing, hence they may strip their clothes off.

These patients often become undernourished and dehydrated because they do not take time to eat and drink and are so very easily distracted. The mouth and tongue can become dry and furred due to dehydration and from talking so much. The excessive amount of energy expended by these patients is not balanced by adequate nutrition and rest, and the result may be complete exhaustion. They become irritable and aggressive if stopped from doing what they want.

Initially their behaviour is infectious, but ultimately it becomes irritating to others and they become unpopular.

Treatment and nursing care

The aim of treatment is to provide the patient with rest and nourishment and to protect him from injury. Sedation is essential; haloperidol has been found to be extremely effective in controlling mania. The phenothiazine group of drugs are also useful in tranquillizing manic patients, and electroconvulsive therapy sometimes dampens their elation.

If the patient is very disturbed he may have to be nursed in isolation. In any event the nurse should try to provide a tranquil atmosphere. She can do this by being particularly quiet, slow and deliberate in her movements and speech; by the use of subdued lights; and by nursing the patient in dull, monotonous surroundings with an absence of noise.

The nurse must use initiative in coaxing the patient to eat. Snacks, sandwiches and high protein drinks should be encouraged throughout the day.

Occupational and recreational activities are an outlet for energy, however manic patients should be given jobs which are quickly done, do not require much concentration and do not excite, stimulate or frustrate the patient. Active activity should not be encouraged. A quiet walk out of doors in open space and fresh air is ideal for these patients.

The nurse can utilize the patient's distractedness to avoid injury or further disruption when the patient becomes aggressive, for example, she can walk him up and down, chatting pleasantly to him all the time drawing his attention away from the irritation. She should avoid struggling with the patient either physically or verbally.

Other patients must be protected from his overexuberance. This may mean that the manic patient requires a special nurse with whom he can build up a relationship and who will keep him away from other patients and from situations liable to excite him.

Clinical features of hypomania

Like a manic patient a hypomanic is extroverted, happy and elated, with lots of drive and energy and a very colourful appearance. He appears interested in everything and everybody and takes on the job of spokesman, leader or organizer of the patient group.

Other patients are at first amused by him and willing to follow his lead. Gradually, however, they become irritated because he is unable to carry out ideas. Eventually they become hostile towards him, seeing him as an interfering individual who tries to ingratiate himself with newcomers. This condition tends to become chronic and the patient may be in hospital for years because he cannot be tolerated in the community outside hospital.

Treatment and nursing care

Treatment is with sedation and tranquillizers. The nurse must protect the patient

Figure 16.8
Hypomania

from other patients, whose tolerance levels may be low, and from overdoing things and exhausting himself. Unlike manic patients hypomanics are often plump because they tend to be greedy; therefore they may need reducing diets.

Schizophrenia

The schizophrenias are a group of illnesses of a psychotic nature characterized by a splitting off of the personality from the refinements of thinking and feeling.

About 45% of mental hospital beds are occupied by schizophrenics. The incidence in the general population is about 0.85%.

The main features of schizophrenia are disturbances of emotion, thought, perception and volition, resulting in abnormal and sometimes bizarre behaviour in which the patient is divorced from reality and living in a fantasy world.

Figure 16.9
Incidence of schizophrenia — at least one of these people is a schizophrenic

Types of schizophrenia

The classical categorization of schizophrenia into four types — simple, hebephrenic, catatonic and paranoid — will be followed here. However, it should be pointed out that this classification is not perfect: there is considerable overlap between the four groups and patients will not fall neatly into one or the other.

Simple schizophrenia first appears in young people and has an insidious onset. A previously intelligent and apparently stable person becomes increasingly solitary and more and more detached from reality. He appears preoccupied, incapable of an emotional response and unable to communicate his thoughts to others. Ultimately he may withdraw completely from society, ceasing to go to work or school, remaining in his room and neglecting his appearance and physical needs until finally he requires hospital care. He may manage to maintain sufficient interest in his health and appearance to live in the community, but he is usually alone and friendless, living at a low economic level and working at unskilled work well below his original capacity.

Hebephrenic schizophrenia also first occurs in young people and is usually acute. The illness generally starts with a period of withdrawal followed by a short phase of wild excitement. The patient will display *incongruity of affect*, flattening of emotion, thought blocking, neologisms (p. 557), *ideas of reference*, strange delusions and hallucinations (p. 557), mainly of an auditory or tactile nature. He usually recovers enough to resume normal life, but relapses are common and flattening of emotion may persist. The personality never quite reverts to its premorbid state and each attack leaves the patient less well than before.

Catatonic schizophrenia is commoner in females and occurs for the first time in young adulthood. Periods of stupor and excitement alternate. Mutism is often a feature, possibly in obedience to hallucinations. The patient may repeat what has just been said to her. She displays resistiveness and negativism and may adopt strange postures and mannerisms. She develops 'waxy flexibility' in that her limbs can be moved into incongruous positions and the pose maintained. During stupor the patient appears to be unaware of what is going on, but afterwards she can relate events quite accurately.

Paranoid schizophrenia first occurs in late life. It is characterized by suspiciousness, delusions and hallucinations of a persecutory nature. The delusions are often plausible and the patient tries to fit his hallucinations into his delusional ideas. The patient behaves as if his delusions were true.

General features of schizophrenia

The cause of schizophrenia is unknown. There is an obvious heredity factor which is thought to be due to a recessive gene.

Commonly the schizophrenic is a day-dreaming, shy, introverted person. Some psychiatrists and psychologists think there is a prepsychotic personality which develops psychotically due to a disturbed family environment that does not allow the individual to mature normally. This fits in with a feature of schizophrenia: the patient seems to retreat from the stresses of reality into the seeming security of a fantasy world.

Certain drugs can produce schizophrenic-type reactions in normal people, for example lysergic acid (LSD), mescaline and amphetamine addiction. This indicates that there is a possible biochemical change in schizophrenia.

Treatment and nursing care

Treatment is palliative to control the symptoms. The major tranquillizers, particularly the phenothiazines, form the basis of treatment. The particular drug of this group that best controls an individual patient's florid and bizarre symptoms is found by trial and error. It is essential that the patient continues drug therapy as long as prescribed; in some cases this will be for life. These drugs have some unpleasant side-effects so that the patient is often reluctant to take them, consequently suffering a relapse. The introduction of the long-acting phenothiazines has helped to solve this problem. Many schizophrenics can now be maintained in the community, attending a Modecate clinic regularly or being visited in their homes by the community nurse who administers their drugs and monitors their effects and the reciprocal influences of patient and environment.

Electroconvulsive therapy is sometimes used, and *leucotomy* may be performed as a final resort. The aim is to reduce the symptoms so that it will be possible to rehabilitate the patient socially.

These patients are emotionally isolated and withdrawn from reality. It is often necessary to retrain them to cope with basic hygiene and nutrition. Group therapy on an occupational, recreational and supportive level helps to socialize an asocial

Figure 16.10
Schizophrenia

patient by ensuring that he spends some time in the company of other people, participating, albeit passively, in activities.

The nurse can help a schizophrenic person to establish and maintain relationships with other people by first establishing a relationship with him. Much perseverance is needed to find a point of contact and to assist the patient to tolerate and later to participate in normal social interchanges. He learns by example to form and sustain interpersonal relationships, and he may need repeated stimulation and prolonged support from a perceptive nurse before he is able to live comfortably with other people.

Care must be taken to ensure that the patient is given suitable work. At first, repetitive, boring and simple jobs may be necessary, but more complex work providing stimulation and some responsibility should be included gradually.

Some patients are able to work out their disturbance through poetry, painting or music. These dimensions may act as a catalyst, opening the flood gates and allowing him to express some emotion.

Difficult behaviour of a violent, obstructive or destructive nature is usually based on fear and is possibly due to the patient's hallucinations and delusions. The nurse should not take such behaviour as a personal affront and should help the other patients and relatives to react helpfully.

If the patient has a secure family environment to go back to, day hospital facilities may be ideal for him. Others may be able to find accommodation and community life in half-way houses or after care hostels.

The prognosis is better for those whose first attack occurred later in life and for those with a stable family background. Most schizophrenics in the long-term need at least the help of the community psychiatric service and benefit from attachment to voluntary organizations that provide them with some form of social life.

Paranoia

Paranoid states have similar features to paranoid schizophrenia except that, apart from the delusions of persecution, the personality is usually normal. Also, the age group affected is usually older.

Paranoid reactions are a feature of most mental illnesses.

Organic psychoses

In the organic psychoses an organic condition is responsible for disturbed cerebral function causing the psychotic symptoms of confusion, memory impairment, disorientation and hallucinations.

ORGANIC PSYCHOSIS	
Causes	
Systemic	*Cerebral*
Infection	Infection
Metabolic disturbance	Tumour
Endocrine disorder	Degeneration
Deficiency disease	Trauma
Drug/alcohol intoxication	Epilepsy
Prominent feature	
CONFUSION	
Treatment	
Correct cause	

Figure 16.11
Organic psychosis

The origin of the cause may be infection, metabolic or endocrine disorder, deficiency diseases or drug intoxication. Cerebral disease including infection, tumours, epilepsy, trauma and degeneration are particularly important.

The nurse in the general hospital will be familiar with delirium and confusion states. In these instances the cause — say, dehydration — is found and treated and the condition is reversed. Sedation provides the patient with rest. Isolation, preferably in a cubicle, provides privacy until the acute stage is over. The presence of relatives and friends at his bedside will help to reorientate the patient. This is one occasion when nurses should try to impress their own identities on the patient so that he can easily recognize individual nurses and not be further disorientated by exposure to numerous faceless creatures in uniform.

Senile dementia

In the mental hospital the nurse will meet many cases of senile dementia, which is a disease of brain cell degeneration.

There tend to be more females than males with this condition and the onset is about 70 years of age. Some conditions with similar effects are known as the presenile dementias, and in these the onset may be as early as 55 years.

The normal changes of old age become steadily more marked. Early signs may be deterioration of memory and social behaviour. Memory for recent events fails but for remote events remains intact. Some physiological disorders, for instance dehydration, may cause symptoms which mimic senile dementia, but these symptoms disappear when the condition is reversed.

The features of the illness are a blunting of emotion, displaying petulant, irritable and childish behaviour. Apathy and depression accompanied by delusions of guilt may also feature. The patient shows obvious intellectual defects, for instance, difficulty in following an argument, perseveration, train of thought easily lost, becoming muddled even with the simplest tasks and mislaying articles.

Eventually talk becomes a mere babble of words and the patient is completely disorientated and unable to comprehend the simplest tasks or instructions. Delusions may be present.

Such people often have a sleep disturbance, turning day into night, and are often found pottering around the house or wandering in the streets during the night. Eating habits become depraved and urinary and faecal incontinence the norm.

When this stage is reached people require hospitalization and need to be separated from the elderly with sound mind, in the interest of the latter. They require intensive, constant care with many precautions for their safety. If at all possible they should be nursed out of bed because they will deteriorate more quickly both physically and mentally if confined to bed.

The patient should be encouraged to do things for himself for as long as possible and should take simple exercise and participate in occupational therapy. If not able to be ambulant the patient should be washed, dressed in daytime clothes and sat comfortably in an armchair with a group of other patients. Care should be taken over the patient's appearance. Many hospitals employ a beautician and hairdresser for this purpose.

These patients are like babies. They can sense approval even though they do not understand what you are saying. The words are unimportant as long as the tone is gentle, kind and approving. They respond to music, particularly the popular music of the era of their youth and the rousing, marching music which has a place in every culture. Small children and domestic animals evoke responses, often long forgotten by these patients, of tenderness and caring. Hands will reach out to touch, caress and offer treats; the names of loved children or pets will be on the smiling lips of someone who cannot name his nearest relative sitting beside him.

Diet should be light, nutritious and soft. Care should be taken in feeding to ensure that sufficient quantities of food and drink have been consumed by the patient.

There is a possibility that incontinence of urine may be psychological, resulting from regression into babyhood. If the patient has been allowed to lie in bed, warm and understimulated, regression to babyhood occurs when excreta was voided auto-

SENILE DEMENTIA

BRAIN CELL DEGENERATION IRREVERSIBLE!

Common features

FAILING FACULTIES

Memory for recent events fails

Disorientation

Blunting of emotion

Lack of comprehension

Simplest tasks muddled

Mislays articles

Perseveration

Confabulation

Talk-Babble

Turn day into night

Eating habits depraved

Incontinence

REGRESSION

Treatment

Clean   Warm   Dry   Fed   Titivated

Companionship   Social activities

L♡VING CARE

Figure 16.12
Senile dementia

matically without the voluntary control of the patient. This can be treated by stimulating the patient, getting him up and dressed, giving him simple occupational therapy and providing toilet training. In conjunction with this, habit training can be introduced in washing, dressing, feeding and toileting. This can be done in small groups with the same activity being practised at the same time each day for each patient and the same series of actions performed on each occasion. This may help to give back to the patient some independence and can help to arrest deterioration.

The nurse should ensure that the patient's bowels are emptied. Use of a commode or toilet is preferable so that he is in the natural position for defaecation. He should also be warm and comfortable. An impacted faecal mass is often a complication and may be masked by apparent diarrhoea. This may be a cause for restlessness and should always be investigated and treated. Often the patient is uncomfortable or in pain. If no cause can be found sedation may be prescribed.

With adequate nursing care and attention deterioration can be arrested and a certain amount of rehabilitation achieved. The greater the amount of activity and interest which can be provided the better the patient will retain his failing faculties.

Anxiety states

The anxiety states are common neurotic reactions which may be treated on an outpatient basis, although many people require treatment in hospital.

Anxiety is a normal, understandable reaction to a threat. Once this stress has been removed the symptoms of anxiety usually abate. Anxiety is a feature of depression, schizophrenia, mild brain damage and some physical diseases, such as thyrotoxicosis, but it can also be a neurotic condition in its own right.

Stress affects individuals differently but always in the areas in which they are already vulnerable. A situation which may seem trivial to one will be overwhelming to another. In an anxiety state the reaction is severe and prolonged and is usually precipitated by difficulties experienced by the individual in coping with a disturbing change in his occupational, social or domestic milieu.

Clinical features

Figure 16.13
Fear

Anxiety is fear, usually of the unknown, which gives rise to recognized physical symptoms affecting all the body systems. These include palpitations, tremors of the hands and feet, profuse sweating, frequency of micturition, diarrhoea, dryness of the mouth, indigestion and unpleasant sensations in the epigastrium, such as 'butterflies in the stomach'. Tension symptoms are frontal headache, mild aching of the muscles and fatigue.

Many anxious people overbreathe and therefore lose excessive quantities of carbon dioxide, which causes alkalosis and tetany.

Anxious people are more responsive to incoming stimuli and the resultant increased distractedness causes the psychological features associated with the condition, namely memory problems, lack of concentration, muddled feeling and fear that they are going mad.

The level of anxiety will fluctuate according to the amount of stress present. Colds and urinary tract infections can make the condition worse. Fear breeds fear and anxiety is habit-forming. An individual can learn to react to stress in a particular way.

An acute exacerbation is described as a 'panic attack' and may occur for little or no obvious reason. The features of a panic attack are palpitations, gasping respiration, unpleasant epigastric sensations, intense fear and a sense of impending death or doom.

Reassurance and sedation form the basis of treatment for such an attack.

Treatment and nursing care

The aim of treatment of an anxiety state is to help the patient recognize and cope with the problem areas of his life. He must be guided into developing insight into his condition.

He may, in common with many of these patients, dwell on physical symptoms to the exclusion of all else. To help him understand the true nature of his illness these symptoms must be fully investigated and, as each cause is eliminated, it is hoped that he will be nearer recognizing that the symptoms will only improve once he resolves his difficulties.

Symptomatic relief for the physical symptoms must be administered. Tranquillizers will be prescribed to help control the anxiety, and hypnotics if there is a sleep disturbance.

The patient must be helped to analyse his problems and this is best done in group, family or marital psychotherapy. Abreaction may help him to uncover the unconscious root of his difficulties. Supportive psychotherapy will encourage the patient to look at his reactions in relation to stress. Occupational and recreational therapy ensures that he is forming relationships with other patients; he can be helped to tolerate stress by being placed in increasingly stressful situations, always provided he has been successful in managing the previous test.

Co-operation from relatives should be sought and the patient should be seen coping with the stressful environment before being finally discharged from care.

The nurse must be sympathetic but firm with this patient to help him face reality.

Other manifestations of anxiety

Anxiety sometimes takes the form of a **phobia** which is an abnormal fear of a particular situation, such as going into crowds. The best treatment for this is behaviour therapy.

Obsessive, compulsive states are another form of anxiety in which the patient is obsessed with a disturbing thought or is compelled to perform repeatedly an act according to a ritual. The previous personality of many of these patients was that of a neat, tidy, punctilious individual who loves order for its own sake. There is often an overlay of depression.

Treatment is with the mild tranquillizers and antidepressants if appropriate. Supportive psychotherapy may be useful.

Hysteria is a way of resolving an anxiety conflict by the production of socially acceptable physical and mental symptoms. It is a common device with the primary aim of modifying the environment to suit the individual; frequently there are secondary advantages, such as gaining much attention. The individual is at least partially unaware of what he is doing.

Treatment is by tranquillizers, abreaction, sedation and analytical psychotherapy.

Anorexia nervosa

Anorexia nervosa is classified by the World Health Organization as a form of neurosis, characterised by starvation and its hormonal consequences. The age of onset is usually between 11 and 35 years. Normally those affected are of above average intelligence and belong to social groups 1 and 2.

There are two recognized types:

Primary anorexia nervosa which is a disturbance in body image concept characterized by the wish for 'thinness' achieved by a refusal to eat. This type commonly occurs in adolescents, mainly girls.

Secondary anorexia nervosa is a ploy of individuals, of both sexes and any age but again mainly women, to manipulate others by losing weight. Every case is different and atypical cases from both these groups are common.

The clinical features are a direct result of starvation. These patients refuse to eat, are emaciated and have serious depression of all vital functions. They present with facial pallor, cyanosis of the extremities, dry skin and head hair, downy growth on face and body, and amenorrhoea in the females. Characteristically they are restless, full of energy and guile.

The aim of treatment is to restore the patient to normal body weight and correct the underlying psychopathological disorder. This is best achieved by bed rest in hospital until the body weight is within normal limits. This allows rapport to develop between the psychiatric team and the patient as well as separating the patient from the family and friends emotionally involved in his/her illness. Treatment is continued in the psychiatric out-patient department.

Alcoholism

Alcoholics cannot control their drinking, which may be continuous or in bouts. Ultimately their physical and mental health is damaged. It is a social disease that disrupts the family and society. Many alcoholics have an underlying depression or anxiety state. By the time the patient comes for treatment it is not always obvious whether the home environment caused the addiction or results from it.

Aversion therapy and group psychotherapy have been used to treat this condition. Neither form of treatment has been very successful in the long term. In response to a government working party some special units were set up in the U.K. specifically for the treatment of alcoholism. Patients had to demonstrate that they were strongly motivated towards cure before being admitted to such a unit. These of course are expensive to run and it is difficult to measure their success rate.

Generally clinical treatment is mainly by sedation and the administration of vitamins to help counteract the withdrawal effects of alcohol. This is known as 'the drying out process' and mainly occurs in the surgical wards of general hospitals following admission from the Accident and Emergency Department.

If further treatment is considered necessary, the patient may be referred to a psychiatrist. His task is to treat any underlying psychiatric conditions although at this stage it is often difficult to gauge which came first — the psychiatric condition or the alcoholism. Other forms of help are given within the social setting, particularly from organizations such as Alcoholics Anonymous. As all the members of Alcoholics Anonymous have been alcoholics themselves they are uniquely able to provide the support and discipline the wavering alcoholic needs.

Alcoholism is now recognized as a social problem affecting people in all walks of life and more help and understanding is being given to the alcoholic at work and in society than ever before.

Moderation in the use of alcohol is advocated and real attempts are being made to make people aware of the unfortunate results of alcoholic abuse while they still have time to change their drink pattern.

Drug dependence

Drug dependence arises from repeated administrations of a drug on a periodic or continuous basis. The clinical features vary according to the drug or drugs involved. Barbiturates, cannabis, amphetamines, morphine, cocaine or LSD (lysergic acid diethylemide) are all examples of preparations which may be misused, either alone or in combination.

People likely to become drug addicts vary from the middle-aged housewife attempting to slim or with an insomnia problem, who becomes addicted to amphetamines or barbiturates, respectively, to the adolescent out for kicks taking LSD or cannabis. Sadly, glue sniffing has become a major problem among school-children.

Figure 16.14
Alcoholism

Figure 16.15
Drug dependence

Basically society is at fault. Drugs are readily available and money can be made from selling them. Taking them adds initial excitement to someone's life. During periods of economic depression when unemployment is common some people are tempted to make money by peddling drugs, or to relieve monotony by experimenting with them.

Increased doses are needed to provide the required effect, and unpleasant psychological and physical symptoms occur when the drug is withdrawn.

Co-operation is necessary for treatment. Hospitalization is best so that the drug can be 'tapered' off slowly. In some cases replacement therapy is given in the form of a synthetic drug, methadone (Physeptone).

The patient's nutritional state is improved and tranquillizers and antidepressants are prescribed if appropriate.

Long-term treatment requires some sort of social support and psychotherapy. Many fall into their old ways. For some death results.

Personality disorders

A psychopathic disorder, according to the Mental Health Act 1959, refers to a persistent disorder or disability of mind resulting in abnormally aggressive or seriously irresponsible conduct by a patient; it is considered to require medical treatment.

These patients are usually devoid of guilt or shame for their actions, are emotionally labile and do not appear to be able to form lasting friendships or respond to social training. They are often in trouble with the law and many are housed in the state mental hospitals.

The aim of treatment is to try to redirect their energies into more socially acceptable channels.

People who practise sexual deviations are also considered to have personality disorders. It is thought that they have regressed or not matured psychologically in their sexual development.

Tranquillizers, psychotherapy and abreaction can all be useful. Aversion therapy is employed to control a perversion such as fetishism.

NURSING IN A MENTAL HOSPITAL

A mental hospital provides a sheltered environment permitting the normal functions of sleeping, eating, work and recreation. In such an environment the patient can be trained — or can relearn — how to cope with everyday living. To meet this function most wards in mental hospitals provide separate sleeping and living accommodation similar to that of the average home.

Patients lead ordered lives: up and dressed for breakfast, off to work, treatment sessions or industrial or occupational therapy by 9 a.m., a break for coffee, more work or therapy before a break for lunch followed by a similar regime in the afternoon. Recreational activities may be confined to evenings or may also be encouraged in the afternoons.

Many patients need to be coaxed to adhere strictly to such an ordered life. Due to their illness many are lethargic and apathetic and much of the nurse's time can be spent in rousing enthusiasm for the various activities. As part of treatment and rehabilitation programmes the nurse participates with patients in all their daily activities therefore she can be found doing domestic work or some routine job in industrial or occupational therapy or perhaps dancing or playing games. By the example of her interactions with people the nurse teaches patients how to relate to others in simple situations, as well as by the part she plays in the various psychotherapeutic treatments. The nurse works, plays, talks and listens to the patient, becoming a confidante and mentor; she helps to develop the patient's potential to live as normal a life as possible by tolerating his eccentricities and by raising his expectations of his own behaviour.

The nurse also participates in discussions on the patient's progress with other members of the therapeutic team. To do this she must be able to report accurately and succinctly significant conversations held with the patient. Similarly, she must observe and report accurately the behaviour of the patient when he is alone and thinks himself unobserved and also his interactions with other patients, visitors and staff.

Many nurses entering mental hospitals for the first time are afraid that they will meet violence and strange behaviour with which they will not be able to cope. Actually, violence in the mental hospital is comparatively rare. Seeming violence is often impulsive behaviour that arises in response to hallucinations. Most patients are so well controlled by drug therapy that outbursts are uncommon, and in most cases a trained nurse is usually able to anticipate such behaviour and distract the patient successfully. Special arrangements are made for the criminally insane.

Nurses and new patients, very quickly become accustomed to the eccentric behaviour displayed by some patients, particularly the rituals of obsessive patients, and once this behaviour is understood it is soon tolerated and accepted as part of a person's individuality.

Boredom is the main complaint of new nurses workng in the field of mental health. Many find it hard to get involved in patient activities, and the quiet, even tenure of life in the mental hospital seems to contrast sharply with the rat race of the world outside the hospital walls. Great enjoyment, job satisfaction and personal development is experienced by the nurse who is able to involve herself in her patients' affairs while retaining a measure of objectivity and who does not allow her professional life to encroach on her personal life.

Mental nursing

All nurses must be able to give basic nursing care so that their patients will be clean, warm, and well nourished. They also require some technical knowledge and skills to be able to administer prescribed treatments. They must also develop the ability to deal with people tactfully and with kindness and understanding so that patients and their relatives will be reassured and trusting relationships formed.

To meet the physical and psychological needs of patients basic skills must be learnt, modified and adapted. For example, while working in a surgical ward the nurse learns how to dress and care for a wound. When working in a medical ward the nurse may meet a patient with a wound. The skills learnt in the surgical area are utilized so that the wound is given the same expert care it would have received if the patient had been nursed in a surgical ward.

Similarly when working with patients with mental illness the nurse has the opportunity to develop her capacity to form professional relationships with patients and staff. The knowledge and expertise which develops out of this experience should be utilized when nursing patients outwith the psychiatric hospital whether it be in the community, the obstetric department, the general medical or surgical wards or areas providing special care.

The psychological care of sick people and their relatives ranks in importance with the physical care required by patients. The nurse prepares herself to provide the physical needs of patients by studying human biology. Knowledge of the normal allows the nurse to understand the requirements necessary to correct any deviation from the normal.

Since nurses deal with people of all ages and circumstances in order to meet the psychological requirements of patients the nurse studies the psychology of: childhood, learning, the maturation process, ageing, bereavement, fear, and guilt. In particular the nurse should develop an understanding of the mental defence mechanisms. This will help her to appreciate the behaviour not only of patients and their relatives but also her own behaviour and that of her colleagues and superiors. Therefore, knowledge of the accepted normal behaviour in a given situation allows the nurse to cope with individual reactions.

This particular skill is one which the nurse will develop and use in her domestic and social life as well as in the work situation. Some may have a natural talent in this direction but all can learn the mechanisms of behaviour and use this knowledge to modify their own behaviour and develop some understanding of the behaviour of others. In her working life it is a skill the nurse will utilize daily wherever she is working and from the first day in the clinical area. She will also learn by observing and following the example set by more experienced nurses.

A period of experience in the psychiatric field gives the nurse the opportunity to consolidate the learning related to this skill. In the group setting she can study and experiment with her own behaviour and observe the behaviour of other members of staff and patients. Psychiatric patients are usually reasonably fit physically, therefore it is possible for both them and the staff caring for them to concentrate on their mental symptoms which usually demonstrate either some deviation from the normal or some exaggeration of the normal. In the environment of the psychiatric hospital the nurse is able to spend time listening to patients and observing their behaviour. Much of what is learnt from this experience can be utilized wherever the nurse is working. For example, anxiety manifests itself in similar ways regardless of whether the cause is real as in childbirth, preoperatively, or as in relatives watching a loved one die, or, with no apparent cause, as in agitated depression. Therefore by learning the responses of psychiatric patients to anxiety the nurse develops an awareness of how everyone reacts to anxiety. She can now work out how to combat or modify these reactions according to individual needs.

If a nurse is to be truly compassionate and at the same time able to offer practical help to patients and their relatives with their emotional needs, it is essential that she develops her skills so that she is able to meet the psychological needs of people as well as the physical needs.

SUGGESTED ASSIGNMENTS

Project

Find out to what extent the following are involved in the social rehabilitation of psychiatric patients in your area:

Halfway houses.
Day centres.
The local community.

Discussion topics

1. Is attempted suicide 'a cry for help'?
2. What do you understand by the term 'blurring of roles' in the context of the therapeutic community?
3. From your own observation does the community psychiatric nurse play a viable role in supporting the mentally ill patient outside the hospital?
4. Alcoholism is the commonest form of addiction in some countries, including Great Britain, and has profound social and psychological effects on the individual and his or her family. How can this problem be tackled nationally?

FURTHER READING

Barker P J 1983 Behaviour therapy nursing. Croom Helm, London
Bluglass R, Rawnsley K 1983 A guide to the Mental Health Act 1983. Churchill Livingstone, Edinburgh.
Brown J A C 1969 Freud and the post Freudians. Penguin, Harmondsworth
Burkhalter P K 1975 Nursing care of the alcoholic and drug abuse. McGraw Hill, New York
Dally P 1979 Anorexia nervosa. Heinemann, London
Department of Health and Social Security 1976 Review of the Mental Health Act 1959. A consultative document. HMSO, London
Drew L R H, Moon J R, Buchanan F H 1974 Alcoholism a handbook. Heinemann, London
Fleming A C, Paterson H F 1969 Mental disorder and the law. Churchill Livingstone, Edinburgh
Fowlie H C, Stokes R F 1972 Psychiatry in comprehensive nursing. Collins, Glasgow
Kneish C R, Ames S A 1974 Mental health concepts in medical surgical nursing. A handbook. Mosby, St. Louis
Kramer J F, Cameron D C (eds) 1975 A manual on drug dependence. WHO, Geneva
Longhorn E 1975 Psychiatric care and conditions. HM & M Publishers, Aylesbury

Maddison D, Day P, Leadbeater B 1976 Psychiatric nursing, 4th edn. Churchill Livingstone, Edinburgh

Mental Health Act 1983 HMSO, London

Mental Health (Scotland) Act 1984 HMSO, London

Mental Health (Northern Ireland) Act 1961 HMSO, London

Pitt B 1974 Psychogeriatrics. Churchill Livingstone, Edinburgh

Saxton D F, Hyland P A 1975 Planning and implementing nursing intervention. Mosby, St Louis

Silverstone T, Turner P 1974 Drug treatment in psychiatry. Routledge & Kegan Paul, London

Thompson S, Kahn J H 1970 The group process as a helping technique. Pergamon, Oxford

Tredgold R F, Wolff H H 1975 UCH notes on psychiatry, 2nd edn. Duckworth, London

WHO 1974 Glossary of mental disorders and a guide to their classification. WHO, Geneva

Section B
Individuals in hospital and community

Chapter Seventeen
The newborn

The birth of a baby is a family event in every culture, race and creed that is generally accompanied by joy and celebration. This precious, new life must be nurtured, protected and watched over with meticulous care.

Present-day obstetric and paediatric practice and improved nutrition and housing have contributed greatly to the reduction of *neonatal mortality* rates so that babies begin life with a much greater chance of survival. During the antenatal period the expectant mother and father attend classes to prepare them for labour, delivery and parenthood. The expectant father is encouraged to remain with his wife during labour and delivery and thus the unique experience of parenthood is shared from the moment of the baby's birth.

PREPARATION FOR DELIVERY

Warmth is essential. The baby will emerge from the uterus as it were from a warm bath — very wet — and so the skin cools rapidly. The delivery room temperature should never be below 25°C and if possible is best kept at 30°C. A cot is prepared with warm blankets, and a specially designed 'baby warmer' is available which provides heat directly over the baby's cot with servo temperature control (Fig. 17.1). The thermo-couple is attached to the baby's skin and the baby's temperature is recorded on a dial on the baby warmer.

A sterile delivery pack must be at hand and resuscitation equipment must be ready for immediate use (Fig. 17.2 A and B)

DELIVERY

When the baby's head is born the midwife quickly feels for the umbilical cord which may be round the baby's neck. The cord is only clamped and cut if it is tight and likely to cause strangulation of the baby during birth. The midwife then wipes the baby's eyelids to remove secretions from the birth canal which might contain pathogenic organisms. With the next contraction, the head rotates and the shoulders are born, followed quickly by the trunk and limbs.

IMMEDIATE CARE AT BIRTH
Airway

It is imperative that mucus extraction is carried out at once to prevent inhalation of mucus and secretions which could seriously endanger the baby's life. When the baby is completely born the head is tilted down for a few moments to allow drainage

Figure 17.1
Baby warmer showing
thermocouple in position

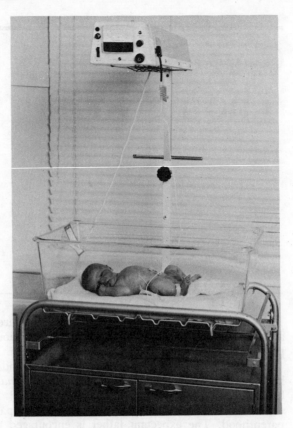

Figure 17.2 A
Resuscitaire with equipment

Figure 17.2B
Resuscitaire in use

Figure 17.3
Mucus extractor in use showing catheter in nasopharynx

of mucus from the trachea and pharynx. Aspiration is carried out by the midwife using a mucus extractor (Fig. 17.3). A healthy baby cries immediately.

Assessment at birth

The baby's general condition is rapidly assessed and care is taken to record the exact time of birth and onset of regular respirations. If the baby's condition gives any cause for anxiety the midwife immediately begins resuscitative measures and sends urgently for the paediatric team.

Apgar score

This is a method of estimating, in numerical terms, the heart beat, respiratory rate, colour, muscle tone and response to stimuli of a newly born baby 1 minute after birth (Table 17.1). It gives an assessment of the total condition and allows comparison of one baby with another. The method was first described by Dr Virginia Apgar. The highest possible score at birth is 10 and a score below 8 would indicate asphyxia. The lower the score, the greater the degree of asphyxia present.

Table 17.1
Apgar score sheet

Name _____ Date _____ Age (in minutes) _____

	0	1	2	Score
Heart rate	Absent	Below 100	Over 100	
Respiratory effort	Absent	Slow, irregular	Good, crying	
Muscle tone	Limp	Some flexion of extremities	Active movement	
Response to catheter	No response	Grimace	Cough or sneeze	
Colour	Blue pale	Body pink Extremities blue	Completely pink	
			Total score	

Sex

The sex is determined and medical aid sought if the genitalia are such that the sex of the infant is in doubt.

Preliminary examination

The baby is quickly examined for any obvious abnormality, but detailed examination is left until later.

The cord

Following cessation of pulsation the cord is clamped with Spencer Wells artery forceps 5 cm from the umbilicus. The second clamp is applied 6 cm from the umbilicus and the cord is divided between the two forceps. The baby is placed in a sterile towel and dried carefully. This towel is then discarded and the baby is wrapped in a fresh sterile towel and placed in the warmed cot until the delivery of the placenta is completed. The cord is finally occluded. There are several different methods in current use for accomplishing this:

1. The application of sterile cord clamps which may be removed in 48 hours or left until the cord drops off (Fig. 17.4).

Figure 17.4
Cord clamp occluding umbilical vessels

Figure 17.5
Application of cord ligatures

2. Ligation. Ligatures must be strong and made of material such as nylon tape which will not cut through the cord; otherwise it will cause immediate and profuse haemorrhage. As the substance of the cord (called *Wharton's jelly*) shrinks, the ligatures may become loose and may need to be reapplied (Fig. 17.5). Cord haemorrhage is a real danger and can have very serious consequences for the baby; therefore frequent examination of the cord must be made during the first 24 to 30 hours. No dressing is applied but the cord may be treated with an antiseptic preparation in surgical spirit.

Identification of the baby

This is an important duty of the midwife. Identification is carried out in the presence of the mother and possibly also the father; ideally it should be checked by them. Various methods are available. One of the most common is a transparent bracelet into which a card is inserted with the baby's particulars recorded on it. The bracelet is placed on the baby's ankle and secured by a special press stud (Fig. 17.6). It can only be removed by cutting it off. On admission to the nursery a second bracelet can be applied to the other ankle as an added safeguard.

Figure 17.6
Identification bracelet in position

The mother

Care of the mother during and after the third stage of labour is described in Chapter 10. It is essential to allow time for the mother to fondle her baby, examine him in minute detail, and put him to the breast if she so wishes. This skin contact, one with the other, is known as 'bonding' and forms the first vital link in the relationship of the mother and her baby. All her thoughts are centred around the baby's safety and physical needs and the mothering and protective instinct is very strong at that time. It is desirable to avoid separation of the mother and her newly born baby and in purpose-built maternity hospitals provision is made to have the baby beside the mother so that she may watch over him and feed him when he demands it (Fig. 17.7). However, rest during the day and sleep during the night are essential for the mother so separate accommodation must be provided to enable the baby to be removed if necessary.

SUBSEQUENT CARE OF THE NORMAL BABY

The baby is left to rest for 1 to 2 hours in his cot in the nursery. Special care must be taken to ensure that the baby's body heat is maintained and that the cord is examined frequently for bleeding. The rectal temperature should be 37°C; the room temperature should be 25–30°C.

Figure 17.7
Rooming in

Detailed examination

This is undertaken by the midwife and the paediatrician. Measurements of length, head circumference and weight must be very carefully checked and recorded as an error can cause great anxiety and distress to the parents.

General inspection, noting the size, cry, colour, limb movements, respiratory rate and chest movement and general reaction to touch, noise and light, is carried out before noting the following particular anatomical details.

The head

This is inspected generally and any swellings such as *caput succedaneum* which may be present from birth, or *cephalhaematoma*, which may develop later, are noted.

The **mouth** must be carefully examined with a good light for cleft palate. A cleft lip is obvious but a posterior cleft in the palate could be missed unless looked for specifically.

An excessive amount of mucus may indicate an abnormality of the alimentary tract and must always be reported immediately.

The limbs

The limbs should move freely. All babies are examined for congenital dislocation of the hips (Fig. 17.8).

The **hand** must be opened out gently to examine the fingers. Occasionally there is an extra digit attached to the little finger (Fig. 17.9). When inspecting the feet the toes are also carefully examined for the same reason. The presence of club foot (*talipes*) (Fig. 17.10) would also be noted.

The back

The back is inspected for *spina bifida* (Fig. 17.11). This condition is described in Chapter 3.

The external genitalia

These are examined carefully. In a male child the urethra may not extend to the end of the penis but open on to the under surface. This condition is known as hypo-

Figure 17.8
Examination for congenital
dislocation of the hips (Courtesy
of Keay and Morgan — Craig's
care of the newly born infant.
Churchill Livingstone, Edinburgh)

Figure 17.9
Extra digit

Figure 17.10
Bilateral club foot (Talipes)

Outline of
normal foot

Outline of
club foot

Bilateral club foot (Talipes)

Figure 17.11
Spina bifida
(Courtesy of
Dr J. B. Scrimgeour,
Consultant Obstetrician
and Gynaecologist,
Western General
Hospital, Edinburgh)

Cerebrospinal
fluid

Skin

Spinal cord

Meninges

spadias. If the urethra opens on to the upper surface of the penis the condition is known as epispadias (Ch. 9). Surgery may be required in childhood to correct either condition.

The anus

Occasionally the anus may be covered with a thin, anal membrane giving rise to an imperforate anus. It can be corrected by incision of the membrane. There may, however, be atresia of the anal canal and if so a colostomy (Ch. 5) will be necessary to relieve the obstruction.

Bathing

It must be borne in mind that the newborn baby's skin is very delicate and susceptible to infection.

Initial cleansing of the skin may be carried out using a diluted solution of an antiseptic detergent such as Phisomed or Sterzac lotion. The prolonged use of the antiseptic detergents can be dangerous but the advantages of short-term use outweigh the risk of staphylococcal infection of the skin.

The temperature control of the newborn is unstable and therefore there is a greater tendency for the body temperature to drop. This must be avoided by ensuring that the bathing area is warm — 25–30°C and the temperature of the bath water is 37.7°C. Infa-Care or a similar preparation which has special cleansing properties may be added to the bath water in place of soap which might not be suitable for the baby's skin. Meticulous attention must be paid to the skin folds of the neck, axillae and groins where there are large amounts of *vernix caseosa*. The cord stump should be treated with an antiseptic such as 0.5% Hibitane in 70% surgical spirit, checked for bleeding and if necessary ligatures applied.

The baby's temperature should always be checked at the end of the procedure. The baby is then dressed in light, simple clothing allowing free movement without constriction.

Feeding

The rate of growth of the baby should continue at much the same rate as it did in the uterus before birth. In order to achieve this and to keep the infant healthy, he must be fed sufficiently often with the correct amount and type of food.

Breast feeding

Breast feeding for the newborn is ideal from both a nutritional and an emotional point of view and every encouragement should be given to the mother to attempt it, even if only for a short period. Antenatal classes will have helped to educate her and she will have had the opportunity to discuss breast feeding at the antenatal clinic and during parentcraft teaching. In preparation for breast feeding advice will have been given regarding a good fitting brassiere and gentle, daily massage of the nipples with a lanoline-based cream preparation.

The baby is usually offered his first feed within a few hours of birth. The early feeds must be fully supervised. Patience and tact are required as this is an unfamiliar experience for the new mother who may become despondent if the baby does not suck readily. Sufficient time must be taken to ensure that she is comfortable and holding the baby correctly (Fig. 17.12). If possible, demand feeding should be encouraged since the baby will feed well when he is hungry.

Colostrum is present in the breasts from the 16th week of pregnancy. It has a higher protein content and a smaller amount of sugar and fat than milk and is easily digested. It also contains immunoglobulins (Ch. 1). During the first 2 or 3 days the colostrum increases in amount and gradually alters in composition and by the fourth day milk is being produced. At this stage the breasts may be tense and feel uncomfortable. Warm bathing will stimulate the flow of milk through the lactiferous ducts

Figure 17.12
Breast feeding

to the nipple and will relieve the tension. A good supporting brassiere should be worn.

Early breast feeds should be of short duration to avoid damage to the nipple. Care must be taken to ensure that the baby draws the nipple back to the soft palate so that the gums exert pressure on the areola, **not** on the nipple itself.

Before and after feeds the breasts and nipples must be carefully inspected, washed and dried. If there is pain associated with feeding, the affected breast is rested, the milk gently expressed by hand and a soothing ointment applied. The mother quickly gains confidence in her ability to feed her baby so long as she has maximum support and reassurance in the early days.

Artificial feeding

If breast feeding is not possible there are many baby milk preparations available.

Prepared feeds

During the last few years a number of firms have produced prepared and sterilized feeds in sealed bottles for use in hospital (Fig. 17.13). A separate sterile disposable teat unit is supplied. This system is costly to use but no milk kitchen or staff is required and there is no risk of the feeds becoming contaminated during preparation. Prepared feeds are coming into production for use at home also, but at the moment they are too expensive for the average household.

Dried milk

Dried milk is used widely. It is reconstituted by adding 30 ml boiled water to one level scoop of powder. It may be necessary to add sugar as recommended on the packet if this has not already been done by the manufacturer. The recommended volume of feed the baby requires should only be used as a guideline; his activity and maturity should also be considered. In 7 to 10 days the baby should be taking 150 ml per kg of body weight divided into five feeds. For example, a baby of 3.5 kg will take 100 ml per feed and five feeds per 24 hours.

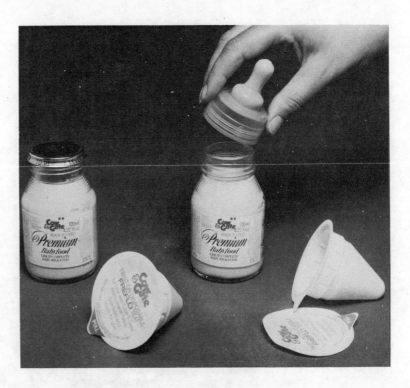

Figure 17.13
Prepared feed and teat unit

It is essential to teach the mother the importance of sterilizing bottles, teats and equipment, how to prepare feeds and the dangers to the baby of faulty technique. The mother must also be taught to hold her baby in the crook of her arm close to her body as she would during breast feeding. It is essential that she gives the baby her undivided attention and maintains 'face to face' contact with her baby throughout the feed.

Daily observations and care

A healthy, thriving baby has a clear, pink skin, moves freely, cries lustily, feeds eagerly and has good muscle tone.

During intrauterine life some antibodies pass across the placenta from the mother to the baby. Most mothers have antibodies to common virus diseases such as measles and chickenpox, so most new born babies have a degree of passive immunity to these diseases. which may last for about 3 months (Ch. 1). Babies are, however, very susceptible to bacterial infection and must be protected by good nursing technique and scrupulous cleanliness of the nursery and equipment. Individual equipment for each baby reduces the possibility of cross-infection. Handling of the baby by friends and relatives must be discouraged.

Accurate recording of all observations is of prime importance in caring for the newborn, and it should be remembered that the paediatrician has to depend upon the nurse to carry out this duty and to rely on her judgements. Some observations are best carried out when feeding the baby or changing him. These include:

Respirations

Any change in respiratory pattern during feeding or crying, particularly if accompanied by a change in colour, is noteworthy and could indicate, for example, respiratory infection or a congenital heart lesion.

Colour

Undue pallor or blueness are always serious signs and should be reported immediately.

Physiological jaundice

The newborn baby has an excessive number of red blood cells. The surplus RBCs are broken down and the iron is stored in the liver and spleen; as the newborn baby's liver cannot cope immediately with conjugating all the bilirubin produced, it accumulates in the bloodstream staining the skin yellow.

This type of jaundice appears around the third day of life and often causes drowsiness and disinclination to feed. The doctor may wish to estimate the serum bilirubin level. In a mature baby the jaundice clears up by the sixth or seventh day and the baby suffers no ill effects. It can however be dangerous to low birth weight babies.

Jaundice occurring during the first 24 hours of life is always of serious significance and jaundice occurring later than the normal physiological type can also be ominous. Thus the time of onset of jaundice must be recognized promptly and recorded correctly.

Vomitus

Records should show when the vomiting occurred in relation to feeding and the character of the vomitus. It may be due simply to poor feeding technique or it may indicate a serious complication.

Urine

Urine is often voided during birth; if so this must be noted as it may not be passed again for 24 hours.

Stools

Meconium is usually passed within the first 24 hours of birth; over the next few days the stools alter to a greenish-brown colour known as the 'changing' stool. After 3 or 4 days the breast fed baby's stools become yellow and soft in consistency and are passed three to four times per day. The artificially fed baby has more formed stools which are greyish in colour and have an offensive odour. The total number of stools must be carefully recorded over a 24-hour period.

Care of the buttocks

The buttocks require thorough cleansing and drying each time the napkin is changed. Zinc and castor oil cream may be applied as a prophylactic measure to the perianal region to prevent soreness. If sore buttocks do occur the cause must be carefully investigated. The soreness may be due to:

1. Faulty washing and rinsing of the napkin. Modern detergents are not suitable for washing napkins and a change in laundering method may produce immediate improvement.

2. Unsuitable feeding. Frequent stools are a source of irritation to the skin. This condition can be caused by too much sugar in the feed or by the feed being prepared incorrectly.

3. Infection. Gastroenteritis also causes frequent loose stools. This is a most dangerous condition in a newborn baby — it results in rapid dehydration and collapse. Speedy diagnosis is vital to the baby's life and any suspicious case must be isolated immediately since the disease readily becomes epidemic. Treatment is directed at removing the cause and restoring fluid and electrolyte balance. Antibiotic therapy is essential. In a severe case the buttocks can be exposed in a warm environment to promote healing. Various soothing creams can be used.

General care of the skin and mucous membranes

From birth until the fourth or fifth day the baby is usually 'top and tailed' in his cot. The technique has already been described for initial cleansing. Special note must be taken of the following points during the procedure:

Eyes

There should be no discharge from a newborn baby's eyes. Tears are not formed during crying in the early weeks and any discharge must be treated as infection.

Mouth

Inspection of buccal mucosa and tongue for thrush infection must be carried out. This condition is most commonly seen in the mouth of an artificially fed baby and seldom in a breast fed baby. It is caused by the *Candida albicans* and is contagious. It can be spread round a nursery by the nurses' hands and equipment. The baby does not feed well and, on examination of the mouth and tongue, there are greyish-white spots which look like milk curd but on gentle examination cannot be removed. Should thrush infection arise the nursery techniques must be carefully investigated, paying special attention to the preparation of feeds and the handling of bottles and teats. The baby will be isolated or barrier nursed with all his equipment including feeding utensils. The doctor may order a course of nystatin oral drops 100 000 units 3 or 4 times daily for 4 to 7 days. Thrush responds quickly to treatment. Early recognition is essential because it can spread very quickly.

Skin flexures

The skin flexures are cleansed, dried and inspected for infection.

Cord

The cord stump and surrounding tissues must be examined for signs of infection and treated at least twice daily with Hibitane in spirit.

Skin

Bathing of the baby is usually permitted by the fifth or sixth day of life. A demonstration is given to the mother who should then be allowed to bath her own baby with guidance from the midwife at least twice before she goes home.

Temperature

The temperature must be taken and recorded at least once daily using a special low reading rectal thermometer (scale down to 25°C).

Weight

This may be recorded daily, but care must be taken to ensure that the mother does not become obsessed with the baby's weight pattern. For the first 2 to 3 days the weight falls mainly due to the passage of urine and meconium and because of a small fluid intake. By the fourth to fifth day it should begin to rise again and a mature and healthy baby will regain his birth weight in 7 to 10 days.

Identification

Identification bands should be checked daily.

The baby should be beside his mother as much as possible and the mother should be encouraged to care for her baby under sympathetic supervision.

SPECIAL CARE OF LOW BIRTH WEIGHT BABIES

If a baby at birth weighs 2500 g or less he is classified as being of **low birth weight**. This may be because:

1. He has been born too soon — **preterm**
2. He has not grown normally before birth — **light-for-dates**.

The preterm baby

In Chapter 10 the method of working out the EDD (expected date of delivery) was described. A baby is considered to be at term if delivered between 37 and 41 weeks. If he is born early, that is before 37 weeks' *gestation* he is known as a preterm baby. The chances of survival are reduced as the gestational period becomes shorter, especially if it is less than 34 weeks. Most maternity hospitals or units have a special care nursery designed to provide the best possible conditions for nursing low birth weight babies under the direction of a consultant paediatrician.

A high standard of nursing care must be maintained with careful attention to detail, and it is crucial that the paediatrician is provided with accurate records. Continuous observation of these babies is essential and in many instances intensive nursing care is required. The survival of special care babies depends on a team effort involving medical and nursing staff.

Modern incubators with an infant servocontrol give a continuous record of the baby's body temperature as well as controlling the incubator temperature to maintain the baby's temperature at a preset level (Fig. 17.14). The baby is nursed naked which makes observation much easier; in particular the colour and respiratory pattern can be readily noted. Oxygen administration must be carefully monitored and regulated and the humidity controlled.

Figure 17.14
Incubator showing apnoea monitor with alarm, which sounds if the baby stops breathing

Feeding

Feeding can be started soon after birth. Human milk is most easily digested but is not always available and it may be necessary to use a special artificial milk preparation for preterm babies. Preterm babies have poor sucking and swallowing reflexes and may need to be fed with expressed breast milk via a nasogastric catheter which can be left in situ (Fig. 17.15). Abdominal distension causing respiratory embarrassment following a feed can occur, and therefore the volume of each feed must be carefully worked out according to the baby's weight and capacity. There may also be problems with the digestion of the feed.

Daily care

Minimal handling with as little disturbance to the baby as possible is essential. The detail of daily care has been already described for the normal baby. All procedures should be carried out prior to feeding, working through the incubator portholes

Figure 17.15
Tube feeding showing use of
incubator porthole

(Fig. 17.15). Weighing may be carried out using a special scale designed for use inside the incubator. The weight usually falls and levels out during the first 7 to 10 days and then slowly rises and the birth weight may be regained in 2 or 3 weeks.

The mother

As the baby must be nursed in a special care nursery some separation from the mother is inevitable. It is vital to the infant-mother relationship that every effort be made to involve the mother as much as possible in the care of her baby. It is now the policy of most paediatricians to allow the mother into the nursery and to encourage her to handle her baby under supervision (Fig. 17.16), even if it only involves holding her baby's hand for a short time.

Complications

Some common complications that are liable to occur in preterm babies include:

Respiratory Distress Syndrome (RDS)

This condition is characterized by cyanosis — rapid respirations with marked indrawing of the ribs and the sternum accompanied by apnoeic attacks which may gradually become more prolonged and severe. This condition manifests itself soon after birth and requires intensive nursing care. High concentration oxygen therapy or the infant ventilator may be required combined with intravenous administration of electrolytes, particularly sodium bicarbonate, via the umbilical vessels. Feeds may be given by continuous drip method via the nasogastric catheter. Many babies do recover but there are a number who die, particularly those of low gestational age.

Oxygen concentration levels must be estimated frequently using a special oxygen analyser. Prolonged administration of a high concentration of oxygen may cause damage to the blood vessels of the retina of the eye causing irreversible blindness. Oxygen should be reduced as soon as the baby's condition shows improvement and discontinued altogether as soon as possible.

Jaundice

Physiological jaundice, which often occurs in the normal full-term baby, tends to be more severe in the preterm baby due to immaturity of the liver. The jaundice

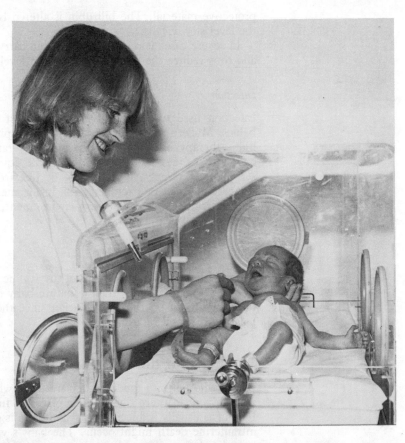

Figure 17.16
Mother making physical contact
with her baby

becomes more intense as the serum bilirubin level rises steadily in the circulating blood. If untreated the baby may suffer permanent brain damage or even die. The serum bilirubin level in the blood is checked twice daily, sometimes even more frequently, and phototherapy may be given (Fig. 17.17).

Phototherapy is exposure of the baby (naked) to fluorescent light which is a source of blue light. Care must be taken to expose the baby for the prescribed number of hours, maintain the body temperature and shield the eyes with a light pad of

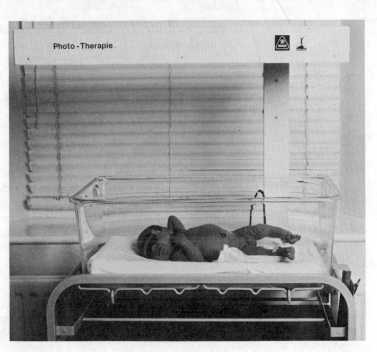

Figure 17.17
Phototherapy

protective material. The bilirubin is altered by the blue light and as it is excreted the level slowly falls.

In severe cases it may be necessary to carry out a replacement blood transfusion and thus reduce the circulating bilirubin level.

Infection

Infection used to be one of the commonest causes of death in low birth weight babies. Modern paediatric practice using improved techniques combined with anti-biotic therapy has cut down the mortality rate. All precautions must be taken to ensure that the nurseries, furnishings and equipment including incubators are kept scrupulously clean. All staff must be free from infection, and visitors other than the parents must be excluded from inside the nursery area. Frequent screening by the bacteriologist of the nursery environment, equipment and staff helps to control infection.

Follow-up

After the baby's initial problems of survival he may be slower to reach the milestones of development (Ch. 18) than a mature baby of the same age. His progress is care-fully monitored by the paediatrician since there is a considerable risk of cerebral palsy and mental retardation.

The light-for-dates baby

Babies who fall into this category are those who have been subjected to inadequate nourishment in utero due to poor placental function, for example in *pre-eclampsia*. Labour is usually induced early when there is evidence of poor fetal growth because intrauterine death might occur. The baby's weight is less than anticipated for the gestational age.

Nursing care

The light-for-dates baby also requires expert care, which is provided in the special care baby unit.

Feeding

Feeding by nasogastric catheter is not usually necessary since the light-for-dates baby can swallow and suck satisfactorily.

Complications

Complications which are likely to occur in a baby which is light-for-dates are the following:

Hypoglycaemia

This condition is liable to occur in the first 48 hours and serious brain damage may occur following convulsions. It may be precipitated by lack of oxygen and chilling.

Prevention is essential. Resuscitation at birth must be prompt and in a warm environment. Early feeding will also prevent the development of hypoglycaemia. Screening may be carried out with Dextrostix and blood specimens examined for glucose every 4 hours during the danger period.

Hypothermia

The light-for-dates baby is lacking in subcutaneous fat and loses heat very quickly. It is an essential part of nursing care to maintain the body temperature and it may be necessary to nurse the baby in an incubator.

Infection

The light-for-dates baby is also at risk, as is the preterm baby.

Follow-up

Follow-up care is carried out by the paediatrician. The outlook for the light-for-dates baby has greatly improved with modern care but he may remain small throughout his life.

MOTHERCRAFT TEACHING

Mothercraft classes in the postnatal period are of great importance (Fig. 17.18). They are more meaningful than those in the antenatal period as the baby is now born and imminent discharge home with the potential problems this involves is almost upon the new mother. Topics covered in these classes may include:

Prevention of home accidents.
Health education.
Demonstration of modern baby 'aids'.
Role of community midwife and health visitor.
Introduction to family planning with leaflets and location of clinics so that the mother can take them home and discuss this important matter with her husband.

A close liaison between the hospital, district midwife, health visitor and general practitioner must be established so that when the mother and baby are discharged home all the relevant information is readily available. Nursing care of the mother and baby in the puerperium is different from general nursing. Patient dependency is minimal: the majority of the new mothers are not ill and are quickly ambulant. The role of the nurse is a supportive one — helping the mother to adapt herself to and accept the responsibilities of motherhood. A great deal of tact, patience and human understanding are essential.

Figure 17.18
Mothercraft teaching

FURTHER READING

Bailey R E, Grayshon J 1983 Obstetric and gynaecological nursing, 3rd edn. Bailliere Tindal, London
Keay A J, Morgan D M (eds) 1982 Craig's care of the newly born infant, 7th edn. Churchill Livingstone, Edinburgh
Jolly H 1981 Diseases of children, 4th edn. Blackwell Scientific, Oxford
Scottish Health Education Group 1980 The book of the child. SHEG, Edinburgh

Chapter Eighteen
Children

This chapter gives an introduction to the special needs of children and outlines the services in the community and in hospital which are designed to meet those needs.

The nurse must remember that children are not small adults; their tolerance of illness and response to treatments cannot be assumed to be in proportion to their size. Indeed their reactions are often markedly different and may bear no relationship to those of adults. In general, children respond quickly and dramatically both to illness and to treatment. Early signs of adverse reactions must be noted and reported with the minimum of delay because a small child's condition can deteriorate so rapidly. For this reason the paediatric nurse must be forever vigilant. A junior nurse should remember that it is better to raise a false alarm than run the risk of irreversible worsening of a young patient's condition through hesitation because of uncertainty.

It is essential to have an understanding of the growth and development of the healthy child so that any deviation from the normal which the sick child may show can be easily and quickly recognized.

GROWTH AND DEVELOPMENT OF THE NORMAL CHILD

Growth refers to an increase in size, development to the processes whereby a child matures physically, mentally, emotionally and socially. The normal rate of growth is not constant throughout the growing years; it is most rapid in the first 2 years of life and during adolescence. Each child has his own pace of development although most children follow the same sequence. The pace is determined by both the child's innate potential and his environment; the physical care and mental stimulation he receives are important influencing factors.

Development depends on the maturation of the nervous system. No amount of teaching will enable a baby to perform a skill before the necessary areas of the nervous system are mature. The direction of development is cephalocaudal, that is from the head downwards through the trunk to the lower limbs. The infant can grasp with his hands before he can co-ordinate with his lower limbs, and he can hold his head up before he can sit. A child learns to sit before he can walk, and the age at which he learns to walk varies considerably from one child to the other.

There is progression from general responses to the more specific. The baby demonstrates his emotions by activity of his arms and legs, increased respirations and by becoming pink with excitement, whereas an older child shows his emotions by facial expression only.

Formulae have been devised from studies carried out on infants and children which provide average standards for growth and development; these are known as milestones or norms.

Stages of growth and development

During the first few months of life activity is instinctive, for example sucking, swallowing, grasping and eliminating. A baby develops an awareness of his surroundings, of being loved and adequately nourished and of security through the care given by his mother. He sleeps most of the time, wakening only for feeds, and he will cry in response to hunger or discomfort. Later crying may indicate fear, anger or frustration.

At 3 months old he sleeps less, recognizes and enjoys his mother's company, smiles and is interested in quiet play. He listens to music and his eyes will follow a moving object which he will attempt to grasp. At 5 months he chuckles and makes babbling sounds, can sit with support for a short time, discovers his fingers and toes and plays by himself briefly, enjoying repetitive play. Also around this time, he can recognize familiar faces and show his pleasure. He may show fear when approached by the unfamiliar.

At 6 months he can determine sound direction and turn his head towards it. He develops a need to bite and, by this time, primary teeth begin to appear, the central lower incisors being the first. At 7 months he can sit unsupported and propel himself in any direction using his arms and hands.

At 9 months he tries to feed himself and can grasp small objects using finger and thumb, often protesting when the object is taken away from him. By now he can raise himself on hands and knees in an attempt to pull himself upright. He speaks in monosyllables and can imitate a variety of sounds. If thumb sucking develops this may signify hunger, distress, tiredness or insecurity.

The toddler is dependent on his mother and a familiar routine. He becomes insecure if the pattern of his daily life is altered. He strives towards independence by attempting to dress and feed himself; these attempts are initially untidy and messy, but with patience and encouragement the child will eventually succeed. At this stage the child is full of curiosity and activity; he sleeps well and requires a nap during the day.

Voluntary control of bowel and bladder begins at the age of $1\frac{1}{2}$ to 2 years. There is extreme urgency initially, but this decreases as he grows older so that by the age of $2\frac{1}{2}$ to 3 years, he attains sphincter control and may demand privacy for toilet purposes.

He lives entirely in the present and time is associated with a familiar routine. He has no concept of sharing. He requires play materials of differing textures and shapes to stimulate co-ordination and learning capabilities. He plays happily on his own, alongside other children, without becoming involved in their play. If disturbed or restricted in his activities, he may display signs of frustration and anger. About this time, too, a child may notice and ask questions about sexual differences. Sibling rivalry may present problems to the 2 to 3 year old who may resent a new baby or the abilities of an older child. Vocabulary increases and he loves repeating simple nursery rhymes or listening to familiar stories.

Primary or deciduous dentition is complete by the third year. From the age of 6 years permanent teeth gradually replace the primary teeth.

Between the ages of 3 and 5 years, improved co-ordination and balance allow the child to run and climb confidently. He becomes socially aware and learns to share and play with other children. He particularly enjoys playing with sand and water, bricks, jigsaws, paint, construction toys and equipment, using imagination to act out domestic activities, pleasant and unpleasant. A greatly increased vocabulary and ability to articulate allow the child to construct simple sentences.

At this stage attendance at a nursery school or preschool group is invaluable; here the child will have the opportunity to increase his social experiences and will be provided with occupations that encourage concentration and learning.

From the age of 5, growth continues at a constant rate until the preadolescent state when there is a marked increase. This is known as the growth spurt. There is rapid growth of the limbs followed by growth of the trunk, and sex differences are demonstrated by the distribution of fat and muscle. These changes and the development of the secondary sex characteristics occur earlier in girls, although they are physically less strong than boys.

During the school years, emotions tend to fluctuate between feeling secure and feeling anxious. Sleep patterns may be disturbed and nightmares are common due to the fears caused by the demands of wider educational experiences. Competition is enjoyed but failure is not easily accepted. Learning continues rapidly, interests widen and the peer group becomes all important.

CARING FOR CHILDREN IN THE COMMUNITY

In the United Kingdom the responsibility for community care is shared by the Departments of Health, Education and Social Services. The facilities they offer are available to all children. The midwifery service takes care of the mother and baby until 10 to 14 days after delivery, whether a baby is born in hospital or at home (Ch. 17).

The preschool child

From this time the main adviser to the mother is the health visitor, unless illness occurs when the family doctor is consulted. The health visitor is concerned with the physical and mental health of the whole family; she has an important role in the prevention and early detection of health problems.

Her work includes visiting homes where there are preschool children. During these visits she advises mothers to attend the local child health centre or group practice 'well-baby' clinics. Such clinics are organized by the health visitors and provide advice on all aspects of mental, physical and social care as the need arises.

Routine medical examinations are carried out by the doctor at the first visit, and at 3, 6 and 12 months, then annually during the preschool years. Physical and developmental assessments are made at these times and the doctor will also be available if the mother or health visitor wishes the child to be seen between routine examinations. When the child is 9 months old, the health visitor carries out routine hearing tests. The clinic provides an immunization service. A sample immunization programme is shown in Table 18.1

Table 18.1
Sample immunization programme

Year	Vaccine/Toxoid	Remarks
1st	(a) Triple antigen (diphtheria whooping cough, tetanus)	(a) At 3 to 6 months
	Poliomyelitis (Sabin)	
	(b) As above	(b) At about 8 months
	(c) As above	(c) At 10 to 12 months
2nd	Measles	May be given in third year to reduce the risk of reactions
5th	Diphtheria/tetanus Poliomyelitis	Booster dose
10th to 13th	BCG	Only if negative on tuberculin testing
11th to 13th	Rubella	Offered to all girls
15th to 19th	Poliomyelitis Tetanus	Usually at school-leaving age

Advice on health education, parentcraft and accident prevention is provided through group discussions, lectures and films. Any special problems such as those of the immigrant family can be dealt with or the family can be put in touch with additional services, if necessary. Welfare foods and vitamins are provided at reduced cost — for instance vitamin drops for the baby and vitamin tablets for nursing mothers. Free milk is available for children in special need. The centre becomes a meeting place where mothers can make friends and have discussions about their families.

Home visiting by the health visitor is continued at regular intervals. The main advantage of home visiting is to see the child in his own environment and thus assess more readily whether adequate care is being given. The health visitor checks that growth and development are proceeding normally. She advises on feeding, clothing, general hygiene and immunization and gives practical guidance on the prevention of home accidents. If she recognizes social or mental stress within the family she will advise and mobilize the relevant services. She maintains a record of progress for each child which is passed on to the school medical service when full time education begins.

Day nurseries for children from 6 weeks up to 5 years are available to families with temporary or long-term social problems. They are open 6 days each week from 8 a.m. to 6 p.m., are staffed by trained nursery nurses and are equipped to meet the needs of the different age groups.

Nursery schools are provided by the Education and Social Services Departments for children between the ages of 3 to 5 years. They may attend for a half day or a full day. Time is spent in constructive play and group activities organized by teachers assisted by nursery nurses. The objectives are to help children become happy, active members of a group, to gain experience with adults outside the family and to prepare them for the wider experience of infant school.

A registered childminder may look after a small group of children in private premises if the facilities have been approved by the Social Services Department.

Private play groups with functions similar to those of nursery schools are supported by the **Preschool Play Groups Association**. Play groups financed by the Save the Children Fund are often sited in socially deprived areas where much of the work is carried out by voluntary help. These, too, must be approved by the Social Services Department.

The school child

In the U.K. it is the responsibility of the school medical service to continue the supervision of the child's health throughout his school years and to co-operate with the education service to help the handicapped child. The health team includes the school doctor, health visitor and/or school nurse. Medical examinations, including hearing tests, are carried out on all children on starting school and at intervals throughout the school years. This includes testing vision when the child is 7 years old. Dental inspection is carried out every 6 months. Reinforcing immunization programmes are continued and BCG vaccination is given to any child leaving school who has a negative response to a Mantoux test.

The school nurse or health visitor carries out regular examinations of the children to ensure that personal cleanliness is maintained. She looks in particular for lice infestation of hair, infections of scalp, skin rashes such as scabies and verrucae of the feet (Ch. 14). Appropriate treatment (which may include the whole family) is initiated as necessary.

The health team assists in promoting health education within the school curriculum and meets with parent-teacher groups. The topics discussed include personal hygiene, dental care, nutrition and eating habits, self-discipline related to the use of leisure hours, sex, smoking, alcohol and drugs.

A school meals service is available and children are provided with lunch at a nominal cost. In cases of need, lunches and extra meals are provided free of charge. Footwear and clothes can be provided when families have financial problems. Children not living within walking distance of school (2 miles for those under 8 years and 3 miles for older ones) are provided with transport to and from school. Representatives of road safety organizations and the police assist in school road safety programmes. To ensure the safety of children crossing busy roads, patrolmen are on duty to control traffic.

The handicapped child

Special care and education are provided by local education authorities for all physically handicapped and educable mentally handicapped children. Some of these services are assisted by voluntary organizations. Disabled children are examined at yearly intervals or more frequently as required. There is close liaison between the school health team, family doctor, parents and teacher to ensure adequate treatment and follow-up.

There are 10 categories of handicap:

Blind.
Partially blind.
Deaf.
Partially deaf.
Educationally subnormal.
Epileptic.
Maladjusted.
Physically handicapped.
Children with speech defects.
Delicate children.

Where possible, these children attend ordinary classes or they are placed in a special class within a normal school, thus enabling them to share in the general activities as far as possible. Others require special schools which may be either day or residential; those with multiple handicaps may be taught at home or in a hospital school. Ideally, all handicapped children should be educated in their home community and should interact with normal children, within the limits of their handicap.

Children whose mental subnormality renders them ineducable are cared for in occupational centres or in hospitals for the mentally subnormal where sociability and independence are encouraged (Ch. 15).

The deprived child

In Britain, the Children's and Young Person's Act of 1963 authorized local authorities to give assistance to deprived children in kind or in cash where necessary and also to work with voluntary organisations. It is an attempt to diminish the need to take children into care. Information about available voluntary and statutory social services can be obtained from the Citizens' Advice Bureau. Voluntary organizations such as Dr Barnardo's and the Woman's Royal Voluntary Service (WRVS) give advice and practical help to families in danger of breaking down. The WRVS helps the overworked mother and provides holiday homes for children.

The incidence of neglect and child abuse is increasing. Child abuse may be referred to as either 'the battered child syndrome' or 'non accidental injury'.

Child abuse takes many forms, from that of extreme physical battering to severe emotional and psychological deprivation. Any age group can be ill-treated though babies of less than 6 months old are especially vulnerable. One child in the family may be singled out for abuse.

In Great Britain approximately 3000–4000 children are deliberately injured each year, of these about 700 die; many suffer permanent injury, brain damage and neurological impairment.

The nature of battering is varied. Common forms include bruising from excessive pressure from fingers on face and trunk, burns from cigarettes or other sources of extreme heat, bite marks and swelling of the upper lip with tearing of the frenulum. Other forms are fractures of the long bones and ribs, head injury and retinal haemorrhages.

Child abuse is most common in families who are physically, financially, intellectually or emotionally deprived, and may occur in any social class. It often takes place when the parents are under stress. They are usually young and have themselves experienced battering in childhood.

The Royal Society for the Prevention of Cruelty to Children works closely with the social services, and the hospital and community health teams to identify and assess 'at risk' families. A multidisciplinary approach is needed to help the whole family and prevent further child abuse.

CARING FOR CHILDREN IN HOSPITAL

When caring for children it is essential to consider their emotional and physical needs. In order to do this account must be taken of each child's background — his family, his home and his environment. Parents are the most important people in the child's life especially when he is sick. They should be helped to feel comfortable in the ward environment and guided to help in the care of their child as much as possible.

Effects of admission to hospital

Separation from family caused by admission to hospital can readily lead to serious psychological trauma; this may be transient or lasting. Signs of psychological trauma in a child are persistent crying and refusal to be comforted, aggression, withdrawal, personality changes and regression in social behaviour such as bed wetting and thumb sucking.

In hospital a child's usual pattern of daily life is disturbed and he must accept a strange routine in unfamiliar surroundings. Nursing and medical care now take precedence and, of necessity, care has to be given by a variety of adults. His 'room' is no longer his own or shared with his family but shared with a number of other unknown children (Fig. 18.1). It is not, therefore, surprising that the majority of children suffer emotionally when admitted to hospital. How much a child suffers depends on his age, his personality and the degree of security previously experienced in his home environment. Predictably the preschool child is the most vulnerable because of his limited ability to communicate and to socialize.

Parents may also demonstrate anxiety when their child requires admission to hospital. They may have feelings of guilt, especially if the child has been involved in an illness or accident that could have been avoided. Loyalties may become divided because the demands of the sick child conflict with the needs of other family members, thus causing friction. Parental anxiety may be shown by the parents' failure to accept explanation or by complaints of a petty nature to other parents or junior staff. Parents require tactful handling, patience and consideration from all staff.

Figure 18.1
Sharing with other children

The adverse effects of hospitalization can be reduced, even in unsuitable buildings, but they are most readily minimized in purpose-built paediatric units.

The paediatric unit

This may be one of several comprising a children's hospital or may be found within a general hospital. In a well-run unit the atmosphere will be kindly and welcoming because the doctors and nurses have a special regard for and understanding of children. The atmosphere is also created in part by the surroundings, which should be cheerful, warm, bright, colourful and safe.

Only in a specially designed unit can the sick child's needs be fully met. Here he can have emotional support, skilled medical and nursing care, opportunity for play and, if old enough, education.

Since emotional support is best given by the mother, accommodation should be available for her to live in the unit. This enables her to be admitted with her child, to help during the 'settling in' period and also to assist in giving care if she is able and willing (Fig. 18.2).

Figure 18.2
A mother helping to care for her child

Play helps the child to relax and allows safe working out of strong emotions such as fear and aggression. The play room should be of adequate size for the number of patients, contain a wide selection of toys and play materials suited to all age groups and be staffed by a play therapist. The play therapist will be able to assist in the rehabilitation of children with special needs. Furniture should be simple, attractive and of sizes suited to the age groups of its users.

Education for the school child is an on-going process and, whenever illness allows, it should be continued. The Department of Education requires that teaching be provided for children who are in hospital for more than 3 weeks (Fig. 18.3). Full-time teaching is an important part of the care of a child who is in hospital for a long time. Part-time teaching is generally sufficient in acute wards.

Most paediatric units provide facilities for day care. This means that a child needing minor surgery or diagnostic tests who does not require elaborate preparation can be admitted in the morning and taken home again that evening.

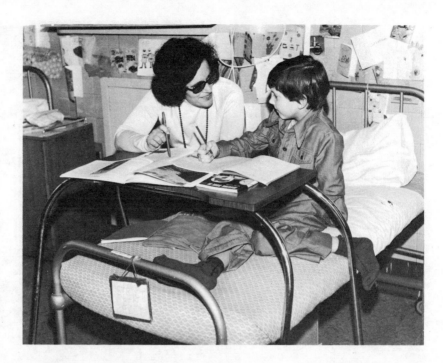

Figure 18.3
Teaching in hospital

General care of the child in hospital

Careful patient care planning is essential to ensure that the child has adequate periods of rest, occupation and play (Fig. 18.4). In this way exhaustion, boredom and frustration will be avoided. Thoughtful care can help to make the child's stay a pleasant experience.

Ward routine should be geared to meet the needs of its occupants and not the other way round, as was so often the case in the past. Open or free visiting is essential in a paediatric unit. If it is not possible for the mother to live in, then she should be encouraged to arrange her home routine in order to be with her sick child as much as she can — especially at meals, play time and bed time when she would normally be closely involved with him. Sometimes the father is able to take a turn (Fig. 18.5), allowing his wife to be free to maintain contact with the home and the other children in the family. Alternatively, he may just look in on his way to or from work.

Figure 18.4
Play

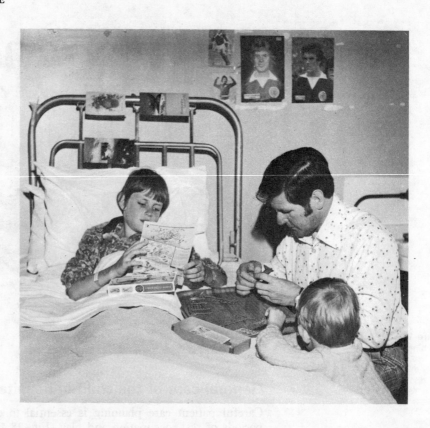

Figure 18.5
Visit from father

The child should have as much freedom as his illness permits; he will be happier and adjust more easily if he is allowed out of bed for meals and play. If he cannot be mobilized he should be dressed in his own clothes and nursed on top of his bed to give greater freedom of movement and maintain a more normal daily routine.

Meal times should be happy, relaxed occasions and free from rush. The food presented should be attractive and suitable for the different age groups of children. After attending to toilet needs and hand washing, children should be comfortably and safely seated at the table where they should be encouraged to remain until the meal is completed. Colourful nursery crockery and suitable sizes of cutlery should be provided and opportunity must be offered to each child to feed himself. He should be encouraged, not forced, to complete his meal. Children enjoy a little play and conversation at meal times. A doll, teddy or story can be used to persuade the reluctant child to finish his food.

Special aspects of care

Special elements of therapy and care merit more detailed consideration.

Admission

Children are admitted to hospital when medical treatment and nursing care cannot be carried out in the home. This may be because home conditions are inadequate, because the care required is highly technical or because special diagnostic tests are necessary. Admission to hospital is usually planned but it may result from an emergency.

Planned admission

This is arranged between the family doctor and the hospital consultant to whom the child has been referred. Visits to a hospital clinic will have preceded admission in most cases, and here full explanations of the reasons for admission, an indication of the date of admission and the approximate length of stay can be given. Good

Figure 18.6
Admission to hospital

relationships develop at this stage if the information provided is clearly understood and the questions asked are fully answered.

The child and his parents should visit the paediatric unit where they will meet the sister. She will give guidance regarding the preparation for admission and make arrangements for the mother to live in with her child if she wishes.

At the time of admission, a welcoming and reassuring approach from the nursing staff will help to allay anxiety. One nurse should deal with the formalities of admission (Fig. 18.6) so that the child can identify with her. She should already know the child's name and the reason for his admission. She should encourage the mother to remain throughout the procedure, since this will calm the child and permit observation of the interaction between him and his mother. Observation should also be made of general health, nutrition and overall cleanliness. An identity bracelet should be made out and checked by the mother before being attached to the child's wrist. Enquiries as to his baptismal state should be made discreetly. If the child is not to be confined to bed, he should wear his own clothing, which must be adequately labelled and cared for. Discussion with the mother should include diet, for example the type of food the child likes and dislikes, and also his sleep pattern and toilet habits.

The following guidelines can be used by nursing staff to elicit information regarding a child during the admission procedure. The information can then be used as a basis for the development of a nursing care plan.

Name of child	Age	Birthday
Pet name	Baptismal status	
Name of brother(s)	Age	
Name of sister(s)	Age	

Does the child require help with
  dressing?
  bathing?
  combing hair?
  cleaning teeth?
Has the child been in hospital previously?
Does the child know why he is being admitted?

Does the child make friends easily?
Has the child a favourite comforter?
   e.g. dummy teat.
       piece of blanket.
       bye byes.
Has the child brought it to hospital?

Diet

Is the child's appetite good?
Is the child breast fed/bottle/spoon/cup?
   Breast feeding
      Regular times?
      Demand feeding?
   Bottle feeding
      Type of milk?
      Amount?
      Number of feeds?
Feeds self alone.   Feeds self with help.
What foods does the child like?
What foods does the child dislike?
What fluids does the child like?
What fluids does the child dislike?
Any food allergies?
Any other food comments?

Toilet habits

Is the child toilet trained
   bowel?
   bladder?
Does the child wear a nappy
   all day?
   night only?
Does the child use a potty?
Does the child use a lavatory?
What words(s) used for bowel movement?
What word(s) used for micturition?
Is the child taken to toilet at night?
What time?

Sleep pattern

Usual bed time?   Hours of sleep at night?
Are naps taken?   What time?
Does the child sleep alone?
Does the child sleep in a bed?
Does the child sleep in a cot?
Any special bed time routine?
   e.g. Dolly's company?
       Teddy's company?
       Saying prayers?

Play/occupation

Has the child a favourite toy?
Has the child a favourite game?
Does the child play alone?
Does the child play with other children?
Does the child play with other adults?
Does the child watch TV regularly?
Does the child have special programmes?
Does the child have a pet?   Name.

School

Does the child attend nursery school?
Does the child attend primary school?
Name of the school.
List special interests
   Hobbies.
   Books.
   T.V.
   Radio programmes.
Any other comments.

A child from a secure, caring home who has been properly prepared for his stay in hospital will adjust more quickly to life in the ward. He is likely to have some impressions of hospital life learned from television, radio and story books. The National Association for the Welfare of Children in Hospital provides booklets, films and slides which are used as teaching aids when visiting schools and mothers' groups. The Association offers advice and practical assistance to mothers with children in hospital by providing baby-sitters and transport if necessary.

Emergency admission

An emergency admission presents difficulties because there is no time for preparation of either child or parents. After the clinical examination of the child, reassurance and explanation is of the utmost importance, particularly if the admission is the result of an accident or sudden illness. Child and parents should be separated as little as possible, for example only during the preparation for operation. In some instances, parents can accompany their child to the anaesthetic room. There are very few situations where parents cannot remain with their child to the benefit of all.

Observation

A normal, healthy child looks bright, happy and interested, is rarely still during the day and sleeps soundly at night.

General observations

In illness the child becomes more dependent on mother. Changes in behaviour are, often, the earliest signs of disease process, e.g. lethargy, fretfulness, loss of appetite, restlessness.

Children adopt unusual postures when in pain and discomfort; for example a child with abdominal pain will lie curled up and flex his knees during bouts of colic and the child with severe cyanotic heart disease adopts a squatting position. Photophobia is demonstrated by turning the head away from the light or burying the head under the bed clothes.

The healthy infant may cry to be lifted up because he is wet, cold or too hot. Hunger is announced by strong, continuous crying accompanied by sucking of the fingers. Episodes of strong crying, accompanied by frowning and drawing up of the legs, may indicate flatulence or abdominal colic. The teething infant often cries with pain, gnaws anything that is hard and cool and has excess salivation and red patches on his cheeks. Head rolling or rubbing of the affected ear and loud crying often indicates earache. The cry of extreme pain and exhaustion tends to be feeble and moaning, and a sharp, shrill, piercing cry is associated with cerebral irritation.

The foregoing are generalizations and included solely for illustrative purposes. It cannot be overstressed that there is no substitute for nursing experience and that the art of observation can only be learned in the practical situation. The value and significance of nursing observations, particularly in relation to children, merit serious consideration. Of necessity doctors spend less time with their patients than do nurses and therefore rely heavily on nursing observations and records. What the nurse sees, hears, feels and smells in relation to her patient may be valuable pointers to his progress. The quick detection and reporting of a sudden change in a child's condition may be the first step in a life-saving measure.

It should go without saying that two of the nurse's most important responsibilities are to observe accurately and record or report faithfully.

Observation and recording of temperature, pulse, respiration and blood pressure

The relationship between temperature, pulse and respiration is important and the three are usually taken and recorded together. In most units this is done routinely twice each day and 4 hourly or more frequently in acute illness. There are two types of thermometers used to ensure the accurate measurement of body temperature:

1. *The standard clinical thermometer*, which is calibrated to record temperatures between 35°C and 45°C.
2. *The low registering thermometer* with a range of between 25° and 40° C.

The type of thermometer used is determined by the age of the child. The standard clinical thermometer is used for children aged 1 year and over and the low registering thermometer is used for all newborn, low birth weight and ill infants. The latter is used so that hypothermia can be recognized. The temperature regulating centre in the hypothalamus is not fully developed in the early years of life and infants are prone to extremes of body temperature if overheated or chilled. A low body temperature in an infant may indicate, for example, that infection is present whereas the older child with an infection will have a pyrexia. These variations are shown in Table 18.2.

The temperature will vary according to the site in which it is taken. The skin temperature, taken in the axilla or groin, is the lowest. The temperature in the mouth is about 0.6°C higher than that of the skin. The temperature in the rectum is about 0.6°C higher than that in the mouth. There is, therefore, a difference of 1°C between the skin temperature and that of the rectum.

To ensure that an accurate record of temperature is kept, the same site should be used each time. To avoid confusion and possible accident due to biting or breaking the thermometer, it is usual to take temperatures of children under 1 year per rectum and for children over 1 year in the axilla or groin unless otherwise instructed. Rectal surgery and enteritis are two examples of situations where taking temperatures per rectum would be contraindicated.

Table 18.2
Variation in body temperature

Body temperature	Range (degrees C)
Normal	36.3–37.2
Pyrexia	
Low	37.2–38.4
Moderate	38.4–39.5
High	39.5–40.6
Hyperpyrexia	Above 40.6
Hypothermia	Below 36.4

When using the rectum, the thermometer should be **held** in position for 1 minute. When using the axilla or groin, the area should first be dried with a towel and the thermometer held in position for 3 minutes. The pulse and respiration are usually in a 4:1 ratio. They vary with the age of the child, being rapid at birth and becoming slower as the child grows older (Table 18.3). They are also affected by physical and emotional activity, which increases the heart rate hence varying the pulse rate. To ensure an accurate record in the young child, pulse and respiration should be

Table 18.3
Normal range of pulse and respiration

Age	Pulse rate per minute	Respiration rate per minute
Birth	150–130	60–30 irregular in rhythm and depth
3 months	130–110	50–30 regular
6 months	120	45–30
1 year	115	30–25
2 years	110–10	30–25
3–6 years	100–90	25
7–10 years	100–80	24–20
11–14 years	90–70	20

counted while the child is resting or sleeping and before he is disturbed to have his temperature taken.

Respiratory activity is assessed by placing the hand lightly on the child's chest. In the baby, observation of the movements of the abdomen will give a more accurate record because of the important role played by the diaphragm and abdominal muscles in respiration. A baby's respirations may be irregular in rate, rhythm and depth. However any irregularity occurring in the older child must be reported immediately.

The sites for locating the pulse are at the anterior lateral aspect of the wrist, over the temporal bone in front of the ear and, in an infant, at the anterior fontanelle. Rhythm and volume are also noted when counting.

The blood pressure is only taken when specifically requested. It is important to ensure that the correct size of cuff and stethoscope is used and that the child is resting and quiet.

Table 18.4
Variation in range of blood pressure

Age	Systolic	Diastolic
Birth	65–95	30–60
2–6 years	60–110	45–75
6–10 years	75–120	50–70

There are two methods of obtaining a reading by:

1. Auscultation. (See Ch. 7. p. 251)
2. Flush method. The cuff is placed on the wrist or ankle and a firm bandage is wrapped round the limb distal to the cuff. The cuff is then inflated to 20 mmHg and the bandage removed. The limb looks blanched and feels cold. The cuff is *de*flated *slowly* until the extremity flushes when the systolic pressure can be read using a stethoscope.

Pre- and postoperative care

Physical and psychological preparation is needed before surgery is undertaken. Some children, especially the older age group, have a fear of being put to sleep and having 'things done to them' so it is important that their preparation is carried out with thoughtfulness. An operation may be elective or emergency. Elective surgery gives time for preparation and ensures that the optimum level of health under the circumstances is achieved.

On admission the child is carefully observed for signs of infection which would contra-indicate surgery. He is weighed and the routine records are maintained. A specimen of urine is collected for ward testing. Bowel preparation is not required unless the child is to have bowel surgery. A bath is given on the day of the operation. Attention should be paid to the cleanliness of hair, nails and skin folds such as the umbilicus, groins and axillae. A detailed medical history is obtained and a physical examination is carried out. The doctor obtains written consent for the operation from the parents.

The immediate preoperative care begins 4 hours before the operation when the older child is given a light meal and told that he must not eat or drink thereafter. An infant is given a half-strength milk feed. A 'nil orally' sign is then placed on the bed or cot. Prolonged periods without food are not tolerated well by children as the blood sugar falls rapidly. The child is encouraged to pass urine, bathed and dressed in an open-backed theatre gown then returned to a clean bed or cot. The hair is secured with a ribbon or cap. The mouth is checked for the presence of an ortho-dontic plate or loose teeth. Premedication is given as prescribed by the anaesthetist and the patient is encouraged to sleep and allowed to have his favourite toy beside him. It is helpful if the nurse spends a little time talking quietly until he becomes drowsy. Case notes, X-rays and drug prescription records are collected and accompany the child when he is taken to the operating theatre. Careful checking is essential to ensure that the correct child and the correct notes are taken to the operating theatre; in particular, identity **must** be confirmed by looking at the arm band.

On return from the theatre, the child has an airway in position and he is placed in a semiprone position. His lower jaw is directed forward to ensure that the airway is adequately maintained. Consciousness is very quickly regained and the airway is usually ejected. He should be observed constantly until fully conscious. Colour, temperature, pulse and respiration are carefully noted and recorded and the wound dressing is inspected for signs of haemorrhage. Analgesia, ordered by the doctor, should be given if the child becomes restless and complains of pain.

The child's first request is usually for a drink; **small** sips can be given unless medical orders are to the contrary; then mouth care should be given to reduce the discomfort of a dry mouth. Hands and face are washed and he is put into his own nightwear and has his hair combed. He is allowed a pillow and encouraged to rest in a comfortable position. The older child can have easily digested food 6 to 8 hours after surgery if he wishes, especially if he is tolerating oral fluids well; normal diet is resumed the following day. The infant is given glucose fluids 3 to 4 hourly following surgery and his normal feeds are gradually reintroduced.

A child is usually anxious to regain his independence and early ambulation presents no difficulty. Parents are invited to be with their child as soon as possible after surgery and to assist where they can in giving care and reassurance.

Maintenance of fluid and electrolyte balance

In health the composition and concentration of body fluids are maintained within very narrow limits, and there is a delicate balance between them (Ch. 4). A child's body weight is composed of 80% water compared with less than 70% in the adult. In the infant the ratio of extracellular fluid to intracellular fluid is greater than in the older child and the adult. The infant also has a greater body surface area and higher basal metabolic rate per unit of weight, the latter being approximately twice that of the adult. The loss of fluid through the skin, lungs, kidneys and alimentary tract is correspondingly greater. The kidneys of the infant are immature so they are less able to conserve and concentrate fluid. To maintain this balance within the body, the fluid requirement for the young child is 150 ml per kg of body weight over a 24-hour period. The fluid requirements decrease as age increases.

Fluid electrolyte depletion occurs when there has been an inadequate intake or an excessive output of fluid, such as occurs in vomiting, diarrhoea or polyuria; the child is then said to be dehydrated.

The signs of dehydration are weight loss, sunken eyes which lack lustre, depressed fontanelle, loss of skin turgor, dry mouth, scanty urinary output, lethargy and poor muscle tone. Fluids can be given orally to correct dehydration provided the child is conscious and not vomiting. Other means of providing an adequate fluid and electrolyte intake are by intravenous or intraperitoneal infusion. The paedia-

Figure 18.7
Scalp vein infusion using butterfly needle

trician will prescribe the type of infusion, the amount and nature of fluid and the rate at which the infusion is to be given (usually in millilitres per hour). He bases his decisions on the clinical signs of dehydration, the results of blood chemistry and the child's weight and needs in terms of fluids and electrolytes.

Common sites for intravenous infusion are the superficial temporal vein (Fig. 18.7), antecubital vein or long saphenous vein. The infusion must be carefully regulated to prevent overhydration and overloading of the circulatory system. To ensure the correct rate of flow the infusion must be checked at quarter to half hourly intervals. Various mechanical aids are available to help the nurse regulate the infusion accurately. Examples are the IVAC pump (Fig. 18.8) and the Holter pump (Fig. 18.9). In the absence of these aids, the following formula may be used:

Figure 18.8
IVAC pump

Drops per minute selector

ON/OFF switch

Start button

Figure 18.9
Holter pump

ON/OFF switch

From giving set

To patient

To patient

Figure 18.10
Microdrip infant recipient set

Figure 18.11
Standard infant recipient set

In the standard recipient set 15 drops equals approximately 1 ml;
ml/hour × 15 = number of drops per hour;

therefore, ml/hour $\times \dfrac{15}{60}$ = number of drops per minute

estimation of rate flow $= \dfrac{\text{ml/hour}}{4}$

= drops/minute

The microdrip recipient set (Fig. 18.10) is calibrated at 60 drops/ml and enables the rate of flow to be more easily regulated; the number of millilitres per hour is equal to the number of drops per minute. The standard giving set (Fig. 18.11) is shown in comparison. It is important to remember that it is **dangerous** to administer intravenous fluids more rapidly than prescribed to the young infant because of the risk of overloading the circulation.

Accurate records of fluids administered and of the child's output are maintained to assist in the estimation of hydration. Other observations necessary are the rates of pulse and respiration. Any significant changes such as restlessness, dyspnoea, cyanosis or the development of oedema must be reported immediately. Should either of the latter occur the nurse should slow the infusion rate and seek medical advice forthwith.

The child should be kept comfortable and his position changed frequently to relieve pressure and prevent chest complications.

Administration of medicines

To ensure that medicines are safely and successfully administered, the nurse must approach the child in a calm, kindly manner. In some instances a great deal of patience and persuasion are needed although older children generally co-operate in taking medicine.

It is essential that the correct drug is given, in the prescribed amount, at the time specified. Careful calculation of the very small amounts of drugs prescribed for children is necessary (Table 18.5). Some drugs, such as phenobarbitone and digoxin, are prepared in doses suitable for children and in a palatable form such as elixirs or syrups, as well as in tablets or capsules.

Table 18.5
Calculation of drug dosage

Formula:	Divide the strength required by the strength available. The fraction obtained is the amount of stock solution of the drug required.
$\dfrac{\text{Strength required}}{\text{Stock solution}}$	= Fraction of stock solution to be given
Example 1	Stock bottle of ampicillin for **oral** use containing 250 mg/5 ml Dose prescribed is 62.5 mg
$\dfrac{\text{Strength required}}{\text{Strength available}}$	$= \dfrac{62.5 \text{ mg}}{250 \text{ mg in 5 ml}}$
Therefore amount required	$= \dfrac{1}{4}$ of 5 ml
	$= \dfrac{5}{4}$ ml
	= 1.25 ml
Example 2	Stock dose of digoxin contains 50 micrograms in 1 ml Dose prescribed is 125 micrograms
$\dfrac{\text{Strength required}}{\text{Strength available}}$	$= \dfrac{125 \ \mu g}{50 \ \mu g \text{ in 1 ml}}$
Therefore amount required	$= \dfrac{125}{50}$ of 1 ml
	$= \dfrac{5}{2}$ of 1 ml
	= 2.5 ml

The child should be fully awakened and given a drink before his medicine is administered. The nurse must ensure that the drug has been swallowed. There are various ploys to aid this, such as crushing tablets and mixing them with drinks, jam or soft sweets, provided these are allowed. The nurse should talk and play with the young child to help him to accept his medicine. It may help to lift the child from his cot and nurse him and place small amounts at the back of the tongue with a spoon.

Young babies may need to be lightly restrained during drug administration and care must be taken to prevent inhalation of the medicine. This may occur if the drug is given too quickly and the baby splutters. Refusal to swallow, resulting in the loss of part or all of the medicine, must be reported and recorded.

Oxygen therapy

Oxygen is given when the child's condition necessitates concentrations of oxygen higher than the 21% found in atmospheric air. Oxygen is supplied to the wards in metal cylinders (black with white top) or through pipes from a central oxygen supply. Oxygen may be administered by using:

1. A disposable polythene mask, suitable for an older child (Ch. 6).
2. An oxygen tent, for a younger or very ill child.
3. An incubator, only suitable for a baby (Ch. 17).

Care of the child in an oxygen tent

Pressure tubing is used to attach the supply of oxygen to the tent, the rate of flow being controlled by a flow meter. Humidification and cooling, by diverting the oxygen supply through distilled water and a container of ice, is necessary to moisten the oxygen as it is very irritant to the epithelial lining of the respiratory tract. The relative humidity can be increased by using a humidifier (Fig. 18.12), atomizer or nebulizer.

When preparing the tent for use, it should be flushed with oxygen, 10 to 20 litres per minute for 20 minutes, and the oxygen content of the tent analysed. The doctor prescribes the concentration required and the flowmeter is adjusted accordingly. To ensure that the concentration is maintained, the rate of flow should be increased when it is necessary to open the tent. Analysis of the oxygen concentration is required 2 to 4 hourly and, if the child's condition does not show improvement, it may be necessary to increase the concentration. Care must be taken to ensure that the inlet and outlet of the tent is not obstructed.

In caring for the child, reassurance is given to help him to adjust to the confined space and it is often helpful if his mother remains with him. The child should be nursed in a comfortable position, supported by pillows. Toddlers and babies are

Figure 18.12
Humidifier and flowmeter

Figure 18.13
Child in baby sitter in oxygen
tent

more easily positioned by using a baby sitter (Fig. 18.13). Over exertion should be prevented and treatment arranged so that he can have adequate rest to increase the effect of therapy. If dyspnoea or cyanosis is present, all care should be carried out in the tent. The child's clothing and bed linen should be changed as often as necessary to prevent chilling by the dampness created by humidification. Fluids should be offered frequently to prevent dehydration. If respiratory distress inhibits the taking of fluids orally, a nasogastric tube may be passed.

When oxygen therapy is initiated, it is important to ensure that the child is observed closely — colour, temperature, pulse, respiration and general behaviour being noted and recorded to determine the child's response. It is also necessary to check the oxygen supply, flowmeter, oxygen concentration, fluid level in humidifier and temperature within the tent, which should be maintained at about 18 to 21°C. Ice is replenished as needed to aid cooling.

The nurse should know how to maintain the equipment to ensure adequate oxygen concentration. She should also be aware of the ignition hazard associated with the use of oxygen and prevent the use of friction toys which create sparks. Paper, grease and oils which are easily ignited must also be kept well away from the tent and the oxygen supply.

Discharge from hospital

'When can I go home?' is the thought uppermost in a child's mind. It does not always indicate that he is unhappy in hospital but rather that he would be happier at home.

Preparation for homegoing must be well planned, particularly if the child and mother have to continue care at home which may involve special diets, drugs or appliances. The special diets could include those peculiar to a child with diabetes mellitus, coeliac disease or with a colostomy or ileostomy. If drug therapy is to be continued, advice must be given on its correct dose, time of administration, storage and disposal of the drug once therapy is complete. Before leaving hospital, the mother and possibly the child should be competent in the use of any appliances such as calipers or colostomy bags. It is also important to ensure that the source of replacement, maintenance and repair of these items is known to the family.

The fact that the child may not readjust to family life immediately should be made clear to the mother so that she will understand the reasons for the child's regression in behaviour. Sleep may be disturbed and it is not uncommon for a child to have nightmares or to sleepwalk following a traumatic experience. On return home, the child may be demanding, perhaps resentful of having been 'left in that place' or unwilling to let his mother out of his sight. However, if the mother has been prepared for this behaviour she herself will avoid feelings of rejection and, with patient understanding, will help her child to readjust and feel secure.

The date and time of discharge should be decided as soon as possible so that transport, either provided by parents or in an ambulance, can be arranged. Any other services needed will be provided by the family doctor and the paediatric community nursing sister. The medical social worker may, if necessary, arrange for the child's education to be continued at home.

Very occasionally, parents decide for one reason or another to take their child home before treatment is completed. They should be encouraged to give a reason for their decision. During discussion with senior members of nursing and medical staff, they should be helped to understand the effects this may have on their child. The parents are asked to sign the relevant form indicating their acceptance of personal responsibility for this action. All possible guidance is given on continuing care. The family doctor is informed of the situation and any request for readmission to hospital is granted.

CARING FOR THE CHILD WITH A TERMINAL ILLNESS

Perception and sensitivity are needed when caring for the terminally ill child and in supporting his parents and relatives. Once diagnosis has been made and prognosis estimated by the doctor, he should talk to the parents in an attempt to help them understand and accept the situation. The ward sister should also be present during this interview so that she will be able to support the parents and answer their questions. The nursing staff must be aware of the need to provide a quiet room where parents can express their grief freely, overcome the initial shock and talk. Often a cup of tea and private discussion is of benefit to parents; the hospital chaplain or family minister may also be involved. The parents may find it helpful to know that staff are always available to talk to them at the time.

The child should be nursed in an area where he can watch the activities of other children. However, when his general condition becomes poor, it will be necessary to move him to a single room. It is essential, at this time, to avoid giving him a feeling of isolation.

It may be possible, in some instances, for the child to be nursed in his own home. This will of course depend on the child's condition, home circumstances, parents' ability and the availability of community care. Parents are assured that the family doctor, district nurse and health visitor will continue to support and assist with the practical aspects of care. Readmission to hospital can be arranged whenever necessary.

Whether the child is cared for in hospital or in the community, the nursing aims are to ensure that the child is kept clean and comfortable with adequate analgesia and sedation to ensure freedom from pain and restlessness. By involving the mother in the nursing care, some of her emotional needs and those of her child are partly satisfied. Parents should be encouraged to maintain their own health, particularly if there are other children in the family who will also need their care and attention.

As the child's condition deteriorates, the nursing staff can help to make the parents aware of the situation by asking if they wish to be informed of any changes, whatever the hour, and to be at the bedside during the final moments. In the absence of parents, a nurse who is familiar to the child should stay quietly by the bedside, talking to him if this is indicated. Parents who choose to stay with their child at this time may also appreciate the presence of a nurse.

After the death of their child, parents should be left at the bedside for a short time and then taken unobtrusively to a side room where they can share their grief and develop some composure before returning home. Any specific wishes regarding the child's belongings should be respected.

The need for support continues after the child's death and can be provided by both hospital and community care teams. Visits from or writing letters to those who have been involved in caring for the child are helpful to some parents while visiting the hospital and assisting in the care of other children is more beneficial to others. Great help may be provided by sympathetic friends and relatives who can give practical and psychological support.

PATIENT CARE STUDIES

The use of a variety of services and the involvement of the parents are illustrated in the following care studies.

Linda — age 7 months

History

Linda was admitted to hospital when she was 7 months old to be investigated for failure to thrive.

At birth she was 2.6 kg in weight having been born at 32 weeks' gestation. She was the third daughter of an unmarried mother who suffered from alcoholism. Although Linda was of low birth weight, her general progress was good and she was discharged home with her mother when she was 3 kg in weight. Her mother was advised to report to the baby clinic in 4 weeks' time so that Linda's progress could be assessed.

Her mother failed to report to the clinic on three occasions and a request for a progress report was made to the family doctor and the health visitor. The family doctor reported that Linda had been in the local hospital with a chest infection on two occasions but was now at home. The health visitor indicated that the home was poor and that Linda's mother showed a limited interest in her child. Linda was difficult to feed and appeared very thin and apathetic. Mother 'fortified' herself very frequently and generally was unable to give adequate care. Assistance had been sought from the Royal Scottish Society for the Prevention of Cruelty to Children (RSSPCC) and a social worker was assigned to work very closely with the family.

A fourth appointment was made, through the social worker, for Linda and her mother to attend the baby clinic. Transport and an escort were provided by the RSSPCC. Her mother was unable to give a complete progress report because of her inebriated state. Admission to hospital was arranged to observe Linda's dietary intake and general behaviour.

On admission she was a pale, pathetic, whimpering little girl of 5.8 kg in weight. She had an irritable cough, was fretful and difficult to comfort. Stools were loose and green.

Among possible reasons for her delay in development were malabsorption and the presence of infection; the appropriate investigations were made. Examination of stools proved negative and it was thought that the alteration in colour and consistency was due to underfeeding. An upper respiratory infection was diagnosed and the antibiotic therapy and physiotherapy were initiated, to which the infection responded well. Development was slightly below average and consistent with maternal deprivation.

Linda's appetite improved slowly, a weaning diet was started and she became very enthusiastic and excited when food appeared. Her general demeanour altered and she became a very attractive, lively and responsive child. Weight gain was slow but consistent.

Linda's mother did not visit her during her 5 week stay in hospital. Her father, however, demonstrated an interest, visited frequently and eventually encouraged her mother to take Linda home as he wished to help to support the family.

Summary

Linda is the third daughter of an unmarried 37-year-old woman in poor social circumstances who suffers from alcoholism. Her income is derived from social security benefit but she works as an office cleaner when able. Linda's father, not necessarily father to the other children, did not show interest or give support until Linda's admission to hospital. Since Linda's return home 6 months ago, the family have remained united but continue to need the support and advice of their social worker.

Peter — age 8 years

History

Peter was admitted to hospital from school complaining of severe abdominal pain, nausea and vomiting. The onset of pain was sudden although Peter had complained of two short episodes of vague abdominal pain a few days previously.

On admission, Peter was a well-nourished, healthy-looking child though rather pale. He appeared intelligent, bright-eyed but anxious. During examination, he was very cooperative and explained how the pain had been 'all over his tummy' and now was present only in his right side. Physical examination revealed guarding and tenderness in the right iliac fossa, and a diagnosis of acute appendicitis was made.

The diagnosis and operation necessary for the removal of the appendix was explained to Peter and to his parents who then gave permission for the operation to be performed.

Peter's mother remained with him until he was taken to the operating theatre 2 hours later. Meanwhile she was asked not to give him any further fluids. She also helped to prepare him for theatre by assisting with his bath and encouraging him to pass urine. An identification band was placed on his wrist. Following the preparation he rested quietly until the prescribed premedication was given.

The operation was performed for removal of the appendix and the wound was closed without drainage. The appendix was acutely inflamed.

Recovery from general anaesthesia was satisfactory and Peter was allowed small amounts of fluids later and a light diet was given the following day. Ambulation started on the first postoperative day and Peter was permitted to sit out of bed and take a short walk. His mother's visits were a great encouragement to him and he was soon moving around easily and playing with the other children.

As his progress was uneventful, he was eating and sleeping well and wound healing was normal, he was discharged home into the care of his parents, the paediatric district nurse and the family doctor. The sutures were removed on the sixth postoperative day as the wound was well healed.

He was visited by the family doctor 2 weeks later and discharged from medical and nursing care.

Summary

Peter developed acute appendicitis for which an operation was performed. Postoperative recovery was satisfactory. Home conditions were good: Peter had his own bedroom and his mother did not go out to work. His mother was advised to restrict his activities for 10 days to 2 weeks and to ensure that Peter had adequate rest and a nourishing diet. She was assisted in caring for her child by daily visits from the paediatric district nurse and supervision by the family doctor.

FURTHER READING

Bates S M 1979 Practical paediatric nursing, 2nd edn. Blackwell Scientific, Oxford
Dennison W M 1974 Surgery in infancy and childhood, 3rd edn. Churchill Livingstone, Edinburgh
Duncombe M, Weller B 1979 Paediatric nursing, 5th edn. Bailliere Tindall, London
Francis D E M 1979 Diets for sick children, 4th edn. Blackwell Scientific, Oxford
Harvey S, Tooke A H 1972 Play in hospital. Faber, London
Illingworth R S 1983 The development of the infant and young child, normal and abnormal, 8th edn. Churchill Livingstone, Edinburgh
Latham H C, Heckel R V 1977 Pediatric nursing, 3rd edn. Mosby, St. Louis
Robertson J 1970 Young children in hospital. Tavistock, London
Wolff S 1973 Children under stress. Penguin, Harmondsworth

Chapter Nineteen
Adolescents and adults

The aim of this chapter is to give a brief overview of human development between the years of childhood and old age and to relate these changes to ways in which adolescents and adults react to illness and hospitalization.

It is emphasized that the patient's behaviour cannot be viewed as if he existed in isolation. The attitudes and actions of his relatives, other patients and members of the care team will have a significant effect upon his perception of his illness and his stay in hospital.

In describing some of the problems which face the patient, his family and the hospital staff, it will become obvious that in many instances there are no unique 'right ways' of dealing with these problems which can be prescribed in the same way as a technical procedure.

Every individual is unique, and illness disability and hospitalization bring problems which differ from one person to another.

Nevertheless some general ideas are suggested which will help the nurse to appreciate some of the many factors involved in caring for adolescents and adults.

A knowledge and understanding of these factors may help the nurse to find the most appropriate solutions to an individual patient's problem.

ADOLESCENCE

Adolescence is the period of transition between childhood and adulthood occurring approximately between 12 and 18 years of age.

It is usually characterized as a period of upheaval, uncertainty and problems, and indeed it is often these aspects of adolescence which feature prominently in any media coverage of adolescents. Juvenile accidents, crime and sexuality have a special fascination in a culture and society which is increasingly youth orientated (see Fig. 19.1).

Yet, despite the popular emphasis given to the problems of adolescence, many young people meet the challenges of adolescence successfully and find much to enjoy during this period of their lives.

Development during adolescence

Physical development

Marked physical changes occur during adolescence. Height, weight and musculo-skeletal development increase during the adolescent growth spurt. This can often affect the adolescent's self image as he may feel ungainly and clumsy. The age of onset of this physical maturity can often cause the adolescent great anxiety if his development is thought to be out of step with that of his friends and peers.

Figure 19.1
A tale of two typical adolescents?

Physical maturation of the sexual organs takes place during puberty and sexual characteristics develop. The most dramatic and occasionally traumatic of these is the onset of menstruation in females and the ability to ejaculate in boys. The latter often occurs as nocturnal emisions or 'wet dreams'. Were either of these events to occur in hospital they could cause serious embarrassment and anxiety for the young person.

Psychosocial development

Adolescence is characterized by a widening of the adolescent's intellectual abilities. He begins to consider abstract and hypothetical problems and attempts to reason out logical solutions to numerous problems and to establish his own system of attitudes and values.

These attempts at exercising their developing mental powers often result in conflict between the adolescent and his parents as he will often adopt views and attitudes to political, social, moral and family questions which are diametrically opposed to those of his parents.

Traditional figures of authority in hospital among the medical and nursing staff may also find their actions questioned and challenged by the adolescent who insists upon discussing all aspects of his care and who demands explanations of tests and procedures.

During middle adolescence there is a return of the egocentrism which was characteristic of the toddler. Elkind suggests that during this phase of adolescence the young person reacts to an 'imaginary audience' and feels that everyone is scrutinizing, criticizing and discussing him (see Further Reading p. 639). The adolescent feels the centre of everyone's attention and interest.

Elkind also suggests that during this phase the adolescent lives out a 'personal fable' where he feels that his experiences and feelings are so unique and so very special. No-one has ever been as deeply in love as he has. No-one has ever cared so passionately about nuclear disarmament, seal culls, injustice, racism, or youth unemployment as he has.

The adolescent will often bemoan the fact that 'no one really understands how I feel'. This egocentrism can often lead to feelings of immunity from life's experiences. The motor cycle accident victim, the young girl with an unwanted pregnancy, the young victim of alcohol, drug or solvent addiction often explain that they were so sure that these were things which happened to other people but that could not happen to them.

Social development in adolescence is characterized by several main features. The desire for independence, the search for identity and the desire to gain peer group approval. Indeed it is often in attempts to 'be somebody' that health problems may arise.

Adolescents are often extremely concerned with how they see themselves in relation to their peers. Any feelings which the adolescent has that he is not developing properly can cause considerable anxiety and unhappiness. For instance it is very common in the 'problem pages' of teenage magazines to find letters from distraught adolescents, concerning personal characteristics which seem to them abnormal. For young people who are patients in hospital this problem may be exacerbated by having to undergo physical examinations and intimate procedures.

Figure 19.2
Which one is the typical adolescent?

YOUNG ADULTHOOD

If we view childhood and adolescence as being times of preparation, then it is the period of life from around 20–40 years of age which is being prepared for. This is a very busy period in the human life cycle when important choices and decisions have to be made about careers, family and life-style.

Development during young adulthood

Physical development

This is the period when full physical maturity and fitness has been reached and is typically the healthiest period of our lives. The greatest threat to health during this period comes not from disease and illness but from accidents, for instance road traffic accidents.

During the latter part of this period future health problems may begin to show such as cardiovascular problems, hypertension, duodenal ulcer and various types of cancer.

Psychosocial development

Intellectual and cognitive functioning is generally at a high level during this period. The abstractions which so preoccupied the adolescent will now make way for more practical ways of thinking which will be needed in the young adult's career and family life.

Early adulthood is also characterized by a greater maturity in relationships. The more transient, sexually dominated encounters of adolescence are now much less important than establishing satisfying, intimate, long term relationships where sexuality, although still very important, is not the overriding concern.

Marriage and family life are still the most common social relationships within which the young adult will function, although there have been dramatic changes within these social institutions.

The idealized picture of the family unit with husband out at work and wife staying at home to look after the 2.2 children is not as commonplace as we might expect.

Many factors have changed the face of family life and these include the increase in the rate of divorce since the late 1960s, the increasing number of one-parent families, the increase in the number of women who wish to work or pursue a career during marriage and parenthood, and the increase in the number of families where the husband is unemployed.

There is also a reaction against the paternalistic view of marriage and family life, where the husband is seen as the 'breadwinner' and 'head of the household', and where the wife is in the submissive role of nursemaid, cleaner and cook. Sharing of responsibility regarding housework, looking after the children and working is now seen as being an essential element of the modern marriage. Some young adults however find these changes difficult to cope with. The husband may feel guilty that he is unable to support his family financially without his wife working. The young working mother may feel that she is depriving her children by taking a job or following her career after having children.

Our society is very materialistic and there is great pressure on young adults to succeed in families and careers and to acquire the trappings of this success: their own home, the new car, a fitted kitchen full of gadgets, a video recorder. Today's luxuries rapidly become tomorrow's essentials.

As well as marriage and work, the other major event in the life of the young adult is parenthood. This brings major changes in the young adult's life-style, roles and relationships with each other. Now they are responsible for the life of another human being and almost certainly their lives will begin to revolve around this new member of the family.

Indeed parents will often remark that caring for a new baby or toddler is a 24-hour job and that they cannot remember how they filled their day before the baby arrived.

Parenthood however rarely resembles the stereotyped image of the baby food advertisement, or the television commercial where the father is always reassuring and supportive, where mother is always looking her best and has the situation totally under control and where baby is pink, healthy and gurgling with contentment.

So pervasive is this image of parenthood, that parents who find the transition difficult or whose baby is constantly crying, sick, or has feeding difficulties often feel that they are failures in this most important of roles.

THE MIDDLE YEARS

Developments during middle age

Physical changes

It is often the changes in appearance which alert the person to the fact that they are no longer as young in years as they may have thought. The grey hairs, the wrinkles, the larger waistline may be accepted as inevitable or be fought by cosmetics, fitness and diet programmes or health farm holidays.

Men may notice a decline in physical strength, agility and perhaps sexual activity. For women the most important biological event during these years is the 'change of life' or menopause. This is caused by a decrease in oestrogen production which ends menstruation and the ability to have children.

It would be simplistic to label the menopause as a purely physical event since it may have emotional and psychological implications which can have a profound effect upon a woman's life. It is not only in areas such as sexuality that our society displays marked double standards. The ageing process provides another example.

Men with grey hair and a few wrinkles are said to look 'distinguished', whereas a woman with such features looks 'old and unattractive'. An unmarried man may be an 'eligible batchelor' whereas a middle aged woman may be a 'spinster' or 'left on the shelf' or perhaps she has been 'selfish' in denying herself the security and pleasures of a husband and children in order to follow her career.

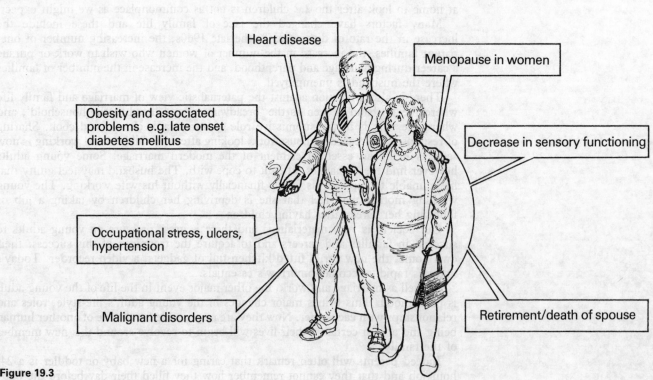

Heart disease

Menopause in women

Obesity and associated problems e.g. late onset diabetes mellitus

Decrease in sensory functioning

Occupational stress, ulcers, hypertension

Malignant disorders

Retirement/death of spouse

Figure 19.3
Health problems of the middle years

Physical health, however, is generally good during the middle years although health problems do occur more frequently as late adulthood progresses.

A variety of minor and more serious illnesses may present in middle age such as high blood pressure, diabetes mellitus, cardiovascular, respiratory and genitourinary problems, psychiatric disorders and problems associated with a decline in sensory functioning.

It is also worth noting that many diseases and illnesses associated with middle age may be linked to elements in the person's previous life-style. For instance if they have been smokers or heavy drinkers, if they have been overweight and have taken little exercise, if they have been exposed to occupational or environmental health hazards or if they have been subject to high levels of stress, they may become aware of features of consequential disorders.

People may react to these changes in different ways. They may choose to ignore early signs of illness, or visit their doctor with every minor symptom, worried that it is the first sign of a serious illness.

Psychosocial development

We sometimes suggest that middle-aged people are deteriorating intellectually. We talk of them 'getting rusty' or of being too old to learn new skills or master new concepts. We adhere to the saying that 'you can't teach an old dog new tricks'.

Yet there is no evidence to suggest that middle age is a time of intellectual or cognitive decline and to suggest this on the basis of age alone without considering the person's past life experience would be very foolish. Indeed some research has shown that middle age is a peak time for activities such as mastering abstract concepts, moral development and creativity.

The career picture in middle age can be variable. The person may have achieved great success in the career which he chose as a young adult and be in a position of power, influence and high status earning an equally high salary.

Alternatively the person may find that the physical and psychological stresses of the job are beginning to tell. It may be that the physical aspects of the work seem more tiring or he feels he is under pressure to prove that he is as capable as the younger members of the workforce and consequently he may work harder and take on more responsibility.

The middle-aged person may also be faced with the fact that he is no longer one of the organization's 'rising stars' or 'whizz kids', and whereas their achievements are marvelled at and applauded, the same achievements are expected from the middle-aged person as a matter of course and may indeed be taken for granted.

There is an increasing number of middle aged people who might say that they would be happy to have these career problems. These are the thousands of people who are unemployed as a result of the decline of many of our older traditional industries. For these people, the prospect of never working again is a very real one as employers in other industries are rather unwilling to employ older people when there are so many younger and often highly qualified people to choose from.

Personal and family relationships are examined and evaluated during the middle years. This 'soul searching' is often interpreted as being a 'midlife crisis', where husband and wife wonder whether they married the right partner, whether they have done as well as they might have in their careers, whether they have raised their children properly, and whether they have any remaining unfulfilled ambitions.

For the family a critical period during the middle years is when grown-up children leave home. Reaction to this event depends to a large extent on the quality of the family relationships in the preceding years.

If parents have been very authoritarian and overprotective, the 'children' may see leaving home as a final break, an escape, and the contact between them and their parents may be slight in the future.

If the parents' marriage has been unhappy, this may be the time when separation or divorce is considered since they may have stayed together 'for the sake of the children'.

For many middle-aged people however, this period is the start of one of the happiest times of their lives. They have privacy and opportunities to re-discover each other and escape from the label of being 'John and Mary's parents'.

During these years another major adaptation of life-style may be undertaken. With the current emphasis on community care and self help within the family, more middle-aged adults are caring for elderly parents often within their own homes. This arrangement may be a good one for all concerned but is not without considerable problems especially if the elderly relative suffers from a physical or mental illness, or if the family do not receive adequate support from community health and social services.

In the later part of the middle years the person may have to adjust to retirement. Many people find this a very fulfilling time when they can indulge in their favourite hobbies and interests. Others however find it a strain to be with their wives or husbands for 24 hours per day.

Sadly, for some people the middle years are marked by the death of a husband or wife. The death of a loved one is always a devastating blow but is perhaps more so during these years. The remaining partner in a marriage may have lost not only a husband or wife but a true friend, a lover and a close companion with whom they have shared the previous 20–30 years.

For this person the prospect of living out the rest of his life in the depths of loneliness may be a very real one.

ILLNESS AND THE EFFECTS OF HOSPITALIZATION

Illness

We tend to view illness as being an abnormal state which is to be prevented or cured. Yet minor illness is a part of all or our experiences. We have all at some time had flu, a sore stomach, a terrible headache or an episode of vomiting and/or diarrhoea.

Thinking of how we felt during these minor illnesses can often give us insight into the behaviours and feelings of our patients in hospital.

For example, think how our mood and feelings change during illness. We may become upset and irritable, angry that this illness is preventing us from doing something that we had planned, worried that the illness may be more serious than we first imagined, uncertain about how long this pain will last, will it get better or worse? We may become snappy with friends and relatives, wanting attention and understanding one moment, the next moment wishing that they would just go away and leave us alone.

Our environment may also affect our mood and feelings. One moment the room is too hot and stuffy, the next moment we feel cold and shivery. Why don't they bring an extra blanket and turn off that glaring room light? And the noise of the kids playing downstairs is terrible; if only I could get to sleep!

Can you think of how changes in mood and feelings may be affected by being in hospital and how the patient's behaviour might reflect these changes?

Attitudes to illness

Our reaction and attitude toward illness is shaped by many factors. Previous experiences of illness in ourselves, family or friends will influence the perceptions of our own illness and its course.

The nature of information which we absorb from the various media sources also has a powerful effect upon how we regard illness and hospitals. However, the quality of this information varies greatly between such sources as women's magazines, television soap operas, documentary programmes and health education material.

People may hold different attitudes towards illness.

Some accept illness as an unfortunate inconvenience which has to be tolerated for a while until recovery is complete and life continues as before.

Others adopt a 'these things are sent to try us' attitude where an illness is something to be fought and conquered. During this process the patient is thought to draw on hidden reserves of character and develop new understandings of his and other people's problems.

For others, illness has a punitive role. The illness affects those who deserve it and have brought it upon themselves, for example people suffering from alcoholism, drug dependence or sexually transmitted diseases. As an extreme example of this kind of thinking the author once read of genital herpes being described as 'God's revenge upon the permissive society'. This is one example of the fact that some illnesses are considered more socially acceptable than others.

Mental illness is much more stigmatizing than physical illness. Sexually transmitted diseases are still thought to be taboo areas for general conversation. People who are scarred or disfigured as the result perhaps of severe burns are often shunned or ignored. Skin conditions are often thought to be infectious and 'dirty'. A young girl in a gynaecology ward who is having a therapeutic abortion may be treated less sympathetically than other patients in the ward who may be trying to preserve a pregnancy or who are undergoing investigations for infertility.

Can you think of factors which make illnesses 'acceptable' or 'unacceptable'?

Anxiety

Patient's anxiety

Being admitted to hospital can be very traumatic, especially if it is the patient's first experience of hospitalization. How anxiety-producing this experience will be depends on a great many factors as is shown in Table 19.1. After studying the table, see if you can think of any other possible sources of worry for a patient.

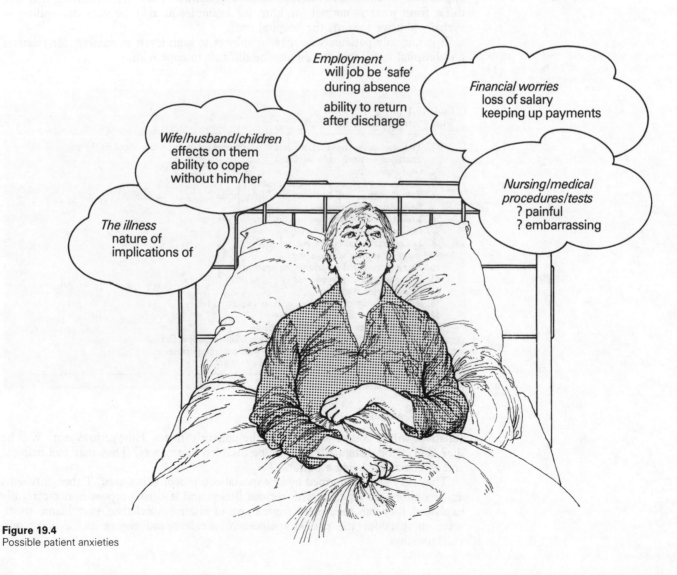

Figure 19.4
Possible patient anxieties

The fact that the illness merits admission to hospital will usually indicate to the patient that his illness is serious. If the admission has been arranged for some weeks previously this may give the patient time to prepare himself psychologically for his stay. However it is also possible that this period may become an interminable wait for the patient who may become more anxious as he thinks the worst about his impending stay in hospital.

Many hospital admissions, however, are not planned weeks in advance but are the results of trauma or serious illness of sudden onset where the patient's anxiety level may be much higher.

Anxiety is not always a bad thing, indeed a mild level of anxiety is an integral part of all of our life experiences. Mild anxiety acts to motivate and alert us. For example, how many people would take the trouble to learn correct driving skills if they were not required to sit a driving test? Would a student nurse study nursing quite so diligently if she were not required to pass module and final examinations? When anxiety becomes excessive, functioning deteriorates. The learner driver may 'go to pieces' and not be able to do a thing right during the test, regardless of the fact that he drives very well with his instructor.

The student sitting her exam may misread questions, omit questions or find that her mind goes blank and be unable to write of things about which she would usually be very knowledgeable.

When patients in hospital experience this high level of anxiety it adversely affects the patient's image of himself, his illness and his immediate environment. He may appear not to understand instructions or explanations fully. His behaviour may also differ from what is normal for him, for example, he may be very demanding or verbally abusive towards the hospital staff.

It is not only patients who may be subject to high levels of anxiety, for relatives and hospital staff, anxiety can also be difficult to cope with.

Table 19.1
What worries a patient in hospital?

1. The immediate stress related to his admission, for example the shock of the myocardial infarction or road traffic accident.
2. Goal frustration.
3 Change of body image/disfigurement.
4. Role change — will he do/say the 'right things'?
5. Being left alone/isolation.
6. Losing control over events in his life.
7. Losing control of body functions.
8. Losing emotional or self control.
9. Being in strange surroundings.
10. Being surrounded by strange equipment.
11. Treatments/tests/procedures.
12. The experience of pain.
13. The possibility of being badly treated or cared for.
14. Death.
15. Being a burden to others on discharge.
16. The possibility of losing his job through illness/hospitalization.
17. How his family/relatives are coping with his illness/absence.
18. Being embarrassed or humiliated.

Relatives' anxiety

Relatives will of course worry about the patient's illness. How serious is it? Will he die? Will he be disfigured? Will he be disabled in any way? They may feel helpless and apologize for being a nuisance.

They may also be alarmed by any special equipment being used. Tubes, infusions and monitors are equated with serious illness and if their purpose is not carefully explained they can seem very frightening to relatives. Relatives may blame themselves in part for the patient's illness or accident and engage in 'if only' self-recrimination.

Anxiety and nurse learners

Staff anxiety in hospitals is common especially in high stress areas such as Accident and Emergency Departments and Intensive Care Units.

Student nurses seem to be particularly prone to stress and anxiety. The student worries about whether she is working satisfactorily, whether she will be able to cope with emergencies, or if she will let everyone down? Whether she will say the right thing to patients and colleagues and whether she will be able to learn the skills necessary for different clinical areas. She will also have the worries related to ward assessments, college exams and final examinations.

The student may also feel anxiety and conflict if her perceived role does not match the reality of her daily work. The student's expectations of her role may be too high or she may find great differences between what is taught in the College of Nursing and what is actually practised in the clinical areas. An American nurse, Marlene Kramer, has written about her personal experience of this, referring to it as 'reality shock' (see Further Reading, p. 639).

The sick role

We all play a variety of social roles in our lives. At work we play such roles as a nurse, doctor, or teacher, at home we play for instance the role of husband, wife or daughter. Within these social roles we display the behaviours appropriate to that role.

Patient's perception of the sick role

These roles are not biologically or genetically determined, they are learned. Just as we learn how to become nurses, a patient learns how to behave as a sick person.

For example the patient may seem to regress in his behaviours and become more dependent upon the nursing staff to help with his daily activities. Here the patient may feel that the nurse's role is to do everything for a patient in hospital and therefore his role as a sick person is a purely passive one.

He is to stay in his hospital bed until the hospital staff have 'made him better'. Only then would it be appropriate for him to revert to his previous role as an independent adult capable of looking after himself.

Nurse's perception of the sick role

Nurses also have expectations of the role which patients should adopt and on this basis often make subjective judgements regarding who is a 'good' or 'bad' patient.

You should try the following exercise with a few of your colleagues. Make up a list of the characteristics of your typical 'good' and 'bad' patient. For instance your good patient might always seem grateful for the care which he is given, whereas the 'bad' patient might always complain about his care.

Do you think that nurses behave differently towards 'good' and 'bad' patients?

Can you think of any reason why these 'good' and 'bad' patients should behave in the way that they do?

After you have come up with your own answers, compare your findings with those of Felicity Stockwell who has examined the question of patient popularity in some detail (see Further Reading, p. 640).

ADOLESCENTS IN HOSPITAL

As with all patients the adolescent will react to his illness and hospitalization in a variety of ways depending on his personality, previous experiences and the nature of his illness.

Some aspects of illness and hospitalization may however affect the adolescent in a more marked way.

Body image

As we have seen, adolescence is a time of great physical and psychological change. During this period the adolescent is acutely aware of his body image and may be constantly 'checking' his physical development against that of his peers whose approval is so important to him. It is not difficult to appreciate the more dramatic examples where the adolescent may experience disturbance of body image: examples are the teenager with a dermatological condition such as severe acne or psoriasis; the physically handicapped teenager; the teenager who is having plastic surgery following burns; the teenager whose growth is either excessive or diminished perhaps due to a hormonal disorder. It is important to realise however, that to an adolescent who is very concerned about his body, any blemish or deviation from the 'normal' as he perceives it may be a source of extreme embarrassment and worry (see Fig. 19.3).

Adolescent reactions to altered body image

How the adolescent may react to changes in body image may depend on several factors, for example his personality, the nature and severity of the changes and how other people react to the changed image.

The teenager may have great difficulty in adapting to adverse changes. He may become sullen and withdrawn, not wishing to talk to other patients or staff. He may also be unwilling to discuss his body or the affected part and refuse to help or co-operate in any related treatments.

If the change in body image has been particularly sudden and traumatic, for example facial scarring from a burn or road traffic accident or amputation of all or part of a limb, then the adolescent may experience almost a state of shock as he is faced with the reality of his new 'impaired' image.

He will be flooded by anxieties, doubts, horrors and many other mixed emotions.

Nursing responses to the adolescent with altered body image

Dealing with these fears and uncertainties requires great empathy and understanding from the nurse.

Being aware of the importance of body image to the adolescent can help the nurse to understand the teenager's moments of anxious embarrassment or seeming bravado.

Accidents e.g. motorcycle

Unwanted pregnancy
Sexually transmitted disease

Alcohol/drug/solvent abuse

Exacerbation of chronic childhood illnesses

Starting smoking

Self-image problems e.g. disfigurement, acne

Figure 19.5
Health problems of adolescents

The nurse's reaction to the patient will be vitally important. If she seems to be embarrassed or disgusted when working with the teenager, this will only reinforce his fears that he is unattractive or repulsive.

It is often difficult when caring for a patient with an altered body image to strike a balance between ignoring the impaired part as if it were insignificant or did not exist, and concentrating all of the nursing attention on to the impaired part, thus exaggerating it. Focusing the nursing care between these two extremes would seem to be the most balanced approach. This impairment may be very painful for the teenager even to recognize, so discussing it and expressing feelings and fears will be much more difficult. The nurse can help here by letting the patient know that she is prepared to listen to him in an accepting and non-judgemental way, and by avoiding giving short definitive answers which can be inaccurate and also tend to stop the dialogue between the nurse and the teenager which may be developing.

Helping the teenager to carry out his own physical care where possible can help to 'desensitize' him to his impairment and can help him to confront his new body image. It is obvious that this process should proceed at a rate determined by the patient. He should not be pushed or forced into facing up to his altered body image.

Privacy needs

The adolescent's need for body privacy is related to the concept of body image. The development of reproductive organs and secondary sexual characteristics produce mixed feelings. The young person may be glad to be maturing and 'becoming an adult', but may also be upset by some consequences of these physical changes, such as menstruation and ejaculation.

The teenager may appear to be very shy and modest concerning body privacy or he may seem to be very brash and unconcerned, with a seemingly wordly wise attitude towards his body. It is important to remember however that displays of machismo, comments of mild sexual innuendo and sexual humour are often masks which hide deep anxieties about the adolescent's body privacy. Procedures which invade body privacy are commonplace in hospital and nurses can easily become blasé as they carry them out so frequently. Bed baths, preoperative shaves, catheterization, helping with elimination and physical examinations all involve invasion of body privacy which will almost certainly be among the adolescent's major anxieties while in hospital.

Will the procedure be painful? Will the nurses think that I am abnormal? Will they have a laugh and giggle at me? Will I blush like a little child? Will I have an erection? All of these anxieties and more will pre-occupy the teenager.

Figure 19.6
Respect for body privacy is important for all patients

It is important therefore that nurses involved in intimate procedures remember the ways to protect teenagers' privacy for instance by ensuring that beds are screened adequately prior to a procedure, that the teenager can bath in privacy or that supervision is as unobtrusive as possible. Careful preparation of all equipment, prior to an intimate procedure helps to ensure that the procedure can be completed as quickly as possible. It is generally agreed that when carrying out intimate procedures the nurse should adopt a more detached 'matter of fact' manner. This helps to place the procedure firmly in the clinical sphere and helps to eliminate sexuality from the procedure. Note however that this is not the same as carrying out the procedure in a cold uncaring silence.

To try to gain an insight into the feelings of a teenager during an intimate procedure, imagine the following hypothetical situation: Your tutor is giving a series of lectures on the reproductive system.

She asks if you would be willing to undress and take the part of a patient undergoing a physical examination. The tutor explains that the class will benefit from seeing the actual anatomical structures involved rather than referring to pictures in a book. She tries to allay your fears by saying that as both you and your 'audience' are nurses and therefore, accustomed to helping patients with intimate functions, being a model in this exercise should not be embarrassing for you.

Would you agree to this request? If you would not, why would you not agree? What would your thoughts and feelings be about being such a model?

Dependence

When admitted to hospital, the patient enters a world of increased dependence on others. He is dressed in pyjamas, put to bed and is no longer in control of his life events. He is expected to get up, eat and go to sleep at the same time as others. He often has to ask permission for the simplest of tasks such as getting out of bed, going to the toilet or eating something. He is no longer completely responsible for his health and physical well-being, doctors and nurses now play the dominant part in these activities.

The adolescent is at the stage in his development where he is becoming more independent and is learning to make his own decisions, friends and mistakes. To be placed in this dependent role is very difficult to accept and initially the teenager may try to show that he has not given up his new found independence by demanding a lot of attention or 'breaking the rules' to try to show that he is still in control of events.

Helping the adolescent maintain his independence

Nurses can help the teenager here by allowing the teenager to participate actively in his care and treatment as far as is possible.

It is common courtesy to explain to patients any nursing activities which you wish to carry out with them. It is also important to ask the patient for his permission and cooperation in treatments or procedures. This can help the teenager to feel less dependent and helpless by giving him some say in his care and by acknowledging that he or she is still a person who is capable of exercising judgement and choice.

The adolescent with a long term condition

The developmental tasks which face the adolescent have been discussed earlier in this chapter. Coping with physical changes, establishing an identity for himself, making vocational choices, learning to cope with his new found sexuality are among the many adaptations he has to make.

These tasks are difficult for the non-handicapped adolescent but are much more so for the adolescent who suffers from a physical or mental disability, a chronic illness, or who is hospitalized for a long period as a result of injuries sustained in, for example, a motor cycle accident.

Chronic illness

The adolescent who has a chronic condition such as epilepsy, diabetes mellitus, or cystic fibrosis may require review and adjustment of his treatment programme during adolescence as this is a period when chronic conditions often become less stable and controlled.

It can often be unnerving and threatening for a nurse to realise that some of these adolescents will have a greater knowledge of their condition than the nurse. Some will take a mischievous delight in correcting the nurse, who 'makes a mistake' in some areas of their care or treatment.

However the teenager's knowledge of his condition can often be used to engage him in discussion about his current hospitalization and future plans. It will also be a boost to the patient's self esteem that nursing staff feel that he is knowledgeable about his condition and can contribute and participate in his own care.

It is important however to listen carefully to the adolescent's accounts and ideas of his condition as he may well have acquired some erroneous information or misconception regarding his condition which staff could help him to correct.

Inactivity/immobility

A major problem which staff face when caring for adolescents over a long period of time is how to occupy teenagers who may be confined to bed, for example with a fractured femur, for a long period of time but who might otherwise be generally healthy. It would be harmful for the adolescent to have no outlet for his energies as he may become very introspective, nurturing and developing fears and anxieties about his illness or injury.

Nursing staff can discuss activities with the patient, identifying necessary limitations on activity and suggest acceptable alternatives. Others involved with the adolescent; the Occupational Therapist, parents, friends or school teacher might be able to help suggest and plan activities.

Adolescent units

The special needs of adolescents have been recognized for many years now in psychiatry and mental handicap and adolescents have been cared for in Adolescent Units. The creation of specialist wards for adolescent patients has not yet become commonplace in our general hospitals. As a result adolescents are often cared for either in general or paediatric wards. Advantages are claimed for placing adolescents in either of these settings.

What advantages and disadvantages would there be in caring for the adolescent in each of these type of wards? What would be the advantages of caring for adolescents in a special adolescent unit?

THE YOUNG ADULT IN HOSPITAL

We can see from Table 19.1 that hospitalization due to illness or injury can be a very stressful event in the life of a young adult, posing as it does threats to his physical and psychological well-being.

It is important therefore that nurses try to meet not only the person's needs related to physiological survival but also the needs related to the person as a patient in hospital and as a member of a family.

Security and safety

Illness or injury confronts the young adult in the most dramatic way with his own vulnerability. He now realizes that it is not only other people who become ill or involved in accidents. The experience of hospitalization can compound these feelings of insecurity.

He may worry about being left alone or that no-one may hear requests for help. He may be afraid of being the victim of a nurse's or doctor's error, for example being given the wrong medication or operation.

Patient's fears often seem illogical or trivial to nurses, but it is important to realize that for the patient they are very real and as such the nurse should carefully consider ways in which she can help to allay these fears.

Reassurance

If there is one cliché which appears with monotonous regularity in nursing it is 'reassure the patient'. With glib ease it finds its way into countless examination questions, nursing care studies and care plans, yet few nurses stop to consider what actions they would take to provide this 'reassurance'.

When we speak of reassurance in nursing we mean those actions which make the patient feel more secure, safe, trusting and confident both in himself and in his treatment and care.

Look again at the worries and anxieties which the hospitalized person may have (Table 19.1). What actions could you take which would reassure the patient and help to reduce these anxieties?

Providing information and explanations

Hospitals seem strange places to the newly admitted patient. They are filled with sophisticated and possibly frightening equipment, unfamiliar people in a variety of uniforms, other patients with a host of unusual illnesses or traumatic injuries and many unusual rituals which are performed.

Thinking of how you feel or felt as a student nurse on your first morning in a new ward can give some idea of how the new patient feels.

He will have a strongly felt need to be informed of plans for his care and to have nursing activities or treatments explained to him in a way which he understands. It is not only discourteous but poor nursing practice to begin to carry out a nursing activity on a patient rather than with him, having neither asked his permission nor explained the procedure to him.

It is important that explanations and information given are truthful and clear. Telling a patient that an injection 'won't hurt a bit' when you both know that it will is far from reassuring. Other responses to patient's questions or anxieties which will not be reassuring include 'palming the patient off'. The question may be one which the nurse cannot answer or perhaps the sentiment which the patient expresses makes the nurse feel uncomfortable. For example, the patient may ask if he is going to die, or if the results of his test were 'bad'. The nurse might tell him not to ask such silly questions and say that 'everything is fine' and that he is 'not to worry'. She may also try to change the subject of the conversation to less uncomfortable matters by asking what the patient had for his lunch, or whether he is expecting any visitors today. She might also try to use banal humour to escape from serious conversation: 'Of course you're not going to die, Mr Smith, we need you to help us in the ward.'

In future the nurse may make a mental note to avoid conversation with this patient as it makes her feel uncomfortable.

Familiarizing the patient with his environment

Making the unfamiliar environment of the hospital more familiar can often help to reduce the patient's fears and anxieties.

The practice of showing patients around the ward on admission and explaining the general routine of the ward is a good one.

These skills of familiarizing patients with their surroundings are often highly developed in, for example, paediatric nursing where it is of even greater importance that the young child is made familiar with his environment in ways appropriate to his level of development.

The adult's environment can be made more familiar by allowing the patient to have personal possessions with him in hospital.

A bedside locker may appear 'tidier' with only a jug of water and a tumbler on top of it but it is hardly the person's own locker unless it has his or her books, photographs and 'get well' cards, on it. It is also important that the patient wears his own clothing in preference to anonymous hospital nightshirts.

Fulfilling the role of the nurse

There are some patients who regard medicine and nursing as areas of mystical and magical power and believe that when they become ill they will enter hospital where doctors and nurses possess the 'commodity' of health which they will pass on to the patient.

Obviously no nurse can be omnipotent and omniscient but patients will expect them to possess certain characteristics such as concern, a willingness to help, knowledge and competence. If a nurse's appearance, attitudes, and behaviours are markedly at variance with the patient's expectations then he may feel insecure in her care.

The young adult as a family member

In recent years there has been much discussion within nursing regarding the need to make nursing care more individual, to concentrate upon the 'whole' person rather than only the diseased or injured part. The phrase 'holistic nursing' is often used in this context although the true definition is wider than this.

The person is not a person in isolation but an important member of a family, whether a son, daughter, husband, wife or mother.

The patient's reactions to hospitalization and his progress while in hospital are closely related to his family and social circumstances.

Financial problems can often be a source of great anxiety for the young adult in hospital. This is often the time in the young adult's life when a family is started and a mortgage taken on. The reduced earning power experienced as a result of illness, especially if it involves a long period of hospitalization, can cause real crises for a patient and his family. Related to this are the patient's anxieties about his job. In the short term perhaps others at work are proving very capable of doing the patient's job. Perhaps he is not as vital or indispensable as he may have thought. If the illness is more long term then his employer may say that 'he will have to find someone else'.

Family roles will also change during the patients' hospitalization especially if it is of long duration. For a young man who sees himself in a dominant role within the family it may be galling to realize that his wife is coping well with being the 'head' of the family and perhaps even the new breadwinner, especially if she enjoys her new role and is unwilling to relinquish it when the patient returns home.

Young mothers in hospital can also experience such feelings if young children are being cared for by their father or by relatives and do not seem to be unduly upset at the absence of their mother.

No-one would expect the ward nurses to be able to solve all of these family and related problems but by listening to a patient's worries with genuine concern they may be able to encourage the patient to talk of these fears and feelings. This exercise itself is often of great benefit to the patient and many will say that they feel much better having had someone to talk to and are grateful for the chance to 'get things off their chest'.

The nurse might also be able to refer the patient to another member of the care team, the health visitor or medical social worker, who could offer help with problems such as these.

ILLNESS IN THE MIDDLE YEARS
Threats to health

It is often said that paediatrics deals with the person as a developing organism whereas adult medicine deals with the person as a degenerating organism. This may seem rather a dramatic statement, nevertheless it is true that degenerative disorders, disorders associated with stress and disorders associated with personal habits and life-style increase in incidence during 40 and 55 years of age.

Stress is typically high in this period related to career, positions of high responsibility or physical work which the person may find increasingly tiring. The financial demands imposed by teenage families, perhaps compounded by problems of youth unemployment may cause the middle-aged worker to take on increased levels of work or responsibility.

Physical factors such as obesity and smoking may combine with these stress factors, increasing the risk of heart disease, hypertension, ulcers and depression. The middle years can be times of increasing dependence on alcohol, tobacco and other drugs such as antidepressants and tranquillisers. The person will often say that he has been smoking heavily since he was a youngster and that it is too late for him to stop now.

It is often during these years that the person may develop illness as a result of environmental or occupational factors, for example if he has been repeatedly exposed to coal dust or asbestos during his working life.

Malignant tumors of the lungs, gastrointestinal tract, genital tract and breasts may develop during these years.

Chronic illness, disability and hospitalization

The onset of chronic illness or disability creates many problems for the older adult. The loss of independence associated with chronic illness or disability may be very difficult for the person to accept. The patient may feel that it is humiliating to be cared for 'like a child' often by nurses who are young enough to be their children or even their grandchildren.

They may react to this situation by either insisting that they do almost everything by themselves without help or they may regress to an almost child like state of dependence, expecting nursing staff to do everything for them as they 'can't manage'.

Chronic illness may also be viewed rather unsympathetically. In the initial stages of an illness, people tend to be very concerned and sympathetic. Family and friends will visit regularly, the 'get well soon' cards and messages will accumulate on the bedside locker. However the illness may soon lose its 'novelty value' and people will find it harder to maintain their initial levels of sympathy and hospital visits. This may cause the patient to become angry, bitter or depressed as he cannot understand why people 'don't care about him anymore'; after all he still has the chronic condition. These feelings of isolation can lead to the person thinking that friends and family no longer care or care for him, that he has become a 'burden' upon them and that perhaps they may not wish to have him home where he may require care and attention. Perhaps they will try to 'dump him in a home or an institution'?

To nurses and the patients' relatives these fears may seem hysterical and groundless yet to the older adult with a chronic disease they may be very real and should be treated as such.

The patient needs to feel that he is still valued as a person and that he still belongs within his family, circles of friends and colleagues.

Nurses can do much to boost this patient's self-esteem by thinking of ways in which they can organize the person's nursing care to suit his particular needs and problems. This may sound like stating the obvious but 'en masse' systems of care where 'the stroke patients' are cared for in one way and 'the rheumatoids' in another still exist and harrowing accounts of thoughtless patterns of care being imposed upon patients can often be read in nursing journals.

It is important also to give sound advice and practical help which will enable the patient to know exactly what he must do in order to cope to the best of his ability with his impaired health or disability.

Trite clichés such as 'pull yourself together', 'you must do more for yourself Mr Smith' or 'take things easy for a while, don't overdo it', are not only meaningless but offensive to the patient as they reduce his serious problems to the level of slogan solutions.

The nurse will not be able to provide all of the answers or advice that the patient will need but it is important that she knows where specialist help can be obtained. This may involve working with other professionals within the hospital such as a physiotherapist or occupational therapist.

It should also involve preparing the patient for discharge from hospital.

Discharge of the patient with a chronic illness should be carefully planned to help alleviate the anxieties which the patient and his relatives may have. These may include worries about how much the person is allowed to do for himself, when he will be able to return to work, will the husband or wife be able to cope with any special care which the spouse needs and who can they contact for help if difficulties arise.

A good liaison between ward staff and community nursing and social services can help to avoid many of these problems associated with discharge from hospital.

SUMMARY

Coping with illness, injury or disability calls for a maturity which allows the patient to make any necessary adaptations which will help him to adjust to his impaired health. Adolescents have many strengths which may enable them to come to terms with these problems. Older adults may find this process more difficult although they may try to give the appearance of being able to adapt.

Nurses will also require to develop a professional maturity if they are to cope with what is an increasingly complex and demanding role.

Many factors conspire to make many different goals difficult for patients and staff to achieve.

A high proportion of those giving care in hospital are still teenagers who are trying hard to cope with all of the adjustments required of their age group.

For many years now nursing has been struggling to rid itself of the stereotypes and myths which have shrouded it, for example that nurses are motivated solely by dedication and have no wish for financial or other rewards. That nurses do not require to be intelligent or to be highly trained, they need only have 'common sense'; that underneath the cool efficient exterior all nurses are obsessed with sexual activity, the 'naughty nurse' stereotype so beloved of the popular press.

No doubt you could think of many other examples of the public image of nursing. How true are these images in relation to yourself and your colleagues?

Yet nurses are only human. The work of a nurse is often stressful and many less experienced nurses find it very difficult to survive let alone deal effectively with the many problems facing their patients.

These can be difficult feelings to admit to. Traditionally nurses have always been expected to 'carry on', regardless of their own feelings and problems and of course to hide these feelings from patients and colleagues. To do otherwise was often taken as a sign that the nurse was 'weak' or 'too emotional' or 'over involved'. Many nurses have paid a heavy price for these feelings, either by leaving nursing, feeling that they were unsuitable or by submerging these feelings under a façade of disillusionment and cynicism.

To show genuine concern for patients' problems without becoming 'over involved'; to adopt a realistic approach without ignoring the problems which you may not be able to help with; to be flexible but not inconsistent or haphazard in giving care; to be an involved and committed nurse while realizing the importance of having a family and social life outside nursing. Can any person live up to all of these ideals and more all of the time?

Perhaps the most important thing for a nurse to realize is that no one person can fulfil all of the varied needs of another, but what will be expected and appreciated is that the nurse should genuinely try, while at the same time realising her individual limitations.

FURTHER READING

Bridge W, Macleod-Clark J 1981 Communication in nursing care. HM&M, London
Darbyshire P 1980 Thanks nurse, you did care more. Nursing Times 76(52): 2223–2224
Elkind D 1967 Egocentrism in adolescence. Child Development 38: 1025–1034
Franklin B L 1974 Patient anxiety on admission to hospital. Rcn, London
Hayward J 1975 Information: a prescription against pain. Rcn, London
Kelly M P, May D 1982 Good and bad patients: a review of the literature and a theoretical critique. Journal of Advanced Nursing 7(2): 147–156
Know your own society 1981 Pan, London
Kramer M 1974 Reality shock. Mosby, St Louis
Millstein S G, Adler N E, Irwin C E 1981 Conceptions of illness in young adolescents. Paediatrics 68: 834–839

Mitchell J R 1980 Male adolescents' concern about a physical examination conducted by a female. Nursing Research 29(3): 165–169

Nursing 1981 Adulthood and ageing. Ist series issue 25 May

Nursing 1981 Ambivalence and adolescence. Ist series issue 24 April

Nursing Mirror 1983 One day you will understand: a 3rd year nurse describes her experience of having an abortion. Nursing Mirror 157(8): xi–xii

Nursing Times 1981 Who am I? Why do I hurt so much? Whatever happened to nursing care? Nursing Times 77(15): 633–639

Pritchard P 1982 Stress and anxiety in physical illness — the role of the general nurse. Nursing Times 77(4): 162–164

Siantz M L 1977 The nurse and the developmentally disabled adolescent. University Park Press, London

Stockwell F 1972 The unpopular patient. Rcn, London

Wilson-Barnett J 1978 Factors influencing patients' emotional reactions to hospitalisation. Journal of Advanced Nursing 3(3): 221–229

Chapter Twenty
The elderly

While this chapter attempts to put normal ageing in perspective, it focuses on the commoner problems encountered by older people living either in hospital or in the community.

Geriatric medicine is concerned with clinical, social, preventive and remedial aspects of illness in the elderly. It has developed as a speciality concerned with old people with health problems and often with additional social difficulties. In geriatric care the emphasis is on supporting the patient to live with his disabilities, whatever they may be. Old age is not always attractive, the therapeutic benefits of treatment are often harder and slower to achieve, relapses are more common and unless steps are taken to ensure otherwise, the patient may return from hospital to unfavourable conditions which militate against the efforts which have been made on his behalf.

Throughout the last 100 years the number of old people has steadily increased and may have reached a peak during the early 1980s. The indications are however that the number of very old, those over 75 years of age will continue to rise until well into the next century (Fig. 20.1). As this group contains many old people who are mentally and physically frail the implication for the provision of nursing care is substantial.

Figure 20.1
Population growth of the elderly
in the United Kingdom (black =
  65+; brown = 75+)

THE AGEING PROCESS

While the study of the ageing process is extremely complex and as a science is still in its infancy, it is necessary for the nurse caring for the elderly to have a working knowledge of the subject.

Who are the elderly?

In the past it was customary to use the retirement age as an indicator, namely 65 years for men and 60 years for women, but ageing and chronological age do not proceed at the same rate. Someone faced with redundancy and with no job prospects may well feel old at 45 years, while others are fit and able to contribute to their family and to society until well into their 70s.

This unfortunate habit of lumping together everyone within an age range of some 30 years is plainly nonsensical and may have perpetuated the stereotype of the elderly as being poor, sick and all alone. Clearly, many are none of these things.

Nurses, especially if they work in hospitals, see only a tiny and very atypical section of the over 65-year-olds, yet it is tempting to believe that they are somehow representative of all old people.

In order to gain a more accurate picture of the elderly, it is useful to consider separately, the **young elderly**, those from 65–75 years and the **older elderly**, those over 75 years of age.

Figure 20.2
The young elderly

The young elderly (Fig. 20.2)

Only about 5% of old people are looked after in institutions, and the number of young elderly thus accommodated is even smaller. In studying this group therefore it is sensible to look at the majority who are living in the community.

The variations within this age group are as great if not greater than in any other. Although it will include the lonely, the chronic sick and the melancholic, an overall picture of despondency is not altogether justified.

While some will have much reduced drive, tending only to bemoan lost opportunities, others will be grateful for the chance to devote more time to their interests and hobbies. For every isolate there may be a valued member of a three generation family (Fig. 20.3) able to contribute to as well as take from those around him. Some will be in receipt of meals on wheels, but still others will be delivering them!

Retirement

In a modern, technological society most old people will have one thing in common, enforced retirement at a specified age. This will inevitably be seen as a major upheaval and a stark reminder to the individual concerned that time marches on.

For many it signals the end of productive life, which in turn is too often associated with a marked lowering of status.

Traditionally, the working class male has found this most devastating, with genuine economic hardship on occasions adding to the void of lost workmates and a great feeling of worthlessness. Women, whether working or not, tend to have a more secure domestic foothold, and are said to make the transition to retirement with far less trauma.

Figure 20.3
The three generation family

Preparation for retirement

Although retirement frequently steals up overnight, (one day you are a worker, the next an old age pensioner) everyone is aware that in time it will happen to him. Most people do therefore try to prepare themselves for the event, however inadequately.

Disengagement is the term coined to describe the unfortunate response of gradual but premature withdrawal by an individual from his environment. This may be marked by cherished ideals, pastimes and friendships being neglected or given up as the ageing person prepares to take a back seat.

On the positive side, many people do plan constructively for retirement, although they may feel that the dice are loaded against them. Inflation reduces the worth of hard-earned savings, while ill health can so easily render impossible the long cherished plans for increased travel, or more time on the golf course.

Thankfully, it is not nowadays left entirely to the individual. A national super-annuation scheme ensures that any financial blow is cushioned and thus the life-style can be partly maintained.

Many companies and local authorities run 'preparation for retirement' classes, often on a day release basis. Here, the young elderly can glean information about financial benefits, adjustment to increased leisure, community facilities available, or avenues open to the voluntary worker. Ideally such schemes will be extended to give everyone the benefit of a planned approach to retirement.

Beyond retirement

The early years following retirement constitute a period of adjustment. Old age is beckoning.

While a small percentage will fail spectacularly to come to terms with the change of status and plummet rapidly towards self neglect or an early death, for most the transition is gradual.

Even for an old person, secure within his family, the death of a spouse can be a savage blow, particularly if it is the man who is left behind.

Offspring, themselves perhaps middle aged, may seem more preoccupied with their own children or problems at work. Grandchildren may be around less often.

Hand-in-hand with these developments may appear the characteristic tendency of the elderly to react in a more rigid manner to their environment. Changes may be less welcome and adapted to poorly.

People in this age group are more likely to be seen by their general practitioners, and physical illness, whether chronic or acute, may manifest itself for the first time.

The older elderly (Fig. 20.4)

Increasing dependency

As the individual ages, the transition to a dependent status, is most likely to be gradual. A crisis such as a cerebrovascular accident (stroke) may herald a complete change of life-style overnight, but only a minority experience a reversal as sudden as this.

The great majority of our elderly population live happily and securely within the community. Many require minimal medical care, while many more never require to be hospitalized. Problems when they do arise, however, may be complicated by a variety of factors, physical, mental or social.

Unlike younger groups who may have a great deal of resilience and a wide circle of potential supporters, the older person's social contacts may be reduced to include only two or three elderly companions.

The retiral home chosen when fit and active may now be expensive to maintain and totally inappropriate, particularly if it is remote from family, remaining friends and amenities.

The way the older person responds psychologically and physically, not only to day to day occurrences but to disease process, can be vastly different from that of younger people.

It is recognized that while no-one escapes the ageing process entirely; individuals, depending on their genetic composition, will show varying rates of deterioration. In other words, it could be said that we have a chronological age and a *biological age*.

Apart from the familiar manifestations of age, complex biological changes take place which result in a general deterioration of the physical performance of organs, systems and the body as a whole.

Multiple pathology

To complicate the position further, many elderly people have accrued a collection of minor ailments and have to contend with the long term results and complications

Figure 20.4
The older elderly

of chronic disease processes such as occurs in diabetes or respiratory disease. It is, therefore difficult for the individual, or indeed the professional to determine whether deterioration can be ascribed to ageing or to disease process.

Many elderly people live from day to day knowing that their independence hangs by a flimsy thread. They may be over anxious and insecure. They deny themselves comforts that often in real terms they could afford, but for fear of debt, they forego. For some the horror of not being able to leave enough money to cover the ever increasing cost of burial predominates.

To complicate matters the elderly generally have low expectations of health and tend to tolerate resolvable problems, attributing everything to advancing years.

NURSING SUPPORT

The nurse has a very positive part to play in caring for elderly people; it is important for her to develop skills to deal with crises when they occur and better still, to detect potential problems at an early stage.

Much of the work of the health visitor to the elderly is directed towards the early detection of problems, thereby avoiding social or physical breakdown. Another important aspect of her role involves teaching the elderly and their relatives to take positive measures to help them live successfully within the limits imposed by their old age.

For any nurse working with the elderly, whether in hospital or the community, it is important to assess accurately the problems which confront them for many problems have at least partial solutions. Ageing is not an incurable disease.

A useful way to do this, and in turn, to determine a nursing strategy, is to consider both the *ageing process and the disease process* as they affect an old person's capacity to carry out the fundamental activities of living.

Breathing

Changes which occur in the respiratory system as a result of ageing include: the calcification of costal cartilages, the reduced mobility of the ribs, a loss of elasticity of lung tissue and a decline in total lung capacity. The strength of the expiratory muscles are decreased, the propulsive effect of the cough is reduced and there is a marked decrease in ciliary activity.

The elderly person is therefore particularly vulnerable to respiratory complaints. For many, superimposed upon these changes may be the fact that for several years they have been the victims of a chronic respiratory disease such as bronchitis or asthma. The increased susceptibility of the elderly to respiratory infection includes the influenzal type of infection so common in winter and measures taken to minimize occurrence should include the protection of the patient from infected nurses or relatives.

Bed rest is potentially dangerous because full expansion of the lungs is more difficult and for this reason is recommended as seldom as possible. There is also an increased risk for the elderly person in undergoing general anaesthesia.

Signs of respiratory infection may be minimal and not perceived until the infection is almost overwhelming.

Typically, respirations slowly increase followed by an increase in pulse rate; body temperature however often remains within normal limits. The patient may merely complain of feeling tired or present with mild confusion. Coughing, if it exists, may be unproductive, and specimen collection may prove difficult.

For the hospitalized elderly, measures taken to prevent problems associated with breathing include plans which ensure the patient is encouraged to be as mobile as possible. When sitting, a chair should be selected which offers support to the back. The patient can be taught gentle breathing exercises ensuring he uses the bases of his lungs. When in bed, the use of pillows and a back rest will promote correct positioning and help prevent slumping.

While it is not always considered appropriate to be too dogmatic about the evils of smoking when dealing with life-long smokers, the nurse should be aware of the horrific mortality associated with the habit.

Eating and drinking

Factors which should be taken into account when considering the importance of eating, drinking and the elderly person, include social, physical and economic constraints which may exist for some of this group.

Biological changes brought about by the ageing process may also influence the nutritional state. The notion that 'apples today don't taste like they used to,' may reflect not so much the quality of the apple but the fact that taste buds are reduced in number with advancing years. Sense of smell too may be dulled.

Recession of the gums and bones of the jaw makes it difficult to fit many older people with dentures which remain comfortable over a period of time. It is not uncommon for old people, once having been fitted with dentures, to fail to maintain contact with their dentist and either suffer from painful ill-fitting teeth, or reject them altogether. With advancing years, there is a marked decrease in the amount of saliva produced, the swallowing mechanism may become impaired and motility throughout the alimentary canal is reduced.

Impaired mobility, coupled with reduced financial status may greatly influence an individual's choice of diet, while for the bereaved or isolated, loneliness may take away the motivation to cook a meal.

The nutritional requirements of the elderly are not significantly altered by ageing. Protein, vitamin and mineral needs remain much the same, although for most people there is likely to be some reduction in energy demand.

Poor eating patterns of youth tend to be exaggerated with age, and knowledge of nutritional factors tends to be limited.

It has been observed that from the age of about 60 years, there is a slow reduction in the overall body weight. It is important however to establish the time span over which weight has been lost, to differentiate between normal ageing and disease process which in the main, occurs over a much shorter period.

The hospitalized elderly and their diet

When caring for the elderly in hospital, the nurse should do much more than merely ensure that her patients are adequately nourished. Meal times should be a special event to which patients look forward.

Facilities can be made available which allow the elderly to attend to their own oral hygiene whenever possible. Well fitting dentures which have been cleaned and rinsed can greatly enhance the individual's ability to enjoy a meal. Today many geriatric hospitals have a dental service.

Maintaining an adequate fluid intake is equally important. The thirst reflex is often suppressed due to ageing, therefore some patients will not ask for a drink, but instead, will have to be encouraged. Variety of choice helps to interest the patient in taking fluids and a selection of hot and cold drinks should be offered at regular intervals.

Feeding aids

When physical disability makes it difficult for a patient to feed himself independently, the selection of an appropriate feeding aid can serve to make the problem less pronounced. A comfortably seated, well-supported patient may be able to feed himself with the help of aids, such as a non-slip place mat, a plate guard and, if necessary, carefully selected, adapted cutlery (Fig. 20.5).

In continuing care wards the patients may become so accustomed to conforming to a routine that unless an alternative is planned, they will eat only what is on offer from the hospital kitchen. It is possible for many of these patients to have a meal out with relatives or friends, or private arrangements can be made to cater for the patients in the ward on special occasions.

Such events, which can be initiated and participated in by the resourceful nurse, help fulfil a social need for the resident, many of whom may regard a fish supper as a rare treat.

Figure 20.5
Special cutlery

In the community, while the majority of the elderly are well able to shop and cook for themselves, there are those who require help.

The *meals on wheels* service, supplies hot meals on a regular basis to the home of the old person. This service has the additional advantage of providing, perhaps, the only human contact, to whom the recipient can look forward.

Some elderly patients will, because of their medical conditions, for instance diabetes, require special diets. These are explained in the appropriate chapters.

Eliminating

Urinary incontinence

One of the most distressing problems facing the elderly and those caring for them is that of urinary incontinence. There can be few situations more demoralising than that which results from the inability to cope with such a fundamental personal need.

Normal ageing brings about changes in bladder efficiency. For many the bladder neither empties nor fills completely. Stress incontinence is common in elderly women due to loss of tone or damage to the muscles of the pelvic floor.

Alteration in nervous control can result in frequency or urgency, which when coupled with impaired mobility can in themselves, be a cause of incontinence.

Neurological changes such as may follow a stroke (cerebrovascular accident) can give rise to incontinence, as may a urinary tract infection. In men, urinary incontinence secondary to prostatic disease is not uncommon, while faecal impaction can also result in loss of bladder control.

Occasionally nocturnal incontinence can be attributed to heavy night sedation, or to alcohol consumption.

Achieving continence

It is important that the geriatrician diagnoses the cause of incontinence. In many instances underlying problems can be treated and the patient relieved of distress. This may involve the eradication of infection, the treatment of faecal impaction, and improving mobility.

In other cases treatment may be more complex, requiring a planned retraining programme for the patient. It is important for the nurse to be aware of the contribution she can make within such a programme.

The use of charts to monitor continence/incontinence can demonstrate a pattern of events around which positive measures may be taken (Fig. 20.6). It may be that encouraging the patient to go to the toilet at set intervals during the day (and possibly even during the night) can achieve continence.

The informed nurse will be aware that the time span between an elderly patient feeling the need to empty his bladder and the point at which involuntary emptying will occur is relatively short. By recognizing the need to deal promptly with such a person's request for toilet facilities many embarrassing accidents can be avoided.

Urinary continence will never again be possible for some old people. For them, there are many aids and appliances available to help to protect skin and clothing and thus to retain dignity. (Urinary incontinence is dealt with more fully in Chapter 9.)

Faecal impaction incontinence

Faecal impaction occurs when a mass of faecal matter is lodged within the lumen of the large bowel. Normally a person becomes aware that the rectum is full, and its contents are expelled at an appropriate time. In faecal impaction this does not happen. The slower onward movement of the intestinal contents allows more time for water to be reabsorbed and the residue becomes abnormally solid. Eventually the constipated faeces which cannot be expelled accumulate in the rectum.

This state may be accompanied by leakage of fluid faecal material, which seeps around the impacted mass and through the anus, an occurrence sometimes called *spurious diarrhoea*. On such occasions however, the faecal mass will be clearly felt on rectal examination, thus differentiating the condition, from 'true' diarrhoea.

HOSPITAL .... UNIT No.

CONTINENCE CHART

NAME

DATE OF BIRTH

DIAGNOSIS

DATE		DAY						NIGHT						REMARKS
		08.00 10.00	10.00 12.00	12.00 14.00	14.00 16.00	16.00 18.00	18.00 20.00	20.00 22.00	22.00 24.00	24.00 02.00	02.00 04.00	04.00 06.00	06.00 08.00	
	U													
	F													
	U													
	F													
	U													
	F													
	U													
	F													
	U													
	F													
	U													
	F													

DATE		DAY						NIGHT						REMARKS
		08.00 10.00	10.00 12.00	12.00 14.00	14.00 16.00	16.00 18.00	18.00 20.00	20.00 22.00	22.00 24.00	24.00 02.00	02.00 04.00	04.00 06.00	06.00 08.00	
	U													
	F													
	U													
	F													
	U													
	F													
	U													
	F													
	U													
	F													
	U													
	F													

IF INCONTINENT, OF URINE, AND/OR FAECES, CROSS HATCH SQUARE, U OR F
AT THE TIME OF THE EVENT

NORMAL URINATION OR BOWEL ACTION MAY BE MARKED BY A DIAGONAL
STROKE IN THE APPROPRIATE SQUARE

Figure 20.6
Continence chart

Figure 20.7
Bathroom aids

Additional indicators which would make the nurse suspect faecal impaction are lower abdominal pain and a distended abdomen.

Once impaction has occurred it can take as long as 3 weeks to clear the bowel completely. The first step will be to empty the rectum digitally.

Mild oral aperients may be prescribed to soften the faeces to allow easier evacuation.

Regular rectal examination is imperative. If there are faeces in the rectum appropriate suppositories or enemeta are inserted. The treatment of faecal impaction involves a great deal of nursing care and patient discomfort. It is an avoidable condition, however, and wherever possible, patients, relatives and nurses should be educated to take measures to prevent its occurrence.

Skin care

Certain changes occur in the hair and skin as a result of the ageing process.

The hair loses its natural colour, gets thinner and starts to fall out; although more common in men and perfectly harmless, women too are affected and may be acutely embarrassed if hair loss is extensive. A wide variety of wigs are available and are frequently worn by women. Some wigs are supplied by the National Health Service. The balding, older man, who regards the loss as a problem, may take to wearing a cap as a solution.

Changes in the skin are also well recognised. Predominantly occurring in the dermis, they bring about, wrinkles, thinning, increased fragility and transparency. The skin now contains less water and the elasticity of the collagen is reduced.

Senile purpura is the name given to haemorrhagic areas, sometimes several centimetres in diameter occurring on the forearms and the back of the hands. This common and benign condition appears to have no medical significance and an assurance of this fact may greatly relieve the old person.

In hospital, bathing will do much to protect the condition of the patient's skin and help to prevent the development of itching or eczema, both of which are prone to occur between skin folds, particularly in the obese. On occasions old people may be admitted in a neglected state, with the corresponding risk of pediculosis, scabies and infected lesions.

Outwith hospital the task of bathing patients unable to look after themselves may fall on the district nurse or in some cases her auxiliary.

Of even greater importance is the propensity of the elderly to develop pressure sores, especially if they are very thin. Although this condition and its important implications for the planning of nursing care have been discussed elsewhere (Ch. 14) the old person's special vulnerability must be considered.

They must, as a priority, be encouraged to remain as mobile as possible. The term 'bed sore', is a misnomer as pressure sores can develop as readily when someone is confined to a hard chair.

The old person should be encouraged to drink plenty of fluids, and nutrients high in vitamins and proteins are desirable, a combination not always to be found in the diet of the elderly, but nonetheless vital for the well-being of the skin.

For the patients confined to bed many familiar aids are available, of which the ripple mattress, the sheepskin and the bed cage, are among the more common examples. Patients nursed in the community should be able to borrow or hire similar devices from their health board on the recommendation of the district nurse.

Temperature control

Tolerance of extremes of temperature is much reduced by age. A less reliable regulating system coupled with a reduced ability to generate heat (often linked to poor mobility), and a diminished subcutaneous layer of insulating fat, make the aged very sensitive to cold. This can range from mild discomfort on the one hand, to the lift threatening state of *hypothermia* on the other. It may be difficult for the hot, busy, nurse to appreciate that her elderly patient will be extremely uncomfortable if radiators are turned down or windows thrown open. Warm drinks, a knee rug, or wool cardigan with windows open at the top rather than the bottom, can result both in fresh air and patient comfort. For the old person living alone, immobility, an inadequate intake of calories, poor heating, and the British climate, increase the risk of hypothermia. The patient's core temperature falls below 35°C, after which pulse and respirations slow dramatically, blood pressure falls and the old person becomes apathetic, drowsy and will eventually lapse into a coma. This situation constitutes a medical emergency requiring hospitalization. Undiagnosed or poorly treated hypothyroidism (Ch. 11) makes an old person particularly at risk.

Measures to prevent hypothermia include educating the elderly on the relationship between nutrition, activity, home insulation and choice of clothing as a means of staying warm in winter. Advice given by the health visitor or other nurses in the community, play a major part in prevention.

At the other extreme an older person can very readily become overheated, for example in a crowded room, or if exposed to direct sunshine. A reduction in the number, size and function of sweat glands together with balding or sparse hair contributes to this. Heat exhaustion does not take long to occur, therefore thought must be given to protecting the old person. Sun umbrellas, straw hats and iced drinks will go a long way to increasing the patient's comfort while allowing him the pleasure of enjoying the sunshine.

Mobility

For man, one of life's initial goals is to achieve the upright position. Every parent can remember with pride the concentrated effort that went into baby's first footsteps, the ability to walk opening up a new and exciting area of independence. It could be said that the fight to remain upright against gravity, is a lifelong struggle, and when we are faced with impaired mobility, the consequences are frightening and far reaching. Again the elderly are the group who are most vulnerable. Reasons for loss of, or reduced, mobility are manifold and it might be useful to consider some common causes under the following headings.

Musculo-skeletal problems

Due to the ageing process, a progressive decline in stature can be noticed. This is brought about by changes in the shape of the spinal column (kyphosis p. 670), and shortening of the spine resulting from narrowing of the intervertebral discs and loss of height of each individual vertebra. There is a slight increase in flexion of hips and knees. In general there is a progressive loss of bone mass over the years (osteoporosis p. 165). The reason for this is not clearly understood but it seems to occur earlier in women than in men and the degree is more marked in the white population. The net result of this is that older women are at greater risk of sustaining fractures following falls.

Immobility greatly increases the rate at which osteoporosis develops.

For some old people degenerative changes of the weight bearing joints (osteoarthritis p. 43) can make walking extremely painful. On the other hand, inflammatory joint disease, (rheumatoid arthritis p. 49) suffered over many years and now quiescent, will nonetheless have left some individuals with restricted movement and deformity of the joints.

Cardiopulmonary problems

Degenerative changes in the blood vessels provide the origin of many problems for the elderly, one of the most devastating being, stroke (Ch. 3). The consequent damage to the nervous system that this produces results in a complexity of problems. For the elderly, the long haul back from such a catastrophe can seem soul destroying. Vascular problems which produce pain can effectively impair the person's ability to walk even a short distance; examples include angina pectoris (p. 267) and intermittent claudication (p. 284) (Ch. 7) The past years have seen a general increase in the number of elderly amputees, the direct result of vascular disease.

Chronic cardiac or pulmonary disease may produce dyspnoea of effort, limiting mobility severely.

However not all factors which limit mobility are dramatic. A corn, or ingrown toenail, affecting an old person who does not know how to summon professional help, can have serious implications, for example if this means they can no longer wear outdoor shoes, they may become housebound and dependent on others. The resulting apathy and isolation may produce consequences far more serious than their relatively simple causes.

Behavioural problems

Not all causes of reduced mobility are physical in origin. It is common to encounter old people who have become extremely apathetic or clinically depressed to the point where getting out of bed or chair is just too much of an effort. On other occasions physical disease may present as a behavioural problem, for example in hypothyroidism when the sufferer's mental and physical functions are slowed to the point of inertia.

There is much to be lost psychologically and physically by prolonged periods of inactivity. A primary objective therefore for those caring for the elderly is to encourage as much mobility as is possible within the limitations disease and ageing impose. This is often difficult for the old person or his relative to comprehend, often they may feel rest has been earned.

A carefully worked out programme which balances activity with rest will be the order of the day. Motivating the elderly person requires a great deal of skill and the nurse must exercise patience, while retaining a positive approach. Members of the multidisciplinary team rehabilitating an old person must work cooperatively towards the common goal of realising the full potential of the individual.

Selection of footwear is extremely important, with well fitting shoes being preferable to slippers. Aids which are available to help combat walking difficulties, should be chosen with the individual's specific needs in mind (Fig. 20.8). The physiotherapist after consultation with the rest of the team, is usually best equipped to make this choice. The actual introduction of the walking aid to the elderly person is vitally important. The nurse must be sensitive to the fact that many people abhor the thought of having to be seen using even a simple walking stick and may even prefer the risk of falling rather than accept such help.

Observation of the person will reveal whether the equipment is being used as was

Figure 20.8
Zimmer aids, tripods, walking
sticks

intended, also whether the patient has progressed to the point when he no longer
requires it. The 'roadworthiness' of all equipment should be checked regularly and
particular attention should be paid to ensure that the rubber ferrules found at the
base of many aids have not worn smooth.

Maintaining a safe environment

Falls in the elderly

It is a well recognized fact that the elderly are prone to falls and accidents. Women,
and particularly women over 75 years old, seem most at risk.

Although thankfully, nurses take their protective role very seriously indeed, in
the community less observation is possible and consequently the individual is at a
greater risk.

When considering why people fall it is important to listen to their own version
of the incident. This led one doctor to the conclusion that most accidents can be
categorised under the headings, 'Trips' and 'Turns'.

Trips (Fig. 20.9)

Figure 20.9
Trips

Trips are more common in the under 75 years age group, who will often blame their
own carelessness for the fall. In fact, a mixture of sensory impairment and environmental factors may be to blame. At home, the old person is faced with a series of
potential hazards: often their environment will have aged with them and frayed carpets, ill fitting footwear, deteriorating floors or stairs can all contribute to an accident.

The health visitor may see many danger areas in any one house, but caution is
essential. Home, however inadequate, is familiar, and hazardous looking bits of
furniture may well act as an orientation cue for the old person. To move them to
the unfamiliar, although safer environment of a hospital, may confuse them
completely and thus make matters worse.

Prevention of accidents

In hospital, the prevention of accidents is a priority. Adequate lighting and
adjustable beds are important. When left in the 'low' position these beds lessen the
likelihood of a serious injury to a patient trying to get up, and reduce the need for
cot sides. These unfamiliar enclosures may alarm a patient and should be used as
little as possible. Facilities such as chairs, toilets, crockery and fires should be
provided and maintained with safety in mind. Electric flexes should not be left where
they can be tripped over and any spills should be wiped up at once. Drugs and
noxious cleaning materials must be locked away. Zimmers or tripod walking aids

must be carefully stacked away after use. Special care is required in high risk areas such as the bathroom, kitchen and stairs.

In trying to strike a suitable compromise between imposing too many restrictions and exposing the patient to avoidable dangers, the nurse should recognise the part played by some well known physical conditions in bringing about trips.

Neurological causes of muscular weakness such as paraplegia (p. 129) or motor neurone disease (p. 124) are important as is Parkinson's disease when considering factors which increase the risk of falling. Conditions such as diabetes or vitamin B_{12} — folic acid deficiency (seen commonly but not exclusively in chronic alcoholics) — may predispose to peripheral neuropathy and be masked by an appearance of simple clumsiness.

Turns (Fig. 20.10)

Turns occur more often in the over 75s and are usually manifested by a feeling of loss of control, with or without a period of unconsciousness. These episodes are normally associated with underlying cerebral or cardiac disease and may either take the form of drop attacks when the person falls suddenly and inexplicably to the ground without losing consciousness and has great difficulty in getting up again, or transient ischaemic attacks. Alternatively, *postural hypotension* (on occasions brought about by prescribed drugs) or a fainting attack, (syncope) may provide adequate explanation for what is always an alarming experience.

What is inexcusable is merely 'writing off' a fall as being due to old age and therefore somehow inevitable. Falls do and will continue to occur with the elderly, but some understanding of the above factors may help minimize the likelihood of their happening.

Figure 20.10
Turns

'Granny bashing'

Yet another form of injury experienced by some old people has led to the invention of the emotive phrase 'granny bashing'.

When a non-accidental injury occurs, (and it is impossible to do more than guess at how common this is) it is almost invariably the end result of months of deteriorating relationships in what may once have been a 'normal' family.

The long term 24-hour nursing care of an elderly relative is more than should be asked of any one person, but unfortunately, this is commonly expected. The potential for violence should be spotted by the health visitor, the social worker (one of whose main concerns is family interactions) or any other member of the health team, but too often the first sign of trouble presents only after the event.

While violence can never by condoned, it is worth mentioning that the perpetrator often acts under great provocation. Nor is 'bashing' a one way process. The elderly have in their number a proportion of individuals who may feel tempted to give vent to their frustrations on the very person who is doing most to help them.

Society must, as a matter of priority, learn to care for the carers.

Sleeping

It is often remarked that old people need less sleep than they did when they were younger. However, the person himself may be unaware that this change is to be expected and may complain of insomnia, when all that is happening is perfectly normal.

Whatever the physiological reasons for sleeplessness (and it seems likely that there is nothing the nurse can do about them), other remedial factors are involved.

It becomes increasingly difficult for many elderly people to spend a whole night in bed without experiencing the need to pass urine. If this is coupled with a fear of incontinence or a disinclination to leave the warm bedclothes, wakefulness will be enhanced and dropping off again may prove difficult.

The control of body temperature is less efficient in the elderly, and small changes in the room temperature may adversely affect sleep.

Many old people complain of leg cramps disturbing sleep, and while simple exercises are sometimes sufficient to alleviate them, medical attention has frequently to be sought. Many of the conditions associated with age involve a degree of pain or discomfort which may be relieved by simple nursing measures or a prescribed analgesic.

Noise and injudicious use of lighting may be features of a hospital at night. Nurses on night duty should perfect the habit of moving around as quietly and unobtrusively as possible. Partially sighted, hard of hearing or slightly confused patients are particularly likely to misinterpret sounds or shadows, thus becoming too frightened to sleep.

Little worries can become exaggerated into a major crisis during the hours of darkness and the perceptive nurse may well become aware of the patient whose psychological stress can be relieved if a little time is spent by his bedside.

Finally, the habit in many hospitals of serving the last meal of the day at a time more suited to the convenience of the catering or nursing staff is unfortunate. Many an insomniac with a well established preference for eating late in the evening has been cured by a cup of tea and a slice of toast.

Sleeplessness in the elderly can often be helped by simple, common sense nursing interventions which are so much more desirable than the prescription of sedatives, which should be a last resort and reviewed frequently.

Dressing

Choosing clothes

The ability to shop for clothes, select an outfit for the day, and dress independently are activities taken for granted by the majority of people. When any or all of this becomes impossible, much distress and frustration can be generated. Features of our personality are often reflected in our choice of clothing and this can be eroded if undertaken by another person.

Choice of clothing may have to be influenced by practical considerations, such as ease of laundering if incontinence is a problem. When there is restricted movement or poor dexterity, loose, easily secured garments may be the best choice. Specially designed clothes for the handicapped are available, with the emphasis once again firmly placed on ease of dressing, to allow for as much independence as possible.

It is all too easy for an elderly person, forced to learn a new approach to independent dressing, to become discouraged. It is equally easy for the well-meaning nurse to run to his assistance. A planned programme which allows such a person to practise the technique in unhurried privacy is more helpful (Fig. 20.11).

In continuing care wards, a policy which ensures that the patient is involved whenever possible in purchasing items of personal clothing is essential. For those who cannot be taken shopping, many local firms are prepared to send a selection of articles on approval, while a mail order catalogue is another possibility bringing, as it does, the added excitement of receiving a parcel.

Personal laundry services are available in many geriatric units, although often the family will choose to undertake this task for their relatives. Careful identification of all clothing with clearly marked labels is extremely important.

Communicating

In the realm of communication, man probably has advantages over other life forms because of his highly developed gift of speech. Diminished intellectual capacity, increased or decreased sensitivity and sensory deficits all render communication difficult. Thought processes may be confused, short term memory unreliable, phonation imprecise and hearing impaired. It must be as frustrating for an elderly person not to be understood as for a nurse to find herself unable to get a message through.

Visual impairment is common. *Presbyopia* (p. 464) the inability of the lens to accommodate or change shape to focus on objects, both near and far, occurs in the

Figure 20.11
Aids to dressing

40s or 50s, and is the reason why almost everyone over that age wears spectacles, at least for close work.

For those with greater handicaps, services like large type library books, especially helpful if delivered to the housebound, or talking books, in the form of cassette recordings are much appreciated. If their condition warrants them being registered as blind (p. 482) additional facilities and concessions may help to maintain independence.

In hospital, if toilets for instance are signposted, the lettering must be large if it is to be at all helpful.

The practice of removing spectacles from people admitted to hospital, presumably in case the spectacles get lost or broken should now be a thing of the past. The nurse who forgets to return and polish her patient's spectacles after a procedure is guilty of thoughtlessness. It is interesting to observe that nurses who are themselves dependent on spectacles seldom make this basic error.

The deaf, or hard of hearing, seem to attract less sympathy than the visually handicapped, nevertheless, their problems are very real.

Most people's hearing acuity diminishes with age, while some become markedly deaf. Simple causes may be found, the most common being wax which can be removed by medically prescribed ear syringing. (p. 501). While not all deafness can be cured, a *hearing aid* is of assistance in many cases, but embarrassment, pride, lack of understanding as to its use, interference or sound distortion may render a hearing aid unacceptable. When the onset of deafness is delayed until old age the skills of sign language or lip reading may be difficult to acquire, however it is helpful if a deaf individual can see the face of the person who is addressing him. A clear, slow voice should be used and the patient asked if he can hear, then the voice should be adjusted as necessary. Shouting is rarely helpful.

People with no hearing problem often accuse those who have of being selectively deaf, that is, hearing when they want to, and being 'deaf' when it suits them. As this frequently infuriates the deaf person and in any case is difficult to prove, the nurse should refrain from making such judgements.

While diminution of sight and hearing may be a normal process, the loss of the power of speech is invariably a catastrophe.

Most commonly as the result of a cerebrovascular accident, (stroke p. 111) involving the dominant hemisphere of the brain, the sufferer may lose a substantial part of his communicating repertoire, with absolutely no prior warning.

It is important that a speech therapist be made available as soon as possible, but the road back is long and not always successful. When normal conversation is impossible, this may cause the patient to withdraw completely, a tendency which may be exaggerated should there be any pre-existing deafness. This can have serious implications on his quality of life.

Figure 20.12
Communication card

Empathy and considerable patience are required: it is sometimes necessary to make use of pencils and paper, a typewriter, (which can be operated by the hand which has retained its function) or one of a variety of communication boards (Fig. 20.12) but all are less than adequate.

When normal communication patterns break down the nurse should be familiar with others available to her. We use **non-verbal communication** all the time, but may be unpractised at interpreting it. Without a word being spoken, the observant nurse may become aware of signals of pain, embarrassment, anxiety, or a need to visit the toilet shown by the patients in her care.

The sense of touch can speak volumes when there is no other way of getting the message across. Holding a dying person's hand, or placing the arm on the shoulder of a bereaved relative, are universally understood and at times can be more appropriate than the most carefully selected words.

For very many people, sex represents a valued and personal means of communication of the highest order. Evidence now exists that some old people may still need or desire an active sex life, a fact that should not be overlooked by the nurse.

Work, play and feeling worthwhile

All of us share the psychological need for acceptance from those around us, security, independence and being seen as somehow useful or productive.

The elderly may find these important needs difficult to fulfil, but the alternative, of sitting around in mindless boredom in a geriatric chair, is unacceptable.

The patient will be fortunate if the hospital is able to provide a planned programme of activities, offering a variety of individual and group experiences, with a positive end result in mind. Such a programme may well be the responsibility of an occupational therapist, but to be successful, must have the enthusiastic support of the nursing staff.

The need for work may be met by performing tasks, such as gluing X-ray envelopes, for other departments in the hospital. These should ideally be broken down to simply mastered stages, capable of being performed in a group setting, and straightforward enough to be done successfully, thus raising the self-esteem. Above all, tasks identified with helping the hospital may be viewed as meaningful, traditional craft work usually is not.

While the average old person in hospital has hours of inactivity, which could potentially be used for leisure, these tend to be spent rather unimaginatively. The diversional therapist's role should perhaps be summed up as being to involve rather than to entertain. Videos, for instance, are entertaining for short periods of time, but too often provide the background music for a cat nap. The aim should be to encourage activities which ensure a degree of participation without belittling the patient in any way.

Individual rehabilitation programmes may go a long way to meet some of the needs mentioned above. For the hemiplegic person to relearn how to make a cup of tea is hard work indeed, but has the definite advantage of being meaningful. If he goes home, he will require to drink fluids, and will also be able to entertain any visitor who may chance to drop by.

As the programme advances, the occupational therapist, either alone or with the medical social worker, will visit the old person's home to try to anticipate any problems, and to work out any adaptations that may have to be made.

The skill of imparting, to their patients, a feeling of achievement and fulfilment is one that nurses must strive to master.

COMMUNITY FACILITIES (Figs 20.13 & 20.14)

The general practitioner (family doctor) who may have known the elderly individual for many years, is in an ideal position to oversee his community care. An increasing number of practices now have district nurses and health visitors attached to them, with the benefits of daily contact between all the members of the team allowing a smoother delivery of care. The provision of an up-to-date age/sex register and at least

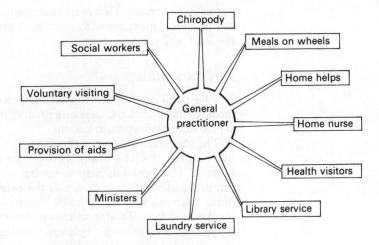

Figure 20.13
Services for the housebound
elderly

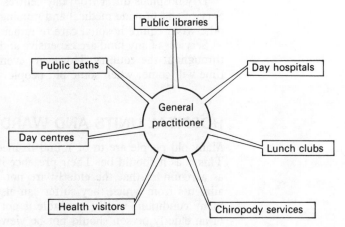

Figure 20.14
Services for the mobile elderly

twice yearly visits to all over 75s, seem worthwhile aims and should be possible where such a team exists.

References have already been made to the value of the meals on wheels service, which is usually run by the WRVS. Home helps provide invaluable support and are organized through the Social Services department. Their job is to do the housework, the washing, shopping, or perhaps cook a meal. A home help may call as often as five times weekly, or as infrequently as once a week, depending on the individual circumstances. They work at weekends only rarely. The home help is a human contact for the housebound elderly and so is not only a physical help, but also, and perhaps more importantly, a psychological and social comfort.

As more specific needs develop in the individual, other community services may be on hand to meet them. In some areas the local authority provides a laundry service for incontinent people being cared for at home. This frequently encourages the family to cope a little longer, and thus reduces the demand on hospital beds.

For the housebound, a mobile library can help break the monotony by providing a varied selection of reading material, while nursing equipment, can also be borrowed by those in need.

The fortunate ones, who live in an area with good facilities, may be aware of the availability of a day centre, which may meet their requirements adequately.

Day centres

The roles of day centres vary from one to another, but generally each provides companionship, warmth, and a midday meal. The staff are frequently volunteers, and since specific medical problems are not dealt with, nurses or doctors will not normally be present. However, beauticians, hairdressers or maybe even a chiropodist can provide a great boost to morale, at prices aimed to be within the reach of even the least well off pensioner.

Day hospitals

Day hospitals are frequently attached to a geriatric or general hospital and allow for medical investigations, assessment and daily supervision of the elderly, without actual admission as an in-patient.

The idea originated some time ago with the psychiatric day hospitals; the geriatric day hospital acts as a bridge between an independent home life, and admission to hospital. Day hospitals help in several ways to preserve, maintain and develop the physical and social competence of the elderly. They ease the load and responsibility of the relatives, who may then be happier to continue with the onerous task of caring for their old folk. Treatment is available which can minimize or resolve the need for hospital admission, while by providing regular follow-ups, those already in hospital may be able to look forward to an earlier discharge. Under the watchful eye of the nurse they provide, for example, good hot meals, access to the geriatrician, facilities for bathing, bowel control and chiropody.

Day hospitals differ from day centres in that they are part of the National Health Service and provide medical and nursing care. They enable many people who might otherwise require hospital care to remain in the community.

Services of any kind are expensive and their provision tends to be spread unevenly throughout the country. However, even when facilities are perfectly adequate, the time will come, when some old people will require to be admitted to hospital.

HOSPITAL UNITS AND WARDS

Many old people are to be found in medical or surgical wards in general hospitals. This is as it should be. Their presence in the mainstream of hospital life should act as a reminder that the elderly are not a race apart and that the vast majority of ailments from which they suffer can also be found in younger patients. Moreover, many conditions will be treatable if not entirely curable; the admission to hospital of an elderly person should not be viewed with pessimism.

Some do however require admission to hospital for reasons mainly connected with their age. Multiple pathology (where several different disease processes may be in evidence) is more common in this age group. Disorientation and physical disorders such as incontinence may demand care and surveillance which hospital staff can provide more readily than a spouse or relative. It would hardly be surprising if, in old age, there was neither spouse nor relative able to offer the unremitting attention required. In those circumstances a geriatrician may be consulted with a view to finding a place in a suitable hospital or unit. Such a referral frequently sparks off a chain of events which differs substantially from any brought about by referrals to other consultants.

The consultant geriatrician will often elect to carry out a domiciliary visit, that is, go to the patient's home to examine him in his familiar surroundings.

This recognizes the fact that some patients will have difficulty in making their way to hospitals or clinics for out-patient appointments. More important, there is the added benefit of seeing the old person function in his normal environment. His performance here may be in stark contrast to the muddled responses, which all to often seem to follow admission to hospital.

The success of any geriatric department depends primarily on its ability to admit, promptly, those who need admission and to make considerate arrangements for the discharge of people no longer requiring its care.

Assessment/rehabilitation wards

These active and busy wards adopt an aggressive therapeutic approach to the investigation, assessment and treatment of a complex variety of conditions.

Figure 20.15
The multidisciplinary approach

A multidisciplinary approach (Fig. 20.15) is common, each professional having specific, though sometimes overlapping, roles to play.

The importance of the fact that many old people suffer from treatable conditions cannot be overemphasized. Vitamin deficiency, constipation, and chest or urinary infections, are common examples, while others, such as diabetes, incontinence, or the effects of a cerebrovascular accident, (stroke) can be modified to a greater or lesser degree. Psychological and personality testing is carried out, and depression, dementia, or frank paranoid states may be discovered and some are amenable to treatment.

If the condition originally requiring admission responds to treatment, or the more lengthy process of rehabilitation, the patient may be discharged home. This is most likely to be possible when he is mentally alert, ambulant and continent.

If relatives can be assured of the continued interest of the geriatric team, and the availability of holiday relief beds and short term admission when things go wrong temporarily, they are more likely to volunteer their care.

It is essential that all comings and goings between hospital and community are seen as two way processes. Admission to hospital should never be allowed to signal the end of hope for an old person, while conversely, discharge should never rule out the possibility of eventual readmission. As a result of this, it has become fashionable to talk of patients being transferred to the community, rather than discharged from hospital. The continuity of care implied in this terminology seems to justify its use.

For those not able to return home, but still capable of a life outside hospital, a place may be found in a private or local authority old folk's home, or in sheltered housing. These combine an appropriate amount of surveillance with a degree of independence.

However, severe difficulty in walking, intractable incontinence, or behaviour disturbances, with or without superimposed dementia, may well result in the need for continuing hospital care.

Continuing care wards

This term is self-descriptive. In many instances care will be required until the patient dies, although the possibility of transfer to more suitable accommodation should rarely, if ever, be ruled out.

The aim in continuing care wards is not to cure the patient, (this is usually impossible) but to maintain and improve the quality of the life that remains.

A patient who requires 24-hour care or supervision and who shows little likelihood of getting better is still entitled to as high a standard of nursing care as anyone else.

Physically, this is not too difficult to achieve, and throughout this chapter we have highlighted nursing problems commonly found among old people, and described how they can be tackled. However, physical care in itself is not enough. When the hospital suddenly becomes home, it is only too easy for the patient to drift into a state of apathy, which may well prove to be the forerunner to becoming institutionalised.

Creating a homely environment

A pleasant, comfortable atmosphere should be created as far as possible, and this frequently means that a compromise has to be reached between furnishings and surroundings which are modern and functional, and those which may be more 'lived in' and acceptable to the older patient.

An ornament, a clock, a photograph, or even an easy chair, brought from home, may act as a comforter, a cue or even a stimulator of pleasant memories. Room dividers, floral decorations and occasional furniture carefully arranged give even the most institutional of buildings an air of informality and their occupants, some social inspiration.

Friends, neighbours and relatives should be actively encouraged to visit at any reasonable hour, with children and babies usually proving very stimulating. Can the patient go for a visit, or a pub lunch? Is it possible for him to be briefly reunited with his pets, or to attend the local church? Is there a newspaper to read, or someone to read it for him?

Can he watch the news, or check his football pools? Is Sunday the same as any other day, or (as it very likely was in his younger days), is it something a bit special? Will his birthday be acknowledged? Will it be celebrated?

Is there a calendar on the wall, or a clock, large enough to be seen?

Ordinary everyday items and occurrences, taken for granted elsewhere, assume great importance in the continuing care ward, particularly if the old person should become forgetful or a bit muddled.

Confusion and dementia

Anyone can become forgetful and slightly confused, but with advancing years memory lapses and sometimes confusion become more common.

Impaired short term memory, a common feature in the elderly, may make them uncertain of time, person or place.

Confusion, which can be caused by many factors, is important for at least two reasons. First because the nurse devotes a lot of time to the tending of the confused patient and second because it is often highly amenable to treatment.

Chest or urinary infections, trauma to the head, drug misuse and sudden environmental changes, as for instance in transfer from home to hospital, are examples which may precipitate acute confusional episodes and which, if recognized, may be treated or prevented.

Dementia (p. 572) on the other hand, is almost invariably progressive and responds rather poorly to attempts at cure. It is common to differentiate between *senile* and *atherosclerotic* dementia. While in practice, the first is more common in women and the second in men, it tends to be rather difficult to distinguish one from the other.

Senile dementia is a result of an accelerated increase in the rate of the death of brain cells, for reasons which are not fully understood. Deterioration of memory, particularly for recent events, is typical, as is impaired intellectual capacity, disintegration of the personality and severe social and behavioural changes. Associated incontinence is common.

Atherosclerotic dementia is caused by a gradual throttling of the blood vessels supplying the brain by atheroma, a porridge like substance found adherent to the walls of arteries. Onset may be gradual, involving 'stroke' like episodes, interspersed with periods of apparent remission.

The rapid downward course of the patient with dementia can sometimes be slowed down if not cured if a determined therapeutic attack is made on the symptoms.

Reality orientation (RO)

This is one type of programme geared towards this end, based on the twin principles of consistency and continuity. The old person is, throughout the day, gently reminded of such things as his name, the town, staff names, and simple current affairs; if he makes a mistake, he is corrected in a friendly but firm fashion. A large, magnetic board, announcing the date, weather, menu, and forthcoming birthdays, acts as a focal point in the ward and a constant reminder of real life. While this feeding of information must be ongoing, it can be augmented by more formal sessions, lasting for about half an hour, perhaps twice daily. This approach using methods of constant reminders including the prominent signposting of all doors, does not achieve miracles, but has a proven value in helping the elderly to keep in touch with their environment.

Care of the dying

Everyone, ourselves included, must die. Perhaps it is this knowledge that has given the subject an air of taboo. A nurse working with the dying is constantly reminded of her own mortality.

It is a common wish of the elderly that they should be allowed to die at home but frequently, this does not happen. Dying, like giving birth, is a natural event, and occurs fairly often in hospital; however care of the dying must never be allowed to become run of the mill.

Most old people, it is said, do not fear death, although many fear the actual process of dying. Their dread is that it may be protracted or painful, or that they will be left alone, with no-one to provide sympathy or reassurance, when it is most urgently required.

The person who is dying is entitled to first class nursing care. It is unpardonable to subject him to unnecessary discomforts which simple nursing procedures can so easily prevent. An alteration of position and the provision of clean bed linen may relieve distress and help to prevent the additional pain which would accompany pressure sores. Mouth breathing frequently occurs in terminal illness, requiring the mouth and lips to be treated as often as necessary. In severe pain, drugs such as narcotics will be prescribed (see below) the timing of which is absolutely crucial.

In fact the nurse may find all this relatively easy, and tend to overemphasize the practical aspects of her care.

The care of the dying can also be psychologically taxing. As the nurse may be unsure of what to say, she may say nothing; because of uncertainty as to what her reply should be, she may not listen but elect to spend her time with fitter patients, who may need her less.

Individual nursing care, as advocated throughout this chapter, will help to establish essential rapport between the nurse, the patient and his relatives. Frequently, it falls on the nurse to allay fears and anxieties. She should listen, look and touch. Being aware of possible cues will enable her to spot when reassurance or factual information is required.

Misplaced cheerfulness and cliches such as: 'Come, come now, don't talk like that,' are unhelpful. Allowing the patient time to express himself is frequently worthwhile. The direct question may catch the nurse unawares, and there are no trite answers to: 'Am I going to die?' As a general principle, tactful honesty, within the limits set by medical and senior nursing staff, has a lot to recommend it. Only experience will prepare the young nurse fully for this difficult situation, for which guidelines, are wholly inadequate.

Patients should not be left to die alone, and in the absence of a relative or clergyman, the nurse will be providing an essential and humane service, by just being there.

The spiritual aspects must always be considered when caring for the dying. For many people, their faith becomes more meaningful with age. Nurses should recognize this and accept that the dying person may find solace and contentment in the words and rituals of religion, whatever his particular faith may be. The relevant clergyman should be informed if the patient or his relatives wish it, and if any doubts exist regarding procedures surrounding death, they are best discussed at this time. A member of the Roman Catholic faith for instance will require to be given the last rites before dying, while an orthodox Jew must not be handled after death by a gentile without permission from a Rabbi.

Bereavement

A death is invariably accompanied by a sense of loss for those who are left behind. This may manifest itself in one of several different ways.

Since hospitals constantly seem to be geared towards cure, a death may result in an unreasonable sense of failure in the nurse. If the patient had been in the ward for a long time, or was well liked, she may suffer a genuine feeling of grief. In the circumstances, this would be perfectly normal.

Relatives will almost certainly be grieving and at this time may be at their most vulnerable. Time spent building an understanding relationship with them in the past will now prove invaluable. They may appreciate a cup of tea, a visit from the clergy, a quiet place to be alone, or conversely, a shoulder to cry on.

It is frequently said that bereaved relatives have to work their way through a sequence of events following the death. First of all, they may refuse to believe it, then they may become angry. A period of depression may follow before finally they can accept, and start coming to terms with what has happened. These stages are not always obvious to the onlooker and may take months, or even years to work through. Relatives' reactions to bereavement are influenced by many factors including age (their age and that of the deceased), kinship and closeness of friendship and understanding (or lack of understanding) that death was impending.

However, a nurse probably upset herself, may be less devastated if subjected to an unjustified angry response from a relative, if she is aware that this is a recognized accompaniment of normal grief.

The hospice movement

The remarkable growth of the hospice movement must be regarded as a significant feature of our time. Hospices are eagerly supported and sought after by the general public, who may see the care they provide as being more personalized than that available from a normal hospital.

Their more recent venture into community care can only increase this popularity, and further enhance their reputations.

Hospices are for those who have little remaining hope of a cure. Consequently, all their energy is devoted towards the relief of pain, emotional security and spiritual peace. The special needs and attributes of the relatives are recognized and acknowledged and the creation of an atmosphere of honesty, acceptance, and tranquillity is the major aim.

Medical staff working in hospices are leading the way in pain relief and their lessons are being learned elsewhere. Carefully prescribed doses and combinations of analgesia have allowed many old people to die, both pain free and mentally alert. With possible addiction no longer a consideration, the drugs should be given before the patient is aware of the onset of pain and at intervals tailored to his individual needs.

The hospice approach with its emphasis on holistic care should not be seen as posing a threat to workers in traditional areas, but rather as an ideal, which can be aimed for.

The nurse and the dying

One of the nurse's unique functions is to contribute to the achievement of a peaceful death for her patients.

The first experience of death for any nurse will usually be traumatic, and need tactful handling. Ideally she should not be required to participate in the care of the dead person, but should be allowed to observe only. Subsequent deaths will be coped with more easily.

On the death of a patient, the nurse must record the time and inform the doctor. Only he is qualified to confirm that the patient has indeed died and to sign the death certificate.

The certificate will be collected by the relatives who must register the death within 3 days and start making the funeral arrangements. A nurse with some knowledge of these procedures can be invaluable to a relative who may never have been in this situation before. Prior arrangements for the disposal of wedding rings, jewellery, and so on should be followed.

When the bereaved relatives are ready to leave the hospital, the nurse should check that they have transport, someone to accompany them, and somewhere to go.

A death cannot and should not be kept a secret from the other patients in the ward, some of whom may have a genuine need to grieve for the deceased. It should be announced simply and without drama, by the nurse as she continues with her duties.

Once the patient has been certified dead, the last offices will be carried out. This should be done in a quiet, efficient and dignified manner.

Although potentially harrowing, the nurse may experience a feeling of satisfaction, in performing this, her last service, to her patient who is now at peace.

FURTHER READING

Blythe R 1979 The view in winter, Allen Lane, London
Bromley D B (ed) 1975 The psychology of human ageing, 2nd edn. Penguin, Harmondsworth
Carver V, Liddiard P (eds) 1978 An ageing population. Hodder and Stoughton in association with the Open University Press
Eliopoulos C (ed) 1984 Health assessment of the older adult, Addison-Wesley, California
Judge T, Caird F 1982 Drug treatment of the elderly patient, 2nd edn. Pitman, Kent
Kenney R 1982 Physiology of ageing, Year Book Medical Publishers, Chicago,
MacHeath J 1984 Activity, health and fitness in old age. Croom Helm, London
  Pitt B 1982 Psychogeriatrics, 2nd edn. Churchill Livingstone, Edinburgh

Glossary

(Abbreviations: F = French; L = Latin; G = Greek)

Abduction (L *abducere* to draw away, separate) Movement of a limb away from the midline of the body.

Adduction (L *adducere* to bring towards) Movement of a limb towards the midline of the body.

Adynamic ileus (paralytic ileus, ileus paralyticus) Ileus resulting from inhibition of bowel motility which may be produced by numerous causes, most frequently by peritonitis.

Aetiology (G *aitia* cause, *logos* discourse) The study of the causes of disease.

After pains Spasmodic painful uterine contractions occurring during the first 48 hours following delivery, most commonly felt by multiparous women. They may be caused by clots in the uterus.

Allergen (G *genein* to produce) A substance capable of producing a specific hypersensitivity in an individual, for example drugs, pollens, eggs.

Allergy (G *allos* other, *ergein* to work) Hypersensitivity to some foreign substance, often certain foods or pollens. These substances, allergens, are usually of a protein nature and can include eggs, strawberries, oranges, pork, cauliflower, fish, dust from feathers or from the hair of horses, cats or dogs.

Alopecia (G *alopex* fox) Baldness. It often occurs in sharply defined patches in disease.

Alpha fetoprotein (AFP) A protein of fetal origin found in liquor amnii (amniotic fluid). In a normal pregnancy there is a small amount which diminishes as the pregnancy develops. In some abnormal conditions of the fetus such as myelomeningocele the level is considerably raised. Maternity units offer a screening test around the sixteenth week of pregnancy.

Amaurosis (G *amauroein* to darken) Complete loss of vision especially that in which there is no evidence of a pathological condition of the eye.

Amaurotic Pertaining to one afflicted with amaurosis. A family idiocy. Term for a group of related familial diseases, marked by dementia, impaired vision and lipid defect.

Amblyopia (G *amblys* dull, *ops* eye) Dimness of vision or loss of sight.

Amnion (G the fetal membrane) The innermost membrane of the fetal sac in which is contained the liquor amnii or amniotic fluid. This fluid acts as a shock absorber to the fetus and allows free movement.

Amyloid disease (G *amylon* starch) A condition in which tissue, especially liver and kidneys, degenerates and becomes waxy in appearance due to deposition of fibrous tissue.

Ankylosis (G *agkylos* crooked) Condition in which a joint is stiffened either by fibrous tissue (fibrous ankylosis) or by bony fusion (bony ankylosis).

Anomaly (G *anomalia* irregularity) 1. Anything contrary to general rule. 2. Any organ or structure which is abnormal with reference to form, structure or position; a malformation.

Anoxia (G *an*, oxygen) A state of deficiency of oxygen in the tissues.

Apnoea (G *a* without, *pnein* to breathe) Temporary cessation of breathing.

Arthrodesis (G *arthron* a joint, *desis* binding together) Fixation of a joint by destruction of the articular surfaces, followed by bony fusion of the bones involved.

Arthrogryphosis (G *arthron* a joint, *gryphosis* a curve) Flexure of a joint — a congenital deformity.

Arthroplasty	(G *arthron* a joint, *plassein* to form) The formation or production of a movable joint by surgery.
Ataxia	(G *ataxia* lack of order or arrangement) Lack of co-ordination of voluntary movements.
Atelectasis	(G *ateles* incomplete, *ektasis* a stretching) A condition in which a lung (or lungs) is incompletely expanded.
Athetosis	(G *athetos* not fixed) Useless, purposeless, disordered movements.
Atrophy	(G *a* without, *trophe* nourishment) Lack of growth and wasting of an organ or limb.
Attention	(L *attendere* to stretch) Power to focus on some phase of consciousness including some aspect of the world of reality.
Autosomes	(G *autos* self, *soma* body) Any of the paired chromosomes other than the sex chromosomes (X and Y). In man there are 22 pairs.
Avulsion	(L *avulsus* torn away) Forcible separation of two parts.
Bougie	(F candle) A solid, cylindrical-shaped instrument used for insertion into a natural orifice such as the urethra, oesophagus or rectum, usually for the purpose of dilatation.
Braxton Hicks contractions	Painless uterine contractions felt on abdominal palpation from the 16th week of pregnancy.
Breech presentation	The term used to describe the fetus lying with its buttocks in the lower part of the uterus. The baby is born with the buttocks coming first, as opposed to the more common vertex presentation (95% of all deliveries), when the baby is born head first. (*See* Vertex).
Bronchography	(G *brogchos* windpipe, *graphein* to record) An examination by X-ray of the bronchi following the introduction of a radio-opaque dye.
Bronchoscopy	(G *brogchos* windpipe, *skopein* to watch) An examination of the inside of the bronchi using a bronchoscope.
Bulla	(L bubble) Large blister.
Calcaneus	(L *calx* the heel bone) In a calcaneus deformity the heel bone becomes abnormally prominent due to acute dorsiflexion of the foot at the ankle joint.
Caput succedaneum	(L head) A localized area of oedema which forms under the baby's scalp caused by vascular congestion from pressure of the cervix during birth. It subsides in 24 to 48 hours without treatment.
Carcinogen	(carcinoma, G *genein* to produce) Any substance which causes living tissue to become carcinomatous.
Carcinoma	(G *karkinos* crab, *-oma* tumour) A malignant tumour which tends to spread, destroying normal tissue as it progresses.
Carina	(L *carina* keel) The area at which the trachea bifurcates.
Cavus	(L *cavum* cavity, hollow) Longitudinal arch of the foot which is abnormally high.
Cephalhaematoma	(G *kephale* head, *haima* blood, *-oma* tumour) A firm, circumscribed swelling on the skull due to an effusion of blood under the periosteum. It most often occurs when there has been a very short labour and rapid delivery and is caused by friction between the baby's skull and the mother's pelvis. No treatment is required but, as it usually persists for 6 to 8 weeks, the mother requires considerable reassurance.
Chondromalacia	(G *chondros* cartilage, *malakia* softness) Erosion of articular cartilage.
Chorion	(G a skin) The outer protective and nutritive membrane covering the fetal sac.
Chromatography	Chemical analysis by which a mixture of substances is separated by fractional extraction or absorption on a porous solid (column of aluminium oxide or filter paper) by means of flowing solvents.
Chromosomes	(G *chroma* colour, *soma* body) Microscopic rod-shaped bodies which develop from the nuclear material of a cell and are especially conspicuous during mitosis; they stain deeply with basic dyes. Chromosomes contain the genes or hereditary determiners. The number of chromosomes is constant for each species, being 46 in man (23 pairs in all somatic cells).
Clinical examination	(G *kline* bed) A physical examination.
Cognitive	(L *cognoscere* to know) A general term covering all the various modes of knowing, perceiving, remembering, imagining, conceiving, judging, reasoning.
Commensal	(L *cum* combined with, *mensa* table) An organism which lives on or within another but which does no harm to the host. Commensals are normally found on various mucous surfaces of the body.
Concept	(L *concipere* to take in) An idea.
Constipation	(L *constipatio* to crowd together) Infrequent or difficult evacuation of faeces; it results from the non-passage of motions for a longer period than is normal for that individual.

Coxa	(L) The hip joint.
Craniotomy	(L *cranium* G *kranion* skull + *tome* cut). Any operation on the skull.
Cubitus	(L *cubitus* to lie down) When reclining on couches during meals, the Romans leaned on their elbows. Hence the present connotation = the elbow, as in cubitus valgus deformity.
Cyto	(G *kytos*, vessel, hollow) Describes relationship to a cell.
Cytology	(G *logos* science) The science of the structure and function of cells.
Dacryocystitis	(G *dakryon* tear, *-itis* inflammation) Inflammation of the lacrimal drainage system, usually an acute painful suppurative inflammation which requires treatment with systemic antibiotics. It tends to occur in the very old and the very young.
Dermatoglyphics	(G *derma* skin, *glyphe* a carving) Study of surface markings of the skin especially those of the hands and feet.
Dextran	A plasma substitute for transfusion purposes which contains complex carbohydrate molecules. Its effect is to exert osmotic pressure, attracting water, thus preventing loss of water from capillaries in shock. Various forms are available, including the low molecular weight Lomodex and Rheomacrodex. Dextran 150 has a higher molecular weight.
Diarrhoea	(G *dia* through, *rhein* to flow) Abnormal (for the individual concerned) frequency and liquidity of faeces. Also described as looseness of the bowels.
DNA	Deoxyribonucleic acid, which is found in the cell nucleus.
Doptone	An ultrasonic device used to monitor the fetal heart. It may also be used to detect pregnancy at an early stage.
Dorsiflex	To flex the ankle or wrist towards the dorsum of the foot or hand.
Dysarthria	(*Dys* + G *arthrun* to utter distinctly + ia) Imperfect articulation of words due to disturbance of muscular control resulting from damage to the nervous system.
Dyscrasia	(G *dys* bad, imperfect, *krasis* mixture) An abnormal state of the body.
Dysfunction	(G *dys* bad etc., L *functio* performance) Absence of completely normal function.
Dysplasia	(G *dys* bad etc., *plasis* forming, shaping) Abnormality of formation or development.
Dystrophy	(G *dys* bad etc., *trophic* nourishment) Abnormal nourishment, therefore imperfect growth.
Eclampsia	(G *ek* centre, *lampein* to flash) An advanced stage of serious pre-eclampsia, characterized by convulsions; the mother's life, as well as the fetus's, is at great risk. Because of the prompt diagnosis and treatment of pre-eclampsia, eclampsia is now rarely seen. (*See* Pre-eclampsia).
Ectropion	(G *ek* centre, *trepein* to turn) Eversion or rolling out of the eyelid. It can result from scarring of the lids or, in the senile form, from loss of muscle tone.
Embolus	(G *embolos* plug) a clot or other substance brought by the blood from another vessel and forced into a smaller one thus obstructing the circulation.
Embolism	(G *en* in, *ballein* to throw) sudden blocking of a blood vessel by a clot or foreign material for example blood, air, fat or infected matter.
Emphysema	(G *en* into, *physema* a blowing) A condition in which the alveoli of the lungs are permanently dilated due to bronchial obstruction.
Encephalopathy	(encephalon, G *pathos* disease) Any dysfunction of the brain.
Endotoxin	(G *endon* within, L *toxicum* poison) Toxic substance produced within bacteria (usually gram −ve). Endotoxins are pyrogenic (produce heat) and increase capillary permiability.
Entonox	Inhalation analgesia consisting of oxygen 50% and nitrous oxide 50%. The United Kingdom Central Council permits the midwife to administer it during the late first stage of labour and during the second stage of labour to relieve pain.
Entropion	(G *en* into, *tropos* a turning) conversion or turning in of the lid margins. It is usually caused by contraction of scar tissue.
Enucleation	(L *e* out + *nucleus* kernel) To shell out whole. The removal of an organ or tumour from its covering. Used in connection with the eye it means removal of the eyeball after the optic nerve and the extrinsic muscles of the eye have been severed.
Epicanthic fold	(G *epi* upon, *kanthos* lip of a vessel) A fold of skin extending from the root of the nose to the median end of the eyebrow, covering the inner canthus and caruncle. It is a characteristic of the Mongolian race.
Episiotomy	(G *episeion* pudenda, *tomē* to cut) An incision made into the perineum under local anaesthesia to allow more room for the delivery of the baby's head and to prevent damage to the pelvic floor and soft tissues.
Equinus	(L *equinus* of the horse) In an equinus deformity the forepart of the foot is plantar flexed in the manner of a horse's hoof.

Ergometrine	Drug used to control haemorrhage following the birth of the baby. Given by i.m. injection or i.v. injection — dose 0.5 mg.
Erythema	(G redness) A rash which appears as a superficial reddening of the skin.
Eschar	(G *eschara* scab) A slough, resulting, from death of tissue due to gangrene or burning.
Eusol	A form of antiseptic containing hypochlorous acid and boric. The name is made up from the initial letters of Edinburgh University Solution of Lime.
Evisceration	(L *e* out + *viscus* the inside of the body) Used in connection with the eye it means removal of the contents of the eyeball leaving the sclera intact.
Exostosis	(L *ex* out of, G *osteon* bone, *osis* a condition of) A condition in which there is a bony outgrowth.
Exotoxin	(G *exto* outside, L *toxicum* poison) Toxic substance formed by bacteria but found outside the bacterial cell or free in the culture medium.
External version	Turning the fetus in the uterus from a breech to a vertex presentation. The manoeuvre is carried out by the obstetrician.
Fetal development	1. The term **embryo** is used up to the 12th week of pregnancy. 2. The term **fetus** is used from the 12th week of pregnancy to birth. 3. After birth, the fetus is known as the **baby**.
Forewaters	The liquor amnii contained in the membranous sac lying in front of the presenting part; it may rupture spontaneously prior to the onset of labour or during labour. (For artificial rupture of membranes, *see* Induction of labour.)
Fructose	(L *fructus* fruit) Laevulose. Fruit sugar.
Galactosaemia	(G *gala* milk, *haima* blood) The presence of galactose (see below) in the blood.
Galactose	(G *gala* milk). $C_6H_{12}O_6$ A monosaccharide or simple hexose sugar. Galactose is an isomer of glucose and is formed along with glucose in the hydrolysis of lactose. Galactose is readily absorbed in the digestive tract; in the liver it is converted into glycogen.
Gene	(G *genein* to produce) The basic unit of heredity. Each gene occupies a certain place on a chromosome.
Genetics	The science that accounts for natural differences and resemblances among organisms related by descent. The study of heredity and its variations.
Gestation	(L *gestare* to bear) Period of intrauterine fetal development from conception to birth.
Glyconeogenesis	(Glyco + G *neoss* new + *gennan* to produce) The formation of carbohydrates from molecules which are not themselves carbohydrates as amino acids, fatty acids or related molecules.
Guthrie test	A means of screening used between the fifth and tenth day of life to detect phenylketonuria and other metabolic disorders. Capillary blood is collected from a heel-prick on to specially prepared blotting paper and allowed to dry before being sent to the laboratory.
Haematocrit	(G *haima* blood, *krinein* to separate) Packed cell volume. When blood is centrifuged and prevented from clotting, it separates into layers. The bottom layer is red cells, which account for 45% of the total volume of blood. In any condition where fluid has been lost from the circulation, as in burns, this figure will be increased.
Hearing Aid	An external appliance which improves the hearing of patients with some types of deafness. Modern hearing aids comprise a small microphone, a transistorized amplifier and a receiver connected to the patient's ear. They are designed to give the best reception for speech.
Hepatolenticular	(G *hepar* liver, L *lens* lentil) Related to the liver and the lenticular nucleus. Hepatolenticular degeneration (Wilson's disease). Progressive lenticular degeneration in cirrhosis of the liver.
Histamine	(G *histos* tissue) A substance found in body tissues. The concentration varies in different organs. In man tissue histamine may be released in response to trauma, antigens, trypsin and bile salts.
Homograft	A portion of tissue removed from a donor to be applied to a recipient of the same species; such a graft survives for a very short period except in the case of cornea, artery, bone, cartilage and perhaps endocrine tissue.
Hydramnios	(G *hydor* water, *amnion* the fetal membrane) Excessive accumulation of amniotic fluid.
Hypernatraemia	(Hyper L *natron* sodium, G haem blood) Excessive amount of sodium in the blood.
Hyperostosis	(G *hyper* above + G *osteon* bone + *osis*) Hypertrophy (overgrowth) of bone; exostosis.
Hypo-	Prefix, from the Greek preposition *hypo*, meaning under, deficient, beneath.
Hypochromic	(G *hypo* deficient, *chroma* colour) A term applied to red blood cells which contain less haemoglobin than normal. It is usually associated with microcytosis and is characteristic of iron deficiency anaemia.

Hypopyon	(G *hypo* deficient, *pyon* pus) Pus in the anterior chamber of the eye. It may occur as the result of a severely infected corneal ulcer.
Hypothermia	(Hypo G *therme* heat) Abnormally reduced body temperature of 35.5°C or less in infants and 35°C or less in adults. Induced hypothermia is used in some types of surgery.
Ideas of reference	A symptom of psychological illness. The patient believes that even the most casual remark and action of others refer in some special way to him. The most obvious example is the paranoid or suspicious individual who is convinced that every time he leaves a room everyone present begins to talk about him.
Ileus	(L; G *eileos* from *eilein* to roll up) obstruction of the intestines.
Incongruity of affect	Display of inappropriate emotion in response to a situation, for instance, to giggle when told of a tragic happening.
Induction of labour	This procedure is usually undertaken in the interests of the mother and the fetus. ARM (artificial rupture of the membranes) is carried out and the uterus may be stimulated to contract by administering i.v. Syntocinon, which is a synthetic form of oxytocin.
Intelligence	(L *intelligentia* perception) The capacity to comprehend relationships. The ability to think. The ability to solve problems and to adjust to new situations.
Intelligence quotient	The measure of intelligence obtained by dividing the individual's mental age (according to the Binet scale) by his chronological age and multiplying the result by 100.
International unit (iu)	A given quantity of a substance having a recognized effect. The active principals of many nutritional compounds have now been discovered, and specific weight equivalents are generally used when discussing intake of these compounds.
Ischaemia	(G *ischo* to restrain, hold back, *haima* blood) Inadequate or deficient blood supply to some part of the body.
Keratin	(G *keras* horn) A protein substance found in the horny layer of the epidermis (keratinize: to make or become horny).
Kernicterus	(G *kern* kernel, icterus = jaundice) A form of icterus neonatorum occurring in infants in which nuclear masses of the brain and spinal cord undergo pathological changes accompanied by deposition of bile pigments within them.
Ketoacidosis	Acidosis accompanied by the accumulation of ketone bodies (ketosis) in the body tissues and fluids as in diabetic acidosis.
Ketosis	A condition characterized by an abnormally elevated concentration of ketone bodies in the body tissues and fluids. It arises when there is insufficient carbohydrate in the diet and increased amounts of fat are used for energy as in starvation or severe vomiting (it can be accompanied by a metabolic alkalosis).
Kyphosis	(G *kyphos* hunch-backed) Forward concave curvature of the spine.
Lanugo	(L down) Fine downy covering of hair on the skin of the premature baby.
Leucotomy	(G *leukos* white, *tomē* to cut) A surgical operation in which the association fibres running from the frontal lobes of the brain to the thalamus are severed. It is performed to alleviate debilitating mental distress when other methods of treatment have failed. The operation can be performed using a variety of techniques. Inevitably personality changes occur ranging from happy-go-lucky attitudes to apathy, emotional blunting and a vegetable-like existence.
Lochia	(G *lochos* childbirth) The name given to the discharge from the uterus following the birth of the baby until the end of the puerperium. (Lochia is pleural, e.g. 'the lochia *are* heavy'.)
Lordosis	(G *lordos* bent with a frontal convex curve) Spinal curvature which is convex anteriorly, e.g. exaggerated lumbar curve.
Low grade intelligence	An intelligence quotient below 25.
Macrocytic anaemia	(G *makros* large, *kytos* cell) This refers to red blood cells of a greater diameter than normal and is found in some types of anaemia, notably pernicious anaemia.
MB tube	Mousseau Barbin tube. A type of plastic catheter with an expanded upper end used to maintain patency of the oesophageal passage in patients with carcinoma of the oesophagus. It can be passed into the oesophagus but requires open operation on the stomach in order to secure it.
Meconium	The first stool passed by the newborn baby. Meconium is dark-green in colour and is present in the intestine from the 16th week of pregnancy.

Mediastinoscopy	(L *mediastinus* midway, G *skopein* to watch) Examination under direct vision of an area on both sides of the carina.
Megaloblastic anaemia	(G *megas* large, *blastos* germ) A type of anaemia in which the red blood cells are of larger diameter than normal and possess an abnormal nuclear structure. It is typical of pernicious anaemia.
Meta	(G among, between, besides, etc.) Used as a prefix, meta implies a change of order, position, kind, shape, etc.
Metastases	(G *stasis* a standing) Transfer of disease from its primary site to distant parts of the body via the circulatory or lymphatic system or by direct invasion.
Metatarsalgia	(L *tarsalis* of the tarsal bones, G *algos* pain) Pain in the part of the foot beyond the tarsal bones, i.e. the metatarsus.
Microcytic anaemia	(G *mikros* small, *kytos* cell) This refers to red blood cells of a smaller diameter than normal such as those found in iron deficiency anaemia.
Moulding	The shaping of the baby's head that occurs as it adjusts to the size and shape of the birth canal.
Movements (active)	Movements of joints which are performed by the patient's own muscles. They may be made with gravity eliminated, e.g. in the hydrotherapy pool, against gravity or against resistance, e.g. weight lifting.
Movements (assisted)	A combination of active and passive movements.
Movements (passive)	Movements of a patient's joints made by a nurse or physiotherapist with no assistance from the patient.
Multigravida	(G *multus* many, *gravidus* pregnant) A pregnant woman who has had two or more pregnancies.
Multipara	(L *perere* to bring forth, produce) A woman who has had two or more pregnancies which resulted in viable fetuses but not necessarily live births.
Myelitis	(G *mylos* marrow, *-itis* inflammation) Inflammation of the spinal cord. (The spinal cord used to be regarded as the marrow of the spinal column.)
Myeloma	(G *myelos* marrow, *oma* a tumour) A locally malignant tumour. Cells are the type normally found in bone marrow.
Myositis	(G *mys* muscle, *-itis* inflammation) Inflammation of voluntary muscle. In myositis ossificans, bony deposits are laid down within the muscle.
Necrosis	(G *nekros* dead, *-osis* condition) The death of a limited amount of tissue, e.g. a group of cells.
Neonate	(G *neos* new, L *natus* born) A newly born child.
Neonatal mortality	Infant deaths occurring in the first four weeks following birth.
Neonatal period	The period of time from birth until the end of the first four weeks of life.
Neuroglioma	(G *neuron* a sinew; later, 2nd century, a nerve; *glia* glue, *-oma* a tumour) A tumour of the special connective tissue of the nervous system.
Neuroma	A tumour involving a nerve.
Nodule	(L *nodulus* little knot) Raised discrete lesion on the skin, deeper and firmer than a papule.
Nystagmus	Involuntary rapid movement of the eyeballs from side to side, up and down or in a rotary manner from the original point of fixation. There are various causes including lesions of the eye, ear and brain.
Oligaemia	(G *oligos* little, *haima* blood) A diminished amount of blood in circulation.
Ophthalmia neonatorum	(G *ophthalmos* eye) Any purulent discharge from a baby's eyes occurring within three weeks of birth. It is a notifiable condition. Micro-organisms causing the condition are the staphylococcus, streptococcus, pneumococcus and still occasionally the gonococcus.
Osteochondritis	(G *osteon* bone, *chondros* cartilage, *-itis* inflammation) An inflammatory condition affecting bone and cartilage. Commonly affects the epiphyses, and the clinical picture is one of degeneration, followed by regeneration, e.g. Perthes' disease.
Osteomyelitis	(G *osteon* bone, *myelos* marrow, *-itis* inflammation) Pyogenic infection of bone and marrow. In 80 per cent of cases the causal organism is *Staphylococcus aureus*.
Palliative	(L *palliare* to cloak) Serving to alleviate symptoms or suffering.
Panophthalmitis	(G *pan* all, *ophthalmos* eye, *-itis* inflammation) A purulent infection of the whole eye. There is a danger of meningitis or cerebral abscess from spread of infection back via the optic nerve or ophthalmic veins to the brain. (The ophthalmic veins empty into the cavernous sinuses.)
Papule	(L *papula*) Discrete lesion raised above the skin surface.

Patch tests	Potential sensitisers are applied to the skin of the patient's back and covered for 24 hours. If positive, a patch of eczema develops at the site 48 to 72 hours later.
Perception	(L *percipere* to perceive) Process of being aware of objects.
Perinatal period	(G *peri* around, L *natus* birth) The period of time from birth until the end of the first week of life. Infant mortality is highest during this period. (Stillbirths are recorded as occurring in the perinatal period.)
Periphery	(G *periphereia* a circumference) The outermost boundary or limit.
Perseveration	(L *perseverare* to persist) Continued repetition of a meaningless word or phrase, or repetition of answers which are not related to successive questions asked.
Pes	(L *pes, pedes* a foot, feet) As in pes cavus — *see* Cavus.
Phthisis bulbi	(G a wasting away) Degeneration, atrophy and shrinkage of the whole eye, following a severe progressive inflammation.
Physiotherapy	(G *physis* nature, *therapeia* treatment) The use of physical measures to correct deformities and restore function after disease or injury.
Plantar/palmar flex	(L *planta* sole of foot, L *palma* palm) Flexion of ankle/wrist towards the sole of foot/palm of hand.
Podophyllin	A caustic chemical used to destroy unwanted tissue.
Post-partum haemorrhage	Bleeding during the third stage of labour or within 24 hours following the expulsion of the placenta. It is a very serious complication of delivery and the mother's life can be in danger.
Pre-eclampsia	A condition peculiar to pregnancy which can adversely affect the survival of the fetus because it causes a reduction in the blood flow to the uterus and the placenta. The three main features of the disease are rise in blood pressure, oedema and proteinuria. Early diagnosis and treatment are essential and the patient may be admitted to hospital with only one of the above signs.
Primigravida	(L *primus* first, *gravidus* pregnant) A woman who is pregnant for the first time.
Proprioception	(L *proprius* one's own, *capere* to take) The awareness of posture, movement and changes in equilibrium, and the knowledge of position, weight and resistance of objects in relation to the body.
Pruritus	(L *prurire* to itch) Severe itching irritation of the skin.
Prosthesis	(G addition) An artificial part which is attached to the patient.
Pseudarthrosis	(G *seudes* false, *arthron* joint) A false joint formed between the fragments of a fractured bone which have failed to unite.
P.U.V.A.	Photochemotherapy treatment for psoriasis using ultraviolet A-type light. The patient is given psoralen to sensitize his skin to sunlight before exposing him to high intensity long wave ultraviolet light.
Quickening	The feeling of fetal movements by the expectant mother. Movements are first felt at about 16 weeks in a multigravid woman and at about 18 to 20 weeks in a primigravid woman.
Retinoblastoma	(L *rete* net, G *blastos* germ, *-oma* tumour) A rare malignant tumour of the eye which occurs in young children (0 to 3 years). It commences in the retina and can spread forwards to involve the rest of the eye and/or back along the optic nerve to the brain.
Retinopathy	(L *rete* net, G *pathos* disease) Any abnormality of the retina, with formation of exudates and haemorrhages. It is associated with general diseases such as diabetes mellitus, atherosclerosis and hypertension.
Retrolental fibroplasia	(L *retro* backward, *lens* a lentil; L *fibra* fibre, G *plassein* to form) A condition, mainly of premature babies, resulting from hyperoxygenation. There is growth of embryonic tisssue, causing the formation of new vessels in the vitreous, which in turn causes retinal detachment. The end result is total blindness. The condition is rarely seen now, because oxygen concentration in incubators is kept below 40%.
Rheumatoid factors	Antigamma globulin antibodies found in the sera of most patients with rheumatoid arthritis and in some patients with other chronic diseases and chronic infections.
Rigor	An attack of intense shivering. The internal temperature rises rapidly and may either remain elevated or fall rapidly as profuse sweating occurs.
RNA	Ribonucleic acid, which is found in the cell cytoplasm and nucleolus.
Salicylic acid	A caustic chemical used to destroy unwanted tissue.

Sarcoma	(C *sarx* flesh, *-oma* a tumour) A highly malignant neoplasm affecting bone tissues.
Satiety	(L *satis* sufficient + *-ety* state or condition of) sufficiency or satisfaction as full gratification of appetite or thirst.
Sinus	(L curve, hollow) An unhealed passage leading from an internal lesion to the surface of the body.
Sofra-tulle	Tulle gras impregnated with Soframycin (framycetin).
Spasticity	(G *spastikos* drawing in) In a state of spasm. The movements of a spastic person show imperfect voluntary control. The muscles relax slowly under continued steady pressure but jerk back when pressure is removed. Tendon reflexes are exaggerated.
Spondylitis	(G *spondylos* a vertebra, *-itis* inflammation) Arthritis of the vertebral column.
Spondylosis	(G *spondylos* a vertebra, *-osis* a condition) Literally an abnormal state or condition of the spine, non-infective in origin, but with some ankylosis.
Stillbirth	The birth of a dead child.
Stimulus	(L *stimulare* to incite) Any agent or factor able to influence directly living protoplasm, as one capable of causing muscular contraction or secretion of a gland, or of initiating an impulse in a nerve.
Symblepharon	(G *syn* together, *blepharon* eyelid) Adhesions between the conjunctiva lining the lids and the conjunctiva of the eyeball and the cornea. It is generally the result of burns of the eye, e.g. lime burns.
Syntometrine	Syntocinon 5 units and ergometrine 0.5 mg combined, given to control haemorrhage during the third stage of labour.
Talipes	(L *talus* ankle) Congenital deformity called, in lay terms, 'club foot'. The deformity is not at the ankle proper, but at the tarsal joints.
Tendovaginitis	(L *tendo* tendon, *vagina* sheath, G *-itis* inflammation) A mild, chronic, non-bacterial inflammation of a tendon sheath prevents free movement of the tendon.
Tenosynovitis	(G *tenon* tendon, *syn* together, L *ovum* egg, G *-itis* inflammation) Inflammation of the epithelial lining of a tendon sheath. There is pain on moving the affected tendons. The cause may be mechanical (overuse) or bacterial (acute or chronic) infection. Commonest site is the flexor tendons of the forearm and hand.
Tetracycline	A broad spectrum antibiotic.
Thoracoscopy	(L *thorax* chest, *skopein* to view) Examination of the pleura under direct vision.
Thoracotomy	(L *thorax* chest, G *tomē* to cut) The operation of opening the chest.
Tomography	(G *tome* section, *graphein* to record) The X-ray of layers of body tissues at any required depth.
Trachoma	(G roughness) A very severe form of conjunctivitis, resulting in many complications. It is associated with hot, sandy conditions, inadequate water purification, flies, poor sanitation and poor living conditions.
Transillumination of sinuses	Inspection of the interior of a cavity by using a light strong enough to pass through its walls. The nasal sinuses can be inspected by placing a lighted torch in the patient's mouth.
Trichiasis	(G *thrix* hair) Turning in of the eyelashes, causing them to scratch against the cornea with the risk of corneal abrasion and ulceration.
Tubigrip	A proprietary name for a form of elasticated leg support.
Ultrasonography	A diagnostic technique using vibrations of the same nature as audible sound waves but of greater frequency. It does not carry the hazards of exposure to X-rays and has therefore largely replaced X-rays in specialities such as obstetrics.
Urticaria	(L *urtica* stinging nettle + *ia*) Vascular reaction of the skin in which there is transient appearance of smooth slightly elevated patches (wheals). These are redder or paler than the surrounding skin and are often attended by severe itching.
Valgus	(L wandering) Divergence of part of the body away from the midline. In coxa valga the angle between the neck of the femur and the shaft is increased. In hallux vulgas the great toe is angulated towards the other toes, i.e. away from the midline of the body.
Varus	(L facing) Angulation towards the midline of the body. In coxa vara the angle between the shaft and the neck of the femur is decreased. Talipes varus is inversion of the foot.
Venous sinuses	Dilated channels for venous blood found within the cranium. They anastomose with each other and run between the layers of dura mater.

Vernix caseosa	(L cheese-like varnish) The greasy substance composed of sebum and shed epithelial cells which covers the skin of the baby at birth. It retains the heat and is protective.
Vertex	(L summit) The area of the fetal head which presents in 95% of all babies born head first.
Vesicle	(L *vesicula* small bladder) A small blister.
Wharton's jelly	The soft, pulpy, embryonic connective tissue forming the basis of the umbilical cord. The umbilical vessels lie within. (Name derived from Thomas Wharton, English physician and anatomist, 1614–1673.)
Whitfield's ointment	A treatment for skin diseases containing 3% salicylic acid and 6% benzoic acid in petroleum jelly base.
Wilson's disease	A rare disease of degeneration of the corpus striatum and cirrhosis of the liver, characterized by tremulous distortion of the muscles, dysarthria, dysphagia and emotionalism. It is thought to be the result of abnormal copper metabolism.

Index